Primary Clinical Care Manual

Developed by the Soweto Trust for Nurse Clinical Training

UPDATED 10TH EDITION

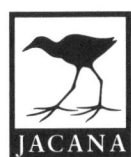

Primary Clinical Care Manual

First Edition 1992
Second Edition 1996, reprint 1997
Third Edition 1999, reprinted new cover 2001, 2004
Fourth Edition 2005, reprint 2006
Fifth Edition 2009,
Sixth Edition 2010
Seventh Edition 2012
Eighth Edition 2014, reprint 2015
Ninth Edition 2016
Tenth Edition 2019

ISBN 978-1-4314-2887-8

Job No. 003433

Published by Jacana Media
PO Box 291784
Melville 2109, South Africa
Tel (011) 628 3200; Fax (011) 482 7280

Printed and bound by ABC Press, Cape Town

COPYRIGHT ©
Copyright subsists in this work. In terms of the Copyright Act, 98 of 1978, no part of this work may be reproduced or transmitted in any form or by any means, electronic or mechanical, including photocopying, recording or by any information storage and retrieval system, without the permission in writing from the publisher.

Notwithstanding the copyright which subsists in the work, and the fact that any person wishing to make copies of the work should contact the publisher, the reader should please note that the publisher will view requests to copy parts of the manual for teaching purposes, especially by persons and institutions who cannot afford to purchase copies of the work, in a sympathetic light. Persons wishing to copy in these circumstances are encouraged to contact the publisher, as this will also provide the publisher with an opportunity of keeping accurate records about who is using the book and in what way, which helps the publisher keep the manual up to date.

The editors, publisher and sponsor do not accept responsibility or liability for either any errors or omissions arising from the use of this manual for any purpose, or for the way this manual, its contents and information are used in caring for patients.

PREFACE

This book represents the collective experiences of more than a decade of nurse - doctor teams, working to meet the needs of the Lillian Ngoyi Training Centre (formerly the Soweto Community Health Centres). The community served ranges from first to third world, from the recent migrant to the multi-generation urban resident and from neonates to geriatrics. The specially trained clinical health care nurses and their colleague doctors thus practice family medicine with all its potential and strengths. As an outreach service of a major teaching hospital, Chris Hani Baragwanath, the clinics have comparable, if different, excellence.

After initial development for Soweto primary health care personnel, the manual has been significantly edited and revised to provide useful, practical and widely applicable guidelines for Southern African usage. Inevitably, local circumstances affect health care delivery, and therefore treatment protocols and delegation of functions may have to be varied and adapted according to individual circumstances.

This manual bridges many disciplines – the common thread being out-patient management. Signs and symptoms are outlined only as a pointer to diagnosis, so that rational management follows. This is not a textbook describing non-essential details of aetiology or pathology, nor does it deal with any in-patient issues.

While the concept of holistic family and whole life care is valued, it is recognised that young children, and particularly neonates, are not simply miniature adults, and that symptomatology and treatment modalities frequently differ. Equally the eight year old and the young athlete are prone to different disorders and may respond differently to the same medication.

Medical students and practitioners may be varyingly familiar with textbooks of Obstetrics, Gynaecology, Paediatrics, Medicine and Surgery, including subdisciplines such as Orthopaedics, ENT and Ophthalmology. The above provide a wealth of background information, but this is the first edition of a health care management manual, ie. a book on "how-to-treat", which brings it all together for those in the front line!

This book is dedicated to the Soweto community, whose health is our primary concern, and also to all those who treat the ambulatory sick, of all ages, wherever they may be.

LUCY WAGSTAFF

Stella and Paul Lowenstein Professor
of Community Paediatrics
University of the Witwatersrand
Formerly a team member of the Soweto Community Health Centres

EDITORS AND CONTRIBUTORS

Editors
The Training Unit, Lilian Ngoyi Community Health Centre, Johannesburg and West Rand Health Region:

Dr L. Pein, The late Dr A. Truscott

Department of Obstetrics and Gynaecology
Professor E. Buchmann

Private: Dr A. Strätling, Consultant Physician

Jacana Media: Sr J. Prangley

Contributors
Zamaguhle Child Abuse Clinic, Zola Community Health Centre, Johannesburg and West Rand Health Region: Dr A. Ilunga

The University of the Witwatersrand, Faculty of Health Science, Chris Hani Baragwanath Hospital:

Department of Surgery
Dr M. Ahmed, Head, Division of Otorhinolaryngology / head and neck surgery
Professor E. Degiannis, Director of Trauma Unit
Dr M. Lakhoo, Senior Surgeon
Professor G. Maclaren, Division of Ophthalmology
Professor R. Valentin, Division of Orthopaedics

Department of Obstetrics and Gynaecology
Professor E. Buchmann
Dr J. Hull

Department of Medicine
The late Dr P. Alexander, Cardiology section

Professor D. Blumsohn

Department of Paediatrics
Contributions co-ordinated by Dr F. Patel

HAST Services, Lillian Ngoyi Clinic
Dr R. Mani

Private
Dr H. Kirby

Tenth Edition 2019
The primary purpose of this revision has been to update and correct the management of conditions, particularly HIV and AIDS. The authors have attempted to incorporate many of the drugs used in the Essential Drug List for Primary Health Care.

References
South African Medicines Formulary, produced by the Department of Pharmacology, University of Cape Town, and published by the Medical Association of South Africa, in co-operation with the Pharmaceutical Society of South Africa, has been used as a reference for drugs and dosage.

Many of the notes have been discussed and corrected by those mentioned in the acknowledgements.

ACKNOWLEDGEMENTS

The manual is the result of years of work, interest and enthusiasm from all the staff of the Lillian Ngoyi Training Centre, Central Witwatersrand Health region (formerly the Soweto Community Health Centres) and many medical workers throughout Southern Africa. It has been inspiring to be associated with many people who have given so freely and generously of their own and their families' time to comment, correct, guide and support this manual.
A list of these people follows. Their contributions are very gratefully acknowledged.

> Dr M A Alli, Dr M Arais, Prof R Ballard, Dr Barnes,
> Mrs Y Bekker, M Bester, Mrs B Bompani, Sr L Bosch, Sr M Bouwer,
> Mrs E du Buson, Sr Campbell, Mrs A Centner, Dr R Chapman,
> Mrs V Charleston, Sr D Charlesworth, Dr P Cooper, Dr D Danelowitz,
> Ms L Deetleffs, Mr B de Wet, Dr C de Wet, Prof D Dimitriades,
> Dr S Donahue, Prof A Dreyer, Dr T Dutkiewicz, Ms P Enslin,
> Dr C Evian, Dr R Farrell, Prof S Fehrsen, Dr T Felhaber, Dr C Ferreira,
> Dr L Floyd, Miss G Fredericks, Dr M Friedman, Miss A Furter,
> Dr T Germond, Sr N Geyer, Mrs P Giemre, Mrs R Hanekom,
> Mrs J Hayward, Prof R Henbest, Dr M Hlalele, Dr J Hodkinson,
> Dr N Hoffman, Prof K Huddle, Dr R Ingle, Dr C Kahl,
> Dr I Kennedy, Dr M Klenovsek, Dr W Kloek, Dr S Knight,
> Sr C Kotzenburg, Mrs L Langley, The late Prof. Lavery, Dr T Leontsinis,
> Dr N Makiwane, Mrs E Malan, Dr J McIntyre, Dr J Marshall, Dr Z Mayet,
> Prof K Mfenyana, Sr M Mofokeng, Ms M Moleko, Sr S Monamode,
> Sr T Nefale, Sr O Ngobeni, Dr C Oettle, Dr T Oosthuizen, Dr A Parrish,
> Dr A Promnitz, Dr Rashid, Dr J Reid, Dr S Reid, Dr W Reid, Dr S Roos,
> Prof S Ross, Mr E Roux, Dr L Russell, Prof D Saffer, Dr H Saloojee,
> Prof Schultz, Prof H Seftel, Dr K Simmank, Mrs Smith, Prof B Sparks,
> Dr G Strang, Sr M Strydom, Dr G Te Haar, Dr M Teichler, Dr R Thom,
> Dr M Tom, Dr C Treadwell, Sr Uys, Dr P Vallabh, Ms B v d Brugghen Klinkenbyl, Dr C van Deventer, Prof G van Gelderen, Dr H van Wyk,
> Mrs O Venter, Dr M Vermaak, J Visagie, Dr P Vos, Sr Wareley,
> E Welmann, Prof D Whittaker

We particularly acknowledge the support, help and guidance of our former superintendents, Dr PJ Beukes and Dr GM Louw, and our former heads of department Dr M Duncan and Dr D Platzky.

The manual has been patiently and enthusiastically supported and nurtured by the entire staff of Jacana Media. Many thanks to them all.

NOTES ON USING THIS MANUAL

The clinical features, drug and non-drug management are based on the needs and limitations in a primary care situation. This means that dosages and drug regimens may differ from those used in hospital practice, eg. antibiotics 4 x daily, instead of 6 hourly.

Sometimes specific reference is made to current practice in Soweto. It may be necessary to adapt this for the user's situation.

Drug trade names may be used where it is thought that this will make it easier for the user. This occurs especially where the generic name is very long, as in the case of contraceptive pills. Sometimes the trade name has been added in brackets.

Note the following:

- **REFER stat,** means urgent referral, ideally by means of an ambulance
- **REFER when convenient,** means non-urgent referral ie.
    - when suitable for the patient and the receiving hospital department
    - probably by appointment
- **Nocte** means at night
- **Mane** means in the morning
- **Stat** means immediately
- **NB.** means important or vital
- **Note** means quite important or only relevant to the section above

> **MANAGEMENT**
> All information inside a "management block" like this outlines the treatment procedures to be followed by all personnel.
>
> Management blocks usually follow this order:
> - Reasons for **REFERRAL**
> - Lifestyle adjustments
> - General measures
> - Medicine management

▼ **Note to doctor**

This heading indicates the start of management guidelines for doctors. These sections begin and end with a triangle ▲

CONTENTS

EMERGENCIES

RESUSCITATION 3
Cardiopulmonary resuscitation (CPR) 3
Airway obstruction (by foreign body) 6
Allergic reactions 7
Drowning 9
Lightning and electric shock 10

BITES, POISONS AND STINGS 11
Animal and human bites 11
Snake bites 11
Poisoning and drug overdose 13
Bee stings 14
Spider bites 14

BURNS 15
Classification 15
Burns in specific areas 16

EAR, NOSE AND THROAT

THE EAR 19
Causes of common symptoms 19
Diseases of the external ear 21
Diseases of the middle ear 25
Diseases of the inner ear 29

THE NOSE AND PARANASAL SINUSES 31
The nose 31
The paranasal sinuses 36

THE MOUTH, THROAT AND LARYNX 39
General clinical features 39
Diseases of the throat 40
Diseases of the mouth 45
Salivary glands 47
Diseases of the gums 47
Diseases of the tongue 48
Diseases of the larynx 49

RESPIRATORY SYSTEM

THE UPPER AIRWAYS 53
Problems of the upper airways 53

THE LUNGS 57
Bronchial asthma 57
Asthma medicine protocol 59
COAD (including chronic bronchitis and emphysema) 61
Pneumonia 62
Haemoptysis 64
Bronchiectasis 64
Lung abscess 64
Tuberculosis 65
Protocol for the treatment of tuberculosis 66

CARDIOVASCULAR SYSTEM

HYPERTENSION 71
Confirmation of hypertension 71
Medicine protocol 72
Management of hypertension in special conditions 76
Management of some drug side effects 78
Hypertension protocol 79
Appendix – example of letters 80

HEART FAILURE AND HEART DISEASE 81
Heart failure 81
Management of heart failure 82
Heart disease 85
Palpitations 87

VASCULAR DISEASE 89
Veins 89
Arteries 90
Cardiovascular disease 90
Management of cardiovascular disease 91

GASTROINTESTINAL SYSTEM

ABDOMINAL SYMPTOMS 95
Abdominal symptoms and their possible causes 95

UPPER GASTROINTESTINAL CONDITIONS 103
Oesophagus 103
Stomach 104
Intestines (small and large) 105

DIARRHOEAL CONDITIONS 107
Diarrhoea and vomiting 107

LIVER, GALL BLADDER, PANCREAS AND SPLEEN 115
Liver problems 115
Gall bladder problems 117
Pancreas problems 117
Spleen problems 118

INTESTINAL INFESTATIONS   119
   Worms   119

ANORECTAL CONDITIONS   121
   Symptoms of anorectal disease   121
   An approach to the physical examination   123
   Anorectal diseases   123

ENDOCRINE SYSTEM

DIABETES MELLITUS   129
   The diagnosis of diabetes mellitus   129
   Short-term complications   129
   Long-term complications   131
   Management of diabetes mellitus   133
   Medicine protocol   135
   Diagram A (Protocol for Type 2 diabetes patients)   138
   Diagram B (Insulin protocol for Type 2 diabetes patients)   139

THYROID GLAND   141
   Thyroid gland problems   141

KIDNEY AND UROLOGICAL DISORDERS

UROLOGICAL PROBLEMS   145
   Urological symptoms   145
   Urological diseases   146

SEXUALLY TRANSMITTED INFECTIONS

HIV AND AIDS   155
   HIV and AIDS in adults   155
   Opportunistic infections (adults)   156
   HIV and AIDS in children   161
   Opportunistic infections (children)   162
   Antiretroviral therapy (ART) in adults   163
   Antiretroviral therapy (ART) in children   166
   Post-exposure HIV prophylaxis   167

OTHER SEXUALLY TRANSMITTED INFECTIONS   168
   Quality care for people with STIs   168
   Urethritis   168
   Epididymo-orchitis   169
   Balanitis   169
   Prostatitis   170
   Genital ulceration   170
   Vaginal discharges   174
   Genital warts (condylomata acuminata)   176
   Molluscum contagiosum   176
   Paraphimosis   176

FEMALE REPRODUCTIVE SYSTEM

GYNAECOLOGICAL SYMPTOMS   179
   Common causes   179
   Abnormal uterine bleeding   183

LOWER GENITAL TRACT DISEASES   **189**
   Infections of the vulva   189
   Swellings of the labia   189
   Vaginal discharge   190
   Diseases of the cervix   191
   Trauma   192

UPPER GENITAL TRACT DISEASES   196
   Diseases of the uterus   196
   Salpingitis/pelvic inflammatory disease (PID)   197

MISCARRIAGE (ABORTION)   199
   Diagnosis   199
   Types of miscarriage   199

ECTOPIC PREGNANCY   201
   Acute ectopic pregnancy   201
   Chronic ectopic pregnancy   201

POST-PREGNANCY COMPLICATIONS   202
   Puerperal sepsis   202
   Perineal lacerations and episiotomies   202
   Breast conditions   203

CONTRACEPTION   207
   Methods of contraception   207

NERVOUS SYSTEM

EPILEPSY   213
   Assessment of seizures   213
   Management of epilepsy   214
   Status epilepticus   217

NEUROLOGICAL PROBLEMS   219
   Headache   219
   Other conditions causing headaches   223
   Weakness   225
   Change in sensation   227
   Mental confusion (and change in consciousness)   228
   Tremor   228
   Dizziness and fainting (syncope and blackout)   228

THE EYE

PROBLEMS OF THE EYE   233
   Indications for referral   233
   Symptoms of eye problems   233
   Diseases of the eye   236
   Eye injury   240

Cataract	242
Eye abscesses	242

THE SKIN

PROBLEMS OF THE SKIN — 245

Assessment of rashes	245
Rashes in neonates and infants	245
Common childhood rashes	247
Nutritional skin diseases	249
Bacterial conditions	249
Viral conditions	251
Fungal diseases	253
Parasites and insects	255
Allergies	256
Miscellaneous conditions	260
Hormonal disorders	261
Pigmentation disorders	263
Common tumours	264
Bullous disorders (blisters of the skin)	265

SURGERY

SURGICAL PROBLEMS — 269

Head injury	269
Shock	271
Stab wounds	272
Open wounds	275
Hand injuries	276
Bruises and abrasions	277
Chest injuries	277
Muscle injuries	278
Infections	279
Leg ulcers	281
Surgical lumps and bumps	282
Inguino-scrotal region	283
Abdominal wall	285
The breast	285

MUSCULOSKELETAL SYSTEM

GENERAL PRINCIPLES — 289

Diagnosis of orthopaedic problems	289
Principles of management of trauma	289

JOINTS — 293

Joint problems	293
Comparison of the clinical features of different types of arthritis	298

BONE DISORDERS — 299

Osteoporosis	299
Osteomyelitis	299

THE SPINE — 301

Spine problems	301

THE ARM — 311

Shoulder problems	311
Elbow problems	312
Forearm problems	313
Wrist problems	314
Hand and finger problems	316

THE LEG — 317

Upper leg problems	317
Knee problems	319
Lower leg problems	323
Foot problems	325

MATERNITY

ROUTINE ANTENATAL CARE — 331

Normal pregnancy	331
The first antenatal visit	331
Antenatal visits	333

ANTENATAL PROBLEMS — 335

Management of common antenatal problems	335

LABOUR AND DELIVERY — 345

Diagnosis of labour	345
Established labour for low-risk women	345
Common labour problems	346
Second stage of labour	347
Third stage of labour	348

THE PUERPERIUM — 351

Routine postnatal care	351
Common postnatal problems	351

NEONATAL CARE — 353

Neonatal conditions	353
Head problems	356
Chest problems	358
Abdomen problems	362
Limb problems	363

TROPICAL DISEASES

MALARIA — 367

MENTAL HEALTH

MENTAL HEALTH — 373

Mental disorder due to a physical illness	373
Aggressive disruptive behaviour in adults	373
Psychoses	374
Mood disorders	375

Adjustment disorder with depressed mood	377
Substance-related disorders	377
Anxiety and stress-related disorders	378

PHARMACOPOEIA 381

ABBREVIATIONS 398

INDEX 400

EMERGENCIES

RESUSCITATION

CARDIOPULMONARY RESUSCITATION (CPR)

MANAGEMENT

C: CIRCULATION
A: AIRWAY
B: BREATHING
D: DEFIBRILLATION
E: EMERGENCY MEDICINES;
   ENDOTRACHEAL INTUBATION;
   ELEVATE LEGS
F: FLUID THERAPY
G: GLUCOSE CHECK
H: HOSPITAL TRANSFER

Check if patient is conscious or not
- Shake the patient gently.
- Shout "Are you OK?"
- If no response, rub the sternum with your knuckles.

Position the patient
- Place the patient supine on a firm, flat surface
  - watch out for, and prevent, spinal injury if patient must be moved.
- Initiate CAB (Circulation - Airways - Breathing) sequence of CPR.

C : CIRCULATION
Check for carotid pulse (in young children brachial or femoral pulse)
- If pulse present and no breathing, ventilate only (see page 4: Airway and Breathing).
- If pulse absent, start with 30 chest compressions at a rate of 100 compressions per minute (compress over the lower half of the sternum).

Ratio for 1 rescuer
- Do chest compressions x 30
- Do mouth-to-mouth x 2
- Do this 30:2 combination x 5
- Recheck pulse
- Repeat 30:2 combination and recheck pulse every few minutes

Ratio for 2 rescuers
- Same ratio as above
- Rescuers switch duties every 5 cycles (or 2 minutes)
  - they should take less than 5 seconds to switch

- Ventilation (breath) rate is 1 breath every 6-8 seconds
  - ie 8-10 breaths / minute
- Compression rate is 100 / minute

Cardiac massage
Assess for a pulse by feeling gently for 5-10 seconds
In adults
- Feel for a carotid pulsation in the neck.
- Place 2-3 fingers on the Adam's apple, and slide fingers sideways into groove between the Adam's apple and the muscle (sternocleido-mastoid).
- Feel for a least 10 seconds (to exclude bradycardia).

In infants
- Feel gently for a brachial pulse on the inner aspect of the upper arm.

Ventilate if pulse is present but patient is not breathing
In adults
- Ventilate 8-10 breaths per minute
- Once every 6-8 seconds

In infants and children
- Ventilate 15-20 times per minute
- Once every 3 seconds

NB.
- Remember to open the airways before attempting inflation.
- Allow time for the lungs to deflate and check the rib cage to see that deflation is taking place.

Compress sternum if pulse is absent
NB. A single precordial thump is only indicated in adults if no pulse is detected, in a cardiac arrest which you have seen happen in front of you.

In adults
- Use the heel of both hands (one on top of the other) placed 2 finger-widths above the xiphisternum (or at least on lower sternum between nipples)
  - keep your elbows straight
  - keep your shoulders directly above your hands
- Compress 30 times to a depth of 4-5 cm at a rate of 100 per minute.
  - use a rhythm of 1 and 2 and 3 etc. up to 30
- Then return to the airway opening, giving 2 slow breaths, then continue 30 compressions (30:2 combination).
- Repeat cycles of 30 compressions and 2 breaths.

In children
- Use only one hand
- Compress to a depth of $1/3$ to $1/2$ the depth of the chest
  - at a rate of 100 per minute
  - using a ratio of 30 compressions to 2 breaths (30:2 combination)

In infants
- Use 2 fingers
    - placed one finger breadth below the inter-nipple line
- Compress to a depth of ½ the depth of the chest
    - at a rate of 120 per minute
    - using a ratio of 30 compressions to 2 breaths (30:2 combination)

NB.
- Do not pause for ventilation if the patient is intubated.
- Check for return of pulse / respiration after one minute (5 cycles of 30 compressions) and after that every few minutes.
- *Never interrupt CPR for more than 7 seconds (unless intubating or defibrillating).*
- For cardiac massage on a baby, see page 359.

A : AIRWAY

- Suction vomitus or manually remove foreign bodies from the mouth.
- Leave dentures in place if possible, as they provide a firm seal when ventilating the patient
    - remove only if they are not fitting well and are causing an obstruction.
- Open the airway by:
    - lifting the bony part of the chin with the fingers of one hand
    - placing your other hand on the patient's forehead and tilting the head backwards
    - this will lift the jaw and tongue off the posterior pharyngeal wall, opening the airway

---

NB.
- **Do not tilt the head backwards if a neck injury is suspected.**
- Instead, place your fingers behind the angle of the jaw on each side
    - push the jaw forwards while opening the mouth with your thumbs (jaw-thrust manoeuvre).
- If the correct size oro-pharyngeal airway is available, this may be inserted.

B : BREATHING

Check for breathing
- Observe the chest wall for movement.
- Listen and feel for air at the nose and mouth.

If there is no breathing, apply artificial respiration
- With Ambubag and face mask

Or
- Mouth-to-mask ventilation

Artificial ventilation
- Cheap, one-way-valve, plastic, mouth protectors for use during mouth-to-mouth ventilation are available from the Heart Foundation of South Africa
    - every person who may need to do CPR should obtain one.
- If patient is not breathing, give 1 **slow** breath into the patient's mouth (lasting 1 second) while
    - keeping the airway open with head tilt / chin lift
    - pinching the patient's nose closed, using the hand which is on the patient's forehead
    - note if the chest wall rises
    - allow 1-2 seconds per breath for the ventilation to be exhaled.
- If the chest does not rise, repeat the head tilt / chin lift
    - give a second breath
    - again watch for the chest to rise
- Mouth-to-nose ventilation may be indicated
    - in the presence of trismus
    - with mouth injuries
    - if a firm mouth-to-mouth seal is difficult to achieve.
- Mouth-to-mouth-and-nose ventilation may be used for small children.

NB.
- If a face mask is being used for ventilation, a tight seal around the mouth and nose is essential
    - while keeping the airway open with a head tilt / chin lift.
- This can be assessed by observing for adequate chest movement when ventilating.
- Oxygen can be connected via a resuscitator bag (eg. Ambu) if available, but initially time should not be wasted looking for oxygen.
- Resuscitator bags are more effective if used by two people
    - one holding the mask firmly on the face
    - the other squeezing the bag adequately
- Slow ventilation decreases the risk of oesophageal and gastric inflation, and therefore regurgitation and aspiration.

D : DEFIBRILLATION, DRIP, DRUGS, DOCTOR

- Defibrillation is essential for ventricular fibrillation
- Drip inserted for intravenous therapy
- Drugs as required
- Doctor's assistance as soon as possible

Defibrillation
- Ensure synchronisation switch is **off**.
- Ventricular fibrillation is the most common mechanism of cardiac arrest in adults
    - therefore, the sooner the patient is defibrillated, the greater the chance of successful resuscitation.
- **In the absence of a doctor, the clinic sister should attempt to do it immediately if there is no pulse.**
- Before placing paddles, put KY jelly or ECG paste on the appropriate areas.

- Place one paddle.
- Place the other paddle just below and lateral to the left nipple in the mid-axillary line
  - press firmly.
- ECG paste, if available, will enhance electrical conduction
  - KY jelly is not as good, but may be used if nothing else is available.

If no pulse is present
- Administer a 200 joules unsynchronised DC shock stat
  - ie. ensure that "synch" button, if present, is switched **off**
  - ensure everyone stands clear before shock is delivered.

If no pulse returns
- Repeat with 300 joules stat

If still no pulse returns
- Repeat with 360 joules stat

NB.
- *3 shocks are administered rapidly and consecutively*
- Check for return of pulse before and after each shock

If still no pulse returns
- Continue CPR
- Set up an IV line
- Administer drugs as prescribed below
  - repeat 3 shocks at 360 joules every minute if no pulse returns while giving the drugs.

Drip and medcines
Adults
NB. Epinephrine is indicated **first** in all cardiac arrests Wnot responding to CPR or defibrillation.
- Set up an IV line of normal saline as soon as possible.
- Give epinephrine 1: 1 000 1 ml diluted in 9 ml normal saline IV immediately as a single dose.
- Repeat every 3-5 minutes during resuscitation
- If no IV line available, it is best to give epinephrine endobronchial through an endotracheal tube
  - give 1 ml epinephrine diluted in 9 ml sterile water or normal saline.

Bradycardia
- Give atropine IV 0.5 mg as a bolus.
- Repeat every 3-5 minutes if no response.
- Maximum dose 3 mg.

Children
- Dilute 1 ml epinephrine to 10 ml using sterile water or normal saline
  - 11-15 years   5 ml
  - 7-11 years   3 ml
  - 5-7 years   2 ml
  - 18 months-5 years 1.5 ml
  - 6-18 months   1 ml
  - 0-6 months   0.5 ml
- Give epinephrine immediately
  - IV or via endotracheal tube
  - repeat every 3-5 minutes during resuscitation if necessary

E : ECG, ENDOTRACHEAL INTUBATION, ELEVATE LEGS
- Do an electro-cardiograph - further management is according to the response
- Intubate if competent to do so
- Elevate legs to counteract shock

Approach to rhythm interpretation
Cardiac arrest rhythms
There are really only two cardiac arrest rhythms:
- Shockable rhythms
  - ventricular fibrillation (VF)
  - pulseless ventricular tachycardia (VT).
- Non-shockable rhythms
  - asystole
  - pulseless electrical activity (electromechanical dissociation, bradysystolic rhythms and pulseless idioventricular rhythms).

▼ Note to doctor
ECG response
Wavy line on ECG with no pulse (ventricular fibrillation) or pulseless ventricular tachycardia
- Defibrillate stat if no pulse detected (200, 300, 360 joules)
- If initial defibrillation is unsuccessful
  - give epinephrine stat (IV or via the endotracheal tube 10 ml (of 1:10 dilution)
  - repeat every 3-5 minutes until the heart restarts.
- Defibrillate 3 times at 360 joules one minute after each epinephrine dose is given (4 joules / kg for children)
  - check for return of pulse before continuing CPR.

Asystole (electrical silence on the monitor)
- Ensure that the electrodes are not dried out / have enough jelly
- This is a non-shockable rhythm
- Remember **CAB**: **C**irculation - **A**irway - **B**reathing
  - confirm asystole
  - give medication ie. epinephrine / atropine
- Consider pacing
- Continue CPR
- If CPR is unsuccessful, give epinephrine stat (IV or via endotracheal tube 10 ml (of 1:10 dilution) (children see dosage chart)
  - repeat every 3-5 minutes as required during resuscitation.
- Give atropine stat (IV or via endotracheal tube) 0.5 mg (children 0.02 mg/kg/dose)
  - repeat dose if no response

Pulseless electrical activity (electromechanical dissociation)
ie. QRS complexes on ECG but no pulses detectable
- Give oxygen
- Control airway
- Continue CPR
- Give epinephrine every 3-5 minutes as required
  - give atropine and sodium bicarbonate
- Look for, and treat, precipitating factors eg.
  - shock from fluid or blood loss (hypo-volaemia)
  - hypoxia
  - tension pneumothorax (see page 274).

Reversible causes of asystole / pulseless electrical activity
The 6 "H"s:
- Hypovolaemia
- Hypoxia
- Hydrogen ions (acidosis)
- Head injury
- Heart block
- Hypothermia

The 5 "T"s:
- Tablets (drug overdose)
- Tamponade (cardiac)
- Tension pneumothorax
- Thrombosis (acute MI)
- Thrombosis (pulmonary embolus)

General comments

- Best success rates are achieved when
    - CPR is started within 4 minutes of arrest
    - advanced life support is started within 8 minutes of arrest.
- Defibrillate as soon as defibrillator becomes available
    - do "blind" defibrillation if no ECG monitor available
    - always check for the absence of pulse **before** defibrillating.
- Epinephrine, atropine and naloxone can be safely and effectively administered via the endotracheal tube if no IV line available
    - but use **double** the IV dose.
- Avoid intracardiac epinephrine if possible (except as a last resort)
- Fixed, dilated pupils may be due to drugs, hypothermia, snake bite, etc. and do not necessarily always indicate irreversible brain damage.
- The use of bicarbonate, calcium and isoprenaline during CPR is uncertain, and may do more harm than good in many cases.
- If not breathing spontaneously but heart still beating, arrange transfer with continued ventilation in the ambulance.
- **If no response,** continue resuscitation for at least
    - 30 minutes in **adults**
    - 60 minutes in **children.**

  This applies particularly if the patient was cold when you started to resuscitate as the brain stays alive longer if the body temperature is cold.

Endotracheal intubation

- Intubate the trachea as soon as practical after cardiac arrest only if
    - competent to do so
    - equipment is in good working order.
- Always oxygenate lungs well before intubating
    - there should be a good seal with Ambubag mask
    - place oropharangeal airway to get the tongue out of the way
    - somebody should apply cricoid pressure to open airway helping to block oesophagus, reducing amount of air entering the stomach
- Intubate using a 7,0-8,0 mm endotracheal tube in adults
- If more than one attempt is required, oxygenate and ventilate patient adequately between attempts.
- Avoid taking too long when attempting intubation
    - hold your breath when intubating
    - when you run out of breath, stop trying to intubate and ventilate with oxygen again ▲

F : FLUID THERAPY
G : GLUCOSE CHECK
H : HOSPITAL TRANSFER

- Fluid therapy
    - see shock on page 271
- Glucose
    - check blood glucose to exclude hypoglycaemia
- Hospital transfer when the patient is stabilised

AIRWAY OBSTRUCTION (BY FOREIGN BODY)

Clinical features

Some of the features indicating obstruction to the airways are

- Inability to talk, breathe or cough
- Patient clutches throat
- Stridor
- Dyspnoea
- Accessory muscles of respiration vigorously (strongly) used
- Marked distension and emptying of jugular veins while trying to breathe
- Intercostal recession
- Cyanosis
- Collapse

MANAGEMENT

In the conscious patient

- Encourage the patient to cough if possible
- *Do not slap the patient on the back*

The Heimlich manoeuvre

- Stand behind the patient and wrap your arms around the patient's waist.
- Make a fist with one hand and grasp the fist with the other hand.
- Place thumb side of the fist against the patient's abdomen in the mid-line just above the navel.
- Administer a series of up to 5 quick, upward thrusts

In the unconscious patient

Finger sweep

- Grab the patient's tongue and jaw, pulling forwards, with the thumb and fingers of one hand.
- Insert the index finger of your other hand inside and along the patient's cheek, down behind the base of the tongue.
- Remove the foreign body with a hook action
    - be careful to avoid pushing it further down.

The Heimlich manoeuvre

- Lie the patient on his / her back (supine)
- Kneel astride the patient's thighs
- Place the heel of your hand in the mid-line just above the patient's navel
    - place one hand on top of the other
- Administer a series of up to 5 quick, upward thrusts
- Repeat the finger sweep

In grossly obese or pregnant patients

If the patient is conscious

- Place your arms around the patient's chest forming a fist over the mid-sternum.
- Apply a series of sharp, backward-directed thrusts

If the patient is unconscious

- Apply chest compressions as with CPR

In small children or babies

- Hold the baby over your arm and resting on your thigh, face down and head down
    - slap on the back between the shoulder blades up to 5 times.
- If the object has come out and the baby is still not breathing
    - turn the baby over and start mouth-to-mouth ventilation.
- If the object has not dislodged
    - give 5 chest thrusts on the mid-sternum (inferior to the nipples).

- If the object is no longer causing obstruction and is now loose
    - remove it carefully with a bent finger, taking care not to push it further down again.
- If not dislodged, turn the baby over and repeat the 5 back slaps as above

NB. *The only situation where a slap on the back helps is where the whole child is held with the head down.*

ALLERGIC REACTIONS

How to decide if a patient is having an allergic reaction or not

- In the working situation a patient who has been given a drug, especially a penicillin injection, may appear to have an allergic reaction.
- It is important to try and decide
    - how serious this reaction is
    - whether it is really due to the drug or the injection.
- The patient may also say if they are allergic to an injection, and with further questioning, they are actually
    - just afraid of the injection
    - **or** have had local swelling or severe pain at the site of the injection, which they thought was an allergic reaction.

MILD ALLERGIC REACTION

Causes

- Allergic reactions are caused by a substance that the person is allergic to (allergen) reacting with the body's defence system.
- This interaction causes cells in the body to release powerful chemicals which are meant to assist the body to protect itself against the foreign antigen.
- In an allergic response there is an over reaction of the body and these normal substances are released in excessive amounts.
- This results in the features of allergy such as
    - dilation of blood vessels and oedema of the area eg. mild cases of local oedema of the skin called a wheal
    - release of histamine and other substances which cause itching and pain.

Clinical features

- It usually starts some hours after an injection or taking a tablet
- Itching which is mild
    - may be generalised
- May have a few wheals on some parts of the body (urticaria)
- Blood pressure, pulse and respiration will be normal
- There will be **no** respiratory symptoms

MANAGEMENT

- Oral antihistamines eg.
    - chlorphenamine 4 mg 3 x daily for adults
    - chlorphenamine syrup 1 mg (2.5 ml) 3 x daily for children 2-5 years
    - chlorphenamine syrup 2 mg (5 ml) 3 x daily for children >5 years

- A wet wrap applied to the rash may help the itch

NB. Supply a sensitivity bracelet warning of the allergy if this is known, or help the patient to apply to "Medic Alert" if he / she can afford it.

MODERATE ALLERGIC REACTION

Clinical features

- Numerous / large wheels on many parts of the body
- Severe itch
- Anxiety
- Flushed and feels hot
- **No** respiratory symptoms
- Blood pressure normal

MANAGEMENT

- **REFER** for observation and possible further treatment.
- Give antihistamine eg. chlorphenamine orally 3 x daily
    - **plus** promethazine (Phenergan) 25-50 mg IM stat
- Arrange for a sensitivity bracelet.
- Observe the patient until you are sure that he / she is improving before sending home.

SEVERE ALLERGIC REACTION (INCLUDING ANAPHYLAXIS)

This is due to the massive release of many different powerful substances/chemicals which results in the following:

- Sudden and great dilation of blood vessels throughout the body which cause acute profound hypo-volaemic shock.
- Localised oedema of some areas of the body especially of the face, lips or tongue, called angioedema
- Swelling of the bronchi and severe bronchospasm.

Clinical features

- Signs of anaphylaxis may occur almost instantly, or may develop progressively over some hours.
- Severe disseminated urticaria and itch
- Sense of impending death
- Upper airways obstruction as shown by
    - swelling of the face, lips, tongue
    - lump in the throat and hoarseness
    - in severe cases progressing to stridor and eventual total upper airways obstruction.
- Lower airways obstruction
    - tightness of the chest
    - coughing
    - wheezing
    - tachypnoea, dyspnoea
    - cyanosis and eventual respiratory arrest.
- Vascular collapse
    - generalised dilation of all blood vessels of the body
    - associated generalised urticaria and wheals as a result of the dilation
    - severe shock due to loss of fluid into the tissues as oedema.
- Followed by collapse, coma and rapid death

Differential diagnosis

Vasovagal attack

- This is common, and it is often misdiagnosed as an anaphylaxis
    - the patient is then labelled "penicillin allergic".
- It is due to anxiety or fear of an injection
- The patient begins to feel faint and light-headed within a minute of the injection.
- They then often faint and collapse
- They have no symptoms or signs of anaphylaxis
- Blood pressure and respiration are normal
- There is **no**
    - rash
    - wheeze
    - swelling of the face.
- The patient recovers consciousness within a minute spontaneously, if left to lie down.

1. ACCURATE ASSESSMENT

- Assess if it really is an allergic reaction or not
- Assess whether it is a mild, moderate or a severe reaction.

2. Place hypotensive or shocked patients in a horizontal position.

- Do **not** sit the patient up.

3. AIRWAY

- Give oxygen 8-10 L/minute via facemask.
- If unconscious, assess if breathing and circulation are intact or if there is a need for CPR
    - call the doctor.

4. EPINEPHRINE

- Give epinephrine 0.5 ml (1:1000) IM into the antero-lateral thigh, provided the patient still has an adequate blood pressure and circulation
- If the patient is severely shocked (child or adult), give epinephrine IV diluted in normal saline.
    - dilute 1 ml epinephrine in 9 ml normal saline (1:10 000) (see dosage chart below)
    - repeat every 5-10 minutes if there is no improvement.
- If an endotracheal tube has been inserted, and if no vein can be found, epinephrine can be injected down the tube through a syringe
    - add 1 ml epinephrine to 9 ml of normal saline or sterile water
    - instil the 10 ml down the tube in an adult.

	Intra-muscular epinephrine undiluted 1:1 000	Intravenous epinephrine diluted 1:10 000	Endotracheal tube epinephrine diluted 1: 10 000
Adults			
	0.5 ml	5 ml	10 ml
Children			
11-15 years	0.5 ml	5 ml	5 ml
7-11 years	0.3 ml	3 ml	3 ml
5-7 years	0.2 ml	2 ml	2 ml
18 months - 5 years	–	1.5 ml	1.5 ml
6-18 months	–	1 ml	1 ml
Birth- 6 months	–	0.5 ml	0.5 ml

5. ADMINISTRATION OF IVI FLUIDS

Put up a drip as soon as possible of normal saline.

6. ANTI-ASTHMATIC AGENTS

If bronchospasm:

- Give bronchodilators by nebulisation (see asthma protocol pages 59-61)
    - **or** give by spray 2 puffs 2 minutes apart eg. salbutamol (Ventolin).

7. ADRENOCORTICO-STEROID

Solucortef

- Give hydrocortisone (Solucortef) 200 mg IV as a bolus as it takes time to start working.

Adult dose

- 100-200 mg = 1-2 amps

Paediatric dose

- 2-3 mg / kg IV (maximum dose 100 mg)
    - 0-3 years   50 mg
    - 3-7 years   75 mg
    - 7-15 years   100 mg

8. ANTIHISTAMINE

If the patient has an itch:

Promethazine (Phenergan)

Adult dose

- 50 mg (= 2 ml) IM or slow IV stat

Paediatric dose

- 0,25 mg / kg body weight IM or slow IV stat
    - 2-5 years   5 mg (0.2 ml)
    - 5-7 years   10 mg (0.4 ml)
    - 7-11 years   15 mg (0.6 ml)
    - 11-15 years   20 mg (0.8 ml)

9. REASSURE THE PATIENT

- Anxiety and stress makes the patient's condition much worse.
- It is important to reassure, support and calm the patient and the relatives
    - this is particularly important with a child.
- Speak to the patient and explain what has happened and what will happen.

10. ADMIT TO HOSPITAL

- All patients with a severe allergic reaction must be transferred to hospital for observation.
- Continue with oxygen and intravenous fluids.
- Record carefully in a referral letter all that has happened including the management given.
- Epinephrine administration may have to be repeated during transport. Close observation during transport is essential.

DROWNING

Near drowning

- Water rushes into the airways
- When it reaches the larynx it often stops, because the water, which is often cold and dirty, irritates the vocal cords.
- The cords snap shut and go into spasm
- This prevents water reaching the lungs
- If untreated, these patients will suffocate, and the heart will stop
- If CPR is started as soon as possible on these patients, they can be saved
- About 40% of drowning deaths would be saved if rescue breathing (mouth-to-mouth / nose) was started in the water, instead of waiting until the patient was removed from the water
- If pulse is absent, chest compressions to start as soon as the patient is on a firm surface.

"Secondary drowning"

- This is not true drowning
- It is the name given to the pulmonary oedema and pneumonia that can result from the aspiration of small amounts of water in cases of near drowning
    - this is before the vocal cords snap shut completely.
- "Secondary drowning" can occur between 30 minutes and 5 days after the immersion.

MANAGEMENT

NB. Always make every attempt to resuscitate, no matter how hopeless the situation seems.

- The hypothermia caused by immersion in cold water protects the brain to some extent from the damage caused by anoxia.
- Cold water in contact with the face also causes a redistribution of blood supply to the heart and brain (the diving reflex).
- Victims can possibly make a complete recovery even after 30 minutes under water.
- ***Do not give up the resuscitation, especially in children.***

Respiration

- If the patient is not breathing, start ventilating **stat**
- Mouth-to-mouth ventilation can be started in the water as you are dragging the victim to the bank.
- Remove victim from the water carefully if there could be any suspicion of neck injury eg. diving accident.

Heartbeat

- After inflating the lungs twice, feel for a carotid pulse or for a pulse in the groin.
- If the pulse is present, continue ventilating the patient until spontaneous respiration returns.
- If there is *no* heart beat, do full CPR (see page 3)
- ***Continue until normal heart beat returns***

Hypothermia

If you are not in a situation where the patient can be properly monitored.

- Do **not** try and re-warm the patient, because the cold protects the brain cells to some extent.

If in a situation where you can properly monitor the patient eg. a hospital

- Check the rectal temperature using a low reading thermometer if available.
- If it is below 35°C, begin active re-warming with **warm IV fluids at 37°C.**
- Give warmed oxygen therapy

General management

- A naso-gastric tube should be inserted to empty the stomach to prevent vomiting and aspiration.
- A fractured neck should always be suspected and a cervical collar should be applied
    - the victim may have fallen into the water as a result of trauma
- Find out why the patient fell into the water
    - ask any witnesses what happened
    - ask relatives and friends if the patient has any medical condition which could cause loss of consciousness eg. diabetes, epilepsy, alcohol intake etc.
- **REFER** for observation for 48 hours, even if the patient seems to make a full recovery, in case he develops "secondary drowning" or pneumonia

NB.

- ***Resuscitate patients continuously until reaching hospital especially in cases of hypothermia.***
- *The results of CPR are very good in such situations because the brain cells are preserved longer.*
- *Fixed, dilated pupils are **not** necessarily a sign of death.*

LIGHTNING AND ELECTRIC SHOCK

With electrical shock the victim may either be thrown away or attached to the power point.

MANAGEMENT
- **Do not touch the victim if still attached to the electric power point or plug**
- If the mains or plug switches are easily reached, then switch them off
- If this is not possible
  - use a non-conducting object such as anything made of wood or glass, or a blanket or newspaper, to pull the victim away from the electric source.
- If the victim has no pulse, start CPR stat
  - results of CPR are good
  - even delayed CPR can have successful results because the brain cells may not die as quickly as expected.

NB. Fixed, dilated pupils are not necessarily a sign of death. Continuous and vigorous resuscitation may reverse dilated pupils.

- Send for help as soon as possible
- **Do not stop resuscitation until at least 2 hours after the event**
- Treat any burns (see page 15)
- **REFER** to hospital for observation in case of cardiac or other damage due to the electricity.

Note.
- The electric shock may cause spinal injury due to muscle spasm.
- Move patients with care

BITES, POISONS AND STINGS

ANIMAL AND HUMAN BITES

- Bites may result in wound infection often due to mixed aerobic and anaerobic infection.
- Human bites can pass on HIV, hepatitis, syphilis, actinomyces and tuberculosis.
- Dog bites can pass on rabies and brucellosis, among other infections.
- Bites of the hands are the most serious because of the high incidence of sepsis
    - tendon sheaths lead into one another
    - therefore infection in one finger can quickly involve the whole hand

MANAGEMENT
REFER

Wound treatment
- Irrigate well and then clean wound with povidone iodine 10% solution (inactivates rabies virus).
- Avoid suturing and local anaesthetic (unless the wound is deep and large) as this may potentially spread the rabies virus.

Rabies vaccine and immunoglobulin (animal bites only)
These are available from the nearest district hospital or community health centre.

Rabies vaccine
- Administer 1 dose on days 0, 3, 7 and 14.
    - in immunocompromised patients, an additional dose must be given on day 28
- Administer vaccine by IM injection in the deltoid region in adults, and anterolateral thigh in infants / young children.

Anti-rabies immunoglobulin, 20 units / kg
- Administer in persons with bites and scratches that penetrate the skin and draw blood.
- Indicated also in persons who are known to be immunocompromised with superficial scratches without bleeding.
- Infiltrate into and around the bite with up to 50% of the dose.
- Administer remaining immunoglobulin into the deltoid muscle opposite to vaccination site.
- It must be given as soon as possible after exposure, but if not available, it must still be administered up to 7 days after the first vaccine dose is given.

Tetanus prophylaxis (animal bites only)
If not immunised within the last 5 years, give tetanus toxoid vaccine IM 0.5 ml.

Pre-emptive antibiotic (only if the hand is bitten or for extensive wounds or human bites)
- Co-amoxiclav for 5 days
    - adults: 875/125 mg 2 x daily
    - children: dosage according to age 3 x daily

- Penicillin-allergic patients
    - adults and adolescents >11 years:
      azithromycin 500 mg daily for 3 days
      plus metronidazole 400 mg 3 x daily for 5 days
    - children: azithromycin daily x 3 days
        - 1-3 years: 120 mg
        - 3-7 years: 200 mg
        - 7-11 years: 250 mg
      plus metronidazole, dosage according to age for 5 days

HIV prophylaxis (human bites only, and only if the patient consents to be tested for HIV and the result is negative)
- Combined TDF + FTC (300 / 200 mg) daily for 28 days

OR
- Combined AZT + 3TC (300 / 150 mg) 2 x daily for 28 days

SNAKE BITES

Bites by snakes that are poisonous are not common. However, all snake bites should be considered dangerous.
Often the damage is caused by incorrect treatment.

- It is impossible to tell by looking at the bite marks whether a person has been poisoned or what type of snake it was
- Venom from poisonous snakes has poisons which are
    - cytotoxic
    - neurotoxic
    - haemotoxic
- Poisonous snakes can be divided into the above *3 groups depending on which type of toxin predominates in the venom*
- Symptoms and signs of poisoning may take several hours to develop
    - do not discharge patients too soon
    - observe for 24 hours in the clinic or hospital

CYTOTOXIC POISONS

These poisons are produced mainly by:

Adders and vipers
- Especially the Puffadder, iBululu (Zulu), iRamba (Xhosa), Lebolobolo, Marabe (Sotho)
    - other examples include the Berg Adder, Gaboon Adder, Night Adder, Stilleto Snake
- Adders have a
    - flat, arrow-shaped head
    - short, stout body
    - often lie in "z"-shaped position

Spitting cobras
- Mozambique Spitting Cobra, Rinkhals

Clinical features
- Local tissue damage
- Severe pain and swelling at the site of the bite
  - may start within 10-30 minutes
- Blisters occur near the bite after a few hours
  - ecchymosis (bruising) and bullous haemorrhagic lesions occur after about 12 hours
- Death may occur due to hypovolaemic shock caused by severe local swelling.

NEUROTOXIC POISONS

Neurotoxic poisons are produced mainly by:

Non-spitting cobras
- Cape Cobra, isiKhotsholo (Xhosa), uPhempethwane (Zulu), masumo (S.Sotho)
- Egyptian Cobra, Forest Cobra

Spitting cobras
- Especially the Rinkhals (cytotoxic as well as neurotoxic) and Black Spitting Cobra.
- The characteristic feature of these is a hood at the back of the neck.
- These snakes may squirt their venom into people's eyes.

Mambas
- Especially Black Mamba, Green Mamba
- IMamba (Zulu and Xhosa), Mokopa (Tswana and Sotho)
- The head is continuous with the body
- They are slender, agile and fast and have large eyes

Clinical features
- There is very little pain at site of the bite
- There is very little swelling
- Weakness (even paralysis) often affecting the eye muscles first
  - this may start within minutes
- Muscle fasciculation (twitching)
- Double vision
- Drooping eyelids
- Difficulty in swallowing (dysphagia)
- Difficulty in breathing (dyspnoea)

Later
- Paralysis of all skeletal muscles
- Death is due to respiratory paralysis
  - **NB.** *Artificial ventilation may keep the patient alive*

HAEMOTOXIC POISONS

Haemotoxic poisons are produced mainly by:

Boomslang
- INambezulu (Xhosa), iNdlondlo (Ndebele), Legwere (Sotho)
- They have large eyes
- They bite deeply and hang on because the fangs are at the back of the mouth

Vine snakes
- The pupil of the eye is vertical like a key hole
- These snakes seldom bite and only a small amount of the venom is injected

Clinical features
- The venom stops blood clotting which leads to bleeding
- There is bleeding from the wound within hours
- Headache that is occipital and severe
- Bruises, epistaxis, haemoptysis and other haemorrhages may occur
- Death is due to internal bleeding

MANAGEMENT
Suspected snake bite
- Examine the area to make sure there are wounds due to the fangs
- It is important to reassure and calm the patient who will often be extremely anxious
- Wipe away any venom left on the skin and clean thoroughly with chlorhexidine 0,05% solution
- Place a clean pad over the wound
- Apply a wide crepe bandage firmly as this slows the uptake of the venom (not for cytotoxic snake bites)
  - apply from just above the bite site up to 10-15 cm proximal to the bite site
  - apply no tighter than for a sprained ankle
- Immobilise the limb with a splint or sling as this
  - makes the patient comfortable
  - slows the uptake of the venom
- **REFER** all patients with bites for observation for at least 24 hours.
- Give tetanus toxoid 0.5 ml subcutaneously.

NB.
- **Never** cut or suck the wound as this causes more damage.
- **Never** apply a tourniquet as this increases damage to the tissues.

If signs of poisoning
Cytotoxic poisons
- Put up a drip of normal saline stat to counteract the shock
- Oxygen is helpful if shock occurs
- Give analgesics eg. paracetamol, ibuprofen or morphine
  - especially for adder bites which are very painful
- **REFER** stat to hospital

Neurotoxic poisons
- If the patient starts to have difficulty in breathing
  - give oxygen if available
  - ventilate if required
- Put up a drip of normal saline or Ringer's lactate
  - **REFER** stat to hospital

Snake bite anti-venom
- It has a high risk of anaphylaxis.
- It should only be used in patients with definite symptoms of poisoning.
- **Note:** Patients with a suspected Black Mamba bite should receive anti-venom before the onset of symptoms.
  - **REFER** patient urgently to hospital

Venom sprayed into the eye
Some snakes, eg. the rinkhals, can spray venom into people's eyes. If this is not attended to, it can cause blindness.
- Wipe venom off the face with a damp cloth
- Wash out the eyes **stat** with **large** amounts of water
- Instil tetracaine 0.5% eye drops into the eye/s and cover with eye pad/s
- **REFER** stat to hospital

Haemotoxic poisons
- Put up a drip of normal saline
- **REFER** for specific Boomslang snake bite anti-venom

POISONING AND DRUG OVERDOSE

Identification of the poison
- If the container is brought to the clinic if may be possible to identify the poison by
    - checking the label or identifying the container
    - smelling any remaining contents may give you a clue (**NB.** petroleum products)
    - send any remaining contents with the patient to the hospital
- If the substance is known, and information regarding specific therapy is required, phone the poison information centre: 0861 555 777

MANAGEMENT

Support vital functions
- Establish and maintain a clear airway
- Ensure adequate ventilation and oxygenation
- Check
    - blood pressure
    - heart rate / rhythm
    - temperature and respiration
    - blood glucose

Prevent further absorption
If there is poison on the skin
- Wash the skin with running water for at least 10 minutes
    - at least 30 minutes for caustic poisons

Gastric lavage
Indications
- This is of value only if the patient has ingested a potentially life-threatening poison and the procedure can be undertaken within 60 minutes of ingestion.

Conta-indications
- Do not attempt gastric lavage if the patient
    - has swallowed strong acids, alkalis or petroleum products
    - is in coma or has decreased level of consciousness unless the airway is protected

Method
- Lie the patient on his / her left side with head down
    - insert a wide bore orogastric tube (36F)
- Instil 300 ml normal saline and suck back
- Repeat until the aspirate is clear
- **NB.** Gastric lavage may be performed only after insertion of a cuffed ET tube in comatose patients

Activated charcoal
Indications
- Where a known poison or drug has been taken in a dose that is likely to be a danger.
- The greatest benefit is achieved if activated charcoal is administered within 1 hour after ingestion of poisonous substance.
- Anti-cholinergics from plants, e.g. stinkblaar and malpitte or from drugs including:
    - anti-psychotics
    - anti-histamines
    - tricyclic anti-depressants, e.g. amitriptyline

Other drugs:
- theophylline
- salicylates and other NSAIDs
- phenobarbitone, phenytoin
- warfarin and superwarfarin
- paracetamol
- sedatives, e.g. benzodiazepines

Contraindications
- Poisoning with corrosives.
- It is of no use after poisoning with metals, e.g. iron or petroleum products, such as paraffin or alcohols, e.g. methanol, ethylene glycol.

Method
- Give activated charcoal to drink (if conscious) or via an oro- or naso-gastric tube (if unconscious).
- Make a mixture of powdered activated charcoal:
    - 6 months-2 years: 10 g in 50-100 ml water
    - 2-5 years: 15 g in 100-150 ml water
    - 5-11 years: 25 g in 200 ml water
    - 11-15 years: 50 g in 400 ml water
    - >15 years-adults: 75 g in 600 ml water
- When mixing add a small amount of water to make a slurry. Then dilute further.
- Stir well and ensure that all the charcoal is fully dispersed.
- If given to a child, it is best put in a cooldrink tin so that the colour of the mixture is not seen.
- This can be given up to 24 hours later if the drug has an entero-hepatic circulation (re-secreted into the bowel from the liver).

Other drugs
- Consider giving naloxone in any patient presenting with
    - CNS depression and constricted pupils
    - even if you are not sure of the cause

SPECIFIC TYPES OF POISON

PARAFFIN POISONING

This is derived from petrol.

Other petrol products are benzene, paint thinners, turpentine

- It is a very common poison, especially in small children
- Paraffin is often kept in cold drink bottles, and children drink it, thinking that it is cold drink
- The most common problem is that the paraffin is aspirated into the lungs causing
    - chemical damage with hypoxia
    - possible direct effects on the brain when absorbed

MANAGEMENT
- Remove any clothes smelling of paraffin and use a damp cloth to wipe away any paraffin left on the skin
- **Never induce vomiting or do a gastric lavage as this makes the aspiration worse**
- Activated charcoal also does not help
- **REFER** all children for observation in hospital, unless the poisoning happened some days before and they are now fully recovered

CARBON MONOXIDE POISONING

- This happens as a result of burning an open fire or brazier in a room with all the windows sealed
- It is common in winter in poorer communities

> **MANAGEMENT**
>
> *If the patient is brought in acutely ill or unconscious*
> - Give oxygen, if necessary by Ambu bag, if not breathing well
>
> *If the patient is conscious*
> - Give analgesics for the headache
> - Advise them about the cause and how to prevent it

ORGANOPHOSPHATE POISONING

- Organophosphates are commonly used as insecticides and pesticides
- Notifiable condition

Clinical features
- Hypersalivation
- Bronchospasm and bronchorrhoea
- Lacrimation. rhinorrhoea
- Miosis / mydriasis
- Bradycardia
- Muscle twitching
- Diarrhoea and vomiting
- Confusion
- Convulsions
- Coma

> **MANAGEMENT**
> - Wear personal protective equipment
> - Intubate and ventilate if necessary
> - Remove clothing and wash affected skin with soap and water.
> - Suction secretions frequently.
> - For bronchorrhoea or bronchospasm
>   - give atropine IV
>   - 5 years and above 1mg
>   - <5 years 0.05 mg / kg / dose
> - Repeat every 10-15 minutes until bronchial secretions are controlled.

BEE STINGS

Generally bee stings only cause local pain and swelling. Stings are dangerous if the person:
- Has multiple stings
- Is allergic to bee stings

Clinical features
The following suggests a genuine allergy to bee stings:
- Swelling of parts of the face or tongue (angio-oedema), not just at the site of the sting
- Urticaria
- Severe symptoms or signs eg. respiratory symptoms
  - wheeze
  - dyspnoea
- Laryngeal oedema or anaphylaxis

> **MANAGEMENT**
> - Pull out the sting or scrape it out with a blade or finger nail **without** squeezing the venom sack
> - Apply a cold compress
> - Give chlorpheniramine
>
> *For allergic patients*
> - If developing the features of allergy, treat as for anaphylaxis (see page 7)
> - If they have definite symptoms of allergy, advise the person to be de-sensitised for bee stings as soon as possible.

SPIDER BITES

Spider bites are quite common, but are often missed and diagnosed as cellulitis or abscesses.

- The most common occurrence is that the person is bitten at night in bed
  - a painful swelling is seen in the morning
  - the swelling is bigger than a mosquito bite
  - careful inspection may show two tiny fang bites

Different species
- Sac spider (*Cheiracanthium*) and violin spider (*Loxosceles*)
  - produce a local necrotic skin lesion
  - ulceration may take months to heal
- Black Widow (button) spider *(Lactrodectus)*
  - black or brown spider with red stripes or dot on top of large abdomen
  - produces increasing local pain that may spread to include the entire limb
  - produces typical target lesions i.e. red ring surrounding a pale centre
  - the venom is neurotoxic, causing nausea, vomiting, sweating, blurred vision, cramp-like pains, difficulty with breathing
  - it responds well to anti-venom

> **MANAGEMENT**
>
> **REFER** *if there is*
> - Severe pain
> - Any symptoms of neurological involvement eg.
>   - breathing difficulty, double vision
>
> *For other bites*
> - Apply a cold compress to the area if bitten within the last 4 hours
> - Give paracetamol when necessary
> - Give re-assurance
> - Apply saline or betadine dressings if an ulcer forms
>   - if the ulcer is greater than 3 cm it may need grafting
> - Antibiotics are not usually necessary

BURNS

CLASSIFICATION

The classification of burns is important as it will determine the management.

CLASSIFICATION OF BURN BY DEPTH

■ SUPERFICIAL BURNS

- Superficial damage to the skin eg. due to sunburn
- There is mild to moderate pain and redness
- There may be mild blistering and later peeling

■ PARTIAL THICKNESS BURNS

- They can be identified by the fact that there is still sensation in the skin and the burns are painful
- The skin appears moist and patchy-red in colour
- The hair follicles are still visible as tiny, dark dots on the skin surface
- There may be blistering and white or yellow slough
- This level of burn heals well, unless complicated by sepsis

■ FULL THICKNESS BURNS

- The important features are:
    - sensation to the area is lost and the burns are painless
    - there is a dry, grey-white, paper-like appearance to the burn
    - there are no hair follicles or sweat glands visible in the burnt area
- Areas greater than 3 cm square will require skin grafting

CLASSIFICATION OF BURN BY EXTENT

This is the most important system of classification in the primary emergency care situation as the extent of the burn affects

- Whether the patient can be treated at the clinic or needs to be **REFERRED**
- Whether shock will occur

The percentage of the body's surface area burnt is calculated by "The Rule of Nine's"

The Rule of Nine's
Adults

Head and neck	= 9%	
Arm	= 9%	(two arms = 18%)
Chest - front	= 9%	
Chest - back	= 9%	
Abdomen - front	= 9%	
Abdomen - back	= 9%	
Leg - upper	= 9%	(whole leg = 18%)
Leg - lower	= 9%	(both legs = 36%)
Perineum	= 1%	
TOTAL	= 100%	

Children
Modified Rule of Nine's for children under 8 years
- For each year below 8
    - deduct ½% from each whole leg
    - and add 1% to the head

Note.
- In scattered burns, use the patient's palm as equivalent to 1%
- Add an extra 20% to the estimated total burnt area if there is
    - a fire burn of the face as this indicates a burn of the airways as well
    - black sputum as this indicates smoke inhalation

MANAGEMENT

- Remove the victim from immediate danger
    - *do not become a victim yourself*
    - *do not do anything that will place you in danger*
- The high temperature in the skin, as a result of the burn, continues to damage the underlying tissue for several hours after the burn has occurred
- **This ongoing damage to the body tissue can be lessened or stopped by cooling the area of the burn as soon as possible**
- This can be done by applying anything cold eg.
    - water, either poured over, or with wet cloths
    - ice wrapped in a cloth
    - or immerse the burnt area in cold water
- Continue with the cold application as long as the patient still feels a burning pain in the area
    - you may need to continue for 30-60 minutes
- It is worthwhile applying something cold to the burn areas at the clinic, even if the patient is only brought in 4 hours after he was burnt
- Examine the patient fully, but rapidly
- Anyone who has been in a burning building, whether burnt or not, has been exposed to smoke and carbon monoxide
    - assess breathing
    - if in doubt give oxygen
- Assess the extent of the burn using the Rule of Nine's

Rule of Nine's management
If the burn covers more than 10% of the body surface area in an adult:
- A drip of normal saline must be put up stat to replace fluid loss
- Give oxygen for shock or smoke inhalation
- Dress the wound with sterile gauze soaked in sterile saline or Tullegras
- Splint for comfort
- Cover the patient with a blanket to prevent, or lessen, hypothermia
- Give morphine 0,1 mg / kg IVI for pain
- **REFER** to casualty stat

If the burns cover more of the body surface than 5% in children (0-2 years) or 8% in children (above 2 years), and do not involve any special areas ie. head, neck, joints, hands, feet or perineum:

If full thickness
- Dress the wound as above
- Splint
- **REFER**

If partial thickness
- Give tetanus toxoid 0,5 ml subcutaneously stat
- Unbroken blisters provide a good dressing
    - preserve blisters as far as possible
- Dress with paraffin gauze dressing and then dry gauze on top.
- **Or** cover burns with a permanent polyurethane dressing
- Splint and elevate if possible
- Give paracetamol and/or ibuprofen for pain
    - or for more severe pain give tramadol
- Check after 3 days
    - check for infection
    - reassess depth of burn
- If infected burn:
    - povidone iodine 5% cream applied daily
- If burns are progressing well
    - blisters can now be removed
    - re-dress and teach how to make up and use home-made normal saline for dressings
    - instruct patient to change dressings every day

BURNS IN SPECIFIC AREAS

HEAD AND NECK BURNS

These can be life-threatening.
- Face burns can be from fire, hot water or chemicals
- In a fire burn of the face, the airways are also burnt
    - these patients are in danger of developing airway obstruction due to severe swelling
    - this swelling can take place rapidly

MANAGEMENT
- Give 40% oxygen at 8 litres per minute
- A drip of normal saline should be put up on all these patients
- Bronchospasm, if severe, may need to be treated with nebulised salbutamol (see Respiratory Protocol page 57)
- Dress the wound with
    - sterile gauze soaked in sterile saline
    - **or** Tullegras
- **REFER** to casualty stat

Airway burns
Airway burns should be referred to a tertiary care hospital ICU as rapidly as possible
- If there is quick access to the tertiary institution, give oxygen until referred
- If arrival in a burns intensive care unit is likely to be delayed by more than an hour
    - give IVI sedation with morphine 0,1 mg / kg IVI
    - then intubate the patient
- Intubation may become extremely difficult once the airways start to swell
    - the patient will need to remain well sedated to enable him / her to tolerate the ET tube
- A doctor or nurse should remain with the patient during transfer, and should ventilate the patient with a bag if the respiration is depressed

Burns of the eyes
For burns involving the eyes (including chemical burns)
- Insert local anaesthetic eye drops (Novesin) if available
    - if not available, insert any local anaesthetic into the eyes
    - **NB.** Never give local anaesthetic for use at home
- As soon as the pain decreases, wash out with water or saline, if available

PERINEAL BURNS

MANAGEMENT
- A urinary catheter should be inserted as soon as possible to prevent urinary obstruction due to oedema
- Dress the wound as above
- **REFER**

HANDS AND FEET

The result of burns on the hands and feet can be severe.

MANAGEMENT
- Dress the wound with
    - sterile gauze soaked in sterile saline
    - **or** Tullegras
- Splint the limb in a position of function especially if it is a hand
    - with the fingers bent gently at all the joints, as if holding a tennis ball
- Elevate the limb
- **REFER**

OTHER BURNS REQUIRING REFERRAL

- Full thickness burns of any size
- Burns over joints especially major joints
- Electrical burns, including lightning injury
- Circumferential burns of the limbs or chest
- Suspected child abuse

Ear, Nose and Throat

THE EAR

CAUSES OF COMMON SYMPTOMS

THE PAINFUL EAR

This may arise from the ear itself, or be referred to the ear from neighbouring structures.

Causes
- A common cause for acute pain in the ear, particularly in children, is acute otitis media.
- Referred pain from the throat, eg. in a tonsillitis, ulcers or tumours in the pharynx and/or larynx.
- Otitis externa
- Ear canal furuncle
- Mastoiditis
- Dental disease
- Foreign body
- Trauma
- Erupting molar teeth
- Parotitis
- Bell's Palsy
- Trigeminal neuralgia
- Ramsey-Hunt syndrome ie. infection with herpes zoster
- Temporo-mandibular joint disease

> If the cause is not obvious **REFER.**

DEAFNESS

This may be classified as conductive, sensorineural or mixed.

CONDUCTIVE

This is due to disturbances in the external or middle ear which prevent sound travelling through normally. Usually it will be possible to see the cause in the canal or drum.

Causes
- Wax
- Trauma eg. injuries to the tympanic membrane
- Middle ear disease eg. acute and chronic otitis media
- Less common causes
    - traumatic disruption of the bones (ossicles) of the middle ear
    - tumours of the canal and middle ear
    - foreign bodies
    - external canal narrowing
    - congenital abnormalities

SENSORINEURAL (PERCEPTIVE)

This is due to disturbance of the cochlea, the neural pathways or the auditory cortex. It suggests more severe disease. The drum will often appear normal.

Causes
- Idiopathic
- Presbyacusis (senile deafness) - deterioration of hearing which occurs with old age
- Acoustic trauma
    - sudden loud noise eg. a blast
    - prolonged loud noises eg. discos, certain occupations
- Head trauma involving the inner ear or eighth nerve
- Drugs such as salicylates, streptomycin, furosemide
- Less common causes
    - acoustic nerve tumour
    - Meniere's disease
    - congenital

> **MANAGEMENT**
> - **REFER** if you cannot adequately diagnose or treat any patient complaining of:
>   - recent onset of deafness
>   - deafness that is getting worse
>   - deafness where the drum is normal
>
> **Children**
> - *In children, especially before 2 years of age, failure to correct deafness may result in permanent speech problems.*
> - If a child does not hear the correct sounds during the critical first 18 months of life, when they are learning to speak, permanent speech problems may occur.
> - It is essential to **REFER** a child if **anyone** suspects that there are hearing problems, even if you:
>   - do not agree
>   - cannot confirm the deafness clinically.
> - **REFER** for assessment.

▼ Note to doctor

Differentiate conductive from sensorineural hearing loss with tuning fork tests.

The Weber tuning fork test
- Place the vibrating tuning fork in the midline of the forehead.
- The patient indicates where the sound is heard.

- In a unilateral conductive hearing loss eg. an acute otitis media, the sound is heard loudest in the affected ear.
- If however the unilateral hearing loss is caused by nerve damage, the sound is heard in the opposite ear.

The Rinne tuning fork test
- This compares air conduction with bone conduction.
- The vibrating tuning fork is first held in front of the ear, and then the base of the tuning fork is placed on the mastoid process.
- The patient then indicates which sound is greater.
- Normally the air conduction (in front of the ear) should be louder ▲

DIZZINESS

This is a very common symptom, especially in elderly people. It is important to decide if the symptom is just dizziness, or whether it is vertigo.

Clinical features
- Usually when the patient says they are dizzy they mean that they:
    - feel unsteady
    - may feel light headed
    - may faint

Causes
- Cardiovascular problems, especially postural hypotension
    - this causes the blood pressure not to respond properly when the person gets out of a chair or out of bed (they have less blood going to the brain)
    - some antihypertensive drugs make this problem worse.
- Gastrointestinal illness especially
    - acute gastroenteritis with fluid loss
    - gastritis due to alcohol or drugs
    - effects of laxatives, purgatives and enemas.
- Abuse of analgesics often presents with dizziness and should be checked, especially in the elderly.
- Stress of any kind is a common cause, especially with associated anxiety eg. fear of having a stroke, or a cancer.
- Acute infections, commonly of the upper respiratory tract should be looked for eg. sinusitis.
- Cerebellar disease
- Alcohol and other drugs eg. sedatives

Differential diagnosis
- Difficulties with vision may be confused with this.
- Orthopaedic problems and muscle weakness may also be confused with this symptom in the elderly.

MANAGEMENT
- Most patients with dizziness respond well to reassurance and advice on how to make the problem less.
- Treat causes that you are able to.
- **REFER** severe dizziness or difficult causes.
- If the symptom seems to be more like genuine vertigo, then the underlying causes are likely to be inner ear disease.

VERTIGO

This is an uncommon symptom.
It usually has more serious causes than dizziness.

Clinical features
- The patient may say "he / she feels dizzy, lightheaded or unsteady"
    - these are vague terms.
- True vertigo is the feeling that objects are moving or spinning, usually in the same direction
    - as if they have just got off a moving swing or roundabout.

Causes
- It may be due to central causes
    - eg. in the brain.
- It may be due to peripheral causes
    - eg. in the inner ear.
- The presence of tinnitus suggests a cause in the inner ear.

Common ear causes
- Infective causes
    - labyrinthitis, viral or suppurative
- Traumatic causes
- Medicine causes
    - aminoglycoside antibiotics especially kanamycin
    - aspirin abuse
    - anti-epileptic drugs
    - quinine
    - chemotherapy drugs
- Meniere's syndrome (see page 29)
- Tumour of vestibular nerve ie. acoustic neuroma

MANAGEMENT
REFER if:
- You suspect true vertigo.
- You are not sure of the diagnosis.

Medicine problems
- Stop the medicine if possible.
- **REFER** if necessary.

DISEASES OF THE EXTERNAL EAR

OTITIS EXTERNA

Otitis externa may be diffuse or furuncular (ie. with multiple abscesses).

Diffuse otitis externa is more common and is usually a mixed infection or a dermatitis.

Furuncular otitis externa is often associated with staphylococcal infections (see ear canal furuncle, below).

Causes
- Trauma caused by scratching or attempts to clean with matchsticks or cotton wool ear buds (this is the most common cause).
- Moisture in the ear
    - allowing soapy water or shampoo to remain in the ears after washing or bathing
    - abuse of ear drops
    - swimming pool chemicals
- Fungi
- Otitis media with otorrhoea
- Seborrhoeic or allergic dermatitis
- Foreign body eg. insects, cotton wool, ear plugs
- Wax

Clinical features
- Itching may be the only symptom in mild cases.
- Pain, increased by jaw movement.
- Discharge – usually scanty.
- Tenderness when pressing on the tragus, and below the pinna. Pain felt on moving the pinna shows that the cartilage of the canal is involved in the infection.
- In mild cases the canal may appear normal or there may be only slight scaling and crusting.
- The canal may appear red.
- Debris may be present.
- The upper drum (attic area) may sometimes be red, however the cone of light is present and normal.
- In more severe cases, especially fungal infections, the canal is oedematous, narrowed and lined with cheesy material (moist debris).
- In severe cases examination may be difficult or impossible without causing the patient acute pain.

MANAGEMENT

In mild cases (itching only, no pain, swelling or discharge)
- Use spirit ear drops (acetic acid 2% in alcohol drops) 3 x daily for 5 days.

In more severe cases (with pain, swelling or discharge)

Adults
- Clean and dry the ear (dry mopping) provided this is not too painful.
- Use spirit ear drops 3-4 x daily for 5 days

plus
- Amoxicillin-clavulanic acid 875/125 mg 2 x daily for 5 days

Children
- Exclude underlying chronic otitis media
- Use spirit ear drops 3-4 x daily for 5 days **plus** (if associated chronic suppurative otitis media)
- Amoxicillin-clavulanic acid 3 x daily for 5 days dosage according to age. See page 27 for treatment.

Eczematous conditions
- May require application of a topical steroid cream / ointment 3 x daily eg. hydrocortisone 1% cream.
- Cream or ointment can be applied by using a clean little finger to push medicament into the canal, followed by several compressions of the tragus.

Fungal infections
- Respond well to cleaning and drying.
- Use spirit ear drops 3 x daily.
- If response is poor use imidazole antifungal eg. clotrimazole cream 3 x daily (applied as above).

Advise the patient
- Not to put drops into the ear unless prescribed.
- Keep the ear clean & dry.
- Not to leave pieces of cotton wool etc. in the ear.
- Not to scratch the ears with matchsticks or other similar objects.

Insertion of ear drops
- It does not help to just prescribe ear drops and send the patient home, without them knowing how to put them in.
- First clean out all the pus and debris from the ear canal
    - see details under perforated otitis media page 26.
- Ear drops cannot easily be put in by the patients themselves
    - if they are going to do any good, someone else needs to do it for them.
- Show the patient how to insert the ear drops by inserting the first drops yourself. They will then know what to tell the person who is going to insert the drops for them.
- Flex the patient's head to one side so that the ear that is to get the drops is facing upwards.
- Pull pinna back and upwards to open meatus.
- Insert the drops.
- Compress the tragus (outside cartilage) of the ear for a few moments so that the drops go deeply into the ear canal.

EAR CANAL FURUNCLE

A boil due to infection of the hair follicles of the canal.

Causes
- This is often as a result of trying to clean the ear with cotton wool buds or matchsticks etc.
- The causative organism is usually Staphylococcus.

Clinical features
- Severe pain - so that the patient refuses to allow the insertion of an otoscope.
- A boil present in the outer part of the ear canal, partially or completely blocking the lumen.
- Marked tenderness on compression of the tragus.

- Swelling of the parts round the ear
    - if it is in the anterior wall, the tissue in front of the tragus is swollen
    - if it is in the posterior wall, the oedema may spread over the mastoid process.
- Swelling of the pre and post-auricular lymph glands may occur.

MANAGEMENT
- Do not attempt to incise the abscess as this may lead to infection of the cartilage.
- Systemic antibiotic should be given
    - flucloxacillin or cephalexin for 5 days
    - **or** azithromycin for 3 days if the patient is penicillin allergic.
- Analgesics are usually needed.
- Advise against the use of ear drops.

WAX

Wax (cerumen) is normal in an ear. It forms a protective layer on the skin of the external ear canal.

- Wax in the ear canal found during a routine examination can be left alone and needs no treatment.
- The only part of the ear canal that needs cleaning out routinely, is the external opening which can be reached by the patient's smallest finger.

Causes of impacted wax
The most common cause of impacted wax is due to attempts to clean the ear canal with a finger or ear bud, resulting in the wax being pushed further into the ear.

Clinical features
- Feeling of fullness (blocked ears)
- Deafness
- Pain occasionally
- Tinnitus - ringing of the ears caused by wax
- Colour of wax may be yellow, brown or black (depending on the degree of oxidation)

The indications for removal of wax
- Hearing loss which could be due to impacted wax.
- Discomfort in the ear for some time due to impacted wax.
- Both these conditions are rare in children, and apply more to adults.
- **NB.** Acute sudden onset of pain in the ear is unlikely to be caused by wax, and otitis media should be considered
    - the presence of otitis media is not excluded by the presence of wax
    - in this case, the wax should not be removed, as any attempt at removal will be extremely painful, and could result in a perforated ear drum.

MANAGEMENT
Do not syringe:
- If the patient has acute pain.
- If you suspect perforation.

How to syringe an ear
- Use a 10 cc or 20 cc syringe or a specific ear syringe.
- Cover the patient with a sheet and have a container available to catch the water coming from the ear.
- Use water at body temperature.
- The nozzle of the syringe must not be allowed to enter too far into the external meatus.
- The plastic canula of an Abbocath or Jelco can be attached to a 10 cc syringe if the wax is difficult to remove.
- Direct the stream along the roof of the auditory canal.
- Re-examine after syringing.
- In most cases the drum will show a degree of redness and infection, particularly on the handle of the malleus
    - however the normal light reflex will be present.
- After removal of the wax, inspect the ear well to make sure that:
    - no wax remains
    - the ear has not been traumatised.
- **NB.** A normal eardrum can usually not be ruptured by irrigation, but it is possible if the drum is infected or scarred.
- Mild trauma to the external canal needs no treatment.
- **REFER** if you are unable to remove the wax with syringing and this is causing symptoms.

If syringing was unsuccessful:
- Send the patient home with ear drops
    - mineral oil, sweet oil, glycerine or sodium bicarbonate if available.
- The following preparations may be useful to soften wax, but should only be left in the ear for 20-30 minutes. They must not be given to the patient to take home
    - dioctyl sodium sulfosuccinate (Waxsol)
    - dichlorobenzene (Cerumol)
    - sodium bicarbonate ear drops

If the ear drops were unsuccessful:
- **REFER** to ENT specialist for manual removal.

EAR CANAL TRAUMA

Causes
- Scratching the itchy ear
- Attempts to clean the ear eg. with matchsticks
- Blows to the ear

Clinical features
- Abrasions of the external meatus
- Possible bleeding

MANAGEMENT

Advice and reassurance
- Advise against any interference with the ear.
- Stop the patient using matchsticks etc. to clean the ears.
- Reassure the patient that the ears do not need cleaning.
- If the ears are itchy, advise them to rub at the canal opening of the ear using the tip of the small finger, and not to put anything into the canal at all.
- Stop the instillation of non-prescribed medication into the ear.
- Use spirit ear drops topically.
- Use oral cephalexin only if infection is present.
- Check whether the ear drum is damaged.
- If the drum is damaged or ruptured, see management of acute trauma to the middle ear (page 28).
- If the damage is due to self-inflicted injury (attempts to clean the ear), then otitis externa may be the result
    - for the management of otitis externa see page 21.

EAR CANAL FOREIGN BODY

Anything small enough to be inserted into the ear can be a potential foreign body (FB) of the ear.
This is a particular problem in children.
There are 3 groups of foreign bodies
- insects
- vegetable material
- non-vegetable material

REFER.

▼ Note to doctor
- **NB.** The two most common causes of severe damage to the ear drum are an unskilled operator and an uncooperative patient.
- First try to get the FB to drop out, by straightening the external meatus
    - pull the pinna posteriorly
    - gently shake the head with the affected ear in the dependent position (downwards).
- Do *not* make many attempts to remove FB in an uncooperative child
    - removal of foreign bodies is not an emergency and it is not worth risking permanent hearing loss by a poor attempt.
- **REFER** for removal under anaesthetic if:
    - the patient is a child
    - the first 2 attempts fail
    - the FB is lying against the ear drum.

Live insects
- The only emergency in terms of an FB is a live insect crawling around in the ear canal, as this can be excruciatingly painful.
- There should be no reason for referring a patient to hospital with a live insect present.
- Try to lure the insect out with a bright light in a dark room
- The insect should be killed with alcohol spirit ear drops or oil (eg. cooking oil or olive oil).
- This usually floats out the insect as well.
- Once the insect is dead, the emergency is over.
- If the FB is superficial in the outer part of the ear canal, and clearly visible, crocodile forceps may be used to try to remove the following soft FBs:
    - insect
    - paper
    - sponge

Note. They should **not** be used for any solid FB eg. a bead, pea etc. as it will only push the solid object through the ear drum.

Solid FBs
- For a solid FB, a curved blunt probe hooked behind the FB may be tried (a Quires hook is the most effective probe).
- Another method is to obtain some dental wax, dip a cotton wool probe into warm wax, attach it firmly to the FB, wait one to two minutes and gently remove the FB.

Metal objects
- Metal objects may be removed with a magnet.

Syringing
- Insert a thin catheter past the FB and attempt to flush the FB out by syringing it from behind.
- Do not syringe vegetable matter as it tends to swell with water.

Note. If the FB has been successfully removed, check the ear canal for trauma:
- if it is traumatised, an otitis externa may occur, particularly if the FB has been present for a few days
- treat as for an otitis externa (see page 21) ▲

DISORDERS OF THE PINNA

HAEMATOMA

Causes
- Trauma to the pinna

Clinical features
- The bleeding takes place between the cartilage and its connective tissue covering (the perichondrium).
- It appears as a spongy swelling, usually of the upper half of the pinna.
- If untreated, the cartilage may necrose, resulting in an ugly changed shape of the pinna (the cauliflower ear).

REFER for formal exploration under anaesthesia.

PROBLEMS WITH PIERCED EARS

■ INFECTION

- This is the most common problem from:
    - using dirty needles to pierce ears
    - keeping the hole open with dirty material eg. straw, cotton, safety pin etc.

MANAGEMENT
- The earring should be removed.
- Clean the area with antiseptic.
- Give an antibiotic
    - cephalexin or flucloxacillin is best.

■ DERMATITIS

- This may occur if the pin of the earring is made from nickel or a mixture (alloy) of metals, as these cause an allergic reaction.

MANAGEMENT
- Replace the nickel earrings with either stainless steel, sterling silver or gold earrings (of at least 9 carat rating - not gold plated).
- Apply topical corticosteroid eg. hydrocortisone cream 1%.

■ TRAUMA

- The earring can be pulled and the lobe lacerated.
- Children should preferably not have their ears pierced.

The laceration may need surgical repair.

■ OTHERS

- Serum hepatitis or HIV may be caused by re-using dirty needles.
- Keloid, thick fibrous scar tissue may form.

MANAGEMENT
- The keloid can be surgically removed but has a tendency to recur (see Surgery Protocol page 283).
- Patients who have had keloids should be advised never to pierce their ears.

DERMATITIS OF THE PINNA

Causes
- Neglect of a discharging ear
- Infection resulting from unsterile perforation of an ear lobe
- Contact dermatitis from earrings (nickel sensitivity)
- Other skin diseases eg. seborrhoeic dermatitis

Clinical features
- Weeping, scaling and crusting lesions
- It may spread from the pinna to the face and neck.

MANAGEMENT
- Identify the cause and manage accordingly.
- Give systemic antibiotic. If infection is present - use cephalexin or flucloxacillin.
- Use azithromycin if patient is penicillin-allergic.
- Clean skin surface with home-made saline.
- Dressings are not needed.
- Apply hydrocortisone 1% cream 3 x daily if the cause is seborrhoeic dermatitis or contact dermatitis.

CONGENITAL ABNORMALITIES

PRE-AURICULAR SINUS

Clinical features
- This is a small blind pit usually seen anterior to the upper pinna.
- It may be unilateral or bilateral.
- It may become infected and form an abscess.

MANAGEMENT
- **REFER** if an abscess has formed for
    - incision and drainage
    - excision of the sinus tract at a later date if infections recur.
- If this is not done the abscess will usually recur.

PROTRUDING PINNAE

- This is a cosmetic, emotional and psychological problem only.
- There are no other associated abnormalities.
- Protruding ears cause no functional problems.

MANAGEMENT
- They are easily corrected by surgery at age 5-6 years.
- Sticking ears back with elastoplast does not help at all.

LOW SET EARS

Clinical features
- The top of the pinna is below eye level.
- It may be normal but it is commonly associated with kidney abnormalities.

Children should be **REFERRED** for paediatric assessment and IVP to exclude renal problems.

PRE-AURICULAR TAGS

- This is a cosmetic problem only.
- There are no associated abnormalities.

Surgery may be done if requested.

DISEASES OF THE MIDDLE EAR

ACUTE OTITIS MEDIA

Causes
- Viral upper respiratory tract infection often complicated by secondary bacterial infection
- Adenoid hypertrophy
- Allergic rhinitis
- Congenital abnormalities
    - cleft palate
    - Down's syndrome
    - eustachian tube abnormality

Clinical features
- Earache is the major symptom
- Loss of hearing
- Symptoms of coryza
- Children may have
    - irritability and difficulty in sleeping (especially in a young child)
    - fever
    - diarrhoea and vomiting
- Rubbing the ear is not a reliable sign
- The appearance of the drum is the main diagnostic feature
- At the beginning of the infection
    - the light reflex is normal
    - the drum is normal
    - the handle of the malleus may be red and more vascular
- Later on in the infection
    - the drum becomes red
    - the drum bulges and loses the normal light reflex
    - it then ruptures leaving a small perforation

Viral infection
- This is the most common cause.
- The typical appearance is a pink drum with a normal light reflex, often associated with a watery (clear) rhinitis.

Bacterial infection
- A high fever, with an acutely tender ear, and a bulging red drum, and a very irritable patient, is more likely to be a bacterial infection.
- It could be caused by any one of the common organisms which occur in the respiratory tract
    - *Streptococcus pneumoniae* (pneumococcus)
    - *Haemophilus influenzae*
    - *Branhamella catarrhalis*
    - Beta-haemolytic Streptococcus.

MANAGEMENT

Medicine management

If a viral cause is suspected - give analgesic only (paracetamol).

Antibiotic
- Use only if there is
    - severe pain or pyrexia
    - a red or bulging drum with loss of light reflex or abnormal light reflex
    - an inflamed perforated drum with a mucoid or mucopurulent discharge

The following antibiotics are to be used in the appropriate dosage and treatment must be given for 5 days:
- Use amoxicillin in all age groups.

Children <10 years of age:

Dosage: 45 mg / kg / dose 2 x daily for 5 days

- 3-6 months	250 mg
- 6-18 months	375 mg
- 18 months-3 years	500 mg
- 3-5 years	750 mg
- 5-10 years	1000 mg

Children >10 years of age and adults:
- 1000 mg 3 x daily for 5 days

- For patients who have a poor response, or those who have received amoxicillin in the last 30 days, use amoxicillin-clavulanic acid (see page 27)
- Use azithromycin in penicillin-allergic patients (see pharmacopoea for dosage).
- Indications for IM ceftriaxone
    - severe pain
    - vomiting in children
    - red bulging drum

Analgesic
- All patients should be given analgesia, preferably paracetamol.
- Avoid aspirin in children.

Note. Antihistamines do not form part of the management for acute OM, unless there is associated allergic rhinitis.

Follow up
- Check after 1-2 days:
    - patients with severe pain and fever
    - babies under 2 months of age.
- Check after 5-10 days:
    - discharging ear/s
    - recurrent otitis media.

REFER
- All patients that return with continuing pain and pyrexia or a persistant bulging drum as they may need myringotomy.
- Sick children who are vomiting, drowsy etc.
- Patients with oedema and tenderness over the mastoid (suspicion of acute mastoiditis).

PERFORATED ACUTE OTITIS MEDIA

Clinical features
- Acute pain which decreases as a discharge appears from the ear (ie. as the drum perforates and the pressure is released).

MANAGEMENT

Dry mopping
- This is the most important part of management.
- The technique must be *demonstrated* to the patient or escort (they cannot just be told to do it)
    - roll a piece of absorbent cloth or paper towel into a wick
    - carefully insert the wick into the ear with a twisting action
    - remove the wick and replace with a clean dry wick
    - repeat this until the wick is dry when removed.

- The patient should:
    - continue dry mopping 2 hourly if possible but at least 3-4 x daily
    - not swim or get water into the ear
    - avoid all applications to the ear eg. Vaseline or oils.

Medicine management
- Antibiotic as for acute otitis media (see page 25) in the appropriate dosage for age.
- Analgesics as necessary.
- Any other disease in the nose, sinuses or pharynx should be adequately treated.

Follow up
- Patients should be checked after 5-10 days.
- If not improving:
    - check that the antibiotic was given in the correct dose
    - if not, repeat the treatment and re-educate on adherence
    - repeat advice about cleaning the ear
    - check again in 5-10 days and **REFER** if not improved.

ACUTE OTITIS MEDIA WITH EFFUSION

An effusion occurs in acute otitis media and usually resolves spontaneously within 14 days. An effusion lasting longer than 14 days and up to 3 months is considered to be subacute otitis media.

Clinical features
- It occurs mainly in children (eustachian tube in children is narrower and more horizontal than in adults).
- Painless hearing loss (mild to moderate).
- White, yellow or amber tympanic membrane that may be inflamed.
- A fluid level or bubbles can sometimes be seen through the drum.
- In adults with persistent unilateral serous otitis media it is important to exclude nasopharyngeal carcinoma.

MANAGEMENT
- In the absence of acute inflammation, antibiotics and antihistamines are not indicated.
- If the drum is inflamed, treat with amoxicillin-clavulanic acid for 5 days.

CHRONIC SUPPURATIVE OTITIS MEDIA (CSOM)

A perforated drum with a mucopurulent discharge that persists for more than 2 weeks.

Causes

- The acute infection was not treated early enough
- Dosage of antibiotics was inadequate or antibiotics were discontinued too soon
- Adenoiditis
- Nasal or sinus infection
- Lowered general resistance, often due to poor socio-economic situation
- Bottle feeding
- Tuberculosis must always be considered, as well as HIV infection

Types of perforation

A perforation is described in terms of its situation in the tympanic membrane and whether it is dry or wet.

- Central
- Marginal
- Apical (attic)

Clinical features

- Deafness is common.
- Pain indicates acute exacerbation / complication.
- The discharge is mucopurulent, intermittent or constant, scanty or profuse and may be offensive.
- The perforation is often large in size and may involve almost the entire drum (subtotal perforation).
- The drum is thickened and opaque.
- Chalky, white patches (tympanosclerosis) may be present on the drum.
- Granulations are sometimes present in the perforation
    - these are bright red and bleed when touched.
- The condition may be dormant from time to time (inactive disease) when examination will reveal:
    - a dry perforation
    - a perforation which has become replaced by thin scar tissue.

MANAGEMENT

- The most important part of treatment is drying the ear (see perforated acute otitis media i.e. dry mopping, page 26).

Children and adolescents:

- Amoxicillin-clavulanic acid 15-25 mg / kg / dose 3 x daily for 5 days
    - 3-6 months   5 ml (125/31.2 mg / 5 ml)
    - 6-18 months   7 ml (125/31.2 mg / 5 ml)
    - 18 months-3 years   5 ml (250/62.5 mg / 5 ml)
    - 3-5 years   6 ml (250/62.5 mg / 5 ml)
    - 5-7 years   7.5 ml (250/62.5 mg / 5 ml)
    - 7-11 years   10 ml (250/62.5 mg / 5 ml)
    - 11-18 years   875/125 mg tabs 2x daily
- If not improved after 5-10 days refer for topical antibiotic ear drops, e.g. ciprofloxacin

Adults

- Ciprofloxacin 500 mg 2 x daily for 5 days
- If there is pain or purulent discharge present (indicating acute exacerbation or complication)
    - prescribe amoxicillin-clavulanic acid instead
    - 875/125 mg 2 x daily for 5 days
- Penicillin-allergic patients: azithromycin once daily for 3 days
    - 1-3 years: 120 mg (3 ml syrup)
    - 3-5 years: 160 mg (4 ml syrup)
    - 5-7 years: 200 mg (5 ml syrup)
    - 7-11 years: 250 mg
    - 11 years and older: 500 mg
- Give analgesic (if necessary)
- Adults and children should be screened for TB and tested for HIV.

REFER

- Any ear discharge still present after 4 weeks
- Any large perforation
- Any attic perforation
- Any perforation not progressively improving after 3 months or closed by 6 months
- Moderate or severe hearing loss

CHRONIC OTITIS MEDIA WITH EFFUSION (GLUE EAR)

This is an otitis media where the eustachian tube remains blocked for a prolonged period (more than 3 months).

Causes

- As for acute otitis media (see page 25)
- Tumours of the naso-pharynx (especially in adults)

Clinical features

- Drum dull, immobile and often retracted
    - opacified white or has a yellowish tinge.

Complications

- Repeated acute suppurative otitis media is the most common problem.
- Poor school performance and delayed speech development due to deafness.

MANAGEMENT

- **REFER** for possible insertion of grommet tubes into the middle ear.
- These will equalise the pressure between the middle ear and the external ear.

▼ **Note to doctor**

- Check mobility of the drum by attaching a small rubber bladder to the otoscope and giving a gentle squeeze.
- A normal drum should be seen to move ▲

COMPLICATIONS OF MIDDLE EAR INFECTIONS

ACUTE MASTOIDITIS

This is an infection of the mastoid air cells ie. an osteomyelitis of the mastoid bone.

Causes
- A complication of acute or chronic otitis media

Clinical features
- Pain which is persistent and throbbing
- Discharge usually gets worse
- Deafness usually increases with the onset of mastoiditis
- It is rare before the age of 2 years
- Very ill patient
- The temperature is elevated
- Tenderness is marked over the mastoid area
- Oedema is often present over the mastoid process
- The pinna is pushed outwards and downwards by the oedema and subperiosteal collection of pus
- Perforation is seen in the drum through which pus may be seen draining
- Sagging of the roof of the canal near the drum

Differential diagnosis
- Ear canal furuncle
    - the drum if visible will be normal
    - marked tenderness on compression of the tragus
    - oedema may be present over the mastoid but no displacement of the auricle.
- Cellulitis of the pinna
    - normal drum
    - acute pain on movement of the pinna may be due to dermatitis of the pinna.
- Lymphadenitis of the post-auricular glands due to
  scalp infection:
    - normal drum
    - enlarged tender glands
    - a site of infection on the scalp
    - patient not very ill

- Set up normal saline IV drip
- Give ceftriaxone 80 mg / kg IM or IV as a single dose
- **REFER** stat to hospital.

OTHER COMPLICATIONS OF OTITIS MEDIA

- As the brain, meninges and lateral sinuses are all close to the middle ear they can all be infected
- Meningitis
- Extradural abscess
- Subdural abscess
- Brain abscess
- Lateral sinus thrombosis
- Osteomyelitis of the petrous temporal bone
- Facial paralysis
- Labyrinthitis
- Neck abscess

REFER.

ACUTE TRAUMA TO THE MIDDLE EAR

Causes
- Cleaning of the ear with matchsticks
- A blow to the ear
- Blast injuries
- Head injury - fracture of the temporal bone
- A foreign body in the ear canal, especially with unsuccessful attempts at removal

Clinical features
- Pain
- Deafness
- Tinnitus
- Look for a tear (perforation) in the drum, blood clots in the canal and bleeding from the ear
- A blueness behind the drum caused by blood in the middle ear
- A clear discharge may indicate CSF leak
    - this will give a positive result when tested with a blood glucose test strip

MANAGEMENT
- **REFER** if:
    - the perforation is very large
    - you suspect an associated skull fracture or CSF leak.
- No specific treatment is needed apart from reassurance and analgesics.
- The patient must be warned not to put anything into the ear.
- The patient must avoid swimming or putting the head under water for about 4 weeks, until the drum is healed.
- Do not clean out the ear or remove the clot.
- Do not put in any drops.
- Do not syringe.
- The ear canal only needs a plug if the patient is working in a dusty environment
    - explain that the plug is not to treat the injury, it is only to keep the dust out
    - it only needs to be inserted when the patient is actually going to be in a dusty area.
- Check the ear at weekly intervals (or sooner if necessary)
    - in most cases the edges of the tear will join rapidly.
- If signs of infection develop, give amoxicillin for 5 days.
- If the tear is not healed after 4 weeks, **REFER.**

DISEASES OF THE INNER EAR

ACUTE LABYRINTHITIS / BENIGN PAROXYSMAL POSITIONAL VERTIGO (BPPV)

This is inflammation or infection of the labyrinth.

Causes
- Unknown, but can follow an upper respiratory tract infection

Clinical features
- Severe vertigo
- Sometimes hearing loss
- Nausea and vomiting
- Postural instability

> **MANAGEMENT**
> - Treat with Chlorphenamine 4 mg 3 x daily
> - If vomiting continues, give metoclopramide 10 mg 3 x daily
> - **REFER** patients not responding to therapy

MENIERE'S SYNDROME

This is possibly caused by increased pressure in the inner ear as a result of a build up of fluid. It is uncommon.

Clinical features
- Episodic vertigo, deafness and tinnitus lasting hours or days.
- There may be associated nausea and vomiting.
- There may be a sensation of pressure or fullness in the ear.
- There is fluctuating hearing loss.
- It is usually unilateral in the beginning.

> **REFER.**

THE NOSE AND PARANASAL SINUSES

THE NOSE

CHRONIC NASAL OBSTRUCTION / MOUTH BREATHING

Causes
- Large adenoids. Suspect if:
  - the soft palate is depressed
  - the soft palate does not move upwards on saying "Aah"
  - the patient has nasal speech
  - there are associated large tonsils (see page 43).
- Allergic rhinitis (see page 32)
- Foreign body (see page 34)
- Nasal polyps (see page 33)
- Deviated septum
- Recurrent sinusitis (see page 36)
- Hormonal
  - sex hormone imbalance ("hay fever") at puberty
  - pregnancy
- Chemical rhinitis
  - prolonged use of vasoconstrictor drops eg. pseudoephedrine may result in severe nasal congestion due to rebound vasodilation ("vasomotor rhinitis medicamentosa")
  - irritating gases in the work situation
  - glue-sniffing
  - snuff
- Drugs
  - alcohol
  - antihypertensive drugs eg. methyl-dopa,
- Vasomotor rhinitis
  - a reaction to outdoor temperature changes causing a blocked or runny nose
- Nasopharyngeal tumours - rare

Clinical features
- Patients may complain of a recurrently or constantly blocked nose.
- Children may breathe through the mouth.
- Severe snoring is an important symptom.
- The nose is often clear and the child may breathe well during the day.
- An older child may have deformity of the palate and front of the mouth due to mouth breathing.
- Halitosis (bad smelling breath) may be present.

Complications of mouth breathing
- With the mouth continuously open, there is no pressure exerted by the tongue on the teeth, therefore the teeth tend to grow inward resulting in malocclusion problems (crooked teeth).
- The most serious danger is obstruction to respiration during sleep.
- This results in anoxia which causes thickening of the pulmonary arteries.
- This may result in irreversible pulmonary hypertension if it is not treated early.

Note: In neonates and infants persistent blocked nostrils interfering with feeding and sleeping should be treated with amoxicillin (see pharmacopoeia for dosage).

RHINITIS

ACUTE VIRAL RHINITIS

Acute viral rhinitis is associated with the common cold (coryza) and is caused by a wide variety of viruses.

Clinical features
- It presents as minor epidemics in the winter months
- There is sudden onset often involving several members of a family at the same time
- Headache
- Watery nasal discharge
- Sneezing
- Blocked nose
- Mild sore throat
- Fever
  - children under 5 years can develop a fever of up to 40°C
- Usually the throat and nasal mucosa are inflamed
- There is crusting around the nose of a child

MANAGEMENT
- Symptomatic treatment only.
- Vitamin B Co or multivitamin is good as
  - a placebo
  - a vitamin supplement.
- Give analgesics if necessary eg. paracetamol
- Encourage fluids and rest.
- Saline nose drops are useful if the blocked nose is preventing sleep or feeding.
- Systemic decongestants (such as pseudoephedrine) are best avoided, especially in young children.
- Antibiotics are not indicated.
- Vaporizers / humidifiers may be of some use.

How to insert nose drops
- The head should be tilted sideways so that the one nostril is higher than the other.
- The drops should then be run in along the lateral side of the nose (ie. the bottom nostril).
- Do not insert with the head tilted backwards as the drops will only run into the pharynx.

ACUTE PURULENT RHINITIS

Usually a bacterial super-infection of the common cold.

Clinical features

- The usual complaint is that the cold is becoming worse.
- There is thick, yellow-green, nasal discharge that persists for several days.
- In children <3 years of age often due to streptococcal infection and is accompanied by fever irritability and anorexia.

Differential diagnosis

- A nasal foreign body usually presents as a **unilateral** purulent discharge.
- In newborns it is essential to exclude syphilis. The features of this are:
    - a sero-sanguinous nasal discharge
    - there may be other signs of syphilis eg. rhagades (fissures at the mouth angles), hepato-splenomegaly, peeling of hands and feet etc.
    - even if there is no obvious evidence of syphilis, any neonate with a persistent nasal discharge must be **REFERRED**.
- Drug abuse eg. glue-sniffing.

MANAGEMENT

- Insert saline nose drops to help wash out secretions.
- Usually does not require the use of an antibiotic.
- In children <3 years of age a mucopurulent discharge should be treated with antibiotics
    - give amoxicillin 2 x daily for 5 days

REFER if:

- There is no improvement.
- You suspect a more serious cause or a foreign body.
- There is a persistent unilateral discharge.
- The discharge is blood-stained or offensive, especially if unilateral, as this may suggest a tumour.

ALLERGIC RHINITIS

This is a common disorder.

The condition mainly arises as an abnormal response on the part of the nasal mucosa to foreign material, known as an allergen.

The response can be produced by a wide variety of allergens, which are often proteins.

The allergens may be classified as:

- Inhalants
    - the most common and important group
    - eg. pollens, house dust, grasses and animal fur
- Ingestants
    - eg. milk, eggs, wheat, sugars, fruit and certain drugs
- Insertion of medicines into the nose
    - eg. Vaseline

Causes

- Hereditary predisposing factors
- Seasonal allergic rhinitis
    - grass, flower and tree pollens
- Dust especially household dust (mites)
- Feathers eg. feather pillows, duvets
- Animal hair (dog or cat fur)

Clinical features

- This usually only occurs after 2 years of age.
- There is a recurrent watery nasal discharge.
- There are recurrent episodes of a blocked stuffy nose.
- Frequent sneezing and it is often accompanied by severe irritation of the nose.
- Conjunctival itching and watering.
- Nasal mucosa is swollen, oedematous and pale grey in colour.
- There is repeated upward rubbing of the nose with the back or palm of the hand (allergic salute) to try to get rid of the itch.
- Commonly they are mouth breathers who snore badly at night.
- A history that it is brought on by a certain situation that the patient can recognise eg. tobacco smoke, or a perfume.

MANAGEMENT

- Avoidance of the allergen
    - it may be possible for the patient to avoid contact with the allergen in the case of feather pillows, certain foods, cats and dogs etc.

For short-term symptomatic use (mild cases):

- Chlorphenamine oral 3 x daily for 7-10 days.
- Oxymetazoline nose drops are useful for the relief of nocturnal nasal blockage
    - use at night for not more than 7 days continuously

- Patients with *severe or persistent symptoms* should be treated with a steroid aqueous nasal spray e.g. Flixonase 50 mcg / spray
    - 1 puff into each nostril 2 x daily
    - direct the spray vertically and **not** to the back of each nostril
    - do not sniff vigorously
    - it may take up to 3 weeks for this treatment to take its full effect
    - **plus** cetirizine oral at night for 4 weeks
    - average period of treatment is 3 months but reassess the patient after the first month.
- Cetirizine is recommended in adults and school-going children because of its less sedating effect
    - give cetirizine oral at night
    - adults and children over 7 years: 10 mg
    - children under 7 years: 5 mg
- NB Avoid the use of antihistamines in children under 2 years of age.
- **REFERRAL**
- Poor response.

NASAL FURUNCLE

An infection of a hair follicle in the anterior nose.

Causes
- This sometimes occurs following interference with the nasal hair.
- It may also occur together with a nasal discharge.

Clinical features
- A small, very tender, red swelling in the anterior part of the nose.

> ### MANAGEMENT
> - As the infecting organism is frequently *Staphylococcus aureus,* give flucloxacillin or azithromycin for 5 days.
> - Prick with a needle only if the swelling is pointing.
> - Warn the patient not to squeeze or incise the furuncle, as this may push pus into the veins draining into the cavernous sinus.
> - Follow the patient up until the furuncle is healed
>   - occasionally the infection can spread fast to the brain, to cause cavernous sinus thrombosis.

NASAL POLYPS

These are pedunculated masses of tissue that consist of oedematous mucosa. They are often difficult to diagnose.

Causes
- They are usually signs of a nasal allergy.
- They also result from chronic ethmoiditis.

Clinical features
- They are fairly rare in children.
- They are generally multiple and bilateral, producing nasal blockage.
- Once polyps become obstructive, the resultant stagnation of secretion is likely to cause sinusitis.
- There is usually some discharge, which may be mucoid or purulent
  - this indicates that the polyps are associated with sinus infection.
- They appear grey in colour
  - occasionally they are more fleshy in appearance and may look like a turbinate.
- They come down into the lower part of the nose from above, but a hypertrophied inferior turbinate protrudes outwards from the lateral side of the nose
  - if in doubt touch gently with an instrument (they are soft and relatively insensitive, but a turbinate is fairly rigid and very sensitive)
  - large turbinates should be treated as for chronic allergic rhinitis (see page 32).

> **REFER** all cases.

EPISTAXIS

Generally this is a benign symptom, except in the elderly. It often, however, causes great anxiety in the patient and relatives.

Causes
Local
- Associated rhinitis is the most common cause but needs no treatment
- Minor trauma
  - common in children and young adults and may follow nose picking or nose blowing
  - often associated with infection
- Severe trauma eg. fracture
- Varicosities or haemangiomas in Little's area (ie. the anterior part of the nasal septum)
- Tumours of the nose and sinuses

General
- Blood diseases
- Cardiovascular (valve) disease
- Hypertension
- Kidney disease
- Liver disease
- Fevers
  - often before the onset of measles, mumps and other childhood illnesses

Drugs
- Chronic aspirin ingestion
- Anticoagulants eg. patients on warfarin
- Alcohol causes liver damage and leads to clotting disorders

Clinical features
- Bleeding usually arises from Little's area.
- Less commonly it occurs far back in the nose from the lateral wall - as seen in epistaxis from hypertension.
- Little's area is usually red with either fresh clots or old crusts.

Note. Recurrent epistaxis should be viewed with concern if:
- There is a history of frequency, from several times a day, to once a month.
- There is associated melaena (black, tarry stools) or haematemesis as this indicates swallowed blood due to severe bleeding.

> ### MANAGEMENT OF ACTIVE BLEEDING
> **REFER** if:
> - Signs of shock or severe anaemia
>   - **REFER** stat
>   - drip if shocked.
> - The bleeding is recurrent.
> - There are other features of disease of the reticulo-endothelial system
>   - eg. hepato or splenomegaly.
> - There is abnormal bleeding anywhere else on history or examination eg.
>   - easy bruising
>   - haematemesis.
> - You suspect a foreign body or a tumour
>   - eg. there is an associated offensive nasal discharge.
> - Bleeding fails to respond to your treatment.
> - No cause can be found for repeated, severe epistaxis.

Clinic management
- Reassure the patient.
- The patient must sit with his / her head flexed slightly forwards
    - pinch the nostrils firmly between finger and thumb for 10 minutes
    - the mouth must be kept open
    - this method usually controls the bleeding.
- If the above is not successful or if the bleeding is profuse
    - advise the patient not to blow the nose
    - **REFER** for nasal packing (see below).
- Check vital signs. BP, pulse, colour, etc.
- If you are worried about possible anaemia, call the patient back the following day for an Hb check (as an Hb measurement done immediately after the bleed may give a false high result).
- Treat the cause eg. alcoholism, hypertension
    - if you suspect alcoholism, liver or nutritional problems, then Vitamin K 10 mg (for adults) can be given IMI.
- The patient should be given normal saline drops and tetracycline eye ointment to apply to the mucosa if crusting is present.

▼ **Note to doctor**
Nasal packing
- If a Merocel tampon is used, drop 1 tiny drop of water on the tip of the tampon to soften it.
- Cover the tampon with a thin layer of KY jelly.
- Insert the tampon parallel with the palate, not pointing upwards towards the brain.
- If the bleeding is coming from far posterior, use a long tampon.
- Check the following day and remove the pack or tampon.

Packing with 2 plugs
- In occasional patients with very wide nostrils, 2 plugs may be needed. If one is long, the other can be short and inserted laterally to the long plug
    - note on the patient's card that 2 plugs have been inserted, so that both are removed!
- If ribbon gauze with BIPP is used, it should not be stuffed in, but carefully placed in layer by layer with nasal forceps
    - it can be left for up to 5 days.
- In those patients who continue to bleed down the back of the throat after insertion of nasal plugs
    - remove the plugs
    - insert a Foley's catheter (large volume, low pressure cuff) into the nose so that the tip slides into the nasopharynx
    - blow up the bulb, and gently pull the catheter forward so that the expanded bulb blocks off the posterior opening of the nose
    - the bulb should be blown up with water, and not with air as this may leak out
    - to stop the catheter from slipping, a thin strip of elastoplast should be wound around the catheter, just outside the nostril to make a tight fit.
- The nose can now be re-plugged. This plugging can be left in place for 2 days and then removed.
- These patients probably need admission to either the short stay ward or to the hospital.
- If dilated blood vessels are found in Little's triangle in the nose, these can easily be cauterised in the clinic.

How to cauterise a nose
- Anaesthetise the nasal mucosa by inserting a cotton wool swab which has been soaked in lignocaine (dental syringe cartridges are convenient).
- Warm up the tip of a straightened out paper clip in a flame (spirit lamp, match or lighter).
- Dip the heated clip into a bottle of silver nitrate crystals
    - a bead of silver nitrate will form.
- This bead can then be touched against the affected area of the nasal mucosa where the dilated vessels are found and a white layer will form.
- Do not cauterise both sides at once because of the danger of a perforated septum.
- Do not try to cauterise while there is active bleeding
    - control the bleeding with a nasal pack first.
- Silver nitrate solution is not ideal as it tends to run and will cauterise the skin around the nose as well.
- Silver nitrate pencils are more difficult to use
    - the plastic covering should be removed on only one side
    - expose only a small area of the stick in order to prevent the edge of the nostril from being inadvertently cauterised ▲

FOREIGN BODIES (FBs) IN THE NOSE

Anything small enough to enter the nose could become a foreign body.
- There are three types of FBs
    - insects
    - vegetable matter
    - non-vegetable matter

Clinical features
- This is especially common in small children who push objects into the nose.
- Usually detected by a parent soon after insertion.
- Occasionally the FB is only detected after some days when there is a unilateral, purulent, offensive or blood-stained nasal discharge.
- Other features may be:
    - epistaxis
    - halitosis
    - nasal obstruction
- Blocked nostril / unilateral

MANAGEMENT
- Clear the nose completely of any secretions by gentle suction.
- There are many possible ways to remove the FB
    - try hard nose-blowing (if the child is old enough)
    - try dental wax stuck on an orange stick which will then stick to the FB
    - pieces of paper or soft objects may be removed with crocodile forceps, but this may push solid objects further back
    - a right angle hook may be passed behind the FB (if there is space) to pull it out.
- If nothing works, **REFER** stat.

Note. Do not struggle to remove FBs in small children who are awake.

REFER if there is any difficulty.

INJURIES OF THE NOSE

FRACTURED NOSE

Clinical features
Most blows on the nose cause swelling.

Suspect a fracture if there is:
- Swelling and discolouration of the skin and subcutaneous tissues covering the nasal bone and in the surrounding area
- Epistaxis, especially if persistent
- Deformity may or may not be present
    - if the patient is seen sometime after the injury, swelling of the soft tissues may hide any deformity
- The chief deformity is usually a deviation of the nose to one side or the other
- Crepitus of the nasal bones
- Obstruction to air passages
- Pain
- The diagnosis of a displaced nasal fracture is a clinical diagnosis
    - the nose will look or feel crooked
    - X-rays are of little use in the diagnosis.

MANAGEMENT
- First treat the epistaxis and any associated injuries.
- A nasal fracture may be a compound fracture and a prophylactic antibiotic must be prescribed eg. amoxicillin 250 mg 3 x daily for 5 days.
- Give analgesia.

Displaced fractures
- Nasal fractures **must** be reduced within 1-2 weeks
- If the patient is seen before oedema has occurred
    - the fracture can be reduced stat
    - **REFER.**
- If oedema is already present:
    - **REFER** as soon as oedema has resolved (usually 3-5 days after the injury).

Undisplaced nasal fractures
- Often due to a fist injury.
- Treat with analgesics and an antibiotic, e.g. amoxicillin.
- **REFER** only if the septum appears to be deviated.

SEPTAL HAEMATOMA

This is a haemorrhage between the layers of the septum.

Clinical features
- It is often associated with a fracture of the septum.
- Haematoma carries the risk of pressure necrosis of the cartilage
    - this can result in a septal perforation.
- There can be severe or complete nasal obstruction
    - nasal passages are blocked by a boggy swelling replacing the septum.

REFER stat.

SEPTAL DEVIATION

This is a common cause of nasal obstruction in the urban community.

Causes
- Developmental
- Trauma

Clinical features
- Nasal obstruction is the main symptom
    - unilateral or bilateral
- Septal deformity is usually obvious on looking into the nasal cavities with a light

Recurrent sinus infection
- This may be due to pressure of the septal convexity on the middle turbinate
    - this results in obstruction of the sinus ostia (where the sinus drains into the nose).
- This may also be due to thickening (hypertrophy) of the middle and/or inferior turbinate on the concave side of the septum
    - this will interfere with sinus drainage.

MANAGEMENT
- If symptoms are minimal and only a minor degree of deviation is present, no treatment is required.
- **REFER:**
    - cases of moderate or severe deviation
    - serious complications from recurrent infections of the sinuses.

SEPTAL PERFORATION

Causes
- Trauma eg. boxers or following a MVA
- Drug use eg. cocaine sniffing
- Following septal operation
- Tuberculosis
- Syphilis
- Leprosy
- Chemicals
- Tumours

Clinical features
- Often there are no symptoms
- Epistaxis and crusted mucus
- Occasionally whistling on inspiration or expiration

REFER.

SEPTAL ABSCESS

Clinical features
- Usually secondary to nasal trauma or furuncle
- It presents with fever, tenderness and a blocked nose
- Fluctuant, grey, septal swelling, usually bilateral

Complications
- Pressure necrosis
- Septicaemia
- Meningitis
- Cavernous sinus thrombosis

REFER stat.

THE PARANASAL SINUSES

SINUSITIS

ACUTE SINUSITIS

Acute sinusitis most frequently starts as an extension of a viral nasal infection eg. coryza, influenza. This viral infection may be followed by secondary bacterial infection.

Causes
- Poor drainage of the sinuses eg. polyps, deviated nasal septum
- Allergic rhinitis
- Overuse of decongestants
- Occasionally infection arises
  - from apical tooth abscesses of the pre-molar or molar teeth
  - after dental extraction

Sinus development appropriate to diagnosis
- Ethmoid sinusitis seldom occurs before the age of 1 year.
- Maxillary sinusitis is unusual before 3 years.
- Frontal sinusitis is unusual before age 10 years.
- The mucous membrane becomes inflamed, oedematous and pus forms.
- The sinus ostia may become blocked.

Clinical features
- Often the symptoms and signs may be mild, unless the infection is severe.
- Two or more symptoms
  - one of which should be either nasal obstruction / blockage or mucopurulent nasal discharge (anterior / posterior nasal drip)
- Facial pain or pressure especially if unilateral
- A reduction in, or loss of, smell
- Pain in the face or headache usually referable to a particular sinus
  - felt especially on bending the head forward
  - the pain is worse in the morning.
- Maxillary sinus pain may be referred to the upper incisor and canine teeth.
- Nasal obstruction - one side may be more blocked than the other.
- Halitosis (bad smelling breath).
- Post-nasal drip - often causing a sore throat and cough.
- The cough is worse at night because of the post-nasal drip.
- Pyrexia may be present.
- There is tenderness over one or more sinuses.
- Maxillary sinusitis - tender over the cheek, just lateral to the alae nasi.
- Ethmoid sinusitis
- tender medial to inner canthus of the eye
  - especially in the young child this may go undiagnosed as a pyrexia of unknown origin (PUO) unless it is specifically looked for
  - a slight redness around the inner canthus may be diagnostic.
- Frontal sinusitis - tender above the supra-orbital ridge.
- A purulent discharge may be seen under the middle turbinate.
- A purulent postnasal discharge.
- The typical cough of a post-nasal drip may be the only sign
  - this is the sound of clearing the back of the throat.

Note. It is important to exclude sinusitis in older children complaining of headache.

Complications
- Osteomyelitis is the most common complication of frontal sinusitis and involves the frontal bone
  - **REFER** stat.
- Meningitis / brain abscess
  - **REFER** stat.
- Chronic sinusitis (see below)

Periorbital cellulitis
- This is relatively rare.
- This follows an ethmoid or frontal sinus infection.
- There is proptosis (the eyeball projects forwards).
- The eye is unable to move.
- Loss of visual acuity.
- Any patient with evidence of sinusitis, peri-orbital swelling and inflammation should be **REFERRED** stat.

Cavernous sinus thrombosis
- This is a rare complication.
- The signs resemble orbital abscess but are usually bilateral.
- This is very serious
  - **REFER** stat.

For management of acute & chronic sinusitis, see opposite.

CHRONIC SINUSITIS

Causes
- The same as for acute sinusitis (see above).
- It may also result from inadequate treatment of the acute infection, or too much use and abuse of antibiotics.
- It is commonly secondary to allergic rhinitis.
- Less commonly due to septal deviation or polyps.

Clinical features
- The mucous membrane lining the sinus becomes thickened and sometimes develops polyps.
- Halitosis (bad smelling breath).
- Nasal and post-nasal discharge.
- Sometimes nasal obstruction.
- Pain is uncommon.
- Chronic cough, usually worse in the early morning.

MANAGEMENT
Medicine management
Antibiotics
The following antibiotics are to be used in the appropriate dosage, and treatment must be given for 5 days:
- Amoxicillin in the recommended dose (see pharmacopoeia)
- For patients who have a poor response, or those who have received amoxicillin in the last 30 days
  - use amoxicillin-clavulanic acid for 5 days (see page 27)
- Azithromycin - use in penicillin-allergic patients.

Nose drops
- Instil oxymetazoline nose drops 3 x daily.
  - 1-2 drops into each nostril for not more than 5 days continuously
- Alternatively get the patient to make the following nose drop solution.

Sodabic nose drop solution
- 1 teaspoon salt
- 1 teaspoon bicarbonate of soda
- 500 ml luke warm water.
- Insert small quantities every 4-6 hours.
- It is better than saline nose drops.
- It dissolves pus to create a thinner and more manageable sinus discharge.

Analgesia
- Paracetamol according to age as required

REFER
- Stat if a complication has occurred eg.
  - periorbital cellulitis with periorbital swelling
  - oedema over a sinus
- If still ill / pyrexial after 24-48 hours
- If not improved after 5 days
- Dental focus of infection is present eg. apical tooth abscess causing maxillary sinusitis.

TUMOURS OF THE MAXILLARY SINUS

The most common malignant tumour of the nose and paranasal sinuses is carcinoma of the maxillary sinus.

Causes
- Chronic abuse of snuff or smoking

Clinical features
- Unilateral nasal obstruction
- Epistaxis
- Pain and swelling of the cheek
- Unilateral offensive nasal discharge
- Swelling or ulceration of the bucco-alveolar sulcus or palate
- Watering eye due to involvement of the naso-lacrimal duct
- Proptosis (eyeball projecting forward) and diplopia (double vision) due to involvement of the floor of the orbit
- Unexplained enlargement of a neck lymph nodes

MANAGEMENT
REFER if:
- There is chronic, unilateral, offensive nasal discharge.
- There is chronic, unilateral, nasal obstruction.
- You suspect a tumour for any reason.
- There is an unexplained lymph node in the neck.

FRACTURED MANDIBLE / MAXILLA

Clinical features
- A fracture is usually due to severe trauma and shows marked bruising and oedema.
- Check also for loose teeth as these occur commonly at the fracture site.
- Trismus or any loss of ability to open the mouth should be viewed as a fracture.
- Inability to clench teeth (bite on a spatula).
- You have diagnosed a fracture if there is
  - a step in the alveolar margin
  - any bony tenderness.

REFER for X-ray and jaw wiring.

▼ **Note to doctor**
- It is rare for a maxilla to be fractured by a blow from a fist.
- In severe facial injuries, eg. from an MVA, or in an uncooperative patient, X-rays may be needed to diagnose a fracture.
- Usually the diagnosis of a mandible or maxillary fracture is a clinical diagnosis.
- Palpate the area of injury, insert a gloved finger into the patient's mouth between the cheek and the teeth, and palpate the alveolar margin in the suspicious area
  - if the tenderness is on the cheek side only, it is a soft tissue injury (manage with paracetamol)
  - if there is bony tenderness along the gum, then it is a fracture ▲

THE MOUTH, THROAT AND LARYNX

GENERAL CLINICAL FEATURES

PAIN ON SWALLOWING

Causes

In children
- Tonsillitis, pharyngitis, herpangina (see page 43)
- Lymphadenitis of the neck lymph nodes
- Foreign bodies should always be considered, especially if
    - the symptoms are acute
    - associated with breathing difficulty
- Moniliasis (thrush)
- Mumps

In adults
- Acute onset - same causes as for children
- AIDS - which causes severe thrush
- Carcinoma of the mouth, larynx or oesophagus
- Avitaminosis and alcoholism
- Severe iron deficiency anaemia

SORES OF LIPS AND MOUTH

Causes

In children
- Thrush in young babies is very common
- Viral infections of the lips and mouth - herpetic stomatitis
- Trauma from eating something too hot
- Tooth or gum disease eg. caries
- Vitamin deficiency
- Bottle feeding and use of dummies

In adults
- Aphthous stomatitis
- Herpes labialis
- Trauma from broken, jagged or malaligned (crooked) teeth
- Vitamin deficiency
- Thrush is strongly suggestive of diabetes or AIDS
- Carcinoma of the lip and floor of the mouth
- Syphilitic chancre and mucous patches

MANAGEMENT
REFER:
- Adult patients with any ulcer of the mouth or lips, of more than 2 weeks duration as this could be due to carcinoma.

HOARSENESS

Causes
- Acute infection, usually viral
- Singer's nodules
    - small nodules of the fibrous parts of the edge of the vocal cords
    - commonly due to vocal strain eg. singing, teaching
- Carcinoma of the larynx and hypopharynx
- Tracheal / laryngeal candidiasis
- Chronic laryngitis
- Vocal cord paresis (paralysis)
- Myxoedema

Hoarseness for more than 3 weeks duration must be **REFERRED**. See chronic laryngitis page 49.

DIFFICULTY WITH SWALLOWING (DYSPHAGIA)

This is the inability to swallow normally.

Causes
- Similar to the causes for pain on swallowing

In children
- Hilar lymphadenopathy due to tuberculosis
- Enlarged heart
- Foreign bodies in the pharynx or oesophagus

MANAGEMENT
REFER:
- Any adult patient with dysphagia for more than 2 weeks, as this could to be due to carcinoma.
- Any child with chronic dysphagia as soon as possible if you can not find a treatable cause.

SWELLING OF THE MOUTH OR JAW

Causes
- Trauma eg. fracture
- Dental disease, especially dental abscess
- Lymphadenopathy
- Mumps (see page 47)

SWELLING OF THE NECK

ACUTE CAUSES

- Acute lymphadenopathy
- Ludwig's angina
- Abscess in a neck gland
- Trauma
- Haematoma
- Salivary gland infections and tumours

ACUTE LYMPHADENOPATHY

Causes
- Infections of the teeth, throat or mouth
- Impetigo of the face and scalp is a common cause in children
    - it is therefore important to check the hair
- Acne and other skin infections in adults
- Abscess formation in the glands

Clinical features
- There will be an obvious source of infection eg. tonsillitis.
- There will be acute swelling with tenderness.

> - Treat the infection with an appropriate antibiotic.
> - **REFER** if the infection does not improve after 2 days.

LUDWIG'S ANGINA

- This is an infection of the sublingual and submandibular area (floor of the mouth)
    - it often follows dental / periodontal infections.
- The infection may spread in the subcutaneous tissue down into the neck.
- If not treated it may result in:
    - respiratory obstruction
    - death.

Clinical features
- Submandibular cellulitis with brawny (thick) oedema
- Swelling below the chin that is getting bigger
- Pain on swallowing
- Difficulty with talking
- Trismus
- Superior-posterior displacement of the tongue
    - pain on sticking out the tongue
- Drooling of saliva
- The patient may develop
    - cellulitis in the neck
    - inability to swallow
    - respiratory obstruction

> - IV drip
> - IV penicillin and metronidazole
> - **REFER** urgently for admission

ABSCESS IN A NECK GLAND

Causes
- This follows infection of a lymph gland.
- It is not easy to diagnose the cause.

Clinical features
- The abscess occurs deep underneath the neck muscles and will not show classical fluctuation.
- Suspect an abscess if there is severe pain which
    - affects sleep
    - is throbbing
    - has been present for more than 48 hours.

> **REFER** stat.

TRAUMA

- The neck contains vital structures.
- After trauma, eg. a stab, it is often difficult to decide if an important structure such as the carotid artery has been damaged.

> **MANAGEMENT**
> **REFER:**
> - Any trauma to the neck for assessment
>   - unless you can be sure it is minor.
> - All stab wounds
>   - unless you are sure it is only a superficial cut.

CHRONIC CAUSES

- Goitre and other thyroid swellings
- Chronic lymphadenopathy
    - TB
    - HIV disease (PGL)
    - carcinoma eg. of head and neck and leukaemias
    - lymphoma
- Thyroglossal cyst
- Chronic mouth infection

> **MANAGEMENT**
> - Chronic lymphadenopathy
>   - **REFER** localised, matted or prominent glands (greater than 3 cm in size) for fine needle aspiration (FNA)
> - **REFER** other causes to doctor unless previously investigated.

DISEASES OF THE THROAT

VIRAL PHARYNGITIS

Causes
- There are many different viral causes of a sore throat.
- It is often associated with nasal infections, influenza and the common cold.

Clinical features
- Sore throat
- Mild dysphagia
- Malaise
- Fever
- Mildly red throat with prominent blood vessels with or without enlarged tonsils

MANAGEMENT
- Antibiotics do not work in viral infections.
- However it is virtually impossible to be clinically sure that there is not a streptococcal infection present which could cause rheumatic fever so
    - penicillin is prescribed routinely for those aged 3-21 years
    - **or** azithromycin if penicillin-allergic
    - treatment is given for 10 days (3 days for azithromycin).
- Salt water gargles may be used
    - 2.5 ml salt in 200 ml lukewarm water
- Antiseptic gargles should **not** be used as they
    - destroy the normal flora of the mouth
    - have no effect on viruses.
- Give paracetamol for pain relief.

ACUTE STREPTOCOCCAL TONSILLITIS / PHARYNGITIS

Causes
- Streptococcal infections are by far the most common cause of definite follicular or membranous tonsillitis.

Clinical features
- Sore throat and dysphagia
- Earache (referred pain)
- Headache and malaise
- Pyrexia often present
- Children may vomit
- The mucous membrane of the pharynx, especially of the fauces, is bright red.
- The uvula may be oedematous.
- The tonsils are red, usually enlarged, and pus exudes from the crypts.
- There may be petechiae on the palate
- The submandibular glands are frequently enlarged and tender.
- The throat signs may be associated with signs of scarlet fever
    - "strawberry" tongue (enlarged red papillae)
    - diffuse, red rash with superimposed fine, papules especially at the base of the neck, face, axillae, groins and inner surface of the thighs
    - rash fades in 2-5 days and is followed by fine peeling most notable in the axillae, groins and finger tips
- Usually halitosis
- The main clinical features that would make you suspect a streptococcal infection are:
    - pyrexia
    - tachycardia out of proportion to the rise in temperature
    - tender, enlarged, submandibular lymph nodes
    - follicles on the tonsils
    - scarlet fever rash
- Follicles are usually large, white, cream-coloured or grey patches on an inflamed tonsil
    - they should not be confused with concretions which are normal tonsillar secretions
- Concretions are cream-coloured, small (pinhead size) and are found on pink non-inflamed tonsils and are often unilateral.
- Follicular tonsillitis may progress to membranous tonsillitis.

Differential diagnosis of membranous tonsillitis includes
- Infectious mononucleosis (see page 43)
- Candida infection

Complications
- Peritonsillar abscess is the most common complication.
- Rheumatic fever
- Acute glomerulonephritis

MANAGEMENT
Antibiotics
Treatment by antibiotics is to:
- destroy the acute infection
- prevent rheumatic fever and glomerulonephritis in susceptible age groups.

Indications
- The presence of follicles
- The presence of a membrane
- Ages 3-21 years
- The presence of a streptococcal rash/scarlet fever
- In a patient
    - with a previous history of rheumatic fever
    - who has confirmed rheumatic heart disease

Oral antibiotic dosage
- Penicillin VK 2 x daily for 10 days
    - <10 years: 250 mg
    - 10 years and older: 500 mg

- Amoxicillin 50 mg/kg/dose once daily for 10 days
    - 6-18 months   400 mg
    - 18 months-5 years   600 mg
    - 5-7 years   750 mg
    - 7-11 years   1000 mg
    - 11-15 years   2000 mg

    - >15 years and adults 1000 mg 2 x daily for 10 days

- If penicillin-allergic, give azithromycin once daily x 3 days
    - 1-3 years   120 mg (3 ml syrup)
    - 3-5 years   160 mg (4 ml syrup)
    - 5-7 years   200 mg (5 ml syrup)
    - 7-11 years   250 mg
    - 11 years and older: 500 mg

Parenteral antibiotic
Benzathine-penicillin (Penilente LA)
- Long-acting intramuscular penicillin that will:
    - kill beta-haemolytic streptococci for 10 days after the injection
    - prevent further infection for 1 month
- Dosage:
    - children <30 kg: 600 000 units
    - children >30 kg and adults: 1.2 million units

Other management
- Analgesics
    - paracetamol (children and adults)
    - soluble aspirin (adults who experience severe pain on swallowing)
- Salt-water gargle

RHEUMATIC FEVER

Clinical features
See under CVS page 86.

PROPHYLAXIS
- Any suggestion of a streptococcal sore throat in the age group 3-21 years should be treated with benzathine penicillin IM or oral penicillin VK for 10 days.
- If the patient has had rheumatic fever, and then gets a repeat streptococcal throat infection, there is a very high chance of getting rheumatic fever again.
- Prophylaxis for all people with confirmed rheumatic heart disease must be treat lifelong with:
  Monthly IM benzathine penicillin
    - children <30 kg: 600 000 units
    - children >30 kg and adults: 1.2 million units
  or oral pen VK 2 x daily
    - children <30 kg: 125 mg
    - children >30 kg and adults: 250 mg
  OR *if penicillin-allergic*
    - children <11 years: (consult with a specialist)
    - adolescents >11 years and adults: azithromycin 250 mg daily
- Patients who have had previous rheumatic fever (but who do not have established rheumatic heart disease):
    - prophylaxis as above for 10 years or until 21 years of age (whichever is the greater)

TONSIL EXAMINATION

Clinical features
- The tonsils are infected if they are more red than the surrounding tissue
    - with or without a membrane or follicles.
- It is *not* an acute infection if they are pink or enlarged
    - with or without concretions
    - and the same colour as the palate and fauces
    - enlargement merely indicates active tonsillar tissue and is a normal finding, especially in children aged between 5-9 years.

Note.
- Causing a patient to gag by placing a spatula into the throat, will draw the fauces together and the tonsils will appear larger and redder than they really are.
- Therefore, if possible, try and examine the tonsils without a spatula by getting the patient to open widely and say "Aah".
- In young children it sometimes helps to get them to stick their tongues out.

RECURRENT TONSILLITIS

Some individuals are subject to recurrent attacks of acute tonsillitis.

Causes
- Sinus infection
- Dental or gum sepsis
- Lowered resistance of the patient eg. malnutrition, alcohol
- Allergy

MANAGEMENT
- Treat each episode as for acute tonsillitis.
- Give antibiotics for at least 10 days.
- Certain patients may benefit from tonsillectomy
    - this is only done once active infection has been cured.

At Chris Hani Baragwanath Hospital one or more of the following conditions must be there before the patient may be considered for tonsillectomy:

- At least 4 infections a year of exudative tonsillitis
    - each episode must have been treated adequately
    - or a first episode with a history of at least 3 other episodes in a year.
- A second episode of peritonsillar abscess (quinsy) because these tend to recur.
- First episode of quinsy with history of recurrent tonsillitis - 4 per year.
- Obstructive symptoms eg. mouth breathing, voice changes.
- Progressive unilateral enlargement of tonsil.

Note. *If there are none of these conditions, the patient will not even be considered for tonsillectomy.*

OTHER CAUSES OF TONSILLITIS / PHARYNGITIS

INFECTIOUS MONONUCLEOSIS

Also known as glandular fever and is caused by the Epstein Barr virus.

Clinical features
- It usually occurs in infancy in low socio-economic areas and is very mild.
- In higher socio-economic areas it usually occurs in adolescence.
- Fever
- Sore throat with or without exudative tonsillitis
- Generalised lymphadenopathy
- Splenomegaly
- It is a self limiting illness
- A maculopapular rash is quite common

Complications
These are infrequent but can include:
- Hepatitis
- Encephalitis / meningitis
- Carditis
- Reye's syndrome (hepatic encephalopathy)

MANAGEMENT
- Symptomatic
    - paracetamol
    - bed rest
- **REFER** for confirmation of the diagnosis if
    - the infection is severe
    - complications are present

HERPANGINA

This is a condition caused by the virus Coxsackie A.

Clinical features
- These are small (2-3 mm) painful ulcers on the folds in front of the tonsils (anterior pillars of the fauces).
- These are sometimes on the soft palate and uvula as well
- Associated fever
- Duration is about 1 week.
- The lesions heal on their own.

NB. It is *not* the same as herpes stomatitis which is found mainly on the anterior part of the mouth ie. gums and tongue, but may involve the pharynx.

DIPHTHERIA

Clinical features
- It occurs in children and adults, but is now rare.
- It begins with a mild, sore throat, fever and malaise.
- Greyish patches of membrane on the tonsils, fauces or folds, and uvula.
- There is often marked cervical glandular enlargement.
- Toxaemia then follows.

MANAGEMENT
- Prevention.
- DPT immunisation is free for all infants.
- Give antibiotics - as for Strep throat.
- **REFER** anybody exposed to this
    - for confirmation of diagnosis
    - **for notification.**

SCARLET FEVER

This is a streptococcal tonsillitis, with added features, caused by a toxin.

Clinical features
- It occurs in children.
- The rash begins on the neck and upper trunk, then spreads over the remainder of the trunk and the extremities.
- The rash is a diffuse, finely papular erythema, and feels like sandpaper to touch.
- It is most severe on the axillae, groins and base of the neck.
- The face may be flushed with circumoral pallor.
- The tongue is coated with the red papillae protruding (white strawberry tongue).
    - later the coating desquamates leaving a beety-red tongue with swollen papillae (red strawberry tongue)
- Petechial spots may be seen on the palate
- Desquamation of the rash occurs after a few days (peeling).

Treat with penicillin or amoxicillin for a **minimum** of 10 days. See also page 247.

PERITONSILLAR ABSCESS (QUINSY)

This occurs as a complication of acute tonsillitis.

Clinical features
- It is especially common in young adults.
- Infection passes through the tonsil capsule into the peritonsillar tissue, where it produces a cellulitis, and then an abscess.
- Patient becomes more ill and dysphagia increases.
- The temperature peaks.
- Trismus is present.
- The soft palate on the affected side will be seen bulging downwards and forwards.
- The uvula is displaced towards the opposite tonsil.

MANAGEMENT
***REFER** for incision if:*
- Abscess appears to be pointing or pus is strongly suspected.
- Suspicion of infective spread beyond the peritonsillar space.
- No response to treatment.

- **Less severe dysphagia:** Co-amoxiclav 875/125 mg 2 x daily for 10 days

Severe dysphagia for fluids and solids:
- IV infusion of 5% dextrose water to correct dehydration and for the administration of IV treatment

If short-stay facilities are available:
- Penicillin G 2 mill units IV 6 hourly

plus
- Metronidazole 500 mg IV 8 hourly
- If dysphagia for fluids is still present the next day, further IV fluids can be given and the patient should be re-assessed for possible Incision and drainage of the quinsy

If short-stay facilities are not available:
- Amoxicillin syrup, 250mg/5ml, 10 ml immediately and repeat 2 x daily for 5 days

plus
- Co-amoxiclav syrup, 250/62,5mg/5 ml, 10 ml immediately and repeat 2 x daily for 5 days
- Analgesic / antipyretic
    - soluble aspirin preferred if unable to swallow tablets

Management follow-up
- Co-amoxiclav 875/125mg tabs 2 x daily to complete 10 days treatment
- Salt water gargle

▼ **Note to doctor**

Unsure of diagnosis
- Attempt aspiration with a syringe and size 18 needle. This can be repeated daily.

Drainage of the quinsy
- Place patient in a sitting position, with a nurse behind the patient, supporting the head from the back.
- It is impossible for a patient to sit still while a quinsy is being drained, and therefore the drainage cannot be performed unless this helper is involved.
- The quinsy occurs at the superior pole of the tonsil, laterally. Beware of the tendency to perform the drainage too far medially, where there is a secondary cellulitis of the palate causing some swelling.
- Spray the mucosa only over the area to be drained, with xylocaine spray.
- Administer morphine 0.1 mg / kg IV.
- Tape a no. 15 BP scalpel blade with strapping so that 2-3 mm only are protruding.
- Make a stab incision through the mucosa directly overlying the abscess.
- It is important only to nick the mucosa enough to allow the forceps in, as the scalpel could damage blood vessels (internal carotid).
- Insert a mosquito forceps through the mucosal incision and thrust it into the abscess cavity.
- Open the mosquito to drain the pus.
- If pus is not obtained on the first attempt, a curved mosquito can be pushed in various directions through the initial incision
    - sometimes large amounts of pus are obtained
    - sometimes very little.
- The patient can then wash out his mouth or gargle with water and spit it into a dish.

- If it is late in the day, reverse the morphine by giving naloxone (Narcan):
    - for an adult 0,4 mg / 1ml
    - give ½ the dose IVI and the other ½ IMI.

Follow up
- Check the patient the next day.
- Antibiotics for 10 days.
- **REFER** for tonsillectomy if a second episode of quinsy occurs ▲

ADENOID HYPERTROPHY

The adenoids form part of the lymphatics of the pharynx. They are situated on the posterior wall of the nasopharynx. They can be very large in children but they usually atrophy at the age of 6-7 years. Little or no adenoid tissue remains after the age of 20 years.

Causes
- Repeated URTI in some children between the ages 1-4 years

Clinical features
- Mouth breathing. Once this is established, it presents with
    - adenoid facies, narrow nose, high arched palate, prominent teeth
- Repeated URTI
- Chronic sinusitis due to impaired nasal ventilation and sinus drainage
- Eustachian tube obstruction leading to
    - recurrent acute suppurative otitis media
    - secretory otitis media (glue ear)
    - chronic suppurative otitis media
- Snoring
- Disturbed sleep (with or without sleep apnoea)
- Adenoids are only directly visible when examining with a mirror
- Large adenoids can be suspected if the soft palate is pushed downwards and forwards

MANAGEMENT

REFER *for adenoidectomy if there are one or more of the following indications:*
- Recurrent suppurative or serous otitis media with associated signs of adenoid hypertrophy
- Persistent nasal obstruction
    - mouth breathing
    - nasal speech
- Disturbed sleep
    - severe snoring
    - with or without sleep apnoea
    - if the cause is related to adenoids
- Cor pulmonale
- Chronic sinusitis
    - not responding to antibiotics
    - with clinical signs of adenoid hypertrophy

▼ **Note to doctor**

Enlargement of adenoids can be seen on a good quality lateral X-ray of head (posterior swelling occluding upper pharynx) ▲

RETRO-PHARYNGEAL ABSCESS

The lymphatic drainage of the adenoids goes via the posterior pharyngeal lymph nodes.

Any infection of the adenoids could potentially cause retro-pharyngeal adenoiditis.

If it goes untreated it may result in posterior pharyngeal abscess formation.

Clinical features
- Fever
- Respiratory stridor
- Dyspnoea
- Dysphagia
- Opisthotonus (hyper-extended neck)
- Prominent swelling on one side of the posterior pharyngeal wall
    - the swelling does not cross the midline because the fascia is fixed to the vertebrae in the midline

Note.
- In some people the one side of the back of the pharynx may bulge slightly more than the other side (this is normal)
- In the absence of signs of infection, do not diagnose an abscess.

MANAGEMENT
- **This is a surgical emergency.**
- Put up a drip (normal saline).
- Give ceftriaxone IV 50-80 mg / kg.
- **REFER** stat to hospital.

DISEASES OF THE MOUTH

APHTHOUS ULCER

Clinical features
- Shallow mucosal ulcer with red margin
    - in the mouth except the gums, hard palate and dorsum of the tongue
    - painful
    - single or multiple
    - heals within 10 days
- It is commonly found in women during times of
    - emotional stress
    - menstruation.
- In HIV/AIDS the ulcer may be large, extremely painful and recur often.

MANAGEMENT
- Chlorhexidine 0,05% mouthwash 3 x daily
- Give paracetamol
- Reassure
- **REFER** to dentist if:
    - widespread ulcers
    - severe and recurrent.

HERPES SIMPLEX

HERPETIC STOMATITIS AND PHARYNGITIS

This is the primary infection of what later can become recurrent herpes labialis.

Clinical features
- It occurs in small children and young adults, but is most common in the former.
- There are shallow, painful, intra-oral ulcers, especially on the gums, tongue and buccal mucosa. These are covered with a yellow-grey membrane.
- There is fever and salivation, and a refusal to eat because of the severe pain.
- It lasts 3-10 days.
- It is self-limiting.

MANAGEMENT
- Small, frequent fluid feeds to correct dehydration.
- Avoid acidic drinks, e.g. orange juice and cool drinks.
- Apply tetracaine 0.5% gel 4 x daily for children >6 years and adults.
- Give paracetamol.
- In severe cases or if dehydrated, **REFER** to hospital.
- In HIV-infected patients and children with extensive oral herpes give:
    - acyclovir, oral, 3 x daily for 7 days
    - use 200 mg / 5 ml suspension or disperse 200 mg tablet in 5 ml water

Dosage:
1-3 months	50 mg	1.25 ml
3-6 months	80 mg	2 ml
6-18 months	100 mg	2.5 ml
18 months-3 years	120 mg	3 ml
3-7 years	160 mg	4 ml
7-11 years	200 mg	1 tablet
11-15 years	300 mg	1½ tablets

HERPES LABIALIS

Clinical features
- The lesions may occur on the lips or on the external nares.
- The lesion consists of a small group of blisters on a red area.
- The condition usually heals on its own within 7-14 days.

Apply zinc ointment.

CHRONIC MUCOCUTANEOUS ULCERATION

This is chronic herpes simplex ulceration in patients with advanced HIV infection (AIDS defining if present for more than 1 month).

Clinical features
- Painful ulcers.
- Occurs in the mouth (hard palate, gums), lips and around the mouth or in the buttock cleft or perianal area.
- May be large with polycyclic edge, or small in size, single or multiple.
- Persists for weeks / months.

MANAGEMENT
- Oral acyclovir 400 mg 3 x daily for 7 days.
- Give paracetamol 2 tabs 3 x daily.
- Keep affected areas clean and dry.
- If pain is severe
  - **REFER** for tramadol 50 mg 6 hourly.

ORAL CANDIDIASIS

Causes
- HIV/AIDS
- Severe alcoholism
- Malnutrition (avitaminosis)
- Oral contraceptives
- Infections, especially in infants and children
- Inhaled or oral steroids (**NB.** asthmatics)
- Unhygienic preparation of bottle feeds in infants
- Prolonged use of broad spectrum antibiotics
- Diabetes mellitus

Clinical features
- White or cream-coloured, curd-like, loosely adherent (sticky) patches anywhere in the mouth
  - these may bleed if scraped.
- Angular cheilitis
  - fissures at the corners of the mouth
  - may be the only feature.

In HIV/AIDS
Specific forms of oral candidiasis may be seen which are strongly associated with HIV infection.

- Erythematous
  - red patches, spotty or diffuse, usually on the palate and / or upper surface of the tongue.
- Pseudo-membranous
  - white patches usually on the palate including the soft palate or buccal mucosa that can be scraped off.
- Hyperplastic
  - white patches on the tongue that **cannot** be scraped off.
- Angular chelitis
  - redness and fissures on the corners of the mouth.
  - fissures lie horizontally.
- In addition, in HIV infection, the candidiasis is often of a severe degree, and the following are commonly seen features:
  - a thick white coating on the tongue either smooth diffuse or irregular patches
  - curd-like patches behind the back molar teeth.

MANAGEMENT
- Remove or treat the cause.
- Infants and children
  - give nystatin suspension 1 ml 4 x daily after each meal or feed
- Adults
  - nystatin suspension 1 ml 4 x daily for 5 days.
- Keep nystatin in contact with the affected areas for as long as possible.
- HIV-infected patients with oral candidiasis and painful or difficult swallowing have oesophageal involvement and must be treated with fluconazole (see page 158).

MUCOUS CYSTS

The cysts may be caused by injury to the salivary gland duct or by a blockage of the duct.

Clinical features
- They are mostly seen on the lower lip but can appear where the salivary gland ducts open into the mouth ie. under the tongue.
- The swelling is about 5-10 mm in size and is painless.

MANAGEMENT
REFER for:
- X-ray to check if a stone is blocking the salivary gland duct.
- Possible surgery.

PRE-CANCEROUS CONDITIONS

LEUKOPLAKIA

- These are white patches which occur on the lips, on the inside of the cheek or on the tongue.
- They are often associated with smoking or chewing tobacco.
- The lesions are painless, hard and look like cracked, white paint.
- They cannot be scraped off the oral tissue.
- If seen as white vertical ridges on the side of the tongue, this is known as hairy leukoplakia and is common in HIV disease.

> **REFER.**

ORAL CANCER

- This is usually present as a chronic ulcer.
- The most common sites for these ulcers are
    - the margins of the tongue
    - the lower lip (because of exposure to the sun)
    - the floor of the mouth

> **REFER**
> - Any ulcer of more than 2 weeks.
> - For possible surgery or radiation therapy.

SALIVARY GLANDS

MUMPS

A viral illness producing inflammation of the salivary glands.

Clinical features
- Painful, swollen salivary glands, usually the parotid glands
- Commonly found in children
- Incubation period 14-21 days
- Fever and malaise are not marked
- May find an inflamed opening of the salivary gland duct (Stenson's duct)

Complications
- Orchitis or oöphoritis
- Pancreatitis
- Aseptic meningitis

Differential diagnosis
- Parotid duct "stones" (calculi)
- HIV disease
- Cirrhosis
- Infection with other viruses eg. parainfluenza

> **MANAGEMENT**
> - Treat symptomatically.
> - Give paracetamol.

> **REFER**
> - Abdominal pain (to exclude pancreatitis)
> - Painful swolllen testis / testes (orchitis)
> - Suspected meningo-encephalitis

DISEASES OF THE GUMS

GINGIVITIS (PERIODONTAL DISEASE)

Clinical features
- Often found in smokers.
- They may or may not be painful.
- There is inflammation and swelling of gum margin.
- Sometimes pus formation.
- There is often gum recession.

> **MANAGEMENT**
> - Promote good oral hygiene, ie. soft brushing and flossing.
> - Chorhexidine 0,2% mouthwash 3 x daily for 5 days.
> - **REFER** if severe.

ACUTE NECROTISING ULCERATIVE GINGIVITIS (ANUG) (VINCENT'S ANGINA)

Causes
- HIV disease
- Poor oral hygiene
- Plaque
- Calculus
- Localised trauma
- Stress
- Vitamin B and C deficiencies
- Smoking

Clinical features
- This condition may affect the gums totally or only partly around single teeth.
- Acutely painful bleeding gums.
- Grey-white membrane between teeth on gums.
- Halitosis is a distinctive feature.
- The lymph glands in the neck may be enlarged.

> **MANAGEMENT**
> - Advice on good oral hygiene.
> - **REFER** to a dentist
> - If a dentist is not available, give metronidazole 400 mg 3 x daily for 5 days
> - Treatment includes a chlorhexidine 0,2% mouthwash 3 x daily for 5 days.

DENTAL ABSCESS (PERIAPICAL ABSCESS)

Clinical features
- Pain (not always present)
- Tenderness on tapping with a spatula or by probing the affected tooth
- Looseness of the tooth (after infection reaches the bone)
- Cheek or jaw swelling

MANAGEMENT
- Give amoxicillin for 5 days
    - or azithromycin for 3 days if penicillin-allergic.
- **Plus** metronidazole 3 x daily for 5 days
    - 12-18 months: 80 mg (2 ml)
    - 18 months-3 years: 100 mg (2.5 ml)
    - 3-5 years: 120 mg (3 ml)
    - 5-7 years: 160 mg (4 ml)
    - 7-11 years: 200 mg (5 ml)
    - 11-15 years: 300 mg (1½ tabs)
    - >15 years and adults: 400 mg (2 tabs)
- Give analgesic.
- **REFER** to the dentist.

PHENYTOIN (EPANUTIN) FIBROMATOSIS

Clinical features
- In this condition the gums are enlarged and appear nodular.
- They have a pale pink colour and are firm.
- The patient's lips may stick out and the teeth may even become displaced.

MANAGEMENT
- A different anti-epileptic drug must be prescribed.
- Promote good oral hygiene
    - rub the gums firmly as this may prevent further development.
- **REFER** for surgery.

PERICORONITIS

This is an infection in the flap of the gum (pericorona) over an erupting tooth.

Clinical features
- It is quite common and tends to occur at the back of the mouth over an erupting molar tooth.
- There is severe pain in the area, made worse by chewing.
- A flap of gum is seen to be swollen and inflamed and very tender on palpation.

- Give paracetamol.
- Saline mouth washes as needed.
- **REFER** to dentist for surgical removal of the gum flap.

ERUPTION CYSTS

Clinical features
- The cysts usually appear on the gums of infants and children when teeth are erupting.
- They present with blue swellings of the gum, usually where the incisors are erupting.

- No treatment is necessary.
- The lesion heals after eruption of the tooth.

DISEASES OF THE TONGUE

FISSURED TONGUE

Clinical features
- This is a developmental abnormality.
- The tongue presents with an irregular fissured pattern.
- Food may collect in the fissures and stagnate causing halitosis.

- Give advice on good oral hygiene.

GEOGRAPHIC TONGUE

The cause is unknown, but stress and allergies may play a role.

Clinical features
- The tongue presents with an irregular pattern.
- There are red areas surrounded by white or yellow borders (rings).

- Give reassurance that:
    - this is a harmless condition
    - it will disappear on its own.

BLACK HAIRY TONGUE

Causes
- Smoking
- Certain foodstuffs
- Spices
- Drugs (penicillins)

Clinical features
- The filiform papillae become very long and look like fine hair on the surface of the tongue.
- A black pigment, produced by fungi, stains the papillae so that the surface of the tongue appears to be covered by fine black hairs.

MANAGEMENT
- Give advice on good oral hygiene including brushing the tongue.
- Give chlorhexidine 0,2% mouthwash 3 x daily for 5 days.

GLOSSITIS

Causes
- Alcohol abuse
- Malnutrition
- Riboflavin deficiency (Vitamin B2)

Clinical features
- It presents as a painful tongue.
- The tongue is reddened.
- The papillae are blunted giving the tongue a smooth appearance.
- Sticking the tongue out is painful.
- The tongue appears small in size.

- Advise to stop drinking alcohol.
- Give Vitamin B complex 1-2 tabs daily.

HAIRY LEUKOPLAKIA

This is seen as white vertical ridges on the sides of the tongue. This predicts progression to AIDS and occurs with declining immunity.

No management is required

DISEASES OF THE LARYNX

LARYNGITIS

ACUTE LARYNGITIS

Acute inflammation of the laryngeal mucosa most often due to viral infection.

Causes
- It may occur singly or in association with an upper respiratory infection eg.
    - influenza
    - the common cold
    - nasopharyngitis
- As a result of inhalation of irritants
- Over-use or mis-use of the voice
- Over-indulgence in alcohol or tobacco

Clinical features
- Hoarseness is the main symptom and it varies from
    - very slight hoarseness
    - to complete loss of voice.
- Occasionally there is pain in the throat.
- Sometimes there are other signs of respiratory infection.

MANAGEMENT
- The voice must be rested.
- Inhalation of steam.
- Decrease smoking and alcohol.
- Avoid decongestants and antihistamines.

CHRONIC LARYNGITIS

This is a chronic inflammation of the laryngeal mucosa.

Causes
- Candida infection especially in HIV/AIDS
- Chronic vocal abuse (nodules)
- Habitual over-indulgence in tobacco or alcohol
- Chronic sinus infection with post-nasal discharge
- Chronic inhalation of irritants eg. chemical fumes
- Allergy
- Tuberculosis
- Syphilis
- Exclude other lesions causing hoarseness eg.
    - vocal cord paresis
    - carcinoma of the larynx

Clinical features
- Chronic hoarseness is the main symptom.
- There may be loss of voice at times.
- Vocal fatigue – the voice may be forced by hard effort to be clear for a short time but it quickly loses power.
- Cough and a constant tendency to clear the throat.

MANAGEMENT
- **Hoarseness of more than 3 weeks duration must be REFERRED to investigate for possible CA larynx unless there is an obvious treatable cause eg. candidia.**
- Treat the cause by:
    - stopping the use of alcohol and tobacco
    - resting the voice
    - taking antibiotics for sinus infection
    - inhalation of steam
    - speech therapy.
- Patients with candidal laryngitis
    - **REFER** to doctor for fluconazole 200 mg daily for 14 days.

RESPIRATORY SYSTEM

THE UPPER AIRWAYS

PROBLEMS OF THE UPPER AIRWAYS

STRIDOR

Stridor is a noise usually heard on **inspiration** similar to snoring. It is caused by air passing through a narrowed or partially obstructed larynx, trachea, or over a swollen epiglottis.
It is a serious symptom usually requiring REFERRAL.

Causes

Common
- Acute laryngotracheo-bronchitis (LTB)
- Foreign body
- Para tracheal lymph node enlargement eg. due to tuberculosis

Less common
- Bacterial tracheitis
- Trauma
- Laryngeal tumours eg. papillomas
- Congenital abnormalities of the upper airways eg. laryngomalacia
- Acute epiglottitis
- Allergy (laryngeal oedema)

Clinical features in children

The degree of obstruction varies.

Grade 0
- Hoarseness (croupy cry)
- Croupy cough

Grade 1
- Inspiratory stridor only
- This is mildest if it is only noticed when the child cries.
- It is becoming more severe if it is also noticed when the child is not crying.

Grade 2
- Inspiratory and expiratory stridor

Grade 3
- Inspiratory and expiratory stridor (active expiration using abdominal muscles).

Grade 4
- Inspiratory and expiratory stridor
plus
- Marked rib retraction
- Apathy
- Cyanosis
- Intermittent apnoea

MANAGEMENT

Children
- **REFER** all children with stridor, but start the following first:
  - prednisone 1-2 mg / kg orally stat (avoid in children with measles and herpes infection)
  - mix 1 ml epinephrine 1:1000 (1 mg) with 1 ml normal saline.
  - nebulise the entire volume with oxygen.
  - repeat nebulisations at 15-30 minute intervals until the stridor stops, or until transport arrives.
- Monitor oxygen saturation, heart rate and respiratory rate.
- Admit urgently if there is no response.

Adults
- **REFER** adults with acute stridor stat.
- Stridor of a more chronic nature can be referred less urgently.

LARYNGOTRACHEO-BRONCHITIS (LTB)

This is an infection of the larynx, trachea and bronchi occurring in young children, usually between 6 months and 2 years of age.

Causes
- Often due to viruses eg. para-influenza, measles, herpes simplex, adenovirus

Clinical features
- There is usually a history of an upper respiratory tract infection for 1-2 days.
- This is followed by inspiratory stridor and hoarseness.
- This may then be followed by expiratory obstruction.
- Stridor becomes softer as the airway obstruction becomes worse.
- Cough is dry, croupy and barking, due to the tracheitis

MANAGEMENT

REFER all patients with stridor.

General measures (children without stridor)
- Small frequent meals, as big meals cause:
  - distension of the stomach
  - pushing up on the diaphragm
  - difficulty with breathing.
- Frequent fluids in small amounts, because children lose fluid from the lungs due to the tachypnoea.

- Avoid undue stress, crying or exertion. The child must be kept as quiet and as calm as possible.
- Humidification. This can be done by placing a boiling kettle or pot in a room where the child is sitting or sleeping.
- Sitting the child up in bed helps the breathing.
- Advise the parents of the diagnosis, the dangers and the prognosis.

Give them specific instructions to bring the child back stat if there is:
- Increasing difficulty with breathing
- Inability to take feeds
- Head retraction
- Increasing anxiety and restlessness
- Drooling and inability to swallow

Medicine management
- As for stridor (see page 53)
- Paracetamol as required for pain or pyrexia
- Amoxicillin for 5 days in the appropriate dosage for age

EPIGLOTTITIS

This is a rapidly progressive infection of the epiglottis and is an extremely dangerous condition.

Clinical features
- It occurs in children aged 2 - 5 years, and is uncommon in children below 2 years.
- A very sore throat and severe dysphagia
    - the child may not be able to swallow at all.
- There is high fever.
- There is rapidly progressive airway obstruction and stridor.
- The child sits with the head held still, and the jaw pushed forward, concentrating on breathing.
- The breathing is shallow, deliberate and slow.
- There may be drooling of saliva.
- The child speaks reluctantly, and the voice is soft.
- The oedema and swelling of the epiglottis may completely obstruct the airway.

NB. Avoid trying to examine the throat or tonsils if you suspect this condition, because the trauma of the examination and the use of a spatula may precipitate total airway obstruction and death.

MANAGEMENT
- **REFER** all children with high fever, dysphagia, sitting up with mouth open and drooling
- Put up a drip (normal saline)
- Give ceftriaxone 80 mg/kg IM or IV as a single dose
- Adrenalin 1 : 1 000 nebulised
    - dilute to 5 ml with normal saline
- **REFER** stat to hospital.

FOREIGN BODY INHALATION

Causes
In children
- They often put objects into their mouths, which can be aspirated, especially if they get a fright
    - the age most affected is 6 months to 4 years.
- Forced feeding causes aspiration and may cause death.
- Peanut inhalation is often fatal in children.
    - ***no young child should ever be allowed to eat peanuts, unless given in the form of peanut butter.***

In adults
- They may aspirate a foreign body, commonly a piece of food.
- The most dangerous foreign bodies are those made up of vegetable matter
    - these swell up from the moisture in the airways
    - they commonly lead to severe broncho-spasm.

Clinical features
- Sudden onset of wheeze, stridor, cough, respiratory distress or choking.
- Beware of a "silent period"
    - ie. after choking, the child may appear to settle, but may collapse later when the foreign body re-obstructs.
- If the obstruction is in the upper airway there will be stridor.
- If there is bronchial obstruction there will be a wheeze, which may be unilateral or bilateral.
- Localised decreased air entry and / or a displaced apex beat suggest collapse of a portion of the lung.
- Pneumonia or lung abscess may be the presenting feature if the condition is not diagnosed initially.
- A child may present with recurrent chest infection.

MANAGEMENT
Prevention
- Advise parents:
    - not to force feed children
    - to prevent children running with objects in their mouths
    - not to give peanuts to young children.

Home management
- Check inside mouth, sweep back of tongue / pharynx with a finger to exclude foreign body there.
- Small children, under one year, should be put over the knee (head and chest down) and firmly banged on the back with a hand until the foreign body is released.
- For bigger children and adults, the Heimlich manoeuvre is best (see Emergencies page 6).

Clinic management
- The above techniques can be attempted at the clinic.
- If you cannot be sure whether the foreign body has been expelled, then it is essential that the patient be **REFERRED** for X-ray.
- Some foreign bodies may not be visible on X-ray and **REFERRAL** for bronchoscopy may be necessary.

TRACHEITIS

Clinical features
- Non-productive cough
- Often retrosternal chest pain
- Temperature usually normal
- Respiratory rate normal
- Clear chest
- Children present with a dry, barking type of cough
- Often there will be a history of a preceding upper respiratory tract infection

Differential diagnosis
- Laryngotracheo-bronchitis (LTB) in children
- Tuberculosis

MANAGEMENT
- Cough mixture
- Paracetamol for pain and pyrexia as required
- Reassurance that the disease will clear spontaneously in a few days

BRONCHITIS

Causes
- Initially a viral infection of the bronchi
    - it commonly follows a viral upper respiratory tract infection.
- This is often followed by a secondary bacterial infection.

Clinical features
- There may be a history of a recent upper respiratory tract infection.
- A productive (moist) cough is characteristic of bronchitis.
- The sputum may be mucoid or mucopurulent.
- There is often retrosternal chest pain.
- Temperature usually normal, when elevated it does not usually exceed 39°C.
- Respiratory rate normal with no signs of respiratory distress.
- Often no abnormal chest signs.
- There may be bilateral rhonchi, wheezes and occasional creps which change or disappear with coughing.
- Children may swallow sputum and may have associated vomiting as a result.

MANAGEMENT
General measures
Advice and reassurance
- The illness should clear spontaneously in a few days.
- The patient should return if:
    - sputum amount increases
    - continuing fever
    - the cough begins to make eating and breathing difficult in children.

Bed rest / off work / off school
- Only if febrile
- Usually for 2-3 days depending on the patient's work or school situation

Medicine management
Analgesia
- Paracetamol as required for retrosternal chest pain.

Antibiotics
- The indications for the use of an antibiotic are:
    - malnutrition
    - chronic chest disease e.g. COPD
    - chronic heart disease
    - infants and small children when pneumonia cannot reliably be excluded or who appear ill
    - elderly patients who appear ill or have mucopurulent sputum
    - no improvement after 5-7 days

Children
- Amoxicillin 2 x daily for 5 days
    - 3-6 months   250 mg
    - 6-18 month   375 mg
    - 18 months-3 years 500 mg
    - 3-5 years   750 mg
    - 5-15 years   1000 mg

- If there is a history of penicillin allergy, give azithromycin once daily x 3 days:
    - 1-3 years: 120 mg (3 ml syrup)
    - 3-5 years: 160 mg (4 ml syrup)
    - 5-7 years: 200 mg (5 ml syrup)
    - 7-11 years: 250 mg
    - 11-15 years: 500 mg

Adults
- Amoxicillin 1 g 3 x daily for 5 days

In penicillin-allergic patients:
- Azithromycin 500 mg daily for 3 days

Bronchodilator
- The indication is wheezing
- If wheezes are prominent, these patients may be suffering from bronchial asthma. They must be managed according to the Asthma Medicine protocol, page 59.

BRONCHIOLITIS

Common cause of wheezing and cough in the first 2 years of life.
- The course of the disease is 4-5 days with the most critical period occurring between 24 and 72 hours.

This is useful to know, because if a child presents:
- **On the first day** with moderate or severe distress
    - then the child needs admission as the disease will very likely progress over the next 1 or 2 days.
- **On the 3rd or 4th day**, and is not severely distressed
    - then the child can be safely treated at home, as the disease will spontaneously improve.

Recurrent episodes of wheeze may occur. Some of these children may develop asthma.

Clinical features

- Occurs in children mainly between 4 months and 2 years of age, but less common in the second year of life.
- Often there is a history of a preceding upper respiratory tract infection.
- Development of symptoms is usually gradual with:
    - tight cough
    - audible wheeze
    - irritability.
- May be difficulty in feeding or sleeping
- Tachypnoea, which is often marked with rates which vary between 60-80 per minute.
- Subcostal recession (lower chest wall indrawing).
- Restlessness which increases with increasing respiratory distress.
- Wheezes, mainly expiratory.
- The temperature is usually normal or only slightly elevated.
- Cyanosis may be present in severe cases.

MANAGEMENT

REFER if:
- Less than 3 months of age
- The heart rate is more than 140 / minute
- The respiratory rate is more than 60 / minute
- Moderate or severe respiratory distress at any stage
- Difficulty in feeding
- Distress when speaking or crying
- Sleep disturbance
- A previous severe episode required hospital admission
- You are unsure of the diagnosis, or suspect bronchopneumonia or asthma
- Oygen saturation <90% in room air

General measures

- Give small frequent feeds and plenty of fluids.
- Bottle feeding may cause aspiration, so encourage breast, or cup and spoon feeds (the child needs to be sat upright for these).
- Use of steam inhalations may help.
- Elevate the child in bed with extra pillows.
- Give advice to the escort on signs of deterioration and to return immediately if any of these are present
    - difficulty in feeding or talking
    - increasing difficulty in breathing
    - increasing restlessness

Medicine management

- Oxygen, humidified, using nasal prongs or nasal cannula at 1-2 l/minute for 10-15 minutes.
- If there is a good response, which is maintained for at least 2 hours, send the patient home.
- If not improved after humidified oxygen:
    - transfer the child to hospital with oxygen to maintain an oxygen saturation > 90%.

Antibiotic
- Because it is often difficult to distinguish bronchiolitis from bronchopneumonia, if the diagnosis is in doubt, it is advisable to treat the child with an antibiotic.
- If the child is **not** being referred for admission:
- Amoxicillin 45 mg/kg/dose 2 x daily for 5 days
    - dosage according to age

THE LUNGS

BRONCHIAL ASTHMA

UNDERSTANDING ASTHMA

- It is important to understand that asthma is a chronic inflammatory disorder of the bronchi.
- In susceptible individuals, exposure to various environmental triggers, allergens, viral infections, weather changes, emotional upsets or other irritants results in inflammatory changes. This then results in:
    - airway hyper-responsiveness
    - increased secretions
    - bronchospasm
- If this is not controlled, eventual bronchial muscle hypertrophy of the airways' smooth muscle may occur.
- There is widespread variable airflow obstruction that is reversible either spontaneously or with treatment.
- Treatment is generally prophylactic (aimed at preventing the inflammation from starting).
    - it must therefore be continued even if the asthmatic patient is asymptomatic.

Clinical features of acute asthma

- Recurrent episodes of coughing, wheezing, chest "tightness" and shortness of breath lasting for some hours or days.
- Symptoms are often worse at night.
- In children coughing and/or wheezing after exercising, or chronic nocturnal cough, is strongly suggestive of asthma.
- Audible wheeze
- Dyspnoea
- Tight cough
- Hyperinflation
- Use of accessory muscles of respiration
- Suprasternal / intercostal recession
- Chest indrawing in children
- Reduced air entry bilaterally
- Scattered or generalised wheezing, dependent on severity
- Reduced peak expiratory flow rate (PEFR) readings

Differential diagnosis

It is vitally important to exclude left ventricular failure as this can look very similar, particularly in patients over 50 years presenting with asthma for the first time.

Clinical features of left ventricular failure

- The dyspnoea and wheeze may last for only a short time and are often relieved by rest
    - this does not occur with bronchial asthma
- There is orthopnoea and exertional dyspnoea.
- There is a forceful and / or displaced apex beat.
- There are bilateral basal creps.
- There is excessive tachycardia, irregular pulse or gallop rhythm.

If in any doubt, **REFER** (see heart failure, page 81).

Classification of asthma severity

Intermittent asthma
- Not more than two episodes of day-time cough and/or wheeze per week.
- Not more than one episode of night-time cough and/or wheeze per month.
- No recent (within the last year) admission to hospital for asthma.
- PEFR more than 80% predicted between attacks.

Mild persistent asthma
- 3-4 episodes of wheeze and/or cough per week.
- 2-4 episodes of night-time wheeze and/or cough per month.
- PEFR more than 80% predicted between attacks.

Moderate persistent asthma
- More than 4 episodes of day-time wheeze, tightness or cough per week.
- More than 4 episodes of night-time wheeze, tightness or cough per month.
- PEFR more than 60%, but less than 80% predicted between attacks.

Severe persistent asthma
- Continuous wheeze, tightness or cough.
- Frequent nocturnal symptoms.
- PEFR less than 60% predicted between attacks.

MANAGEMENT OF CHRONIC ASTHMA

Aims of management

- Remove the symptoms.
- Restore normal, or best possible long term function of the airways.
- Reduce the number and severity of acute attacks.
    - it is easier to prevent an attack than to break it once it has started.
- The peak flow readings should remain within normal limits at all times for children
    - some adults may be found to have persistently low readings which cannot be improved.
- Find out which precipitating factors might be making the asthma worse and try and help the patient to find ways of avoiding these.

Patient education and training

Patients or parents should be made aware of the following:

- The nature of the disease
- The need to observe for precipitating factors eg. cigarette smoke, pollens, emotional stress
- The importance of regular treatment ie. for those patients who have frequent symptoms
- The difference between relieving an acute attack and treatment of bronchial inflammation by using anti-inflammatory medicines

- The prognosis ie. that there is a good chance that childhood asthma will improve after puberty
- The danger signs of a severe attack
    - inability to talk or eat
    - failure to respond to the usual treatment

Patients must be given instructions on how to respond to worsening asthma
- They need to know about increasing the dosage of inhaled steroids.
- They need to know where to obtain urgent medical attention, should this be required.

Parents must be advised about the following:
- They must not over-protect asthmatic children. The child must live a normal life as far as possible, and not be stopped from joining his or her friends in whatever they may be doing.
- Babies may be protected to some extent from asthma and allergy if:
    - they only have breast milk for the first six months
    - proteins such as cow's milk and cereals are only introduced after 6 months.

Patients should be trained
- Patients on inhalation therapy should have training in the proper use of inhaled drugs and the correct inhalation methods.

Avoidance of precipitating factors
Find out which precipitating factors might be affecting the patient and stress their avoidance as far as possible and practical.
- Allergens
    - dust - put plastic over mattresses and feather pillows
    - wash blankets in hot water
    - avoid heavy, linen curtains and thick carpets which retain dust
    - mop floors with a wet mop or vacuum the house regularly
    - avoid flowers inside if they seem to cause attacks
    - keep animals outside the house and avoid cats as household pets
- Drugs may be the cause eg.
    - aspirin and other NSAIDs
    - beta-blockers
- Preservatives such as sodium benzoate, tartrazine and sulphur dioxide.

- Occupational sensitising chemicals that may be found at work.
- Smoking is harmful to asthmatics and should not be allowed in the home of any asthmatic.
- Emotional stress.
- High levels of atmospheric pollution.

Follow-up visits
These should include the following:
- Check the frequency of symptoms (especially nocturnal).
- Ask about any interference with normal activities (eg. work loss).
- Enquire about the frequency of use of the bronchodilator inhaler.
- Check if the patient understands asthma and its management.
- Check the patient's skill in the use of inhalers.
- The patient must know the action to be taken if signs of deterioration develop.
- Do peak flow recordings to assess if the asthma is controlled or not.

PRINCIPLES OF MEDICINE MANAGEMENT
Intermittent therapy
- Indication is intermittent asthma (see page 57).
- Treat only if symptomatic using a beta-2 stimulant inhaler eg. salbutamol (Ventolin).

Exercise induced asthma
Asthma brought on by exercise is fairly common particularly in children and young adults.
- It is best prevented by advising the patient to use:
    - a beta-2 stimulant inhaler 15-20 minutes before exercise.

Continuous therapy
- Indication is persistent asthma – all grades (see page 57).
- Treat with:
    - an anti-inflammatory drug, ie. inhaled steroid
    - **and** a beta-2 stimulant bronchodilator.
- The anti-inflammatory drug must be used **continuously** as it prevents and suppresses inflammation which leads to mucosal swelling.
- The beta-2 stimulant is used to treat episodes of bronchospasm
    - it should preferably only be used when the patient is symptomatic
    - it should not be used continuously.

Follow up
Patients on continuous therapy must return 4 weekly for medication and follow up.

Bronchodilators
The safest and most effective way to give medication in asthma is by inhalation.

Inhalers in children
- Children, especially small children, struggle to use inhalers correctly.
- The use of a spacer for an inhaler makes this much easier.
- Allow the child to breathe slowly in and out of the spacer continuously for 30 seconds.
- While still breathing, release one puff from the inhaler into the spacer.
- Continue breathing for 4-5 breaths.

■ ASTHMA MEDICINE PROTOCOL

1-6 YEARS
- **REFER** to doctor / paediatrician for assessment and for confirmation of the diagnosis.
- In acute asthma:
    - nebulise 2,5 ml salbutamol nebule (2,5 mg) diluted in 2,5 ml normal saline
    - prior to referral.
- Children referred to clinic for continuation of chronic maintenance therapy should use a spacer device eg. Aero-chamber for all inhaled medication (with a mask attachment in children under 3 years of age).

6-14 YEARS
Mild infrequent symptoms (intermittent asthma)
- Inhaled salbutamol
    - 1-2 puffs (100-200 micrograms) 3 x daily as required until relief is obtained (2 puff dose 10 years and older).

More frequent or severe symptoms
Step 1
- Inhaled corticosteroid (budesonide, beclomethasone 50 mcg / puff)
    - 2 puffs (100 micrograms) 2 x daily.
- **Plus** inhaled salbutamol
    - 1-2 puffs 3 x daily as required (2 puff dose 10 years and older).
- A spacer device is advisable if the child is having difficulty with the co-ordination of inhaler activation and inhalation.
- If asthma is controlled for 6 months or more
    - reduce dose to 1 puff (50 mcg) 2 x daily.

Step 2
- Inhaled corticosteroid
    - 4 puffs (200 micrograms) 2 x daily (doctor initiated).
    - reduce to 2 puffs 2 x daily after 1 month if the condition has improved
- **Plus** inhaled salbutamol
    - 1-2 puffs 3 x daily as required (2 puff dose 10 years & older)

14 YEARS AND OVER (AND ADULTS)
Mild infrequent symptoms and no sleep disturbance (intermittent asthma)
- Inhaled salbutamol
    - 2 puffs 3 x daily as required.

More frequent or severe symptoms, or nocturnal symptoms
Step 1
- Inhaled corticosteroid (budesonide, beclomethasone 100 mcg / puff)
    - 2 puffs (200 micrograms) 2 x daily.
- **Plus** inhaled salbutamol
    - 2 puffs (200 micrograms) 3 x daily as required.
- If asthma is controlled for 6 months or more
    - reduce dose of corticosteroid to 1 puff (100 mcg) 2 x daily.
    - stop inhaled steroid if controlled for at least 6 months on 100 mcg 2 x daily

Step 2
- Inhaled corticosteroid
    - 4 puffs (400 micrograms) 2 x daily
- **Plus** inhaled salbutamol
    - 2 puffs 3 x daily as required.
- If patient is well and stable after 6 months
    - reduce the dose of corticosteroid by 200 mcg every month until a dose of 200 mcg (1 puff) 2 x daily is achieved.

Step 3
- Stop inhaled corticosteroid
- Add LABA / corticosteroid combination e.g. salmeterol / fluticazone inhalation
    - 2 puffs (50/250 mcg) 2 x daily (doctor initiated)
- If symptoms are still not adequately controlled and adherence and inhaler technique are not considered to be a problem:
    - **REFER** for consultant opinion.

Short-term oral steroids (pulse dose)
- Prednisone 30-40 mg daily for 7 days in adults
    - 1 mg/kg/day for 7 days in children up to a maximum of 30 mg daily.

NB. Administer the initial dose early in a severe attack.

Indications for pulse dose oral steroids:
- Any asthmatic requiring nebulisation
    - i.e. any severe attack treated at the clinic.

- If symptoms are not adequately controlled despite good inhaler technique and adherence
  - and referral to a consultant is not immediately possible.

Note.
Patients needing repeated courses of corticosteroids (more than twice over 6 months or more than 3 x in a year) should be **REFERRED**.

Antibiotics

When to use an antibiotic

- Asthma may be brought on by respiratory infections, particularly in children.
- Usually the respiratory infections are viral, and an antibiotic is **not** indicated.
- If there is evidence of bacterial infection, an antibiotic should be used eg.
  - bronchial breathing
  - fever with localised crepitations
- *In bronchial asthma yellow or green sputum may not be indicative of bacterial infection and by itself is **not** sufficient reason to prescribe an antibiotic.*
- Antibiotics are indicated if a child:
  - has localising chest signs
  - is ill-looking or febrile.

Which antibiotic to use

In children
- Use amoxicillin in a dose appropriate for age.

In adults
- Use amoxicillin 1 g 3 x daily for 5 days
- *If penicillin-allergic give:*
  - azithromycin 500 mg daily for 3 days

Chest infection with bronchospasm

In patients where asthma has not been confirmed eg. "wheezy bronchitis" (not including bronchopneumonia), use the following:

- Salbutmol inhaler 3 x daily as required.
- An antibiotic as above to cover for possible bacterial infection
  - dosage according to age.

Unilateral wheeze in small children
- Consider a foreign body, tuberculosis or congenital abnormalities of the airways.
- **REFER** the child.

Bilateral wheeze in small children
- Administer inhaled salbutamol eg. by nebuliser.
- If there is an immediate response:
  - asthma should be considered
  - the diagnosis will be supported by associated allergic rhinitis, eczema or family history of allergic disorders
  - **REFER** the child for assessment of severity of disease and appropriate commencement of chronic maintenance therapy.
- If there is a poor response and the child is under 2 years of age:
  - consider acute bronchiolitis
  - manage child accordingly.
- If there is no response and the onset of the wheeze was sudden:
  - **REFER** child immediately to exclude the inhalation of a foreign body.

MANAGEMENT OF ACUTE ASTHMA

Indications for REFERRAL

- A severe attack (see below - recognition of severe asthma in children and adults)
- Repeated attacks despite good adherence (i.e. "difficult" asthma)
- Any patient having an attack who is on treatment with
  - oral steroids
  - **or** full-dose inhaled steroids

Recognition of severe asthma in adults

- Not able to complete sentences in one breath
- Restless, drowsy or confused
- Respiratory rate greater than 30
- Pulse rate greater than 120
- "Silent" chest, i.e. markedly reduced air entry
- PEFR less than 50% predicted

Recognition of severe asthma in children

- Respiratory rate greater than 40
- Chest indrawing / recession
- Too breathless to talk
- Too breathless to feed
- Absence of wheezing
- Impaired consciousness
- PEFR less than 50% predicted

Oxygen

- Use the highest concentration facemask available (usually 40% for adults).
- Set the correct flow rate for each particular facemask
  - 6-8 L/min for 40% facemask
- In older children the best method of administration is via nasal cannulae.

Nebulisation
- The nebuliser should preferably be oxygen driven.
- Use salbutamol or fenoterol alone, or (in more severe cases or a repeat nebulisation)
    - use in combination with Atrovent

Adults
1 ml salbutamol 0.5% solution diluted in 4 ml normal saline, or 2 x salbutamol nebule 2.5 mg/2.5 ml, undiluted
or
2 x 0.5 mg/2ml fenoterol nebule undiluted
or (more severe cases / repeat nebulisation)
Salbutamol nebule 2.5 mg/2.5 ml or fenoterol nebule 0.5 mg/2 ml + 0.5 mg Atrovent UDV.

Children 6–14 years
1 ml salbutamol 0.5% solution diluted in 4 ml normal saline, or salbutamol nebule 2.5 mg/2.5 ml diluted with 2 ml normal saline
or
Fenoterol nebule 0.5 mg/2 ml diluted in 2 ml normal saline
or (more severe cases / repeat nebulisation)
Salbutamol nebule 2.5 mg/2.5 ml or fenoterol nebule 0.5 mg/2 ml + 0.25 mg Atrovent UDV.

Children < 6 years
0.5 ml salbutamol 0.5% solution diluted in 2 ml normal saline or salbutamol nebule 2.5 mg/2.5 ml, undiluted
or (more severe cases / repeat nebulisation)
0.5 ml salbutamol 0.5% solution or 1 ml salbutamol nebule 2.5 mg/2.5 ml + 0.25 mg Atrovent UDV.

Immediate treatment
- Do a baseline peak flow if possible.
- Oxygen
    - by 40% facemask in adults
    - via nasal cannulae in older children
    - via funnel in small children.
- Nebulise as per schedule above.
- Prednisone
    - 40 mg orally in adults
    - 1 mg / kg orally in children (max dose: 30 mg)
- If very distressed start IV therapy:
    - use 1 litre 5% dextrose water
    - run the drip to maintain a state of normal hydration (do not overhydrate)
    - give Solucortef directly via the IV line
    - 100 mg IVI stat in adults
    - 4 mg / kg IVI stat in children (max dose: 100 mg)
- No sedation of any kind.
- If no nebuliser available:
    - give salbutamol 4-8 puffs by inhaler (use a spacer in small children).

If the patient has not improved after 20-30 minutes
- Continue oxygen administration.
- Repeat nebulisation and every 2 hours thereafter if needed.
- Do a chest X-ray (if facility available) to look for other pathology which might account for the poor response
    - eg. spontaneous pneumothorax, heart failure.

If the patient is still not improving
- Arrange transport to hospital with oxygen
- Keep IV line open
    - run drip at a slow rate to avoid overhydration
    - adults 100 ml / hour
    - children 2.5 ml / kg / hour

Subsequent management (if the patient is improving)
- Check peak flow.
- Give prednisone
    - 40 mg daily for another 6-7 days in adults
    - 1 mg / kg daily for another 6-7 days in children.
- **Plus** steroid inhaler
    - 2 puffs (200 micrograms) 2 x daily in adults
    - 2 puffs (100 micrograms) 2 x daily in children.
- **Plus** salbutamol inhaler
    - 2 puffs 3 x daily as required in adults and children 8 years and over
    - 1 puff 3 x daily as required in children.

COAD (INCLUDING CHRONIC BRONCHITIS AND EMPHYSEMA)

Clinical features
- It is more common in middle aged or elderly patients.
- It is especially common in smokers.
- There is a typical history of a chronic productive cough for years.
- Dyspnoea, usually slowly progressive.
- Often evidence of barrelling of the chest.
- Air entry diminished.
- There may be prolonged expiration and wheezing.
- There may be scattered, coarse creps, mainly at the lung bases.
- There is a reduced PEFR.

MANAGEMENT

Indications for REFERRAL

REFER patients with any of the following
- Signs of respiratory distress eg.
  - cyanosis
  - use of accessory muscles
  - dyspnoea at rest.
- Very low PEFR (below 150 L / minute).

Referral will not be necessary
- If any of the above have been previously assessed by the doctor.
- And provided the situation is not worse.

Lifestyle management

- The patient must not smoke at all
  - give advice and educational material to help the patient stop.
- REFER for physiotherapy if available
  - request education for improved breathing techniques and a graded exercise programme.
- Note: If there is any suspicion of pulmonary TB, this must be excluded.

Medicine management

Bronchodilators

These are indicated in all patients:
- Who are wheezing or are dyspnoeic
- With a low PEFR of less than 50% below the predicted value.

First visit
- In a stable patient, do a baseline PEFR.
- Then give a test dose of salbutamol - 2 puffs.
- Repeat PEFR 15 minutes later.
- If there is a 15% or greater improvement in peak flow
  - treat as for asthma.

Patients failing to respond to the test dose:
- Give salbutamol 2 puffs 3 x daily as required.
- A careful explanation of how to use the inhaler must be given to the patient.
- If the patient is unable to use the inhaler correctly, provide a spacer.
- Check at monthly intervals and assess progress both clinically and with a peak flow meter.

Subsequent visits
Increase treatment if:
- Persistent wheezing / dyspnoea
- Low PEFR ie
  - less than 250 L / minute (males)
  - less than 200 L / minute (females)

Step 1
- Inhaled salbutamol 2 puffs 3 x daily as required

Step 2
- Add inhaled LABA / corticosteroid combination
  e.g. salmeterol / fluticazone inhalation (doctor initiated)
  - 2 puffs (50/250 mcg) 2 x daily
- If there is symptomatic or objective benefit (improved effort tolerance or PEFR), continue the above as maintenance therapy.
- If no improvement is found REFER patient to pulmonologist.

Antibiotics
- These are indicated for episodes of respiratory infection which are associated with sputum increase or a change in sputum colour to yellow or green.
- Amoxicillin and doxycycline are the antibiotics of choice
  - they should be given for 5-7 days.

Acute exacerbation / attack management
- *This is an acute episode with*
  - *significant wheezing or dyspnoea*
  - *deterioration in PEFR*
- It is commonly associated with a secondary bacterial infection.
- Give oxygen with care (preferably by 24% or 28% facemask, if available)
  Plus
  - nebulise with salbutamol and Atrovent as per Asthma Protocol
  - give pulse dose oral steroids
- If acute infective exacerbation
  - treat with amoxicillin / doxycycline as above
- If infection is not the likely cause of the exacerbation
  - give pulse dose oral steroids
  - omit antibiotic

N.B. If there is any suspicion of TB, this must be excluded.

PNEUMONIA

LOBAR PNEUMONIA

Clinical features

The typical features are:
- Fever, rigors, pleuritic chest pain and cough with rust-coloured sputum.
- Tachypnoea, intercostal recession, flaring, splinting of the chest on the affected side.
- Initially decreased air entry and creps on affected side may be present.
- Later the classical signs of consolidation appear:
  - bronchial breathing
  - increased vocal resonance
  - dullness on percussion.
- A pleural friction rub may occasionally be heard.
- During resolution, the signs of consolidation are replaced by creps.
- However, in elderly patients or patients with lowered resistance such as diabetes or AIDS, the clinical picture will be less obvious.
- Suspect pneumonia in any adult with a cough, raised respiratory rate, pleuritic chest pain and who is ill, even though no chest signs are found on examination.

BRONCHOPNEUMONIA

Clinical features
- The patient will be ill with physical signs such as:
    - fever
    - cough
    - tachypnoea (age dependent - see below)
    - recession
    - lethargy and irritability
- Initially no localising or adventitious sounds
- Later scattered crepitations and wheezes appear, affecting one or more lobes.
- The presence of a cough in a neonate, even in the absence of other physical signs, is sufficient evidence to diagnose bronchopneumonia.
- **In small infants, less than 2 months old**, clinical features may be minimal. Bronchopneumonia should be suspected if there are **any** of the following:
    - a cough on history or examination
    - respiratory rate above 60 / min
    - subcostal recession / chest indrawing (of the lower chest wall)
- **In infants 2-12 months**, the diagnosis of bronchopneumonia is suggested if:
    - respiratory rate is above 50 / min
    - subcostal recession / chest indrawing
    - nasal flaring
- **In small children 1-5 years**, the following are important features:
    - respiratory rate above above 40 / min
    - intercostal recession
    - flaring nostrils

Severe pneumonia
- Infants less than 2 months of age with rapid breathing
- Lower chest wall indrawing
- Nasal flaring
- Auscultatory sounds, i.e. crepitations, bronchial breathing
- Grunting or intermittent apnoea

Other causes of a raised respiratory rate in children

High temperature
- Check this by reducing the temperature.
- If the respiratory rate now drops, it was only due to pyrexia.

Acidosis
- This occurs particularly if the child has gastroenteritis and dehydration or has been given aspirin.
- **REFER** if you suspect aspirin poisoning or if there is severe acidosis in association with gastroenteritis.

Crying or exercise
- This will also raise the respiratory rate.
- Recheck the respiratory rate when the child is quiet.

Blocked nostrils
- This may produce recession and a raised respiratory rate.

MANAGEMENT OF PNEUMONIA IN ADULTS

REFERRAL
Urgent REFERRAL for admission
If a patient has two or more of the following:
- Confusion or decreased level of consciousness
- Hypotension (systolic BP less than 90 mm Hg, or diastolic BP less than 60 mm Hg)
- Dehydration
- Respiratory rate above 30 / min
- Over 65 years

While awaiting transfer:
- Give oxygen
- Set up an IV drip to run **slowly**
- Give ceftriaxone 1 g IVI or IMI stat

Other indications for REFERRAL
- Severe cyanosis
- Multilobar involvement
- Poor socio-economic background
- No access to immediate transport
- Unlikely to comply with treatment

General measures
- Bed rest.
- Encourage high fluid intake.

Medicine management
- Give amoxicillin 1 g 3 x daily for 5 days.
- **Plus** paracetamol 2 tabs 3 x daily

Penicillin-allergic patients
- Moxifloxacin 400 mg daily for 5 days.

Patients over 65 years or with underlying medical conditions that include:
   - heart failure
   - COPD
   - HIV/AIDS
   - alcoholism
   - diabetes
   - chronic kidney disease
- Give co-amoxiclav 875 / 125 mg 2 x daily for 5 days

Investigations
- A chest X-ray is advisable in most cases if this is available.
- If there is any suspicion of TB, eg. TB contact, weight loss, night sweats or haemoptysis
    - do a sputum smear or Xpert MTB PCR.

Follow-up
- Advise ill patients to come back after 1-2 days.
- Other patients to be checked in 4-5 days, but instruct the patient to return sooner if not improved.

REFER if:
- Poor response to treatment after 48 hours.

MANAGEMENT OF PNEUMONIA IN CHILDREN

REFERRAL

Danger signs indicating urgent admission
- Inability to drink
- Impaired consciousness
- Cyanosis or intermittent apnoea
- Grunting
- Age less than 2 months

Other indications for REFERRAL
- Children with bronchopneumonia **and**:
    - nasal flaring
    - chest indrawing or marked intercostal recession
    - auscultatory signs of bronchopneumonia eg crepitations (i.e. not merely a cough)
    - malnutrition eg. kwashiorkor
    - failure to thrive
    - other diseases eg. heart disease, TB, AIDS
- All children with lobar pneumonia identified by bronchial breathing
- Recurrent episodes of bronchopneumonia
- If in any doubt about the diagnosis

General measures
- Ensure adequate hydration.
- Continue feeding:
    - babies should be breast fed if possible
    - give frequent small feeds

Medicine management
- Give amoxicillin 45 mg/kg/dose 2 x daily for 5 days
    - 1-3 months: 200 mg
    - 3-6 months: 250 mg
    - 6 months-18 months: 400 mg
    - 18 months-3 years: 500 mg
    - 3-5 years: 750 mg
    - 5-10 years: 1000 mg
    - Children 10–15 years of age: Amoxicillin 1000 mg 3 x daily for 5 days
- **Plus** paracetamol 120 mg / 5 ml 3 x daily
    - 0-6 months: 2.5 ml
    - 6 months-3 years: 5 ml
    - 3-5 years: 7.5 ml
    - 5-11 years: 10 ml
    - 11-15 years: 1 tablet

Management of severe pneumonia
- Oxygen 1-2 L/min via nasal prongs

Initial doses before referral:
Ceftriaxone IM / IV
- 0-1 month: 225 mg
- 1-3 months: 300 mg
- 3-6 months: 440 mg
- 6-12 months: 625 mg
- 12-18 months: 750 mg
- 18 months-3 years: 800 mg
- 3-5 years: 1 000 mg
- 5-15 years: 1 500 mg

NB.
- Don't inject more than 1 g (1 000 mg) at one injection site.
- Contraindicated in neonates who are severely jaundiced (palms or soles yellow).
- Not to be used in neonates who are not severely ill.

In infants 2-6 months, consider PCP
- Add co-trimoxazole, 5 ml, oral

REFER
- Very ill patients to hospital on oxygen.
- If poor response to treatment.

HAEMOPTYSIS

Causes
- It is important to exclude causes such as epistaxis, a bleeding tooth socket, a bitten tongue etc.
- The most common respiratory cause in adults and children is tuberculosis.

All patients must be **REFERRED** unless you are sure it is due to another cause eg. epistaxis.

BRONCHIECTASIS

Clinical features
- A diagnostic feature is a cough with large quantities of sputum
    - made worse by lying in some positions
    - relieved by other positions.
- Chronic cough with purulent, sometimes offensive sputum
- Clubbing
- Weight loss
- Basal creps, unilateral or bilateral
- It may be associated with COAD

MANAGEMENT
- **REFER** to exclude tuberculosis ie. chest X-ray
- Physiotherapy is of great value
    - treatment must be arranged if possible
    - family members must be taught postural drainage.
- Antibiotics are indicated for acute cases ie. with increased sputum production or mucopurulent sputum
    - if not severely ill, use amoxicillin-clavulanic acid 875/125 mg 2 x daily for 10 days
    - use moxifloxacin 400 mg daily for 10 days if penicillin-allergic.

REFER severely ill patients for admission.

LUNG ABSCESS

Clinical features
- Chronic cough with profuse, purulent and offensive sputum
- History or evidence of
    - alcohol abuse in adults
    - foreign bodies in children
- Often pyrexial
- Severe halitosis is often characteristic
- Clubbing
- Weight loss
- Signs of consolidation may be present
- Localised chest pain
- Usually ill patient

REFER for X-ray and admission.

TUBERCULOSIS

Note.
The primary methods of pulmonary TB diagnosis in adults and older children are sputum smear microscopy, PCR assay and culture.

- Although chest X-rays are very useful in suggesting the possibility of tuberculosis, they are most often not diagnostic. Assessing children's and adult's X-rays with possible tuberculosis is also often difficult.
- A good clinical history and examination is of great importance.
- Tuberculosis may be difficult to diagnose
    - often there are **no** physical signs
      to be found on examination.

Clinical features of pulmonary TB

In children

- Weight loss for more than one month
- A drop or levelling off on the pre-school record card (road to health card)
- A cough for more than 2 weeks
- Close contact with an infectious TB case
- Child less playful or complains of feeling tired
- Wheeze or stridor
- Night sweats
- Lymphadenopathy especially of the neck

In adults

- A cough for more than 2 weeks
- Haemoptysis
- Weight loss of more than 5 kg which is not due to
  deliberate dieting
- Sputum
    - may be absent
    - initially mucoid
    - later mucopurulent
- Night sweats
- Loss of appetite, fatigue, weakness
- Chest pain (non-specific or pleuritic)
- Shortness of breath (advanced disease)
- Poor socio-economic circumstances
    - overcrowded living conditions
    - close contact with an infectious source case
    - other features of generally lowered
      resistance such as alcoholism,
      malnutrition or HIV disease
- Clubbing may be present.
- Anaemia and pedal oedema may be present.
- Pulse is usually rapid.
- Chest signs may be absent or there may be:
    - crepitations (common) / or bronchial
      breathing (particularly important
      if present in the apices)
    - or localised wheeze.
- There may be evidence of previous disease such as:
    - deviated trachea
    - percussion dullness
    - diminished air entry at one
      or other lung apex

DIAGNOSIS OF TUBERCULOSIS IN CHILDREN

The most useful tool in the diagnosis of TB in children under 5 years of age is the tuberculin PPD skin test.

Mantoux test

- This is the most accurate skin test for diagnosing TB.
- It tests the child's response to the intradermal injection of purified protein derivative (PPD).
- If the result of the MonoTest or Tine Test is uncertain, then the Mantoux test should be done, especially in under 5 year old children.

Method

- A 26 gauge, short needle or diabetic syringe should be used.
- The RT 23 brand of PPD is ready to use.
- The injection should be given **intradermally,** not subcutaneously.
- The test is read after 72-96 hours

Reading

- The amount of palpable swelling is measured (ignore the redness around the swelling).
- The transverse and longitudinal diameters are measured.
- The reading is taken as the average of the two measurements.

Results

Positive reaction

HIV negative	HIV positive
10 mm or more	5 mm or more

Negative reaction
Either no reaction or any reaction less than the positive for each category.

Interpretation of results

Check if BCG immunisation has been given. Find a scar or record of vaccination on the immunisation card.

No reaction
If never immunised:

- **REFER** for BCG immunisation.
- If patient is a TB contact, withhold TB immunisation until infection excluded
    - for TB contacts in infants (see page 67).

If previously immunised

- This is often a false negative test.
- A common cause for this with the Mantoux test is that the test was not done properly due to the PPD having been injected subcutaneously
    - if this is considered to be the reason,
      and if clinically indicated, repeat
      the Mantoux test.

Other possible causes for a false negative response are:

- Expired Mantoux solution or the solution not kept in the fridge after mixing.
- Development of tuberculin sensitivity only occurs 3-6 weeks after infection, so tests before this time will be negative, although the patient is infected.
- Overwhelming infection eg. miliary TB or any other severe infection.
- Post measles and after measles vaccination (up to 6 weeks).
- Malnutrition.
- Immunological deficiency eg. HIV disease, kwashiorkor.
- Acute febrile illness.
- Patient on steroid therapy.
- Some patients just fail to produce a positive response even to a natural infection.

If there is clinical suspicion of TB:
- **REFER** for chest X-ray and opinion.

If the child is recovering well, e.g. from a chest infection, not malnourished and growing well:
- No action need be taken.

Some reaction (but not positive)
- Usually a normal hypersensitivity immune response
- If there is clinical suspicion of TB:
  - **REFER** for X-ray and opinion
  - if the child is also a TB contact (close contact), **REFER** to start TB treatment
- If the child is clinically well / growing well:
  - no action need be taken.

Positive reaction

Children under 5 years:
- If there is clinical suspicion of TB:
  - **REFER** for chest X-ray and to start TB treatment
- If the child is clinically well / recovering well from chest infection:
  - **REFER** for INH prophylaxis

INVESTIGATING PULMONARY TUBERCULOSIS IN ADULTS

The most important part of the diagnosis of pulmonary TB in adults is the finding of TB bacilli in the sputum, either by PCR or by smear microscopy. A sputum specimen is stained and examined under a microscope to look for TB bacilli or submitted for PCR of MTB DNA (molecular technique).

Method of sputum collection
- The sputum collection should be performed outside in a well-ventilated area.
- Explain the steps fully and slowly.
- Demonstrate with deep breathing followed by a deep cough.
- Supervise the collection, but do not stand in front.
- Give the patient the container without the lid. Hold the lid yourself, ready to replace it immediately.
- Store in a cold place, preferably in a fridge.
- Send to the laboratory as soon as possible.

Molecular techniques (GeneXpert, Line Probe Assay)
- This is more sensitive than sputum-smear microscopy.
- Only a few organisms are necessary to give a positive result.
- Both detect rifampicin resistance. The line probe assay (LPA) detects INH resistance as well.
- There is therefore a short turnaround time for the detection of MDR-TB.
- It cannot be used for monitoring treatment because it does not distinguish between dead and live bacilli.

TB cultures
- Highly sensitive for Mycobacterium species identification.
- Used for diagnosing smear or PCR negative pulmonary TB, and TB from specimens obtained from extra-pulmonary sites.
- Also used for determining drug susceptibility especially in MDR and poly-resistant TB.
- Used monthly together with smear microscopy for monitoring in MDR-TB.
- Slow turnaround time - takes several weeks before a result is available.

Chest X-rays
- Chest X-ray findings can in most cases only suggest active disease.
- Confirmation of the diagnosis will usually depend on finding TB bacilli in the sputum.
- Chest X-rays are necessary in patients:
  - who cannot produce sputum
  - who have negative Xpert results and are HIV positive
  - where extra-pulmonary TB, (such as pleural effusions and pericardial TB) or miliary TB is suspected.
- While chest X-ray is non-specific for TB, the presence of infiltrates, lymph nodes or cavities is highly suggestive of TB.

DIAGNOSIS OF PULMONARY TUBERCULOSIS IN ADULTS

General information
- Take a comprehensive history. It is important to find out if the patient was ever previously treated for TB or has been in close contact with a confirmed case of pulmonary TB.
- Do the necessary clinical examination.

Send one sputum specimen for Xpert MTB/RIF:
- If Xpert MTB/RIF is positive, treat for TB and send a sputum specimen for smear microscopy (the smear is used for reporting, not for diagnosis).
- If Xpert MTB/RIF is positive and demonstrates resistance to rifampicin, commence MDR treatment and send sputum for drug susceptibility testing (DST) to confirm MDR-TB.
- If Xpert MTB/RIF is negative and patient is HIV positive, send sputum for culture and do a chest X-ray if available:
  - if the X-ray findings are consistent with TB, treat as drug-susceptible TB
  - if the X-ray findings are normal, treat with an antibiotic and monitor response
  - follow up and review LPA/culture results
- If Xpert MTB/RIF is negative and patient is HIV negative, treat with an antibiotic and consider further investigations only if symptoms persist.

PROTOCOL FOR THE TREATMENT OF TUBERCULOSIS

This protocol for the treatment of tuberculosis is in accordance with the National Tuberculosis Control Programme of the Department of Health.

WHAT IS AN ACTIVE CASE OF TUBERCULOSIS?

Adult TB suspect
- One positive sputum Xpert MTB/RIF or one positive smear microscopy.

- One positive sputum culture
- Suggestive symptoms of tuberculosis which may include failure of response to treatment with a broad spectrum antibiotic
    - **and** chest X-ray abnormalities consistent with active TB
- Extrapulmonary TB

Child TB suspect

- Any child presenting with symptoms of TB is regarded as a case of TB if there is:
    - a history of exposure to an infectious TB case or confirmed infection (positive Mantoux) **and/or**
    - an abnormal chest X-ray suggestive of TB
- Any child presenting with a history of exposure to an infectious TB case or with confirmed infection (positive Mantoux) is regarded as a TB case if:
    - there are symptoms of TB **and** (if available)
    - an abnormal chest X-ray suggestive of TB

TREATMENT REGIMENS
ADULTS

- New patients with age above 8 years and adults (smear / PCR positive and smear / PCR negative and extrapulmonary TB).
- Treatment should be given daily, every day of the week.

Intensive phase 2 months
Rifampicin / INH / Pyrazinamide / Ethambutol
Combination tablet (RHZE)

Dose	30-37kg	38-54 kg	55-70 kg	>71 kg
150/75/400/275 mg	2	3	4	5

Continuation phase 4 months
Rifampicin / INH
Combination tablet (RH)

Dose	30-37kg	38-54 kg	55-70 kg	>71 kg
RH 150/75 mg	2	3	–	–
RH 300/150 mg	–	–	2	2

NB. Miliary TB, TB meningitis and bone TB treat for 9 months (add 3 months to continuation phase).

CHILDREN
- Children with uncomplicated pulmonary TB

Intensive phase 2 months
Rifampicin / INH / Pyrazinamide

Dose	5-7.9 kg	8-11.9 kg	12-19.9 kg	20-24.9 kg	25-29.9 kg
RH 60/60 mg	1	2	3	4	5
PZA 500 mg	½	½	1	1½	2

Continuation phase 4 months
Rifampicin / INH (RH)

Dose	5-7.9 kg	8-11.9 kg	12-19.9 kg	20-24.9 kg	25-29.9 kg
RH 60/60 mg	1	2	3	4	5

A baby born to a mother with active TB
- The baby should not receive BCG at birth.
- If the baby is symptomatic, **REFER** to hospital for evaluation and treatment.
- If the baby is asymptomatic, give INH preventive therapy 10 mg / kg / day for 6 months.
- BCG is administered after completion of preventive treatment.

CHILDREN >8 YEARS AND ADOLESCENTS
Intensive phase 2 months
Rifampicin / INH / Pyrazinamide / Ethambutol
Combination tablet (RHZE)

Dose	30-37 kg	38-54 kg	55-70 kg	>71 kg
150/75/400/275 mg	2	3	4	5

Continuation phase 4 months
Rifampicin / INH
Combination tablet (RH)

Dose	30-37 kg	38-54 kg	55-70 kg	>71 kg
RH 150/75 mg	2	3		
RH 300/150 mg			2	2

MULTIDRUG-RESISTANT (MDR) TB

This means resistance to both INH and rifampicin.

- Because of the low cure rate associated with this form of TB, early detection is very important.
- All close contacts of MDR patients must be screened for signs and symptoms of TB.
- If active disease is suspected, the contact should have sputum sampling done by PCR assay or microscopy, culture and drug susceptibility testing.

Medicine treatment
- Treatment of MDR TB should preferably be started by a specialist.
- Treatment should be coordinated and monitored by the dedicated provincial MDR TB treatment centres.
- Those with severe disease or recurrent MDR should be hospitalised in a dedicated MDR TB hospital.
- Prolonged treatment for up to 2 years or more is required in patients diagnosed with MDR TB.

Standardised regimen for treatment of MDR TB

Drug	<33 kg	33-50 kg	51-70 kg	>71 kg
Kanamycin	15-20 mg / kg	500-750 mg	1 000 mg	1 000 mg
Ethionamide	15-20 mg / kg	500 mg	750 mg	750-1 000 mg
Moxifloxacin	400 mg	400 mg	400 mg	400 mg
Pyrazinamide	30-40 mg / kg	1 000-1 750 mg	1 750-2 000 mg	2 000-2 500 mg
Terizidone	15-20 mg / kg	750 mg	750 mg	7 500-1 000 mg

There are two phases of treatment:

Intensive / injectable phase

- Treatment with the 5 drugs above including daily injection with kanamycin / amikacin.
- Treatment given daily.
- Duration is guided by culture conversion but should be continued for a minimum of 6 months and for at least 4 months after culture conversion.

Continuation phase

- Treatment with 4 drugs excluding the injectable.
- Duration is a minimum of 18 months from culture conversion.

Monitoring

- Close monitoring of patients is essential to assess treatment response and detect and manage adverse events early.
- Patient's weight, sputum smears and cultures are performed monthly.
- Conversion is defined as 2 consecutive negative smears and cultures taken 30 days apart.

TB PREVENTIVE THERAPY (IPT)

This has shown to decrease risk of TB disease in those individuals with latent TB infection.

IPT is part of the package of care in HIV-positive individuals, prior to starting ART.

Eligibility for IPT

All HIV-positive people with:
- No signs and symptoms of TB
- No alcohol abuse
- No active liver disease
- Not currently taking TB treatment

NB. Exclude active TB by checking for symptoms:
- Cough >2 weeks
- Fever >2 weeks
- Drenching night sweats
- Weight loss >5 kg body weight in last 4 weeks

Clients with one or more symptoms should be investigated for TB.

Note.
- IPT is not contra-indicated and can be started at any time during pregnancy.
- IPT can be started after successful completion of TB treatment.
  Remember that active TB disease must be excluded in both.

Recommended regimen

- Adults: INH 5 mg / kg / day (maximum 300 mg / day)
- Children: INH 10 mg / kg / day (maximum 300 mg / day)
- Pyridoxine (Vitamin B6) 25 mg / day prevents occurrence of peripheral neuropathy
- Duration: 6 months of continuous treatment

Cardiovascular System

HYPERTENSION

CONFIRMATION OF HYPERTENSION

*The treatment of hypertension often requires the lifelong taking of medication. For this reason, it is **very important** that the diagnosis is confirmed with reasonable certainty.*

Blood pressure recording
- This often produces incorrect or unreliable results
- Due to a number of factors
    - the patient not being able to relax in the presence of a health worker
    - anxiety brought on by the procedure itself
    - wrong size cuff
    - calibration error or faulty blood pressure recording equipment
- When taking the BP, try and get the patient to relax as much as possible
    - then take a minimum of two readings at each visit

Reasons for an artificially raised blood pressure

Sharp rises in blood pressure may be caused by alcohol, stress, pain or infection. The rise may occur in spite of the fact that the patient is receiving drug therapy for hypertension or that the blood pressure had been previously controlled.

If stress is considered to be the cause of an increase in blood pressure
- Reassure the patient
- If the problem is severe, **REFER** him / her to the social worker
- Do not increase drug dosages unless the blood pressure elevation is prolonged and / or severe
- If anxiety is severe, especially if physical manifestations such as palpitations or sweating are present
    - prescribe a beta-blocker drug
      eg. atenolol 50 mg daily

If the rise in blood pressure is caused by pain or infection
- This will decrease following
    - control of the infection
    - control of the pain
- Therefore drug treatment for hypertension should be avoided in such patients (unless severely elevated), until the infection has cleared up, or the pain controlled

If alcoholism is found to be the cause of an increase in blood pressure
- Educate the patient on the dangers of alcohol
- Do not increase the dosage of the drugs unless the BP elevation is severe
- Prescribe Vitamin B Co and/or thiamine if necessary

NB. Remember that alcohol withdrawal often presents with symptoms and signs of acute anxiety.

CARDIOVASCULAR DISEASE RISK FACTORS

The risk of cardiovascular disease in patients with hypertension is increased in the presence of one or more of the risk factors listed below.

Major risk factors
- Diabetes mellitus
- Hypertension
- Smoking
- Central obesity: waist circumference (men >94 cm; women >80 cm)
- Dyslipidaemia
- Physical inactivity
- Family history of early onset of cardiovascular disease (men <55 years; women <65 years)
- Age: (men >55 years; women >65 years)

CLINICAL SIGNS OF TARGET ORGAN DAMAGE / CLINICAL CARDIOVASCULAR DISEASE

- Left ventricular hypertrophy (displaced forceful apex beat)
- Angina or prior myocardial infarction
- Left ventricular failure with or without right ventricular failure
- Evidence of previous stroke
- Transient ischaemic attacks (transient minor strokes)
- Chronic renal impairment (proteinuria with or without haematuria)
- Peripheral vascular disease
- Microalbuminuria or proteinuria

MANAGEMENT

Advice
- Explain to the patients that the disease is a chronic one and that they must be prepared to look after themselves for the rest of their lives
- Inform them honestly but gently about some of the complications of hypertension eg. cerebro vascular accidents, kidney failure
- Find out if patients expect to have difficulty in obtaining time off work to come for treatment
    - where necessary supply them with a copy of the letter to the employer (see page 80)
- Elderly patients who have hypertension, who may experience problems with adherence, should be given the special letter for a relative, spouse or friend (see page 80). This letter
    - informs these people about the patient's condition
    - asks them to assist them with the taking of drugs and lifestyle management

Lifestyle management

- Explain that non-drug measures are particularly important in the treatment of this condition
    - should these not be sufficient to control the blood pressure level, then drug treatment will have to be added
- Advise patients to restrict their intake of salt as much as possible, by using very little salt in cooking and avoiding extra salt for flavouring
    - salty foods are to be avoided entirely - chips, salty biscuits, etc.
- Advise patients to restrict their fat intake.
- Encourage them to eat foods which have a high potassium content. eg. fresh fruit
- Advise patients to eat foods with a high fibre content such as rough maize, brown bread, green beans, and to increase diet roughage
    - encourage them to eat natural, unrefined, unprocessed foods
- Supply the diet sheet hand-out
- If patients are overweight, encourage them to lose weight
    - supply a special diet sheet
    - patients must be weighed at each visit
- If the patients smoke cigarettes, give them advice on how to stop smoking and supply an advice hand-out
- If the patients drink, advise them to stop drinking alcohol and supply an advice hand-out
- **REFER** them to Alcoholics Anonymous (AA) or South African National Council on Alcoholism and Drug Dependence (SANCA)
- Try to identify causes for anxiety or stress
    - these are frequently of a psychological, social or economic nature
    - try to advise and assist, or **REFER** to a social worker, psychologist or an organisation which may be able to help
- Encourage relaxation and promote relaxing activities eg. gardening, hobbies
- Advise the patient to avoid preparations which may make hypertension worse eg.
    - cough, cold and flu remedies
    - nasal drops
    - NSAIDs (non-steroidal anti-inflammatory drugs) eg. aspirin
    - oral contraceptives
- Encourage regular moderate physical activity eg. 30 minutes walking 3-5 times a week

Medicine management advice

- If patients are given tablets, it is important to stress the need for them to be taken regularly and in the correct dosage
    - advise the patients that the tablets are packed in units for 28 days
    - they must return on their appointment date for further supplies
- Tell patients to take their morning dose on the day of each visit
- Encourage the patients to bring back their tablet packets each month even if they are empty
    - the number of unused tablets is noted and these are returned to the pharmacy
- If patients inform you that they are going away for more than a month, or if they are leaving the area permanently, they must be given a letter
    - this must explain the treatment so that the patient can continue treatment elsewhere
- If indicated, discuss with the patients some of the side effects which they may experience from taking the prescribed drugs
    - eg. that ACE-inhibitors may cause swelling of parts of the body such as the lips
    - inform them that this should be reported immediately
- Sometimes when patients are made aware of the cost of the drugs their adherence is better

Subsequent visits

- In patients who are overweight, check if they are gaining or losing weight and record any significant loss or gain
    - if they are losing weight, compliment them and encourage them to continue
    - if they are gaining, try to establish the reason for this, repeat the dietary advice and stress the importance of losing weight
- If the patients have not stopped alcohol or smoking, or reduced their use of salt, then discuss this with them again
- If they remain anxious, continue to reassure them
- Check on all of the above advice and management
    - re-educate as needed
- Check the medicine adherence
    - check if the patients are returning on their appointment dates
    - count any unused tablets brought back by the patients
    - establish that the patients are taking their tablets correctly
    - re-educate if adherence is poor

Note.
- Any side effects of drug therapy experienced by the patients
- Advise them on measures that can be taken to prevent these effects
- If the side effects are considered to be serious
    - reduce or change drug treatment
    - **or REFER**

■ MEDICINE PROTOCOL

GENERAL PRINCIPLES OF MEDICINE MANAGEMENT

- Increased drug dosages and "next step" drugs should not be prescribed at intervals of less than 4 weeks
- Before changing the prescription, ensure that
    - the drug has been taken regularly
    - stress is not the cause for the increase in BP unless the BP is severely elevated
- Continue with health education at each visit, especially if the blood pressure is not satisfactorily controlled
- Any patient with moderate or severe hypertension complaining of severe headache must be **REFERRED**, on the same day, unless some obvious cause for this is

found eg. sinusitis
- Avoid frequent increases or decreases in the dosages of drugs as this
  - may confuse the patient
  - could lead to problems with adherance
- If the treatment previously received (from local or other sources) is not appropriate or in agreement with this protocol
  - then prescribe the protocol treatment which is most appropriate or **REFER**

Defaulters

The term defaulter applies to patients who have had very little, or no treatment, over a 2 week period before coming to the clinic

If the patient has defaulted
- Try to establish the reasons why the patient defaulted. It may be due to
  - drug side effects
  - difficulty in getting off work to come for treatment
  - financial problems
- Advise and try to help by
  - making appointments at a more convenient day and time
  - providing the patient with a letter to the employer etc.
- Re-educate the patient on the importance of drug treatment and non-drug treatment

Reasons for REFERRAL

***REFER** if any of the following features are present:*
- Heart failure with:
  - severe dyspnoea at rest
  - intercostal recession
  - cyanosis
  - respiratory rate >30/minute
  - gallop rhythm
  - profuse basal crepitations
  - right-sided failure
  - no response to antifailure treatment
- Very irregular pulse not previously investigated
- Pulse rate
  - more than 120/min
  - less than 50/min
- Proteinuria if the spot urine protein–creatinine ratio is >0.1 g/mmol and heart failure, infection or menstruation have been excluded
- Chest pain suggestive of angina pectoris or myocardial infarction
- Severe headache associated with either moderate or severe hypertension
- Serious side effects of drug therapy e.g.
  - angioedema
  - bradycardia
- Any patient on drug treatment that you do not clearly understand
- Patients with kidney disease with worsening proteinuria or GEFR <60 ml/min

TREATMENT STEPS

If one or more medicines used in the following steps are contraindicated or not tolerated proceed to the next recommended step.

Step 1
- Use hydrochlorothiazide (HCTZ) 12.5 mg daily
- Contraindications: gout, pregnancy, albinism, prior skin cancer and kidney failure (eGFR < 30).

Step 2
- Add a long-acting dihydropyridine calcium antagonist e.g. amlodipine, and increase to the maximum dose if necessary (preferred in black hypertensive patients).

	Initial dose	Maximum dose
Amlodipine	5 mg daily	10 mg daily

Or
- Add an ACE-inhibitor e.g. enalapril, and increase to the maximum dose if necessary (preferred in nonblack hypertensive patients)

	Initial dose	Maximum dose
Enalapril	10 mg daily	20 mg daily

- Contraindications: pregnancy, aortic valve stenosis, history of intolerance to an ACE-inhibitor or ARB e.g. angioedema.

Note: Should a woman become pregnant while receiving an ACE-inhibitor, the treatment must be stopped immediately.

Step 3
- Add either enalapril or amlodipine to the medicine used in Step 2, whichever has not already been used, and increase to the maximum dose if necessary.

Step 4
- Increase HCTZ to 25 mg daily (contraindicated in gout)

Step 5
- Add spironolactone 25 mg daily (Dr initiated)
- Contraindications: hyperkalaemia, kidney failure (eGFR < 30).

MEDICINE DETAILS

THIAZIDE DIURETIC
- Contraindicated in patients with uncontrolled gout.
- Patients who develop gouty arthritis while on hydrochlorothiazide can be managed with:
  - a calcium antagonist
  - an ACE-inhibitor (in non-black patients)
- Strongly indicated in heart failure and post-stroke.
- Increased risk of non-melanoma skin cancer with prolonged therapy especially in light-skinned individuals

CALCIUM ANTAGONISTS
- Very effective in patients with more severe degrees of hypertension
- Important side effects are:
  - oedema of the legs
  - palpitations
  - gum hypertrophy

ACE-INHIBITORS
- In black hypertensive patients, the addition of a diuretic is usually necessary to obtain an adequate response.
- Important side effects are:
  - persistent dry cough
  - angioedema
  - dizziness
- They have a compelling role in the treatment of heart failure, post-stroke, diabetes and chronic kidney disease

SPIRONOLACTONE
- Aldosterone antagonist used in patients with resistant hypertension.
- Routine serum potassium monitoring every 6 months is recommended.
- Increased risk of significant hyperkalaemia in patients on ACE- inhibitors, potassium supplements and in the elderly (> 65 years).
- Contraindicated in patients with kidney failure (eGFR < 30)
- Adverse effects are:
    - hyperkalaemia especially if combined with ACE-inhibitor potassium supplement
    - oestrogen-like side effects such as decreased libido, erectile, dysfunction, gynaecomastia (in higher doses and usually reversible).

MEDICINE MANAGEMENT

GOAL BLOOD PRESSURE
- *In adults < 60 years the goal BP is < 140 / 90*
- *In adults > 60 years the goal BP is < 150 / 90*
- *In hypertensives of all ages with diabetes or target organ damage e.g. chronic kidney disease, the goal BP is less than 140 / 90*

MILD HYPERTENSION
- SBP 140-159 mm Hg;
- or DBP 90-99 mm Hg

First visit (not previously treated)
- Repeat BP measurements monthly for 2 months to confirm the diagnosis.
- Start lifestyle modification and patient education immediately.

Patients with no other major risk factors, no target organ damage or associated clinical conditions
- If the BP is still at this level after 3 months
    - continue lifestyle changes
    - give HCTZ 12.5 mg daily
    - check BP at 4-week intervals

Patients with other major risk factors, target organ damage and/or associated clinical conditions
- Initiate treatment after confirmation of diagnosis
- Give HCTZ 12.5 mg daily.
- Check BP at monthly intervals.

Subsequent visits
- Increase the treatment to the next step if the BP is still at this level after 1 month and adherence to treatment has been good

Defaulters
- Restart previous treatment and re-educate on the importance of good adherence.
- Check BP monthly.

MODERATE HYPERTENSION
SBP 160-179 mm Hg;
or DBP 100-109 mm Hg

First visit (not previously treated)
- Start lifestyle modification.
- Check BP within 2 weeks
    - a minimum of 2 readings must be taken at this visit
- If the BP is confirmed at this level
    - give HCTZ 12.5 mg daily
    - plus a calcium antagonist e.g. amlodipine 5 mg daily, or an ACE-inhibitor e.g. enalapril 10 mg daily (see Medicine details page 73)
- Check BP at 4 week intervals.

Subsequent visits
- Increase the treatment to the next dose or step after 1 month if adherence to therapy has been good and the BP is not at target level.
- Continue monthly BP checks

Defaulters
- Restart previous treatment and re-educate on the importance of good adherence.
- If the previous treatment is not known, treat as outlined above.
- Check BP after 1 month.

SEVERE HYPERTENSION
- SBP 180 mm Hg or higher; or DBP 110 mm Hg or higher;

First visit (not previously treated)

Note: A minimum of 3 BP readings must be taken at the first visit (two at the beginning of the examination, and one at the end)

Asymptomatic severe hypertension
- *This includes patients with mild non-specific symptoms such as mild headache or dizziness.*
- The BP should be lowered gently with oral agents
    - give HCTZ 12.5 mg daily
    - plus amlodipine 5 mg daily
- Give triple therapy (HCTZ + amlodipine + enalapril) if the patient was previously on triple therapy or is uncontrolled on dual therapy.
- Administer stat doses at the clinic.
- Check patient after 1 month (after 1 week if BP >200 / 120 mm Hg).

Subsequent visits (for patients on treatment for 4 weeks or more)
- Increase the treatment to the next dose or step if the BP is not at target level provided adherence to therapy has been good.

Defaulters
- Restart previous treatment and re-educate on the importance of good adherence.
- Check BP after 1 month (after 1 week if BP >200 / 120 mm Hg).

- **REFER** patient to Dr if BP target level is not reached at maximum doses of 4 antihypertensive medicines and provided adherence has been good.

Urgent situation
- The patient may present with symptomatic very severe hypertension (BP often >220 / 120) with no life-threatening neurological or cardiac complications, e.g. mild or moderate heart failure, severe headache or epistaxis
- The aim is to lower the BP to 160 / 100 gently over 48-72 hours.

Patients not in heart failure
- **REFER** to clinic doctor
    - nurse clinician to manage if there is no doctor available
- Administer stat doses of hydrochlorothiazide 12.5 mg
    - **plus** amlodipine 5 mg
- Monitor patient (see below)

Patients in heart failure
- **REFER** to clinic doctor
    - if there is no doctor available, nurse clinician to start management
- Administer stat doses of oral / IV furosemide 40 mg
    - **plus** amlodipine 5 mg
- Monitor patient

Monitoring
- Observe the patient for 1-2 hours if possible, and check BP ½ hourly.
- **REFER** patient to doctor / hospital for admission.
- All patients to be admitted unless there has been substantial improvement in the patient's condition or there is only a mild degree of urgency, e.g. mild heart failure (doctor's decision only).
- If the patient is not admitted, discharge on the above treatment and check patient after 1-2 days.

Emergency situation
- It may present with:
    - acute and severe pulmonary oedema
    - hypertensive encephalopathy (severe headaches, visual disturbances, confusion or seizures)
    - unstable angina or myocardial infarction with a very high BP
    - dissecting aortic aneurysm (severe chest pain radiating to the back)
- The BP is often greater than 220/120 mm Hg

This is an acute hypertensive crisis, an uncommon but life-threatening condition, requiring IMMEDIATE lowering of the blood pressure.

- Summon the clinic doctor.
    - if no doctor available nurse clinician to commence management
- Administer oxygen therapy, especially if the patient is in heart failure.
- Give amlodipine 10 mg orally stat.
- **Plus** if pulmonary oedema is present, give isosorbide dinitrate 5 mg sublingually immediately and repeat every 5-10 minutes if required
- **Plus** furosemide 40 mg IV immediately as a single dose (see page 85)
- **REFER** to hospital urgently.

WHEN TO REDUCE TREATMENT
- Patients should have maintained their target level for a minimum of 6 months before they may be considered for a dose reduction.
- Reduce the dosage by one dose or step.
- Should this be successful (i.e. BP stays at target level)
- Continue to reduce the dosage but not more frequently than every 3 months.
- Take care not to reduce or stop medicines that are being used for treatment or prevention of other conditions e.g. enalapril for treatment of heart failure or atenolol for prevention of recurrence of myocardial infarction.
- If the BP rises again and remains elevated for 2 consecutive visits, it will be necessary to increase the dosage again until the BP is controlled.
- Thereafter, should the BP remain controlled, further attempts to reduce the dosage can be tried.

MANAGEMENT OF HYPERTENSION IN SPECIAL CONDITIONS

PATIENTS BELOW 25 YEARS

MANAGEMENT

If the BP is greater than 160 / 100 mm Hg
- **REFER** for investigation for a possible secondary cause for the hypertension.
- Treatment should follow the normal protocol guidelines.
- Once investigated and treatment has been started, the nurse clinician may take over the monthly follow-up care.

If the BP is less than 160 / 100 mm Hg
- Manage according to protocol

▼ **Note to doctor**
- Exclude common causes of secondary hypertension.
- Ask about medication e.g. NSAIDs, oral contraceptives.
- Examine for the presence of:
  - anaemia
  - endocrine disease e.g. hyperthyroidism, Cushing's syndrome
  - a renal bruit (renal artery stenosis)
  - radio-femoral pulse delay (coarctation of the aorta)
- Do urine dipstix
  - if proteinuria is 1 plus or more, send blood for creatinine concentration and urine for protein-creatinine ratio
- Chest X-ray
- If all normal, continue with treatment ▲

ELDERLY PATIENTS

- In elderly patients > 60 years with no target organ damage or co-existing disease e.g. diabetes, start medicine treatment only when the systolic BP is above 150 mm Hg or the diastolic BP is above 90 mm Hg.
- The goal BP is systolic BP <150 mm Hg and diastolic BP <90 mm Hg.

HEART FAILURE

MILD LEFT VENTRICULAR FAILURE (LVF)

MANAGEMENT
- Initiate treatment with:
- HCTZ 25-50 mg daily (maximum 25 mg daily in diabetics)
  - **plus** enalapril 5 mg 2 x daily
  - **or** perindopril 4 mg daily (see management of heart failure page 88)
- Plus if BP greater than 180/110 mm Hg - amlodipine 5 mg daily

MODERATE AND SEVERE FAILURE (LVF OR CCF)

MANAGEMENT
- Use furosemide (therapy started by doctor) 40 mg daily or 2 x daily
  - **plus** enalapril 5-10 mg 2 x daily
  - **or** perindopril 4 mg daily
  - **plus** if BP greater than 180/110 mm Hg - amlodipine 5 mg daily
- Thereafter follow steps as given in Heart Failure Protocol, page 83
- The nurse clinician may continue the treatment of patients stabilised on the above treatment.

KIDNEY DISEASE

- Any patient with proteinuria of 1+ or more in the absence of infection, heart failure or menstruation should have urine sent for spot PCR (protein-creatinine ratio).
- If the spot PCR is >0.1 g / mmol
  - prescribe an ACE-inhibitor
  - send blood for serum creatinine concentration and eGFR or calculate the patient's creatinine clearance
- If the creatinine clearance/eGFR is below 60 ml/min, **REFER** patient to specialist to develop a care plan.

MANAGEMENT
- Patients who have kidney disease, and have a confirmed BP of 140 / 90 or greater should be treated with medicines.
  - **REFER** to doctor to start treatment
- Furosemide is the preferred diuretic drug
- ACE-inhibitors have been shown to slow progression of kidney failure and are strongly indicated except in advanced disease (eGFR < 30).

- Other medicines that can be used relatively safely are amlodipine and atenolol.
- **REFER** patients with:
  - eGFR below 60 ml/min
  - no resolution of proteinuria with ACE-inhibitor therapy
  - uncontrolled hypertension / fluid overload

ANXIETY

When this is prominent, especially in young individuals, the treatment of choice is a beta-blocker drug eg. atenolol 50 mg daily.

PREGNANCY

Hypertensive disorders of pregnancy can be classified as:

Chronic hypertension:
- Hypertension diagnosed before pregnancy or < 20 weeks of pregnancy.

Gestational hypertension:
- Hypertension without proteinuria, diagnosed ≥ 20 weeks of pregnancy.

Pre-eclampsia:
- Hypertension with proteinuria, diagnosed ≥20 weeks of pregnancy (high risk patients include: nulliparity, obesity, multiple pregnancy, chronic hypertension, kidney disease, diabetes, pre-eclampsia in a previous pregnancy, advanced maternal age or adolescent pregnancy).

Eclampsia:
- Generalised tonic-clonic seizures in women with pre-eclampsia.

Chronic kidney disease:
- Proteinuria with/without hypertension, diagnosed at <20 weeks of pregnancy.

LEVEL OF HYPERTENSION	BP LEVEL mmHg		
	Systolic		Diastolic
Mild	140-149	or	90-99
Moderate	150-159	or	100-109
Severe	≥160	or	≥110

Referral
- Chronic hypertension
- Severe gestational hypertension
- Pre-eclampsia (all levels of severity)
- Chronic kidney disease

CHRONIC HYPERTENSION

- Stop ACE-inhibitors when pregnancy is planned or as soon as pregnancy is diagnosed, change to methyldopa and refer for assessment and management.

Medicine Treatment
- Methyldopa, oral, 250 mg 3 x daily.
- Intermediate dose: 500 mg 3 x daily
- Maximum dose: 750mg 3 x daily.

GESTATIONAL HYPERTENSION: MILD TO MODERATE

General Measures
- May be managed without admission before 38 weeks of gestation, provided no proteinuria.
- Educate on signs requiring urgent follow-up (headache, epigastric pain, visual disturbances, vaginal bleeding, etc).
- Review BP and urine analysis weekly

Medicine Treatment
- Methyldopa, oral, 250 mg 3 x daily
- Titrate to a maximum dose: 750 mg 8 hourly.
- When using iron together with methyldopa, ensure that iron and methyldopa are not taken concurrently. (Take 4 hours apart from each other).

Referral
- All patients with gestational hypertension at 38 weeks for delivery
- Pre-eclampsia (all levels of severity)
- Poor control of hypertension.

GESTATIONAL HYPERTENSION: SEVERE

Description
- A systolic BP ≥ 160 and/or a diastolic BP ≥ 110 mmHg, with no proteinuria.
  (Always measure BP in the left lateral and not supine position).

Medicine Treatment
Aim to reduce BP to 140/100 mmHg.
- Nifedipine, oral, 10 mg (not sublingual) as a single dose.
- May be repeated after 30 minutes if diastolic BP remains ≥110 mmHg.

Referral
- Urgent. All cases

PRE-ECLAMPSIA

Description
- A systolic BP ≥140 and/or diastolic BP ≥90 mmHg with proteinuria, after 20 weeks of pregnancy (significant proteinuria defined as ≥ 1+ proteinuria).
- Severe pre-eclampsia is acute severe hypertension (systolic BP ≥ 160 and/or diastolic BP ≥ 110) with ≥ 1+ proteinuria, or any level of hypertension with 3+ proteinuria.
- Imminent eclampsia is pre-eclampsia with severe persistent headache, visual disturbances, epigastric pain (not discomfort), hyper-reflexia or clonus.

General Measures
- Advise all pregnant patients to urgently visit the clinic if severe persistent headache, visual disturbances, epigastric pain (not discomfort).

Medicine treatment
- If severe pre-eclampsia or imminent eclampsia:
- Magnesium sulphate, IV, 4 g as a loading dose diluted with 200 mL sodium chloride 0.9% and infused over 20 minutes.

AND
- Magnesium sulphate, IM, 10 g given as 5 g in each buttock
- Then IM, 5 g every 4 hours in alternate buttocks.

CAUTION: USE OF MAGNESIUM SULPHATE
Stop magnesium sulphate if knee reflexes become absent or if urine output <100 mL/4 hours or respiratory rate <16 breaths/minute.

If respiratory depression occurs:
Calcium gluconate 10%, IV, 10 mL given slowly at a rate not > 5 mL/minute.

AND

If systolic BP ≥ 160 and/or a diastolic BP ≥ 110 mmHg:
Nifedipine, oral, 10 mg (not sublingual) as a single dose.
May be repeated after 30 minutes if diastolic BP remains
≥ 110 mmHg.

Referral
- Urgent
    - Severe pre-eclampsia and imminent eclampsia
- Non Urgent
    - All women with pre-eclampsia (within 24 hours).

POSTNATAL PATIENTS

MANAGEMENT

140 / 90
- Continue antenatal treatment
- Review monthly

140 / 90 – 159 / 109
First visit
- Methyldopa 250 mg 3 x daily
- Titrate to a maximum dose: 750 mg 8 hourly.
- Check BP at weekly intervals until BP controlled

Currently on treatment
- Increase dose of either methyl-dopa or amlodipine.
- Check BP at monthly intervals

160 / 110 or greater
- **First visit**
- Amlodipine 5 mg immediately and then daily
  (Dr initiated if patient breastfeeding, unless
  hypertensive urgency)

Currently on treatment
- If poor adherence not considered to be the cause of
  the elevated blood pressure:
    - initiate treatment with amlodipine unless
      already prescribed.
    - all other patients to be **Referred**.

MANAGEMENT OF SOME DRUG SIDE EFFECTS

GASTROINTESTINAL UPSETS

This may be overcome by advising patients to take their medicines with food.

PERSISTENT COUGH

This is a common side effect in patients on treatment with an ACE-inhibitor.

MANAGEMENT
- Exclude other causes of persistent cough eg. heart failure, sinusitis, reflux oesophagitis.
- **REFER** if assistance is required to exclude other causes.
- Stop the medicine if the ACE-inhibitor is assessed as the cause of the cough.
- Alternative medicines that can be used are:
    - amlodipine
    - spironolactone

ANGIOEDEMA

This is a common side effect in patients on treatment with an ACE-inhibitor. It most commonly involves the lips or tongue.

MANAGEMENT
- Stop the ACE-inhibitor immediately
- Give immediate and urgent management. See page 256 management of acute urticaria and angio-oedema
- Alternative medicines that can be used are
    - amlodipine
    - spironolactone

BRADYCARDIA

Slow pulse rate is a complication which may result from treatment with beta-blockers eg. atenolol or methyldopa.

MANAGEMENT
- If the pulse rate is less than 50/min - **REFER**
- Alternative medicines which can be used are:
    - an ACE-inhibitor
    - amlodipine

PEDAL OEDEMA

This is a common side effect in patients being treated with a calcium antagonist

MANAGEMENT
- Exclude other causes of pedal oedema, especially heart failure which is common in hypertension.
- Reduce the dose of the calcium channel blocker, if possible to do so without risking a significant rise in blood pressure.
- Increasing the dose of the thiazide diuretic to 25 mg daily may also help lessen the problem.

HYPERTENSION PROTOCOL

Confirmation of hypertension (minimum of 3 BP readings)

BP < 160/100

HCTZ 12.5 mg daily
(Contraindications: gout, albinism or kidney failure)

↓ If uncontrolled

ADD
Amlodipine 5 mg daily
(preferred in black hypertensives)
Or
Enalapril 10 mg daily
(preferred in non-black hypertensives or if compelling indication, e.g. diabetes, previous stroke)

Contraindications:
Pregnancy, history of ACE-inhibitor intolerance, e.g. angioedema

↓ If uncontrolled

Increase the dose of the second antihypertensive

Note:
- **Intolerant to ACE-inhibitor** (e.g. enalapril) ie. cough or angio-oedema – substitute ACE-inhibitor with next step drug i.e. amlodipine.
- Patients on spironolactone require routine potassium monitoring every 6 months.
- **Gouty arthritis**: Patients with active gout or who develop gouty arthritis whilst on hydrochlorothiazide may be managed with amlodipine or an ACE-inhibitor as sole therapy.

BP ≥ 160/100

HCTZ 12.5 mg daily
PLUS
Amlodipine 5 mg daily
(preferred in black hypertensives)
Or
Enalapril 10 mg daily (preferred in non-black hypertensives or if compelling indication, e.g. diabetes, prior stroke, chronic kidney disease)

↓ If uncontrolled

Increase the dose of the second antihypertensive chosen in the first step

↓ If uncontrolled

ADD
Starting dose of the alternative second antihypertensive not used in first step (third antihypertensive)

↓ If uncontrolled

Increase the dose of the third antihypertensive

↓ If uncontrolled

Increase HCTZ dose to 25 mg daily
Plus **ADD** Spironolactone 25 mg daily
(Dr initiated)

BP ≥ 180/110

HCTZ 12.5 mg daily
PLUS
Amlodipine 5 mg daily

↓ If uncontrolled

Increase amlodipine dose to 10 mg daily

↓ If uncontrolled

ADD
Enalapril 10 mg daily
(provided not contra-indicated and patient not intolerant e.g. cough, angioedema) and increase to 20mg if necessary

↓ If uncontrolled

Increase HCTZ dose to 25 mg daily
Plus **ADD**
Spironolactone 25 mg daily
(Dr initiated)

Contraindications:
hyperkalaemia, kidney failure
(eGFR <30 ml / min)

APPENDIX – EXAMPLE OF LETTERS

Letter To Spouse, Relative or Friend

CLINIC ....

TEL ....

DATE ....

Dear Sir / Madam

.... has agreed that you should know

that he / she suffers from ....

This means that he / she must take tablets every day.

If this is done, he / she can live and work like a normal person. If the pills are stopped, he / she may become very ill.

Please help him / her to take the pills at the right time every day.

Please help him / her to lose weight.

Please remind him / her to come for a check-up every 4 weeks.

Yours sincerely

_____

HEART FAILURE AND HEART DISEASE

HEART FAILURE

Heart failure results when the heart is unable to produce an output of blood, sufficient for the needs of the body, provided the venous return to the heart is adequate.

- In the mildest forms of heart failure, cardiac output is:
    - adequate at rest
    - becomes inadequate only during exercise.
- In most patients, however, it is possible to notice at least some features of heart failure even when the patient is examined at rest.

Factors which may precipitate heart failure or make an existing heart failure worse:

- Poor drug adherence
- Poor dietary habits eg. excessive calorie and salt intake
- Infections eg. respiratory, infective endocarditis, septicaemia
- Excessive alcohol intake
- Excessive fluid intake in patients with severe heart lesions
- Strenuous exercise
- Emotional stress
- Environmental stress eg. hot weather
- Hypertension
- Arrhythmias - certain types
- Heart block (bradycardia)
- Thyrotoxicosis
- Anaemia
- Pregnancy
- Pulmonary embolism
- Drugs eg. beta-blockers
- Cardiac valve disease
- Myocardial infarction
- Altitude

LEFT VENTRICULAR FAILURE (LVF)

Clinical features

- Dyspnoea (shortness of breath) is the most common symptom and may be:
    - mild eg. when walking uphill or climbing stairs
    - moderate eg. when walking a moderate distance on level areas or doing routine housework
    - severe eg. at rest or on walking a very short distance, even slowly.
- Orthopnoea (breathlessness which occurs when the patient is lying flat). This is a very important symptom of left ventricular failure. However, there are conditions which may be symptomatically difficult to distinguish from the orthopnoea of left ventricular failure such as:
    - bronchial asthma attack. In this condition the patient finds the sitting position the most comfortable because it allows for a greater respiratory effort
    - extreme obesity, all forms of ascites and abdominal distension may produce dyspnoea when lying, which may be confused with orthopnoea
    - COPD
- Cough (due to pulmonary oedema)
    - frequently worse at night
    - initially dry, then later watery and frothy
- Haemoptysis - usually pinkish, blood-stained, sometimes frank blood
- Wheezing ("cardiac asthma"), which is often worse at night
- Palpitations follow exercise or anxiety
- Dizziness / syncope (fainting) especially when occurring on exertion
- Exertional fatigue and weakness
- Recession
- Tachypnoea (fast respiratory rate)
- Tachycardia
- Forceful and displaced apex beat
- Gallop rhythm (third heart sound)
- Crepitations first found at the lung bases at the back, then later extending to the sides and the front
- Mitral incompetence murmur
    - if left ventricular dilatation and / or valvular disease present
- Cyanosis
    - usually only present in severe heart failure
- Cold extremities
    - due to poor perfusion

Diagnosis of left ventricular failure

- The number and severity of the symptoms and signs may be few and are very variable.
- It is necessary to be able to make a diagnosis of left ventricular failure with only a minimum of symptoms and signs
    - orthopnoea and exertional dyspnoea are the important symptoms
    - any patient with these should be considered to be in left ventricular failure and **REFERRED,** unless another definite cause for the symptoms is found.
- The presence of physical signs is very valuable in helping to confirm the diagnosis
    - however these signs may be easily missed.
- The following are the most important signs of LVF, but none are essential for diagnosis
    - a displaced apex beat
    - gallop rhythm
    - basal crepitations
- The presence of basal crepitations in particular is important but it must be realised that the diagnosis can be made in the absence of this sign
    - eg. the combination of a displaced apex beat and an increased respiratory and / or pulse rate could indicate left ventricular failure.
- A displaced apex beat or a mitral incompetence murmur frequently remain, even when a patient is out of failure, and so cannot always be used as signs of failure.

Note. LVF may sometimes not be associated with a displaced apex beat eg. mitral stenosis.

RIGHT VENTRICULAR FAILURE (RVF)

Clinical features

- Swelling of the legs, is the most common symptom.
- Anorexia, feeling of fullness in the abdomen.
- Right hypochondrial pain, due to stretching of the liver capsule.
- Decreased urine by day (oliguria).

- Increased urine at night due to improved renal blood flow during bed rest (nocturia).
- Raised jugular venous pressure (JVP).
- Oedema of the lowest parts of the body
    - initially ankles or sacrum (if confined to bed)
    - later thighs, scrotum, abdomen (anasarca).
- Enlarged liver (may or may not be tender).
- Left parasternal heave (lift)
    - this is especially found in cor pulmonale.
- Tricuspid incompetence murmur.
- Proteinuria and/or haematuria
    - this is mild and is due to renal congestion.
- Ascites
- Pleural effusion

Diagnosis of right ventricular failure

- The most important signs of right ventricular failure are:
    - a raised jugular venous pressure
    - the presence of oedema of the lower parts of the body.
    - usually both are present together
- It may sometimes be difficult to be sure about the presence of an elevated JVP and these cases must be **REFERRED** for confirmation.

MANAGEMENT OF HEART FAILURE

Indications for REFERRAL

Anti-failure treatment may be started or continued by the nurse clinician, provided none of the factors listed below are present ie. REFER if there is

- Dyspnoea present at rest or on mild exertion
- Intercostal recession
- Cyanosis
- A diastolic blood pressure of 130 mm Hg or greater
- An elevated jugular venous pressure (definite or suspected)
- A pulse rate
    - more than 120 / min
    - less than 50 / min
    - less than 60 / min in patients on digoxin
- Very irregular pulse not previously investigated
- A respiratory rate of more than 30 / min
- Markedly displaced apex beat for which the patient was not previously referred
- A murmur present (and not previously investigated)
- Gallop rhythm
- Profuse basal crepitations
- Active rheumatic carditis, (tachycardia, murmur, pericardial friction rub), chronic rheumatic valvular disease or infective endocarditis
- Haemoptysis
- Severe dizziness or syncope
- Chest pain suggesting angina pectoris or myocardial infarction
- Significant side effects to drug therapy eg.
    - weakness
    - calf muscle cramps
    - nausea and vomiting
- An unsure diagnosis eg. basal creps with chronic obstructive airways disease (COAD) and apex beat not palpable

GENERAL MEASURES

Bed rest
- If tachycardia or tachypnoea are present, bed rest with extra pillows is necessary
    - this decreases the workload of the heart
    - it increases renal blood flow resulting in improved diuresis
    - it should be continued until clinical improvement has occurred (usually for about 1 week).

Relief of stress
- Stress and anxiety play an important part in making heart failure worse.
- Give psychological support and advice to those patients who require it.

Diet
- Small frequent meals will help to decrease heart workload.
- Salt intake must be restricted.
- Fluid intake should be restricted only in patients who are fluid overloaded
    - ie. in patients with oedema which does not respond to the use of diuretics.
- Obese patients must try to lose weight.
- Intake of foods rich in potassium should be encouraged eg. oranges, bananas or tomatoes.

Exercise
- Patients are to avoid strenuous activity of any kind
    - book off work in an acute situation
    - average period needed is 4-7 days.
- Once the condition has improved, encourage them to have regular graded exercise.

Smoking and drinking
- Patients must make every effort possible to stop smoking and to avoid drinking alcohol
- They should be warned that alcohol has a direct toxic effect on the heart muscle.

REFER to
- Physiotherapy to
    - teach graded exercises
    - help the patient develop a suitable exercise programme for the heart
- Occupational therapy to give guidelines
    - for coping at home
    - on how to function adequately in the work situation with the heart failure
- Social workers to
    - counsel patients and their families about the medical problem
    - help with financial matters
    - assist with work problems

Indications for investigations

- Chest X ray
    - at diagnosis of heart failure or if heart failure is suspected
    - in patients not responding to anti-failure therapy
- Urine check for protein:
    - urine to be checked annually for protein
    - any patient with proteinuria 1+ or more in the absence of uncontrolled heart failure, infection or menstruation should have urine sent for spot PCR (protein-creatinine ratio) - see page 150, kidney disease.
- Serum urea and electrolytes (U&E) and creatinine tests:
    - previous abnormal U&E and creatinine results
    - abnormal urine PCR results >0.1 g/mmol
    - 6 monthly in patients with known chronic kidney disease

- Echocardiography
    - if cause of the heart failure is obscure
    - more severe degrees of heart failure
    - in patients not responding to anti-failure therapy

*The following patients must be **REFERRED** every 6 months for review:*
- On digoxin therapy
- On treatment with furosemide
- Patients with chronic kidney disease

How to assess if the failure is improving
On history ask about the following
- Improvement in the degree of dyspnoea and orthopnoea
- If there is less cough or wheeze at night
- Adherence with drug and non-drug therapy

On examination check for the following
- Presence of signs of respiratory distress eg. dyspnoea at rest, intercostal recession
- Respiratory and pulse rates returning to normal
- Fewer basal creps
- Decrease in jugular venous pressure
- Oedema decreased
- Weight decreasing is a valuable and easy sign to check
- Blood pressure control in hypertensives

MEDICINE MANAGEMENT
Mild heart failure
Treatment may be started or continued by the PHC sister:
- Hydrochlorothiazide (HCTZ) 25-50 mg daily

Plus
- An ACE-inhibitor
    - **either** enalapril 5 mg 2 x daily
    - **or** perindopril 2-4 mg daily
- Patient to return in 4 weeks for check-up, or sooner if not feeling better

Hypertensive patients
- If they are on treatment with hydrochlorothiazide 12.5 mg daily, they should have the treatment increased to hydrochlorothiazide 25-50 mg daily.
- Add an ACE-inhibitor drug if patient not already on this treatment.
- Any other treatment being taken should continue unchanged, except for beta-blockers, e.g. atenolol, which should be stopped.
- **REFER** if an adequate response to treatment has **not** been achieved after 4 weeks.

Note
The presence of **profuse** crepitations is an indication for the use of furosemide. The persistence of a few basal crepitations **only**, is not a sign of failure to respond to therapy.

If the patient has improved symptomatically
- Then continue with the above as maintenance therapy provided:
    - there are no signs of respiratory distress
    - both heart and respiratory rates are within normal limits

Moderately severe heart failure
(LVF or biventricular failure)
To be initiated by doctors **only.**
Step 1
- Give furosemide 40 mg daily or 2 x daily
- **Plus** enalapril 5-10 mg 2 x daily
    - **or** perindopril 2-4 mg daily
- Check after 4 weeks or sooner if not improved

Patients who are well controlled
- Reduce the dose of furosemide to the lower dose
- Check in 4 weeks
- If there is no recurrence of the failure
    - substitute furosemide with hydrochlorothiazide 25-50 mg daily
- If the patient is on the lower dose already
    - substitute furosemide with hydrochlorothiazide immediately

Step 2
*If an adequate response to treatment has **not** been achieved after 4 weeks e.g. patient still has effort dyspnoea, basal crepitations:*
- **Add** spironolactone 25 mg daily (only if serum potassium can be monitored)
- **Note**: Spironolactone can cause severe hyperkalaemia
    - do **not** use together with potassium supplements
    - do **not** use in kidney failure (eGFR < 30 ml / minute)

Step 3
Provided the patient is not severely fluid overloaded or hypotensive, or has bradycardia:
- Commence carvedilol dosage build-up
    - starting dose 3.125 mg / day
- Increase after 2 weeks to 3.125 mg 2 x daily
- Increase at two-weekly intervals by doubling the daily dose until a maximum of 25 mg 2 x daily, if tolerated.
- If not tolerated, i.e. worsening of heart failure manifestations, reduce the dose to the previously tolerated dose.
- Up-titration can take several months.
- Carvedilol build-up must be complete and the patient's condition stable before the patient can be down-referred to the PHC sister for follow-up.
- **Note**. It may be considered preferable to **REFER** the patient for cardiologist assessment and stabilisation at this stage.

Step 4
Still symptomatic despite above therapy:
- **Add** digoxin, oral, 125 mg daily (specialist initiated)
- **Note**: plasma digoxin levels should be monitored in the following patients:
    - the elderly
    - patients with poor renal function
    - hypokalaemia
    - low body weight

Defaulters
- Check defaulters for recurrence of failure.
- If failure has recurred, restart the previous treatment.
- **REFER** if the failure is severe.
- If failure has not recurred, despite the patient defaulting for a long period
    - restart the previous treatment
    - omit the diuretic if the patient is not fluid overloaded

Diuretics
The use of a diuretic is essential in the treatment of heart failure until the condition is well controlled and the patient is free of fluid overload. All diuretics increase the urinary excretion of salt and water.

The main effects of this are a reduction in:
- Oedema, both in the lungs and in the limbs.
- The amount of blood reaching the right and left ventricles (ventricular preload), which lessens the workload of the ventricles.
- The pressure in the arteries (left ventricular afterload), as a result of a vasodilating effect, which also helps to improve cardiac function.

Use of diuretics in special conditions
Gout
- Thiazide diuretics are not to be used.

- Furosemide is the preferred diuretic drug.
- **REFER** (for treatment of gout, see page 295).

Diabetes mellitus
- Thiazide diuretics should be used with caution (max 25 mg daily) as they can raise the blood glucose level
    - they are therefore suitable for treatment of very mild failure only.
- Furosemide is the preferred diuretic.
- **REFER** unless the failure is very mild.

Impaired kidney function
- This can be shown by:
    - persistent proteinuria with or without haematuria
    - abnormal U & E results
- Thiazide diuretics are contra-indicated in patients with impairment of renal function (eGFR < 60 ml / minute).
- **REFER** for furosemide, the preferred diuretic drug

Vasodilators
- These drugs are used in heart failure to reduce the heart workload.
- Vasodilators may be:
    - venodilators (reducing the preload) eg. isosorbide dinitrate (Isordil)
    - arterial dilators (reducing the afterload) eg. diuretics
    - both pre- and afterload reducers eg. perindopril, enalapril (ACE-inhibitors).

Angiotensin converting enzyme inhibitors (ACE-inhibitors)
- They act by blocking the renin-angiotensin-aldosterone mechanism, and are strong vasodilators.
- They are used commonly in the treatment of patients with LVF, or biventricular failure / CCF due to:
    - cardiomyopathy
    - hypertension
- They are not used in pure right-sided failure.
- In most cases they are used together with diuretics in the management of heart failure.
- In moderate or severe failure, therapy with vasodilators must be started by the doctor as they are usually prescribed together with furosemide.
    - the nurse clinician may continue the treatment after that.
- Because of the potassium-sparing properties of ACE-inhibitors, when these drugs are used together with furosemide, Slow-K can be omitted, or its dose can be substantially reduced.

Enalapril
- Initial dose 5 mg 2 x daily
- Average dose 10 mg 2 x daily.
- Maximum dose 10 mg 2 x daily.

Perindopril
- Initial dose 2 mg daily
- Average dose 4 mg daily.
- Maximum dose 8 mg daily.

Note. Patients who develop a persistent dry cough as a result of ACE-inhibitors intolerence, must be **REFERRED** to a specialist for initiation on an angiotension receptor blocker e.g. Losartan, Telmisartan

Carvedilol (doctor initiated)
Indicated for all stable patients or those not well controlled on the above treatment.

Contraindications
- Severe fluid overload
- Hypotension
- Bradycardia or heart block
- Asthma

Build-up
- Starting dose: 3.125 mg daily.
- Increase after 2 weeks to 3.125 mg 2 x daily, if tolerated.
- Increase at 2-weekly intervals by doubling the daily dose until a maximum of 25 g 2 x daily, if tolerated.
- If not tolerated, i.e. worsening of heart failure manifestations, reduce the dose to the previously tolerated dose.
- Up-titration can take several months.

Spironolactone (doctor initiated)
- This may be used **only** if serum potassium can be monitored.
- It must not be used together with potassium supplements.
- Dose: 25 mg daily.

Digoxin (specialist initiated)
- This is a cardiac muscle stimulant which improves the contraction of the ventricles.

Indications
- Used in patients with symptomatic CCF due to systolic dysfunction.
- It is also used in the treatment of fast atrial fibrillation, when this occurs together with heart failure.

Dosages
- Patients at high risk for digoxin toxicity:
    - the elderly
    - patients with poor renal function
    - hypokalaemia
    - low body weight
    - recommended dose is 0,125 mg daily
- Digoxin treatment should not be initiated if the patient is hypokalaemic.

Toxicity
At each visit the patient should be checked for any toxic effects from digoxin therapy.

On history
- Anorexia and nausea are early symptoms of toxicity, and are important to recognise.
- They may be due to other drugs used by the patient eg. potassium chloride (Slow-K).
- Vomiting, diarrhoea, altered colour vision may occur later.

On examination
- Early signs are:
    - heart rate less than 60/minute
    - occasional irregular (ectopic) beats, unless these were present prior to digoxin therapy.
- Later more complex arrhythmias may develop.

Management of patients on digoxin
- PHC sisters may continue the management of patients on digoxin. They should **REFER** every six months for review of treatment.
- Should symptoms or signs of toxicity occur, **REFER.**

ACUTE PULMONARY OEDEMA

Clinical features
- Dyspnoea / tachypnoea
- Orthopnoea
- Restlessness / anxiety

- Productive cough with pink, frothy sputum
- Wheezing
- May be hypertensive or shocked
- Gallop rhythm
- Basal crepitations
- Signs of RVF may be present eg.
    - raised JVP
    - pedal oedema

Note: It is important to distinguish this condition from that of acute bronchial asthma as both may present with acute bronchospasm tight chest and respiratory distress.

MANAGEMENT
- Place patient in a sitting or semi-Fowler's position (in bed propped up at 45 degrees)
- Give oxygen by 40% ventimask at a rate of 6-8 L per minute.

AND

- Isosorbide dinitrate (Isordil), 5 mg beneath the tongue (sublingual) immediately. Repeat every 5-10 minutes, if needed
- Do not administer if hypotensive

AND

- Furosemide, IV, 40 mg
- If no response after 30 minutes
    - Give furosemide, IV, 80-100 mg

To treat hypertension:
- ACE - inhibitor, e.g. enalapril 10 mg, oral, as a single dose.
- Record urine output.
- Monitor vital signs and record them.
- **REFER** to hospital with oxygen.

▼ Note to doctor
- Furosemide 80-100 mg IVI may be given slowly to those patients taking oral furosemide (especially in high doses) or those in kidney failure ▲

HEART DISEASE

HYPERTENSIVE HEART DISEASE

Clinical features
- Left ventricular hypertrophy (forceful localised apex beat or displaced lateral to the mid-clavicular line).
- Symptoms and signs of heart failure, either LVF or congestive heart failure (CCF).
- Hypertension

Note. Mild hypertension may occur in heart failure from other causes (reactive hypertension) which may be difficult to distinguish from hypertensive heart disease. A previous history of hypertension suggests this to be the cause of the heart failure.

MANAGEMENT
- Treat heart failure if this is present.
- Treat hypertension (Hypertension Protocol pages 72-75).
- An ACE-inhibitor eg. enalapril is indicated at the first visit.
    - preferably given 12 hourly
    - starting dose 5 mg 12 hourly increasing to 10 mg 12 hourly if necessary

- Avoid beta-blockers eg. atenolol (Tenormin)
    - as they may make the heart failure worse
    - if the patient is already on a beta-blocker
    - this should be stopped

CARDIOMYOPATHY

Causes
- Chronic alcoholism associated with chronic malnutrition is a common cause.

Clinical features
- Usually not diagnosed before heart failure has occurred.
- It presents initially as LVF.
- Progresses to biventricular failure, when the symptoms and signs of RVF are usually the more obvious.
- Oedema and ascites are often prominent.
- Often a large heart is found together with a poor volume pulse.
- Functional incompetence of the mitral and / or tricuspid valves is frequently present.
- Arrhythmias are common eg. atrial fibrillation.
- The blood pressure is usually normal or low.

MANAGEMENT
- **REFER** for anti-failure treatment.
- Advise patient to:
    - take an adequate diet
    - avoid alcohol totally.
- Give Vitamin B Co 1 tab 3 x daily.

▼ Note to doctor
- This form of heart failure is commonly associated with poor left ventricular function which is best assessed by means of echocardiography
    - **REFER** to cardiologist ▲

BERIBERI HEART DISEASE

Causes
- Thiamine deficiency

Clinical features
- Commonly found in alcoholics who have had a high consumption of alcohol over a period of a few weeks.
- The patient often appears to be well fed.
- There is ventricular failure (high output type) as shown by:
    - obvious oedema
    - severe palpitations and breathlessness
    - a good volume pulse (bounding)
    - **warm** extremities.
- Occasionally Shoshin or acute fulminant cardiovascular beriberi occurs. This is evidenced by:
    - mental confusion or impaired consciousness
    - hypotension with poor volume pulse
    - biventricular failure
    - severe acidosis.

MANAGEMENT

- **REFER** for anti-failure treatment.
- Advise patient to take an adequate diet and that alcohol has a severe damaging effect on the heart.
- Give Vitamin B Co
    - 1-2 tabs daily.
- Give thiamine 100 mg daily.

RHEUMATIC HEART DISEASE AND RHEUMATIC FEVER

ACUTE RHEUMATIC FEVER

Clinical features

- Age of greatest incidence of the first attack is 3-15 years.
- Rheumatic fever is very rare before the age of 4 years.
- Repeated attacks of rheumatic fever can occur up to about 30 years of age but it is very rare for a first attack to occur after 15 years of age.
- Rheumatic fever only follows Group A beta-haemolytic streptococcal infections of the throat and upper airways
    - it is *not* a complication of impetigo.
- The disease is more common in low socio-economic areas.
- The latent period between the streptococcal throat infection and rheumatic fever is about 10-21 days.
- Low grade fever.
- Fatigue and malaise.
- Joint pains (arthralgia) or joint inflammation (arthritis)
    - mainly affecting big joints eg. knees, elbows, shoulders, wrists
    - central joints of the hips and spine not affected
    - flitting ie. one joint improving as another becomes worse.
- Palpitations
- Lower anterior chest pain
- Abdominal pain
- Heart involvement is common and is shown by:
    - tachycardia (unrelated to the rise in temperature)
    - heart murmurs
    - pericardial friction rub
    - possible cardiomegaly and heart failure.
- Chorea
    - involuntary, purposeless, fidgety movements of the limbs, trunk and facial muscles
    - eg. facial grimacing, difficulty in holding the protruded tongue still (jack-in-box tongue).

CHRONIC RHEUMATIC HEART DISEASE

Clinical features

- History of rheumatic fever (joint pains and swelling) in childhood
    - symptoms of recurrent sore throats are not a reliable guide.
- Presence of murmurs and cardiomegaly.
- Possible symptoms and signs of
    - heart failure
    - sub-acute bacterial endocarditis (SBE).

MANAGEMENT OF RHEUMATIC FEVER AND RHEUMATIC HEART DISEASE

REFER if you suspect rheumatic fever.

Primary prevention (to prevent rheumatic fever)

All patients with streptococcal throat infections must receive prompt treatment with:
- Pen VK 2 x daily for 10 days
    - <10 years: 250 mg
    - >10 years and adults: 500 mg
- or benzathine penicillin IM, single dose
    - <30 kg: 0.6 million units
    - >30 kg and adults: 1.2 million units
- or if penicillin-allergic: azithromycin daily for 3 days
    - 1-3 years: 120 mg (3 ml)
    - 3-7 years: 200 mg (5 ml)
    - 7-11 years: 250 mg
    - >11 years and adults: 500 mg

Secondary prevention (to prevent repeated attacks of rheumatic fever)

- Benzathine penicillin IM 1.2 million units if >30 kg, **or** 0.6 million units if <30 kg every 28 days
- **or** Pen VK 2 x daily
    - <10 years: 125 mg
    - >10 years and adults: 250 mg
- If penicillin-allergic:
    - <11 years: consult with a specialist
    - >11 years and adults: azithromycin, oral, 250 mg daily
- Patients with no rheumatic valvular disease
    - prophylaxis is given for 10 years or until the age of 21 years, whichever is longer.
- Patients with rheumatic valvular disease, treat lifelong.

Note: To reduce the pain of injection, lignocaine 1% should be used as a diluent for benzathine penicillin.

Tertiary prevention (to prevent infective endocarditis)

- Before dental extraction give amoxicillin 2 g as a single oral dose (1.5 g <10 years)
    - 1 hour before the procedure.
    - repeat dose 6 hours later
- If penicillin-allergic, use clindamycin, oral, 600 mg
    - as a single oral dose
    - 1 hour before the procedure
    - repeat dose 6 hours later

REFER if the patient:

- Has not been previously investigated, as he / she may require surgery to valves.
- Is in heart failure (either to start or increase anti-failure treatment).
- Is not responding to medical treatment, as he / she may need surgery.
- Has evidence of:
    - active carditis (tachycardia, changing murmurs)
    - arthritis
    - chorea
- Has evidence of infective endocarditis (SBE) ie:
    - fever
    - anaemia
    - clubbing
    - splenomegaly
    - haematuria
    - conjunctival haemorrhage
- Appears ill for any other reason.

COR PULMONALE

Clinical features
- History of chronic bronchitis, smoking, mining or bronchial asthma.
- Clinical features of COAD eg:
    - polycythaemia
    - barrel-shaped chest
    - hyper-resonance
- Cyanosis
- Right ventricular enlargement is usually prominent as shown by a parasternal heave (lift) and/or a palpable pulmonary second sound.
- Symptoms and signs of RVF.

MANAGEMENT
- **REFER** for anti-failure treatment.
- Use a diuretic to releive fluid overload.
- Use bronchodilators eg. beta-2 stimulant inhaler, (see COAD management page 62).
- Give antibiotics for episodes of acute bronchitis (when sputum is purulent).
- Encourage the patient to stop smoking.

REFER for:
- Physiotherapy if available to:
    - increase lung expansion
    - increase removal of secretions
    - strengthen respiratory and heart muscles
    - reduce bronchospasm.
- Occupational therapy to
    - assist with the work and home situations
    - advise about alternative work if needed.

OTHER CAUSES OF HEART FAILURE

- Ischaemic heart disease
- Thyrotoxicosis
- Anaemia
- Pericarditis
- Congenital heart disease

REFER for investigation if you suspect any of these causes.

PREGNANCY AND HEART FAILURE

- Pregnancy will make heart failure worse.
- Heart murmurs are often heard in normal pregnant women as a result of increased blood flow
    - functional murmurs are likely to change in loudness with change in position of patient.
- These murmurs do not necessarily mean heart disease is present, unless other evidence of this is found.

MANAGEMENT
- **REFER**
    - heart patients who become pregnant
    - if in any doubt about a heart murmur.
- Advise heart patients to attend the family planning clinic.

PALPITATIONS

- Palpitations (awareness of heartbeats) alone, do not indicate heart disease.
- These are common in healthy people particularly:
    - if anxious
    - after exertion
    - in smokers.

Causes
- Usually due to anxiety and stress
- Thyrotoxicosis
- Heart failure
- Arrythmias
- Any acute illness
- In young people, undiagnosed rheumatic heart disease must be carefully looked for on history and examination.
- Drugs eg. tea and coffee
- Anaemia

MANAGEMENT
- Inquire about domestic, social, work or financial stress.
- Also ask the patient about diet
    - coffee and cheese can cause palpitations
    - tea can also be a cause in sensitive people.
- Make sure that the cause is not heart disease, anaemia or thyrotoxicosis.
- If pulse beat feels irregular this may be due to
    - changes with breathing (sinus arrhythmia)
    - extra beats (extrasystoles).
- Reassure and advise if:
    - the patient is generally well and nothing abnormal is found
    - stress is considered to be the cause.
- If symptoms are severe, prescribe a beta-blocker eg. atenolol 50 mg daily.
- **REFER** if:
    - you suspect serious disease
    - many extra beats are present
    - the pulse is slow or rapid
    - stress is severe, to the social worker for counselling and help with stress problems.

VASCULAR DISEASE

VEINS

SUPERFICIAL VENOUS SYSTEM

VARICOSE VEINS

MANAGEMENT

Discuss with the patient the choice between conservative and operative treatment.

Conservative treatment
- **REFER** for
    - elastic stockings preferably pantihose

Operative treatment
- Surgery is needed if there is incompetence of a major venous system eg. from the groin down, or from the back of the knee down
    - this will show itself as large varicose veins which cause pain and discomfort to the patient.
- Surgery is also needed if there is persistent pain in any incompetent bunch of veins.
- The patient will need to wear elastic stockings post operation for some time.
- Surgery in a woman is best left until after she has completed her family.

BURST VARICOSE VEINS

When a varicose vein bursts, there is a sudden gush of blood from the leg, which may be frightening, but is usually not serious.

MANAGEMENT
- Elevate the leg
    - the worst thing to do is for the patient to sit in a wheel chair.
- Apply a firm, compression bandage over the bleeding point, to apply local pressure.
- Suturing is usually not necessary.
- In a few days
    - the wound usually heals up
    - the involved vein often thromboses.
- Discuss with the patient the possibility of surgery at a later date, to strip out the veins.

SUPERFICIAL THROMBOPHLEBITIS

This is less serious than a deep venous thrombosis (DVT). Often there is no obvious cause for this.

Clinical features
- A tender cord-like induration (hardened area) with redness occurs
    - this happens along the course of a subcutaneous vein
    - commonly affects veins at drip sites and varicose veins.
- Oedema of the leg and deep calf tenderness are absent unless deep thrombophlebitis has also developed.
- Chills and fever suggest septic phlebitis.

MANAGEMENT
- This can be managed as an out-patient.
- Give ibuprofen 400 mg 3 x daily for 1 week.
- Anticoagulation is not indicated unless the disease is rapidly progressing or if there is extension into the deep system.
- **REFER** for possible investigation if the vein affected is not a varicose vein or at a drip site.
- **REFER** patients with septic thrombophlebitis.

DEEP VENOUS SYSTEM

DEEP VENOUS THROMBOSIS (DVT)

This condition is the formation of a blood clot (thrombus) in the deep veins. It is also known as phlebothrombosis.

Causes
- It may occur
    - after a debilitating illness
    - after surgery
    - spontaneously
- Patients at risk include
    - those over 35 years old
    - obese patients
    - smokers
    - women taking the oral contraceptive pill
    - bedridden patients
    - patients with heart disease (eg. heart failure)
    - post operative patients
    - pregnancy and post partum

Clinical features
- The calf veins or pelvic veins are commonly involved
    - pieces may break away and pass through the right side of the heart to lodge in the lungs
    - this results in a pulmonary embolus, which may be fatal.
- Unilateral, tender, swollen calf strongly suggests a DVT (unless there is another obvious cause eg. trauma)
    - even if the swelling and oedema appear to be mild
    - a useful sign is that the calf is harder and more tender than the normal calf, even though the swelling may not be obvious
    - the tenderness is felt when the muscles are gently compressed against the bone.
- Homan's sign (pain in the calf if the foot is dorsiflexed) should **not** be checked for
    - it is not a reliable sign
    - it can be dangerous by causing the clot to become dislodged.
- If the whole leg is painful, swollen and congested it suggests the pelvic and femoral veins are affected.

REFER if suspected, even though you may not be sure of your diagnosis.

VENOUS ULCERS

MANAGEMENT
- The most urgent treatment is to get rid of the oedema.
- This is more important than treating the wound.
- See Surgery page 282 for topical treatment and pressure bandages.

ARTERIES

Clinical features of arterial disease
- The arterial supply of any organ is vital for its function.
- Arterial disease causes a lowered blood flow (ischaemia) and this will affect that organ's function.
- An important guide to arterial insufficiency will be that the symptoms get *worse* as the function of the organ *increases*
    - this is clearly shown with muscular tissue (see below).

Heart muscle
- Blood flow obstruction (myocardial ischaemia) causes chest pain (angina).
- This pain is:
    - made worse by exercise when the heart muscle needs more blood
    - relieved by rest.

Muscles of the leg
- Poor arterial flow causes pain (claudication).
- This pain is:
    - made worse with exercise
    - relieved by rest.

Gastrointestinal system
- The pain of ischaemia to the bowel is made worse after a meal.

CARDIOVASCULAR DISEASE

CARDIOVASCULAR DISEASE (ATHEROSCLEROSIS)

Any of the following may be involved:
- CNS - cerebro vascular disease (see also Nervous System, cerebro vascular accident, page 220).
- Limbs - peripheral vascular disease.
- Heart - angina and myocardial infarct (see coronary artery disease pages 91 and 92).

For more information on each, see the sections which follow.

PERIPHERAL VASCULAR DISEASE

Blood supply to the periphery, particularly the lower limbs, is reduced because of atherosclerosis.

Clinical features
- Intermittent claudication, which is pain in the calf muscles
    - made worse by exercise
    - relieved by rest.
- Pain in the thighs and buttocks, if the iliac and femoral arteries are affected.
- Absent pulses. Check the posterior tibial, dorsalis pedis, popliteal, femoral, radial and brachial pulses as far as possible.
- Trophic skin changes as a result of inadequate blood supply to the skin. There will be:
    - thinning of the skin
    - a shiny appearance to the skin
    - loss of hair
    - dryness of the skin
    - skin peeling off (flaky)
    - dry and flaky nails
- Coldness of the limb, especially the feet due to poor circulation.
- Poor perfusion of the feet with postural change
    - the soles go white when the legs are raised above the body
    - they are slow to regain their colour when the legs are lowered again.
- Gangrene, especially of the toes.

MANAGEMENT
- Stop smoking.
- Advise good foot care
    - the same guidelines should be observed as for diabetic foot care
    - see Diabetes Protocol page 132 under diabetic foot.

- Gradually increased exercise
    - patients should walk as much as possible.
- Avoid beta blockers
- Control associated disorders e.g. diabetes, hypertension

REFER if:
- signs of gangrene
- cold limbs with absent pulses
- not previously investigated.

MANAGEMENT OF CARDIOVASCULAR DISEASE

PAIN BELOW THE LEFT BREAST

This is a very common symptom, particularly in women.

Causes
- Stress and anxiety
- Reflux oesophagitis which is:
    - related to food
    - relieved by antacids
    - without any cardiovascular symptoms or signs
- Fibrositis of the chest muscles made worse by:
    - movement of the arm
    - direct palpation
- Inflammation of the joint between ribs and costal cartilages (costochondritis)
    - tender on direct palpation of the affected joint
    - made worse by chest movement eg. deep breathing
- Lung diseases eg.
    - pneumonia
    - pleurisy
    - adhesions from old diseases such as tuberculosis
- Heart disease, particularly angina, myocardial infarction, and rheumatic fever in children and young adults
    - usually there will be specific cardiac symptoms or signs.

MANAGEMENT
REFER
- Any patient with chest pains
    - who has any heart symptoms or signs
    - who has any irregularities of the pulse
    - unless previously investigated.
- For an ECG if there is any suspicion of heart disease especially in middle-aged or older patients
    - as myocardial infarction may have different symptoms from those usually expected
    - eg. they may have pain mainly in the epigastrium.
- Anxiety disorder
    - counsel on stress prevention and management
    - an antidepressant drug eg. amitriptyline can be used if depressive symptoms have developed.

CORONARY ARTERY DISEASE

ANGINA PECTORIS

Angina pectoris is chest pain resulting from myocardial ischaemia.

Clinical features
- Feeling of tightness or constricting pain.
- Retrosternal chest pain. It may radiate:
    - to the left shoulder
    - frequently moving down the inner aspect of the left arm as far as the tip of the little finger
    - less commonly to the right shoulder and distally
    - to the neck and lower jaw
    - to the back
- The pain is started by exercise, heavy meals, lifting heavy weights, stress, anxiety or cold weather.
- Rest relieves the pain:
- The pain lasts from a few seconds up to 10 minutes
- A worsening of the condition is indicated if the episodes of angina become "unstable" ie.
    - increase in frequency and severity
    - increase in duration (± 10-20 minutes)
    - occur at rest
    - not relieved by sublingual nitrates.
- On examination of the cardiovascular system there are usually no abnormal findings.

MANAGEMENT
General Measures
- Stop smoking
- Weight reduction in overweight patients (BMI > 25)
- Reduce alcohol intake
- Reduce intake of sugar and sugary rich foods, animal fats.
- Encourage high fibre and unrefined carbohydrates with adequate fruit and vegetables.
- Regular moderate exercise e.g. 30 minutes brisk walking 3–5 x a week.
- **REFER** for ECG.

Medicine management
- Aspirin, oral, 100 mg daily
- Nitrate, short acting e.g. isosorbide dinitrate (Isordil) sublingual, 5 mg every 5–10 minutes as required
    - maximum 4 tabs per episode
    - this reduces venous tone and preload, and lowers the oxygen demand of the heart.
- Beta-blocker e.g. atenolol 50 mg daily
    - this reduces heart rate, blood pressure and myocardial contractility
    - If a beta-blocker cannot be tolerated or is contraindicated use a calcium channel blocker e.g. amlodipine 5 mg daily
- Organic nitrate e.g.
    - isosorbide mononitrate, 10-20 mg 2 x daily at 8h00 and 14h00 in order to provide a nitrate free period to prevent tolerance.
- Statin therapy e.g. simvastatin 10 mg at night.

REFER
- If not previously assessed by a doctor.
- For reassessment if frequency and duration of pain increase.
- Stat if the pain lasts for more than 20 minutes, as this strongly suggests a coronary thrombosis.
- Pain not relieved by sublinqual nitrates.

Follow up
The PHC sister may continue the above treatment once the patient's condition has stabalised.

MYOCARDIAL INFARCTION
(HEART ATTACK)

Severe coronary atherosclerosis may result in complete blockage of a coronary artery (a coronary thrombosis). A myocardial infarction (death of some of the heart muscle) will result.

Clinical features
- Risk factors as for atherosclerosis.
- History of previous myocardial infarct.
- History of previous angina pectoris.
- Sudden onset of a very severe, prolonged episode of angina for more than 30 minutes.
- The pain of a myocardial infarct
    - is more intense than angina and the patient is aware that it is different
    - it is described as squeezing or constricting
    - is characterised by holding a fist over the mid-chest
    - often radiates to the neck and jaw
    - may radiate from the chest to the epigastrium
    - may occur only in the epigastrium.
- The patient may break out in a cold sweat and feels weak.
- Dizziness, syncope (fainting), dyspnoea (breathlessness), cough, wheezing, nausea, vomiting may be present in any combination.
- The heart rate may vary from marked bradycardia (slow pulse) to tachycardia (fast pulse).
- Pallor
- The blood pressure may be
    - high, especially in former hypertensives
    - low, in patients with shock.
- Confusion
- Distant heart sounds
- Gallop rhythm (S4)
- Cardiac murmurs

Differential diagnosis
- Reflux oesophagitis is the most common (see upper GIT on page 103). The pain:
    - is related to food
    - is relieved by antacids
    - radiates more to the back than to the side
    - is worse at night and after bending
    - is more common in women and the obese
- Fibrositis of the chest muscles
- Inflammation of the costal cartilages
- Disease of the lungs

MANAGEMENT
This is an emergency. If there is a cardiac arrest, start cardiopulmonary resuscitation (CPR) stat (see resuscitation page 3).

- Place patient in semi-Fowler's position (unless hypotensive or shocked.
- Give oxygen via mask 6-8 L / minute.
- Put up a drip of 200 ml normal saline, to run **slowly.**
- Aspirin oral, 100 mg immediately (exclude allergy to aspirin).

Pain relief
- Morphine IVI
    - 10 mg diluted in 9 ml water for injection or normal saline
    - administer 1 mg per minute until pain relieved.
- Pain not responsive to this dose:
- Isosorbide dinitrate (Isordil) sublingual 5 mg every 5–10 minutes as required to a maximum of 4 tablets.

Thrombolytic therapy
- Streptokinase IVI 1,5 million IU diluted in 100 ml dextrose 5% or normal saline, and given over 30-60 minutes
    - only for confirmed ST elevation, myocardial infarction or new left bundle branch block, if patient presents within 6 hours of onset of pain
    - discontinue streptokinase if patient shows manifestations of impending shock (not merely a drop in blood pressure).

Monitor
- Ongoing chest pain
- Development of pulmonary oedema
- Signs of shock
- Development of arrhythmias

REFER as soon as the condition has been made as steady and safe as possible.

POST-MYOCARDIAL INFARCTION

Patients with a previous history of myocardial infarction are at risk of a repeat infarction.

MANAGEMENT
General measures
- Progressive increase in physical activity (walking, climbing stairs).
- **REFER** for:
    - physiotherapy
    - occupational therapy
- Prevent patients from thinking of themselves as invalids by encouraging them to continue to lead as normal a life as possible.
- Sexual relations should continue as before
- Control of underlying associated conditions
    - hypertension
    - diabetes
    - obesity
- Advice on a healthier lifestyle
    - stop smoking
    - reduce fat in the diet
    - increase roughage in the diet.

Medicine management
- Aspirin oral, 100 mg daily.
- For post infarct angina:
    - isosorbide dinitrate (Isordil), sublingual, 5 mg immediately
    - may be repeated every 5-10 minutes for 3 or 4 doses
- Beta-blockers, e.g. atenolol 50 mg / day
    - if heart failure develops replace atenolol with carvedilol
- Simvastatin, oral, 10 mg nocte.

REFER
- Ongoing chest pain or post infarct angina
- Signs of heart failure
- Irregular pulse as it is suggestive of heart dysrhythmia

Gastro-Intestinal System

ABDOMINAL SYMPTOMS

ABDOMINAL SYMPTOMS AND THEIR POSSIBLE CAUSES

ANOREXIA, NAUSEA AND VOMITING

- This is usually due to disease in the upper gastrointestinal tract.
- It may also be due to non-intestinal diseases:
    - within the abdomen
    - involving other organs of the body eg. neurological system, genito-urinary system.

ANOREXIA (LOSS OF APPETITE)

Many diseases are associated with anorexia and are very often occult (hidden) diseases which lead to loss of weight. Anorexia leads to diminished food intake.

Causes

Overt causes

- Acute infections
    - meningitis
    - pneumonia
    - gastroenteritis
- Chronic illness
    - chronic obstructive pulmonary disease
    - chronic liver disease
    - congestive heart failure
    - neurological disease
    - autoimmune / inflammatory disease
    - chronic kidney disease (uraemia)

Occult causes (hidden causes)

- Chronic infections
    - HIV
    - tuberculosis
    - endocarditis
- Cancer
    - hypercalcaemia (malignancy hyperparathyroidism, sarcoidosis)
- Endocrine
    - adrenal insufficiency
    - hyperparathyroidism
- Psychiatric / neurological
    - anorexia nervosa
    - depression
    - Alzheimer's / other dementia
- Pernicious anaemia

NAUSEA AND VOMITING

Causes

- Acute abdominal emergencies
    - associated with inflammation of a viscus (appendicitis / cholecystitis) or obstruction
- Infections of the intestinal tract
    - often accompanied by diarrhoea
- Acute systemic infections
    - especially important in children
- Central nervous system disorder
    - raised intracranial pressure
    - migraine
    - meningitis
- Heart
    - acute myocardial infarct
    - congestive heart failure
- Metabolic / endocrine disorders
    - uraemia
    - diabetic ketoacidosis
    - hypo- / hyperparathyroidism
    - adrenal insufficiency
- Medicines
    - digitalis / morphine / theophylline / phenytoin
- Toxins
    - food poisoning / some herbal toxins
- Pregnancy
    - hyperemesis gravidarum

In children

- Acute gastroenteritis is one of the most common causes
- Any systemic disease may give these symptoms

In neonates (severe vomiting)

- Bile-stained vomiting in a neonate or young infant indicates bowel obstruction until proved otherwise.
- Consider the possibility of pyloric stenosis, especially if the baby appears to be very hungry, but losing weight
    - visible peristalsis or a mass may be noted on examination.

HAEMATEMESIS (VOMITING BLOOD)

This usually means serious disease.

Causes

Common (not related to GIT)

- Swallowed blood from bleeding mouth or nose.

Serious

- Peptic ulcers
- Carcinoma stomach
- Oesophageal varices
- Acute gastritis (alcohol / aspirin / non steroidal drugs like indomethacin)

Mallory Weiss syndrome
- This is tearing of the mucosa of the lower end of the oesophagus due to severe vomiting.
- It is a common cause of haematemesis in Soweto, and is caused by:
    - repeated forceful vomiting
    - the use of medicines and herbs as an emetic
    - self-induced vomiting / retching
    - hyperemesis gravidarum in pregnancy

Note. Haematemesis is sometimes confused with haemoptysis (coughing blood) which also needs **REFERRAL**.

> **REFER** all serious causes.

ABDOMINAL PAIN

EPIGASTRIC PAIN

Causes
- Gastritis - commonly caused by abuse of drugs eg. alcohol, NSAIDs, laxatives
- Hepatitis
- Peptic ulceration
- Pancreatitis
- Pneumonia should also be considered
- In susceptible adults, coronary artery disease (especially acute myocardial infarction) may present with epigastric symptoms
- Cholecystitis
- Tonsillitis and dental disease in children
- Muscular pain

RIGHT UPPER QUADRANT PAIN

Causes
- Diseases of the liver
- Disease of the lower lobe and pleura of the right lung eg. pneumonia
- Amoebiasis causing a liver abscess
- Subphrenic abscess
- Kidney disease
- Peptic ulceration, especially with complications such as perforation
- Cholecystitis
- Heart failure may cause distention of the liver

LEFT UPPER QUADRANT PAIN

This is less common.

Causes
- Colonic disease eg. amoebiasis and other forms of dysentery
- Laxative or enema abuse
- Disease of the left lung eg. pneumonia
- Kidney disease
- Pancreatitis
- Splenomegaly

UMBILICAL PAIN

This is generally due to disease of the small bowel.

Causes
- Gastroenteritis
- Drug and laxative abuse
- Early appendicitis
- Urinary tract infections
- Anxiety and stress, especially in children
    - often called "chronic bellyachers"
    - manifests by recurring central abdominal pain
- Hernia especially if strangulated

RIGHT ILIAC FOSSA PAIN

*Any child or adult with acute pain in the right iliac fossa should be assumed to have an **appendicitis** until proved otherwise.*

Causes
- Appendicitis
- Salpingitis, and other gynaecological disease
- Renal disease eg.
    - kidney stones
    - urinary infection
- Colitis of other causes eg.
    - worms
    - typhoid
- Orthopaedic conditions of the hip or spine
- Hernia
- Disease of scrotum or testes

LEFT ILIAC FOSSA PAIN

Causes
- Sigmoid volvulus (very common!)
- Amoebiasis
- Enema or laxative abuse
- In older people
    - diverticulitis
    - carcinoma colon
    - constipation
- Kidney disease
- Salpingitis and other gynaecological diseases
- Orthopaedic conditions
- Hernia
- Disease of scrotum or testes

SUPRA-PUBIC PAIN

Causes
- Disease of the bladder
- Disease of the genital system

COLICKY PAIN

This is a cramping pain which comes and goes.

Causes
- An obstruction or inflammation of a muscular tube causes increased peristalsis which is painful.

Affected organs
- Gall bladder eg. with cholecystitis
- Uterus eg. labour pain, abortion
- Ureters eg. when passing a kidney stone

- Excessive peristalsis of bowel in
    - gastroenteritis
    - bowel obstruction

BURNING PAIN

Causes

- It is an important symptom of disease of the upper bowel when present epigastrically, and is related to gastric acid secretion:
    - peptic ulcer disease
    - gastritis
    - reflux oesophagitis.
- Patients may have this symptom present suprapubically when passing urine. This would suggest:
    - disease of the urinary tract, especially of the urethra
    - infection of related structures such as vulva and vagina.

VAGUE ABDOMINAL PAIN

■ IN CHILDREN

Causes

- Worms
- Tuberculosis
- Urinary tract infections
- Stress and anxiety
- Lymphadenitis
- Constipation
- Food intolerance or allergy
- Abuse (physical / sexual)
- Bilharzia

Clinical features

- Small children cannot explain abdominal pain, and it is therefore poorly localised.
- A small child may also feel pain elsewhere, and just point to the abdomen as the site of the pain.
- Pain due to disease is more likely to:
    - be severe, localised and may be related to meals
    - wake the child from sleep.
- Pain due to stress (psychogenic pain):
    - is vague, poorly localised, not related to meals
    - never wakes the child
    - may have a history of previous attacks
    - these attacks last 5-30 minutes
    - there may be tenderness, but there is no muscle spasm.

Warning signs which indicate that the cause of the pain could be dangerous

- Pain lasting longer than 1-2 hours
- Pain with persistent vomiting
- Pain with diarrhoea lasting longer than 24 hours
- A raised temperature
- Getting worse

Note.

- Checking the urine and a PR examination may help in diagnosing the cause of abdominal pain.
- Always check the scrotum in boys to exclude testicular torsion or a hernia.
- The diagnosis is *clinical,* investigations do assist, but they may be misleading.

MANAGEMENT

- Observe the patient and see what happens
    - it is important to see if the symptoms get worse or better
- **REFER** for investigations
    - blood for white cell count (WCC)
    - stool - microscopy for parasites / blood (intussusception)
    - abdominal X-ray may show right iliac fossa appendicolith or impacted stool
- Treat for possible worm infestation.

■ IN ADULTS

Causes

- Laxative and enema abuse
- Drug abuse eg. alcohol or analgesics
- Gynaecological disease
- Constipation
- Worms
- Kidney disease
- Bilharzia
- Prostatic disease
- Aortic aneurysm
- Tuberculosis
- Cancer
- Psychogenic
    - fear of impotence
    - fear of cancer or AIDS
    - stress and anxiety
- Spastic colon

Note.

- Always check the scrotum in men to exclude testicular disease.
- Checking the urine and a PR examination may help in diagnosing the cause of abdominal pain.

MANAGEMENT

- Usually it can be treated symptomatically at the clinic.
- **REFER** if:
    - there are any signs of significant disease
    - there is a significant unplanned weight loss (ie. more than 5% of the total body weight).

SEVERE ABDOMINAL PAIN

Usually this will mean there is severe disease and needs
REFERRAL.

Causes

- Intestinal obstruction
- Perforated peptic ulcer
- Carcinoma of the bowel
- Volvulus of the bowel (the bowel is twisted on itself)
- Severe infection of the intestinal tract
- Peritonitis
- Strangulated inguinal or other hernia
- Aneurism (defects in vessel walls which can rupture)
- Severe urinary tract infection
- Renal calculi
- Obstetric or gynaecological disease eg.
    - ectopic pregnancy
    - labour pains
    - strangulated ovarian cyst
    - infection and inflammation

Causes outside the abdomen
- Pneumonia / pleurisy
- Coronary thrombosis (ie. myocardial infarction)
- Spinal or neurological disease
- Acute closed angle glaucoma (see page 239)
- Increased intracranial pressure

MANAGEMENT
REFER
- Patients in severe pain unless an obvious treatable cause can be found.
- If on examination there are findings of an acute abdomen (see page 105).

CHRONIC AND / OR RECURRENT ABDOMINAL PAIN

This may be due to recurrent episodes of minor disease. Generally it suggests an important cause. Usually severe disease will show progressive deterioration and other symptoms and signs eg. weight loss, anaemia etc.

Causes
In children
- Worm infestation
- Anxiety, stress and abuse (including sexual abuse)
- Urinary tract infection
- Food intolerance and allergy
- Drug abuse, especially laxatives, enemas and emetics
- Irritable bowel syndrome (IBS)
- Chronic or recurrent tonsillitis
- Diabetes
- Hepatitis
- Other infections eg. amoebiasis, tuberculosis

In adults (as in children above plus the following)
- Carcinoma
- AIDS
- Peptic ulcer disease
- Cholecystitis
- Vascular disease
- Genito-urinary
- Pancreatitis
- Gastritis secondary to alcohol, NSAIDs, laxatives
- Colitis due to laxatives / enemas
- Diverticulitis
- Amoebiasis
- Constipation
- Bilharzia

MANAGEMENT
REFER
- Unless you can treat the cause.
- If there are any associated signs such as:
    - anaemia
    - tachycardia
    - significant weight loss
    - associated chronic diarrhoea
    - constipation.

ACUTE CONSTIPATION

Causes
In neonates
- Bottle feeding
- Infrequent stools in breast fed infants may be mistaken for constipation
    - breast fed babies may only have a stool once a week or less often
    - the normal breast fed stool will be soft in consistency (the constipated stool is hard and dry)
- Rectal fissure causing severe pain on passing stool
- Intestinal obstruction

In children and adults
- Abuse of laxatives
    - diarrhoea is followed by constipation as the bowel recovers
- Travel, recent stress or change in environment
- Bowel obstruction from any cause
- Drugs such as
    - diphenoxylate (Lomotil)
    - antacids eg. aluminium hydroxide
- Low roughage diet
- Hormones in pregnancy
- Decreased bowel peristalsis in old age
- Colon carcinoma can present with alternating constipation and diarrhoea.

MANAGEMENT
Infants and small children
- Babies who are breast fed generally have normal bowel function, so encourage breast feeding and stop bottle feeding if possible.
- Increase fluids, either plain water or sugar water
    - ½ teaspoon sugar or honey in 15 ml of water 1 x daily
    - alternatively give pure fruit juice.
- Multivitamin syrup also softens the stool
- **Any neonate with bile-stained vomiting must be REFERRED stat as a possible intestinal obstruction.**

Older children
- Increase fluids
- Increase fibre (roughage) in the diet
- Glycerine suppositories may be used (stool softener)
- If constipation is very severe, **REFER** for a fleet enema

Note. Other stool softeners and purgatives are contra-indicated in children.

Adults
- Re-establish regular bowel habits
    - ensure that there is time set aside for regular defecation once the regular habits are re-established (don't rush!)
- Stop laxatives and enemas as they interfere with the normal bowel reflexes
    - in a person who has used them for a long time a milder laxative can be used temporarily.
- Ensure adequate intake of foods with high fibre content eg.
    - unpeeled fresh fruit, vegetables, brown bread, coarse mielie meal, oats, bran, etc.
- Ensure adequate fluid intake
- Encourage moderate physical exercise

Medicine management
- Lactulose, oral, 10-20 ml daily
  or
- Sennosides A and B, oral, 15 mg (2 tabs) at night 3 x a week

CHRONIC CONSTIPATION

This is an important symptom and needs investigation and **REFERRAL** *unless you can be sure of the cause.*

Causes

In neonates and young children
- Congenital bowel diseases
- Child abuse
- Behavioural problems

In the elderly
- Carcinoma of the bowel must be considered
  - especially if associated with alternating diarrhoea

Treatable causes
- Abuse of laxatives and enemas
- Low fibre diet
- Chronic use of drugs eg. morphine in terminal carcinoma.

ACUTE DIARRHOEA

Causes

In children
- This is usually due to a viral infection
- Any other systemic diseases
- Initially the breast fed infant may have frequent, loose but not offensive stools. Check that the child is well and is maintaining weight and hydration
  - if so, continue with breast feeding
  - it not, then **REFER.**
- Bacterial disease
- Parasites
- Purgatives and enemas
- Food poisoning

In adults
- Viral infections
- Medicines
- Infected food (food poisoning)
- Stress
- Bacterial infection
- Some traditional medicines / enemas (remember to ask patient).

CHRONIC DIARRHOEA

This is an important symptom.

Causes

In children
- AIDS
- Malnutrition
- Drug and enema abuse
- Normal breast fed stool mistaken for diarrhoea
- Amoebiasis
- Tuberculosis
- Worms
- Malabsorption
- Lactose intolerance
- Chronic infections such as urinary tract infection

In adults
- Carcinoma of the bowel
- GIT lymphoma
- Tuberculosis of the bowel
- AIDS
- Malnutrition
- Abuse of drugs and enemas
- Chronic stress
- Irritable bowel syndrome (IBS)
- Food intolerance (especially to milk)
- Overflow diarrhoea due to chronic constipation in elderly patients.

REFER for investigation, unless an easily treatable cause can be found.

INCONTINENCE OF FAECES

This is a surprisingly common problem.

Causes

In children
- Physical causes such as congenital abnormalities of the bowel.
- Mental retardation.
- More commonly it is due to behavioural disturbance.
- Child abuse, especially if anal sexual abuse.

In adults
- Severe constipation, especially in the elderly with overflow diarrhoea.
- Trauma due to obstetric or gynaecological disease.
- Neurological disease affecting anal tone eg. myelopathy (spinal cord damage).
- Laxative abuse.

Clinical features
- The patient and / or parents are usually embarrassed to admit to this problem.
- Direct questioning may be necessary to get details.
- The incontinence may:
  - be severe
  - only occur during the stress of coughing or laughing
  - occur only with loose stools.
- It may be primary ie. they **never** had control.
- It may be secondary ie. they had control, but for some reason control is lost.
- Stool retention may be associated with abdominal pain.

In children
- They may pass stools daily but it is an incomplete stool.
- As the problem progresses the nerve (sensory) feedback to the brain may fail and the child may be unaware of passing a stool.
- The stool retention causes increased water absorption by the large bowel, making the stools harder and harder.

Overflow incontinence
- This may occur when there is severe constipation.
- Abnormal bowel habits cause a build up of stool in the large bowel until it is over-full and starts "leaking out".

Examination

It is important to do a careful physical examination
- Exclude palpable faeces in the sigmoid which would indicate severe constipation.
- A rectal examination is vital to:
    - exclude local pathology, especially carcinoma in adults
    - check for anal tone to exclude neurological disease
    - check for constipated faeces.
- The diagnosis may be confirmed by an X-ray abdomen.

MANAGEMENT
- Treat the cause
- If you suspect it is due to a physical or psychological problem
    - **REFER** for further management
- Reassure the patient, and explain the problem
- **REFER** to special organisations
    - these help the handicapped and paraplegics
    - they have considerable experience and knowledge with this type of problem

---

ENCOPRESIS

This is the inappropriate passing of normal stools by a child. Soiling must occur at least once a month for at least 3 months, and the mental or chronological age of the child must be at least 4 years.

Causes
- Usually due to a severe behavioural disturbance.
- Physical abnormality.

Clinical features
- Typically occurs during the day.
- Associated with a conduct disorder.
- Retentive encopresis is characterised by a cycle of several days of retention, a painful expulsion, and another period of retention.
- While the faecal mass is growing, there may be leakage around the mass. A soft poorly-formed stool leaks out.
- Non-retentive encopresis is when a large well-formed stool is deposited in inappropriate places.

Etiology
- Retentive – painful defecation, inadequate or punitive toilet training, fear of school bathroom or toilet-related fears.
- Non-retentive – may be a deliberate attempt to bring about a change as a means of avoiding stressors or communicating anger.

MANAGEMENT

The investigation into the cause and the short and long term management of the problem is very involved and will need **REFERRAL** (to a special team).

A short summary is as follows:

Establish the cause
- Physical abnormality
- Emotional stress

Long-term management
- Try to find out if there are any emotional stresses and try to solve them.
- Education about bowel functioning with both parents and child.
- Treatment with laxatives – initial bowel purge, after which the child receives a daily dose of laxatives.
- Start regular bowel habit training in a firm but gentle way eg.:
    - every morning the patient must have a bowel action before going to school
    - if parents are rushed at this time, then use a time that is comfortable for everyone as long as it is the *same time every day.*
- Follow up and check progress
- Carry on until the patient has been "accident free" for about 1 year.

THE BABY WITH COLIC

Colic, like regurgitation, is commonly found in small infants, usually between the ages 10 days and 3 months.

Causes

The recurrent, sudden, abdominal pain of colic may be caused by any of the following
- Bottle feeding if the milk flow is too slow or too fast.
- Crying
    - the baby swallows air
    - this causes further crying.
- A hungry baby will suck fingers and swallow air.
- A distended breast (engorged) which means the baby cannot fix onto the nipple to release the milk from the areola. This can be managed by:
    - encouraging frequent feeding
    - expressing if the breasts are hard.
- Emotional stress which makes the colic worse eg.:
    - family tension
    - stressed mothers.
- Food intolerance:
    - this may be associated with a family history of lactose intolerance
    - some foods the mother is eating may affect the baby, eg. wheat/chocolates
- Many medications and food breakdown products are excreted in breast milk eg. laxatives and iron supplements
    - check what the mother is drinking / smoking / eating
    - check what pills she is taking.

Clinical features

There is a characteristic pattern
- There is a sudden onset of severe crying
    - this is loud and continuous
    - it usually starts soon after a feed
    - it often occurs the same time every day
- There is a distended abdomen and the legs are drawn up over the abdomen.
- The face may be flushed and the fists clenched.
- It usually stops only when the baby is exhausted.
- There is often a history of apparent relief after passing flatus or a stool.
- The baby is generally well and thriving.
- The parents may be exhausted, anxious and upset.

MANAGEMENT

Ensure there is no serious physical cause.

Treat the acute attack
- Release swallowed air by burping the baby
- Soothe the baby - rocking, walking etc.
- Keep the baby as vertical as possible
- Carry the baby on the back as this will:
    - soothe the baby
    - automatically burp the baby by the vertical position and the bouncing

Advice and reassurance
- Support and reassurance to the parents is most important
    - reassure them that it is nothing serious
    - tell them it will get better in time
- If the mother is not coping, there is a danger that she might assault the child
    - ask her if she sometimes feels like hitting the child
    - counsel her if this is a problem
- Try to help the mother to get good rest as regularly as possible
- Give advice about breast feeding methods
- Give advice about the mother's diet

Prevent further attacks
- In bottle fed babies check that the teat holes are not too small or too large
    - if a bottle of milk is held upside down, then 1 drop each second is the correct flow rate
- Suggest feeding on demand, to prevent periods of excessive hunger which causes swallowing of air.
- Educate parents on burping techniques
- Check on and correct any other causes of colic
- Avoid medication with a high sodium content (a lot of salt).
- Repeated changes in the kind of milk given to the baby is common but is usually of little help.

GASTRO-OESOPHAGEAL REFLUX DISEASE (GORD) IN CHILDREN

- If the only symptom is frequent small vomits, no investigation or treatment is needed.
- Recurrent vomiting or regurgitation requires investigation and treatment if associated with any of the following:
    - respiratory symptoms, such as recurrent wheeze or cough, recurrent aspiration, pneumonia
    - failure to thrive
    - abnormal posturing or opisthotonus

HICCOUGHS (HICCUPS)

This is due to irritation of the diaphragm.

It is usually a benign condition which lasts at most for a few hours.

If the patient has persistent hiccups, serious disease must be considered

Causes of persistent hiccups
- Subphrenic abscess
- Pancreatitis
- Abdominal distention from any cause.
- Diaphragmatic hernia.
- Infection of the diaphragm eg. due to tuberculosis.
- Carcinoma involving the nerves to the diaphragm.
- Kidney failure
    - any older adult with severe hiccups should have investigations to exclude kidney failure.
- People undergoing "Twasa", or who are traditional healers, may have hiccups as part of their practice.
- Structural lesion or infection of central nervous system.

MANAGEMENT
- The basic technique to stop hiccups is to stretch the diaphragm
    - breathe in
    - push out the stomach
    - hold the breath
- Sometimes drinking fluids may help
- Metoclopramide, oral / IM 10 mg 6 hourly as needed
- **REFER** for investigation if:
    - the hiccups persist and do not respond to simple remedies
    - serious disease is suspected.

UPPER GASTROINTESTINAL CONDITIONS

OESOPHAGUS

OESOPHAGITIS

Causes
- Candidiasis
  - **NB.** immuno-compromised patients
- Alcohol
- Reflux oesophagitis (see below)
- Corrosives eg in poisoning

Clinical features
- Odynophagia (pain on swallowing) or dysphagia of varying degrees of severity
- Retrosternal chest pain
- Heartburn - a burning sensation extending from the epigastrium to varying levels behind the sternum
- Patients with candidal oesophagitis usually also have oral thrush

---

MANAGEMENT
- Remove or treat the cause
- Candidal oesophagitis
  - give fluconazole (doctor initiated) 200 mg daily for 14 days.
- **REFER** any patient with difficulty in swallowing for more than 2 weeks, who is not obviously immuno-compromised, to exclude a carcinoma of the oesophagus.

GASTRO-OESOPHAGEAL REFLUX DISEASE (REFLUX OESOPHAGITIS)

Clinical features
- Most frequently occurs in middle aged or elderly people
- Usually obese people
- Common in pregnancy and smokers
- Heartburn is the most characteristic symptom
- There is epigastric or retrosternal pain which may radiate to
  - below the left breast
  - the back
  - the left shoulder
- Symptoms are brought on by
  - bending or lifting
  - large meals
  - lying down at night
- History of relief by antacids
- Sour taste in the mouth

MANAGEMENT
Lifestyle management
- Advise patients to sleep with the head of the bed elevated or to use extra pillows.
- Obese patients to be given a weight-reducing diet.
- Recommend small, frequent, dry meals
  - it is important that patients should avoid lying down immediately after meals.
- Advise patients to avoid bending as much as possible
  - it is important to squat when lifting heavy objects.
- Discourage the wearing of tight clothing around the stomach area.
- Smoking must be stopped

Medicine management
- Proton pump inhibitor (PPI) e.g. lansoprazole 30 mg daily for 14 days

REFERRAL
- **REFER** if no response within 7 days of starting PPI treatment.
- Presence of warning symptoms and signs:
  - weight loss
  - dysphagia
  - anaemia
  - haematemesis
  - palpable abdominal mass
- Young patients who are PPI dependent and will require life-long treatment

---

CARCINOMA OF THE OESOPHAGUS

This is a common condition and should not be missed.

Clinical features
- There may be retrosternal pain or only a feeling of retrosternal fullness.
- There will be progressive difficulty with swallowing (dysphagia)
  - firstly for large solids (ie. pieces of meat)
  - later for soft foods (porridge, mince meat)
  - finally even for liquids and saliva (late stage)
- There may be coughing on drinking liquids
  - this is a more serious sign as it indicates the development of a fistula (hole) between the oesophagus and the trachea
- Loss of weight or wasting is a late sign

REFER if
- You suspect this disease
- No acute cause for dysphagia can be found

STOMACH

GASTRITIS

Causes
- Alcohol
- Drug usage
  - salicylates particularly, but also other anti-inflammatory drugs such as indomethacin
  - Slow K
  - antibiotics (doxycycline in particular)
  - theophylline
  - iron salts
  - laxatives
  - emetics (to cause vomiting)
- Viral infections
  - viral gastroenteritis
    (particularly important in children)
  - influenza
  - viral hepatitis
- Food poisoning, particularly meat products
- Bacterial infection with Helicobacter pylori

Clinical features
- Anorexia, nausea and sometimes vomiting.
- Burning epigastric pain, not well localised
  - made worse by food
  - relieved by alkalis
- Diarrhoea is common with toxins, infection and alcohol.
- Epigastric tenderness and guarding may be present.
- Succussion splash (see page 107) will suggest
  - spasm of the pylorus
  - retained fluid in the stomach
- Chronic gynaecological or urinary disease can give referred epigastric pain, and may need to be excluded by vaginal examination and urine testing.
- Often no definite abnormal physical signs are found.

Differential diagnosis
- Consider peptic ulceration if:
  - intermittent symptoms of gastritis have been present for months or years (symptoms that come and go)
  - alcohol or drug effects have been excluded.
- In patients over 40 years, consider carcinoma of the stomach

MANAGEMENT
- Advise to stop alcohol, salicylates, laxatives and emetics.
- Other medicines should be taken with or after meals unless stated otherwise.
- Proton pump inhibitor (PPI) e.g. lansoprazole 30 mg, daily for 14 days.
- **REFER** if no response within 7 days of starting PPI treatment.

SUSPECTED PEPTIC ULCERATION

Clinical features
- Often a family history of the disease
- Well localised epigastric pain which may radiate to
  - below the costal margins
  - the back
- Relationship to food, with the onset of
  - duodenal ulcer pain, 2-3 hours after meals
  - gastric ulcer pain, within 1 hour after meals
- Duodenal ulcer pain often wakes the patient at night, usually between midnight and 02h00.
- Episodic symptoms with pain recurring at intervals of weeks or months (symptoms that come and then go away).
- Pain is usually relieved by
  - food
  - antacids
  - vomiting
- Epigastric tenderness and guarding
  - these may, however, be absent
- Alcohol and smoking make the condition worse
- Melaena stools (black tar-like stools), perhaps with features of anaemia if long-standing.

Precipitating factors
- Psychological stress
- Drug treatment
  - salicylates and other anti-inflammatory drugs
- Infection with *Helicobacter pylori*

MANAGEMENT
REFER if
- Recurrent problem
- The patient is over 40 years of age and has not been investigated
  - carcinoma of the stomach is common at this age and must be excluded by special investigations
- **No improvement after one week on treatment**
- Melaena or haematemesis is present
- Persistent vomiting
- Severe abdominal pain
- Significant weight loss
- Palpable abdominal mass

All other patients
- Advise to stop alcohol and smoking
- Avoid anti-inflammatory drugs, including aspirin
- Proton pump inhibitor (PPI) eg. lansoprazole 30 mg, daily for 14 days
- Advise regular meals
- Encourage adequate rest and recreation
- Assess psycho-social problems

CARCINOMA OF THE STOMACH

Clinical features

- Usually older than 40 years
- Upper gastrointestinal symptoms, eg. epigastric pain, anorexia, nausea, vomiting.
- Weight loss
- Palpable abdominal mass (a late sign)
- Signs of metastatic disease which include
    - hard, nodular liver
    - enlarged left supra-clavicular (Virchow's) node

REFER for admission to hospital.

INTESTINES
(SMALL AND LARGE)

THE ACUTE ABDOMEN

Any patient with an abdominal complaint and any of the following symptoms or signs should be suspected of having an acute abdomen until proved otherwise.

Clinical features

- Severe pain
    - colicky in nature
    - getting worse
- Severe vomiting
- Anorexia
- Severe constipation or obstipation (no stools passed)
- Not passing flatus
- Haematemesis or melaena
- Decreased urine output
- The patient is ill, distressed, pale or shocked
- High fever, high pulse and rapid respiratory rate
- Evidence of acidosis (tachypnoea, dehydration, restlessness)
- Tongue dry or coated suggests significant bowel disease
- Abdominal distension
- Guarding, rigidity and rebound tenderness
    - if a patient is markedly tender on light palpation of the umbilicus, it suggests peritonitis
- Bowel sounds decreased or absent.
- Stools with changed blood or significant amounts of blood.

Note.
- *PV, PR and urine testing may often give valuable information in a suspected acute abdomen.*
    NB. Exclude a strangulated hernia.
- *Young children and the elderly often show minimal symptoms or signs of an acute abdomen.*
- *Even minor symptoms or signs in these groups should be viewed with great care.*

- Put up a drip
- **REFER** stat

APPENDICITIS

Inflammation of the appendix is a common problem in children and young adults.

The cause is not clear but appears to be related to a low fibre diet.

Clinical features

- *It is the most common intestinal problem of childhood that requires surgery*
- The usual age is 4-12 years but it can occur at any age
- In babies, small children, pregnant women and old people, the signs may not be typical
- Pain starts peri-umbilically
- After a few hours to a few days, the pain moves to the right iliac fossa where it persists
- Vomiting usually not severe
- Nausea and malaise
- Constipation is usual
- Fever
    - low grade 37,5° - 38,5°C
    - a higher fever is suggestive of a perforation of the appendix with peritonitis
- The patient often walks doubled up with pain
- Guarding with localised tenderness over McBurney's point (right iliac fossa - RIF)
- Psoas sign where extension of the right hip joint causes RIF pain
- Obturator sign where external rotation of the hip joint causes RIF pain
- PR may be very tender on the right side of the rectum

*NB. **Any** patient with pain or tenderness in the right iliac fossa must be considered to have an appendicitis until proved otherwise*

In pregnancy, diagnosis is more difficult.

- The appendix is carried high as the uterus enlarges
- As localization of the pain in the RIF may **not** occur, look for
    - Murphy's triad - pain, fever and localised abdominal tenderness means appendicitis
    - pain shifts, made worse by movement
    - pain wakes patient from sleep or prevents sleep
    - vomiting
    - anorexia
    - guarding

Causes of missed appendicitis

- Signs not in the right iliac fossa
- Tissue interposition
- Patient younger than 5 years old
- Retarded patient
- Pelvic, retrocolic or retrocaecal positions of the appendix
- Pregnancy
- Elderly patient

Differential diagnosis

- Mesenteric adenitis
- Pyelonephritis
- Pneumonia
- Gastroenteritis
- Primary peritonitis
- Ectopic pregnancy
- Salpingitis
- Ruptured ovarian cyst
- Ovarian torsion
- Deep iliac lymphadenitis

> **MANAGEMENT**
>
> *If appendicitis is suspected*
> - Put up a drip of 5% dextrose water
> - Keep patient nil per mouth
> - **REFER** stat for possible surgery
>   - the prognosis is excellent with early surgery

IRRITABLE BOWEL SYNDROME

This is motility disturbance of the entire GIT. Also known as spastic colon.

Clinical features

- It presents in children as well as in adults.
- It may start as early as 1 year old but is more often seen in teenagers.
- Characterised by some combination of:
    - abdominal pain
    - constipation and / or diarrhoea
    - flatulence and excessive mucus in the stools
    - dyspeptic symptoms (bloating, nausea)
    - varying degrees of anxiety or depression.
- Variable abdominal tenderness, particularly along the course of the colon.
- Often mild abdominal distension.
- Children usually gain weight and grow normally.

Differential diagnosis

- Food intolerance
- Urinary tract infection
- Abuse (physical / sexual)
- Pelvic inflammatory disease (PID)
- Carcinoma
- Diverticulitis / diverticulosis
- Enema or laxative abuse
- Worms (see page 119)
- Stress and anxiety
- Alcohol / drug abuse

> **MANAGEMENT**
>
> - Do a full urinary and GIT examination.
> - Try to remove any possible emotional stress.
> - A high-fibre diet may help in patients with constipation.
> - Hyoscine butylbromide (Buscopan) 10 mg 3 x daily may be used for relief of spasm if required.
> - Laxatives only for those who are constipated.
> - Give anti-diarrhoea medication only for those who have diarrhoea.
> - Give reassurance that the symptoms are not due to an organic disease.
> - Anxiety or depression should be treated appropriately
>   - **REFER** if this is a significant problem.
> - Tricyclic antidepressants may be used as additional therapy
>   - amitriptylline 25-75 mg nocte
>   - titrate dose as appropriate
> - Eliminate any food suspected of contributing to the symptoms and monitor the response.

DIARRHOEAL CONDITIONS

DIARRHOEA AND VOMITING

Children commonly present with diarrhoea and vomiting.

Causes
- The usual cause is a viral infection
    - however other serious diseases also present with these common symptoms eg. meningitis
    - it is therefore essential to look for these before you diagnose the child as having gastroenteritis
- Other important aspects which should be evaluated are the nutritional status. If a child is failing to grow well, this means
    - the resistance will be lower
    - the effects of the gastroenteritis will be more devastating
- Beware of a child with recurrent gastroenteritis. This may be due to:
    - lowered resistance
    - AIDS
    - the child being in the dangerous situation of recurrent infection, decreasing nutrition and lowered resistance.
- In neonates, virtually any illness may present with diarrhoea and vomiting

All systems of the child should be fully examined to exclude causes outside the intestine.

Note. *Mothers who bring children in with gastroenteritis often say that there is blood and mucus in the stool. Generally this is not serious.*

FEATURES SUGGESTING A SERIOUS CAUSE

- Severe colicky pain suggesting
    - intussusception
    - intestinal obstruction
- Profuse, watery diarrhoea with evidence of shock suggesting
    - cholera
    - toxins
    - shigella
- Evidence of moderately heavy blood-staining of the stool suggesting
    - intussusception
    - toxins
    - amoebiasis
- Fresh blood may be due to a local colitis, or an anal fissure (see page 123)
- High fever suggests Salmonella or Shigella infection which may be associated with
    - fits
    - evidence of severe dehydration
    - an obviously ill child
- Blood-staining of the stools with a lot of mucus which could be
    - intussusception
    - amoebiasis
    - damage due to enemas
- Localised tenderness or guarding suggests
    - local peritonitis eg. due to perforation and should be **REFERRED**
- Chronic or persistent diarrhoea which may be due to
    - AIDS
    - tuberculosis
    - malnutrition
    - lactose intolerance
    - urinary tract infection

Succussion splash
- To test for this, place your ear close to the child's abdomen and gently shake the abdomen.
- If there is a large amount of fluid in any part of the gut, due to delay in peristalsis or absorption, you will be able to hear it splashing.

ACUTE DIARRHOEA IN CHILDREN

MANAGEMENT
Prevention
- It is very important to have a good knowledge of ways in which gastroenteritis (GE) can be prevented.
    - this forms an essential part of the education of all mothers with babies and young children.
- The most effective way of preventing gastroenteritis is to ensure that the baby is given only breast milk for at least the first 4 months.
    - breast fed babies are *not* subjected to unhygienic food preparation methods.
    - breast milk contains antibodies that protect babies against infection.
- Beware of the "Triple Nipple Syndrome" This is when the mother is supplementing the breast with water by means of bottle or cup in a normal healthy baby
    - *there is no need for water supplementation, and this practice should be **strongly discouraged.***
- Personal, food and toilet hygiene should be encouraged as far as is possible. Be careful not to make the mother.
    - feel that it is all her fault
    - feel inadequate
    - spend a lot of limited money on expensive hygiene methods.
- It has been shown that adequate intake of Vitamin A helps prevent infections, including gastroenteritis.
    - this is found in yellow vegetables.

If breast feeding is not possible
- If for some reason breast feeding is not possible and the child is being bottle fed, encourage the best hygiene possible in the mother's circumstances.
- As a general rule it is safer and more hygienic to feed a baby with a cup and spoon rather than a bottle.

Sterilising bottles and teats
- Milton is useful for sterilising
    - but it allows Candida overgrowth

- The following is an acceptable method
  - wash the bottles and teats
  - rub the teats with salt
  - boil the bottles and teats in boiling water for 10-15 minutes

HOW TO MAINTAIN HYDRATION AT HOME

- Encourage mothers to start with homemade sugar and salt solution (SSS) as soon as the child starts vomiting or has diarrhoea
  - this will prevent dehydration and serious illness
  - tell her that SSS will not **stop** the diarrhoea.
- The normal course of the illness is 4-5 days, and she only needs to worry if:
  - the child's condition becomes unsatisfactory
  - the illness persists
  - there is persistent vomiting.
- Milk (especially breast milk) is excellent as a rehydration fluid.
- Encourage the mother to give fluids by cup and spoon, and not by bottle.
- Milk intolerance is not common and is over-diagnosed. Lactose intolerance is not usually dangerous in a PHC situation. It needs no special treatment, as the child will usually recover the enzymes in a few days provided you:
  - ensure adequate hydration
  - give the child adequate nutrition during the diarrhoea.
- The children most at risk are those with chronic diarrhoea, malnutrition or lowered resistance eg. AIDS.
- Continue with small frequent meals of any foods that the child will accept.

SUGAR SALT SOLUTION (SSS)

Constituents

Fluid

- This is to replace the water lost from the body.

Sugar and salt

- This is vital for the absorption of water.
- Without sugar and salt the bowel lacks the energy to actively absorb any fluid, no matter how much water is given.
- It is therefore better to have too much sugar, rather than too little, in the SSS.
- *But too much salt is dangerous.*

Orange juice

- Add freshly squeezed orange juice if possible
  - it is rich in potassium, which is one of the most important electrolytes lost
  - it makes the fluid taste much nicer, and encourages the child to drink more
  - it supplies glucose and vitamins

SSS can easily be made up using the following recipe

- *1 litre water*
- *8 level teaspoons of sugar or honey*
- *½ teaspoon salt*

This can be mixed with some freshly squeezed orange juice if available.

It is unnecessary to boil the water if it is:

- Tap water from a municipal main supply
- Water from a protected source
- Water from a well

If the water is not clean:

- To purify water domestic non-perfumed bleach can be added.
- This takes 2 hours
  - add 5 ml bleach to 25 litres of water
- However, if this is not available, the mother must *not* withhold water
  - even if she suspects it is contaminated
  - what is needed is the fluid!
- **The child may die from dehydration if fluids are not given**

The rural alternative to this recipe, if no utensils for measuring are available:

- 1 cup water
- 2 level teaspoons of sugar
- 1 pinch salt

Mix with freshly squeezed orange juice (if available).

Teaching method

- The best way to teach the mother how to make up the SSS and give it to her child, is for her to do it *herself* while you are watching.
- If possible have the constituents available in your clinic.
- If you have a written hand-out to give the mother, this can be a great help, especially if it has pictures.
- Fluid that is too salty will cause vomiting
  - *rehydration fluid should never be more salty than tears.*
- Too much sugar is **not** likely to make diarrhoea worse, so do not worry about it.
- The fact that the SSS does not **stop** the diarrhoea will often make the mother anxious
  - reassure her that the diarrhoea will take time to improve
  - explain that the SSS will **prevent** dehydration if she uses it properly.

How much and how often

- Fluids should be given as often as the child will tolerate them.
- **A recommended amount of 10 ml / kg should be given with each loose stool.**
- If the child cannot take much fluid at a time, encourage the mother to give a small amount as often as possible.

HOW TO REHYDRATE A CHILD AT A CLINIC

Assess hydration

Severe dehydration (2 of the signs below)	Some dehydration (2 of the signs below)
• lethargic or unconscious	• restless or irritable
• eyes sunken, dry mouth	• eyes sunken, dry mouth
• drinks poorly or not able to drink	• thirsty, drinks eagerly
• severe decrease in skin turgor – skin pinch returning over 2 seconds or more	• moderate decrease in skin turgor – skin pinch returning in less than 2 seconds

Fluid management

Severe dehydration
- Give rapidly:
    - normal saline, IV, 20 ml / kg
    - repeat up to twice if radial pulse is weak or undetectable
- Continue with 20 ml / kg every hour for the next 5 hours.
- **REFER** urgently for continued management unless the child is reclassified as "Some dehydration" (see below).
- As soon as the child can drink, also give ORS eg Sorol solution 5 ml / kg / hour.
- If IV administration is not possible, insert a nasogastric tube.
- While waiting and during urgent transfer give:
    - ORS, 20 ml / kg / hour via the nasogastric tube
- If only oral administration is possible and the child is not improving, transfer the child urgently giving ORS during transfer 20 ml / kg / hour.

Some dehydration
- Give:
    - ORS eg Sorol solution, 80 ml / kg over 4 hours (10 ml / kg every 30 minutes)
    - give more if the child wants it
- If the child vomits, wait 10 minutes and then continue more slowly
- Show caregiver how to give ORS with a cup and spoon using frequent small sips.
- Encourage caregiver to continue feeding the child (especially breast feeding).
- Encourage caregiver to give 10 ml / kg after each diarrhoea stool until the diarrhoea stops.
- Continue at home and instruct caregiver on how to make the SSS at home.

Indications for IV infusion
- Severe dehydration
- The child is unable to take oral fluids
- The condition is deteriorating, despite oral fluids
- Symptoms or signs suggesting ileus
    - severe vomiting
    - distended abdomen
    - no bowel sounds heard

SOLID FEEDING
- Solids should **not** be stopped even if the gastroenteritis is severe.
- Children, particularly if they are malnourished, desperately need whatever food and nutrition they can get, even though some is lost in the diarrhoea
    - the child needs the food to have the energy to fight the diarrhoea
    - not giving food may delay healing.
- Give any type of solids that the child will tolerate
- Solids which are good are
    - carrots and any yellow vegetable as Vitamin A may help with viral diseases
    - apples
    - bananas
    - *any* available foods should be given.
- Encourage the mother to give small, frequent feeds.

MEDICINE MANAGEMENT
NB. "Anti-diarrhoea" agents such as loperamide (Imodium) or kaolin-pectin do not stop gastroenteritis.

- Anti-diarrhoea agents only *stop* the diarrhoea stools from being passed
    - the water and electrolytes are still lost to the body as they are pooled in the intestine
    - ie. these medicines do not put the fluid back into the body
- *These medicines can cause a false sense of security*
    - *you think the diarrhoea is better, therefore, rehydration fluids are stopped*
    - *but the fluid is still lost into the lumen of the gut resulting in continued dehydration*

Antibiotics
- More than 90% of gastroenteritis is caused by viral infections
    - so avoid antibiotics, unless you suspect a bacterial infection, eg. Shigella or Salmonella
- Antibiotics may aggravate diarrhoea
- In all children who are able to take oral medication, give zinc acetate
    - <10 kg 10 mg / day
    - >10 kg 20 mg / day

WHEN TO ALLOW A CHILD HOME
The child can go home when:
- Taking the calculated volumes of fluids adequately.
- The hydration is satisfactory or improving.
- Vomiting has stopped.

The mother should bring the child back:
- If the condition does not steadily keep improving.
- If the diarrhoea gets worse or carries on longer than one week.
- If the child is malnourished and needs regular follow up
- If the vomiting recurs.
- If the mother is worried.

PERSISTENT DIARRHOEA IN CHILDREN

MANAGEMENT
- Prevent dehydration, using sugar salt solution (SSS) - see page 108.
- Counsel mother regarding feeding
    - if breastfeeding, give more frequent, longer feeding
    - if replacement feeding, replace milk with fermented milk products such as amasi, yoghurt, or lactose-free milk formula
- Continue with solids
    - give small, frequent meals at least 6 times a day
- Follow up after 1 week.
- **REFER** if diarrhoea persists.

ACUTE DIARRHOEA IN ADULTS

MANAGEMENT

The management of gastroenteritis is by fluid replacement to treat and prevent dehydration

- Give oral rehydration formula eg Soral powder to prepare at home or instruct the patient how to make sugar and salt solution (SSS) at home (see page 108).
- For more severe diarrhoea, especially if prolonged
    - give loperamide, orally, 4 mg immediately
    - then 2 mg as required after each loose stool (maximum 12 mg daily)
    - **NB Do not give in dysentery.**
- Solids can be given if the patient can tolerate them.
- Consider antibiotics if you suspect a bacterial cause (dysentery-blood and / or mucus in the stool).
- Give metoclopramide IV / oral 10 mg 6-8 hourly
    - for significant nausea and vomiting

REFER if:
- The patient is unable to take oral fluids adequately
- You suspect a serious underlying cause eg. cholera, typhoid
- Significantly dehydrated ie.
    - poor volume pulse
    - low BP
    - decreased tissue turgor
    - shock
    - acidosis
    - very low urine output
- There is severe vomiting
- Significant amounts of blood in the stools
- There is peritonism
- There is a distended abdomen
- The patient is vomiting bile

Severe dehydration
- Start IV therapy
    - normal saline
    - **or** dextrose saline

CHRONIC DIARRHOEA IN ADULTS

This is diarrhoea lasting more than 2 weeks. The majority may be HIV related. Giardiasis is a common cause (see opposite).

MANAGEMENT
- Send a stool sample for microscopy for ova, cysts and parasites.

HIV negative
- Give empiric treatment for giardiasis unless this has already been done (see page 111).
- Give loperamide, oral 2 mg 3-4 x daily as required
    - maximum 8 mg (4 tablets) daily
- **REFER** all cases with
    - no pathogen identified and significant diarrhoea

HIV positive
- See page 158.

INTUSSUSCEPTION

Clinical features
- Age 3-18 months
- It is slightly more common in males
- There is sudden abdominal colicky pain
    - the child screams and draws up the knees for 1-2 minutes
    - the child then becomes quiet for about 15 minutes
    - then there is a repeat episode of screaming etc.
- There may be abdominal tenderness and bile-stained vomit
- The child may pass red-currant jelly-like mucus.
- The child may show systemic signs of illness eg.:
    - tachycardia
    - pallor
    - signs of shock
- The abdomen may be distended
- Sometimes a palpable mass may be felt in the epigastric or left colonic areas.
- Rectal examination may occasionally reveal a protruding mass of intestine through the anus.
- Bowel sounds

MANAGEMENT
- *If you suspect this diagnosis, **REFER** stat as early correction has an excellent prognosis.*
- **Delay can result in the child's death**
- Put up an IV drip of normal saline at a rate of 120 ml / kg in 24 hours (ie. 5 ml / kg / hour).

ENEMA ABUSE

There may be damage or perforation of the bowel due to enema abuse.

Clinical features
- The mother may or may not admit to using enemas or traditional medicines.
- Damage or perforation should be suspected if:
    - the child is more ill than expected
    - there are any signs of an acute abdomen
    - there is profuse fresh rectal bleeding.

- **REFER**
- Put up an IV drip of normal saline at a rate of 120 ml / kg / 24 hours.

TYPHOID

Clinical features

An ill patient for no other reason
- High fever with no apparent cause
- Severe headache, especially in adults
- There may be mental confusion or convulsions

- Cough may be an early symptom
- Abdominal pain
- Early intestinal symptoms may include constipation (especially in adults) or diarrhoea that is mild (in children)
- Muscle and joint pains
- Recent contact with a known typhoid patient, or recent return from an area where there is typhoid
- A comparatively slower pulse than would be expected for the temperature, particularly in adults
- There may be a red macular rash in the first week known as "rose spots"
- Hepatosplenomegaly is usually present
- Signs of an acute abdomen (due to perforation) are late
- Typhoid is a difficult diagnosis to confirm clinically
    - often it is only confirmed on blood tests

> - **This is a notifiable disease.**
> - Treat dehydration if present.
> - **REFER** if you suspect it.

DYSENTERY

This is diarrhoea with blood and/or mucus.

Causes
- Shigella
- Salmonella
- Campylobacter
- E. coli

Clinical features
- Sudden onset of diarrhoea with blood or mucus in the stools
- Fever
- Lower abdominal pain and tenderness especially left iliac fossa
- In children meningism and convulsions may occur.

NB. It is important to exclude intussusception in children. Evidence of this includes:
- Pain and abdominal tenderness
- Bile-stained vomitus
- Red-currant jelly-like mucus in stools
- Appearance of the intussusceptum at the anus

> ### MANAGEMENT
> - Treat dehydration if present
> - If not severely ill:
>   - *adults:* ciprofloxacin 500 mg 2 x daily for 3 days
>   - *children over 1 year old:* ciprofloxacin 15 mg / kg / dose 2 x daily for 3 days
>   - 12-18 months: 150 mg
>   - 18 months-3 years: 200 mg
>   - 3-5 years: 250 mg
>   - 5-7 years: 300 mg
>   - 7-15 years: 500 mg
>
> ### REFER
> - Severe illness
> - Severe dehydration
> - Acute abdominal signs (severe pain and tenderness, bile-stained or persistent vomiting)
> - Failure to respond within 3 days
> - Children less than 12 months of age

GIARDIASIS

Clinical features
- May be asymptomatic but upper intestinal manifestations are common.
- Diarrhoea, abdominal pain, bloating, belching, flatulence, nausea and vomiting.
- This infection is more common in children with lowered resistance
    - eg. malnutrition
- The stools are grey in colour, bulky, greasy, frothy and smell offensive as there is malabsorption.
- The burping may also be offensive (sulfurous).
- It causes a prolonged diarrhoea in adults and children which does not respond to normal conservative management.

> ### MANAGEMENT
> Giardiasis may be difficult to diagnose on stool microscopy therefore empiric treatment is recommended.
> - Give metronidazole 2 g daily for 3 days
>   - or 400 mg 3 x daily for 5 days.
> - Children 7,5 mg / kg / dose 3 x daily for 5-7 days
> - **REFER** is there is no improvement.

CHOLERA

Clinical features
- Occurs in epidemics
- Acute onset of very severe diarrhoea with frequent, watery stools (up to 1 litre per hour).
- The liquid stool is grey, without faecal colour, blood or pus ("rice water stool").
- Severe dehydration and shock
- No major systemic signs, and no marked abdominal signs.
- The diagnosis is confirmed by laboratory investigation.

> ### MANAGEMENT
> - **This is a notifiable disease.**
> - Replacement of fluids is the most important part of treatment.
> - In mild cases, **oral** rehydration may be adequate.
> - In severe cases or patient in shock, intravenous rehydration is necessary
>   - put up IV line (normal saline) at the clinic.
> - **REFER** for admission.
>
> ### Medicine management
> *Adults*
> - Ciprofloxacin, oral, 1 g as a single dose
> - **NB** Loperamide is contraindicated as it may result in toxic megacolon.
>
> *Children*
> - Ciprofloxacin, 20 mg / kg, oral, as a single dose

MALNUTRITION

- *There are many syndromes of malnutrition depending on the type of deficiency in the diet ie.*
    - energy (or calorie) deficiency
    - protein deficiency
    - both energy and protein deficiency
- These syndromes are the most common cause of failure to thrive.
- In children, malnutrition occurs typically in pre-school (6 months-5 years)
    - but it can occur in any age
- These children are prone to infections, especially of the respiratory and gastrointestinal systems.

Risk factors
- Low socio-economic status or poverty
- Broken homes
- Large number of children in the family
- Poor education
- Expense of high protein foods
- Cheaper refined carbohydrate foods
- Drought or famine

PROTEIN ENERGY MALNUTRITION (PEM)

■ UNDERWEIGHT

This is the most common presentation and most frequently missed.

Clinical features
- Underweight and undersize but with normal proportions (weight : height ratio)
- No other specific clinical signs, except prone to infections
    - gastroenteritis
    - respiratory disease
    - tuberculosis
    - measles

Differential diagnosis
- It is important to look for other causes of the drop in weight
    - unless these are treated, diet alone will not correct the problem
- These causes may be
    - tuberculosis
    - urinary tract infection
    - HIV / AIDS
    - heart disease
    - child and sex abuse

Investigations
Useful investigations are PPD test and urine test for nitrites, blood and protein to detect possible urinary tract infection or sexual abuse.

MANAGEMENT
REFER any child with the following:
- Not responding to clinic treatment
- Severe weight loss below the 60% expected weight line
- Where you feel the child needs more than clinic management.

■ KWASHIORKOR

This is a severe form of PEM.

Causes
- It occurs often after weaning from the breast / bottle (9 months-2 years) if the diet is deficient in milk or other protein.

Clinical features
- Anorexia (loss of appetite)
- Low weight
- Muscle wasting
    - the child is unable to walk, sit or hold head up
- Oedema of dorsum of feet or over lower tibia
    - beware of false chubby appearance
- Skin lesions
    - pellagra-like
    - pigmentation, desquamation (peeling), depigmentation, ulceration
    - can look similar to burns if severe
    - occur in **both** exposed and unexposed areas
    - perineum and buttocks affected in toddlers
- Mouth
    - reddening
    - smooth tongue
    - fissures at mouth corners (angular stomatitis)
- Hair
    - sparse, thin, easily pulled out
    - colour change (reddish or grey)
- Eyes - xerophthalmia
- Mental and neurological changes
    - irritability
    - apathy (not playing)
    - occasionally parkinsonian-like tremors
- Hepatomegaly
- Paleness (anaemia)
- Diarrhoea
- Infections
    - pneumonia
    - septicaemia
    - gastroenteritis

Poor prognosis if the following are present
- Severe infection
- Hypothermia
- Hypoglycaemia
- Jaundice
- Dehydration with collapse

MARASMUS

Causes
- This occurs when the diet is deficient in energy foods
    - ie. the child is not getting enough food (starvation)
- Insufficient breast milk or dilute bottle feeds

Clinical features
- Common during the first year of life
- Irritability or apathy
- Diarrhoea, acid stools
- Children are usually very hungry, but some are anorexic
- Child has a shrunken appearance (no subcutaneous fat)
- Less that 60% of weight for age
- Muscles are weak
- Skin, hair and mucous membrane lesions and oedema **not** usually present.

Differential diagnosis
- HIV
- Tuberculosis
- Syphilis
- Tropical infestations

MARASMIC KWASHIORKOR

This term is used to describe those children with a variety of clinical features typical of both marasmus and kwashiorkor.

MANAGEMENT OF MALNUTRITION
- **REFER** severely malnourished children (ie. many clinical features present).

Mild cases of malnutrition
- They can be treated at the clinic
- These are the children who are found to be underweight, but are not ill enough to need admission.
- They are at risk from infections (eg. gastroenteritis).
- These children need adequate amounts of protein and energy foods.
- The normal diet should be gradually increased by adding extra meals (one or two) per day, as the child may be unable to tolerate a large meal at one time.
- Staple food such as maize, bread or rice should be supplemented by milk, meat, egg or fish if available.
- Otherwise vegetable proteins can be used to supplement the staple food eg. beans, peas, lentils, peanuts (peanut butter).
- Protein intake required
    - full cream milk is good to cover a child's basic protein requirements
- Encourage foods with high calories such as
    - margarine, butter or any oil eg. fish, olive, sunflower
    - fried foods
    - peanuts
- Give Vitamin A orally
    - infants 0-5 months: 50 000 units
    - 6-12 months: 100 000 units
    - 1 year and older: 200 000 units

LIVER, GALL BLADDER, PANCREAS AND SPLEEN

LIVER PROBLEMS

JAUNDICE

Many conditions of the blood, liver, gall bladder and pancreas present with jaundice. For guidelines on neonatal jaundice see Neonatal conditions (page 354).

There are three types: *pre-hepatic, hepatic and post-hepatic.*

■ PRE-HEPATIC

Causes
- Haemolysis ie. Increased destruction of red blood cells (usually associated with marked anaemia) due to:
    - infections such as septicaemia and malaria
    - inherited disorders like sickle cell anaemia
    - drugs
    - auto-immune conditions.

■ HEPATIC

Causes
- Liver infections such as viral hepatitis
- Congenital abnormalities
- Alcohol-induced hepatitis
- Drug-induced hepatitis e.g. INH, methyl-dopa, nevirapine
- Kwashiorkor - if a child with kwashiorkor has jaundice as well, it is a very poor prognostic sign
- Cirrhosis with liver failure
- Hepatoma - end stage

■ POST-HEPATIC

Causes
- Obstruction in the biliary tree (cholangiocarcinoma)
- Gallstones
- Carcinoma of the pancreas
- Vanishing bile duct syndrome (HIV/AIDS)

Clinical features
- Jaundice usually presents as a yellow discolouration of the skin, sclera, nails and mucous membranes.
- The best place to detect early or mild jaundice is:
    - under the tongue
    - on the floor of the mouth.
- As jaundice progresses, the skin of the nose and the sclera of the eyes also show evidence of jaundice.
- Severe jaundice covers the entire body
- Pale stools or dark urine may also be noticed by the patient

MANAGEMENT
Jaundice is an important sign, and generally means the patient needs **REFERRAL**.
Note. All patients with jaundice **must** be **REFERRED** to exclude serious causes.

VIRAL HEPATITIS

This is an acute contagious inflammation of the liver, often associated with jaundice, caused by a number of specific viruses.

The well-known viruses causing hepatitis are:
- Hepatitis A virus (HAV)
- Hepatitis B virus (HBV)
- Hepatitis C virus (HCV)
- Hepatitis E virus (HEV)

Clinical features
The following are common features to all types
- Symptoms of upper respiratory tract infection ("flu"-like)
- Fever, chills, malaise, headache and joint pains
- Anorexia, often severe
- Nausea, sometimes vomiting
- A dislike of cigarette smoke and fatty foods
- Right hypochondrial tenderness and pain
    - may only occur a few days after the onset of symptoms
- Pale stools and dark urine
- Often hepatomegaly
- Jaundice
- With the onset of jaundice
    - the *stools* usually become *pale* grey-white due to a lack of bile pigment
    - the *urine* becomes *dark* with bilirubin and urobilinogen
    - pruritis (itching) of the skin

Differential diagnosis
- Other infections such as amoebiasis, cytomegalovirus, glandular fever etc.
- Toxins eg. alcohol
- Drugs
- Obstructive disorders of the bile ducts (eg. gallstones)
- Neoplasms
- Congenital abnormalities
- Malaria

Complications
- Bleeding disorders, because the liver is unable to make sufficient prothrombin.
- Liver failure
- Chronic hepatitis (HBV and HCV viruses)
- Cirrhosis (HBV and HCV viruses)
- Hepatoma (primary carcinoma of the liver) due to HBV virus

Investigations
- Liver function tests to demonstrate elevated bilirubin and transaminases
- Hepatitis antigens and antibiotics:
    - to identify the viral type
    - and later to determine if the patient is recovering or is developing chronic hepatitis and a chronic carrier state

MANAGEMENT

All cases must be notified.

The following measures should be taken for viral hepatitis

- The patient usually knows what foods will make him nauseous and he should be allowed to choose what he wants to eat
    - in general, fruit, fruit juices and fat free soups, such as chicken soup, are fairly well tolerated
- Avoid drugs metabolised in the liver such as sedatives, analgesics, methyldopa, oral contraceptives.
- Careful disposal of faeces and washing of hands after handling excreta.
- Bed rest
    - if febrile
    - in the elderly
- Give Vitamin B Co. and multivites
- Avoid alcohol
- **REFER** for investigation

REFER for admission if

- Patient has signs of liver failure e.g. drowsiness, confusion
- There is severe vomiting
- There is severe abdominal pain
- Any patient who has mild hepatitis but is not improving after 2-3 weeks of observation.

NB. Hepatitis B can be prevented by immunisation. Try to ensure that all children are fully immunised.

- Recommended also for spouses of hepatitis B carriers if they are sero-negative

Hepatitis in children

- In children, the most common cause is hepatitis A
    - exclude other serious causes
- Hepatitis A can be treated at home unless it becomes complicated
- Tell the family to bring the child back if:
    - child becomes worse
    - child has severe vomiting
    - child becomes confused
    - there is severe anorexia
    - the jaundice persists more than 10 days.
- Give vitamins
- Encourage a high calorie diet if possible, and avoid excessive protein, fats and oils.
- Encourage good hygiene to prevent spread to other family members.

▼ **Note to doctor**

Interpretation of hepatitis investigations

Hepatitis A
- anti-HAV IgM positive

Hepatitis B
- Acute hepatitis
    - HBsAg (hepatitis B surface antigen) positive
    - HBcAb (hepatitis B core antibody) IgM or HBcAb total (i.e. IgM + IgG) positive during and for approximately 6 months after acute infection.
- Recovery from infection
    - HBsAb (hepatitis B surface antibody) positive
    - HBcAb IgG positive
    - HBsAg negative
- Late acute and chronic hepatitis
    - HBcAb (predominantly IgG) positive
    - HBsAg positive
- Immunisation
    - HBsAb positive (protective antibody)

Hepatitis C
- HC antibody positive ▲

CIRRHOSIS

Cirrhosis of the liver is a chronic destructive process of the liver.

Causes

- Chronic alcohol abuse
- Complication of hepatitis B or C
- In childhood as a result of certain biochemical disorders (this is rare)

Clinical features

- More commonly found from middle age
- Gastritis / epigastric pain, anorexia, nausea and occasionally, vomiting
- Dark pigmentation of the skin in sun-exposed areas
- Palmar erythema
- Impotence
- Peripheral neuropathy
- Mentally dull (if liver failure)
- Weakness, fatigue, weight loss and wasting
- Right hypochondrial abdominal pain
- Diarrhoea is frequently present
- Jaundice occurs late
- Digital clubbing
- Hepatomegaly (firm to hard and with a blunt or nodular edge)
- Splenomegaly may be present
- Ascites
- Pedal oedema
- Distended abdominal veins
- Testicular atrophy and gynaecomastia
- Spider naevi (in less pigmented patients)
- Bruising / bleeding tendency
- Liver failure, encephalopathy, flapping tremor, confusion
- Haematemesis is often a presenting symptom

MANAGEMENT

Cirrhosis of the liver is a permanent destruction of liver tissue and there is no effective treatment.

- The PHC sister should explain to the patient
    - the nature of the disease
    - that drinking alcohol **must stop** to prevent further hepatic destruction
- Nutritional advice may be required
- Vitamin supplementation is often needed
- If ascites is present
    - **REFER** for prescription of spironolactone (Aldactone) and furosemide (Lasix) and low dose beta-blocker
- Encourage them to go to Alcoholics Anonymous (AA) or South African National Council on Alcoholism and Drug Dependence (SANCA).

REFER
- All newly diagnosed cases
- Any patients in whom the condition deteriorates (such as gastrointestinal bleeding or liver failure)

GALL BLADDER PROBLEMS

- The most important disease is cholecystitis (ie. inflammation of the gall bladder) which is often secondary to gallstones.
- Many people have gallstones which are asymptomatic
- However, one of these may block the cystic duct and infection develops behind the obstruction.

CHOLECYSTITIS

Clinical features

- Patients are often fat, female, and about 40 years of age
- There is right hypochondrial pain often radiating to the interscapular area
- Nausea
- Vomiting
- Fever
- Fatty intolerance
- Flatulence
- Shoulder tip pain
    - due to irritation underneath the diaphragm
- Dark urine with bilirubin and urobilinogen on urine dipstix
- Right hypochondrial tenderness, worse with palpation during inspiration.
- Jaundice usually not present

> **REFER** for investigation and possible cholecystectomy.

BILE DUCT STONES

Clinical features

- Characterised by biliary colic
- Frequently recurring attacks of right hypochondrial pain
- Severe pain that persists for hours
- Pain may radiate to interscapular area
- Chills and fever
- Jaundice
- Right hypochondrial tenderness
- Hepatomegaly may be present

> **REFER**

PANCREAS PROBLEMS

ACUTE PANCREATITIS

Clinical features

- Epigastric pain
    - generally abrupt in onset
    - following alcohol
- Pain characteristically radiates through to the back
    - but may radiate to the left or the right
- Pain often made worse by:
    - lying supine
    - walking
- Pain relieved by:
    - crouching (kneeling down)
    - leaning forward
- Nausea and vomiting are frequently present
- May be shocked in severe cases
- Upper abdominal tenderness
- Guarding, rigidity and rebound are often mild though pain is severe
- Abdomen may be distended and bowel sounds may be absent in associated paralytic ileus.
- If it is severe:
    - the patient will be distressed, sweating and anxious
    - severe pain, guarding, rebound
    - vomiting and anorexia
    - pyrexia, tachycardia, hypotension
    - may be shocked with cool, clammy skin.

> **MANAGEMENT**
>
> *If mild*
> - Advise nutritious well balanced diet.
> - Advise strict alcohol avoidance.
> - Proton pump inhibitor (PPI) eg. lansoprazole 30 mg daily for 14 days.
> - Give paracetamol 2 tabs 3 x daily.
> - Hyoscine (Buscopan) 10-20 mg IMI stat (if available) to decrease pancreatic secretion and as an antispasmodic, but it may worsen the ileus.
>   **and/or**
> - Hyoscine 10 mg orally 3 x daily for 3-5 days
>
> *If moderate or severe*
> - Place naso-gastric tube to drain gastric secretions
> - Start IV therapy
> - Give morphine, slowly IVI, 10 mg
> - **REFER**

CHRONIC PANCREATITIS

Clinical features
- Persistent or recurrent episodes of:
    - epigastric pain
    - left hypochondrial pain.
- Pain characteristically does not respond to antacids.
- Attacks may last only a few hours, or as long as two weeks, and may eventually be continuous.
- Anorexia, nausea, vomiting, constipation, flatulence
- Weight loss
- Steatorrhoea (frequent, bulky, offensive, pale, fatty stools) due to malabsorption.
- Tenderness over the pancreas with mild guarding
- Glycosuria may be present
- Anaemia secondary to Vitamin B12 malabsorption

> **MANAGEMENT**
> - Treat acute attacks as for acute pancreatitis (see page 117)
> - Treat associated diabetes
> - Advise strict alcohol avoidance
> - Small frequent meals and restricted fat intake reduces pancreatic secretion and pain
> - **REFER**
>   - if not previously assessed
>   - for prescription of pancreatic enzymes (these may reduce pain by negative feedback on pancreatic secretion)

CARCINOMA OF THE PANCREAS

Clinical features
- Emaciation (very thin)
- Upper abdominal pain with radiation to the back
    - slightly relieved by leaning forward
- Fatty intolerance with pale, fatty stools and dark urine
- Possible history of chronic pancreatitis
- Jaundice accompanied by pruritis (late finding)
- Palpable gall bladder may be present (50% of patients)
- Signs and symptoms suggesting diabetes
- Possibly an epigastric mass palpable

> **MANAGEMENT**
> - **REFER** all cases
> - Terminal patients need
>   - narcotic analgesics eg. morphine
>   - **REFERRAL** to Hospice if available

SPLEEN PROBLEMS

SPLENOMEGALY

Causes
- Malignancy (infiltration or due to extra medullary haematopoeisis)
    - leukaemia
    - lymphomas
- Infections (due to immune hyperplasia)
    - viral infections (especially in children) including HIV infection
    - infective endocarditis
    - TB
    - typhoid fever
    - malaria
    - bilharzia
- Cirrhosis (portal hypertension)
- Collagen vascular diseases (disordered immunoregulation)
- Infiltration of the spleen by deposits (amyloid, hyperlipidaemias etc.)

> **REFER** any patient with an enlarged spleen unless it has been previously investigated.

INTESTINAL INFESTATIONS

WORMS

- Worms are extremely common in children.
- Often one has to treat on suspicion, when the diagnosis can not be confirmed on stool microscopy.
- Often the child is infected with more than one worm species.

Clinical features
- Vague abdominal pains
- Itching anus
- They may actually see the worm in the stool.
- A mass of worms may sometimes be palpable, often in the right iliac fossa.
- Any child with recurrent wheezing should have a course of worm treatment as Ascaris larvae in the lungs can cause this.
- Other children in the family may have worms too.

Prevention through education
- Use toilets
- Good personal hygiene
- Beware of under-cooked meat
- Clean, hygienic playing areas for children

In pregnancy
- The drugs used for the treatment of parasitic infestations are contra-indicated in pregnancy.
- Treatment must be withheld until after delivery
    - mebendazole can be used while breast feeding
- An exception is niclosamide (Yomesan) which is used to treat tapeworm.

ROUND WORM (ASCARIS)

- This is the most commonly diagnosed worm
- It is a white or pink-coloured worm with pointed ends (20-40 cm in length)
- It may be:
    - coughed up
    - vomited
    - seen in the stool.
- Early in its life cycle the worm migrates to the lungs
- There it develops and then migrates to the
    - oesophagus
    - small bowel where it lays its eggs
- The escort may bring the worms in a bottle, to make identification easy.

Clinical features
- Vague, ill-defined abdominal pain
- If the worm load is severe, the worms may form a mass in the right iliac fossa
    - this is often palpable as an irregular mobile softish mass
    - this may cause intestinal obstruction and the child will then present with vomiting and colicky abdominal pain (or acute abdomen)

- Worms themselves are not an important cause of weight loss, but the children who are undernourished have
    - lowered resistance
    - therefore a higher worm load

MANAGEMENT
- Give mebendazole (Vermox)
    - children 1-2 years 100 mg (5 ml susp) 2 x daily for 3 days
    - adults and children over 2 years 500 mg (5 x 100 mg tabs) or 25 ml susp orally stat
- Or albendazole (Zentel)
    - children 1-2 years 200 mg (10 ml susp) orally stat
    - adults and children over 2 years 400 mg (1 tab) or 20 ml susp orally stat

WHIPWORM

These are 3-5 cm in length.

Clinical features
- Usually only diagnosed on stool microscopy
- Most infections are asymptomatic
- May have abdominal pain with sometimes bloody / mucoid diarrhoea
- Rectal prolapse in children with massive infestation

Manage as for round worm opposite.

HOOKWORM

- These occur in patients from other parts of Africa and from Limpopo Province.
- People are infected by the larvae entering through the skin, particularly of the feet.
- They reach the intestine via the bloodstream and then the lungs.

Clinical features
- Chronic abdominal pain (initially epigastric)
- Weight loss
- Anaemia (iron deficiency) and all the symptoms of anaemia
- The diagnosis is usually only confirmed when the hook worm ova are found in the stool on microscopy.

MANAGEMENT
- Albendazole 400 mg (1 tab) or 20 ml susp orally stat for adults and children over 2 years
- **Or** mebendazole 500 mg (5 x 100 mg tabs) or 25 ml susp orally stat
- Treatment for iron-deficiency anaemia
- Improve sanitation
- Encourage the community to wear shoes to prevent the hookworm larvae entering through the skin of the feet.

PINWORM

- These worms are tiny (3-10 mm in size)
- They live in the large bowel
- The female worm lays its eggs in the skin around the anus
- The disease is spread via the contaminated fingers of the affected person

Clinical features
- Itchy anus causing scratching (often worse at night)
- Diagnosis can be made by applying sticky tape to the anal margin and pulling it off again
  - the eggs will be sticking to it
  - send for microscopic examination

- Management as for round worm on page 119.
- It is important to treat the whole family.

SANDWORM (CUTANEOUS LARVA MIGRANS)

- Usually caused by a hookworm of dog or cat
- The larvae in the soil penetrate skin through the feet, legs, buttocks or back.
- It causes creeping eruptions or winding thread-like trail of inflammation with itching and scratching.
- Secondary bacterial infection may occur.

MANAGEMENT
Albendazole
- Adults and children over 2 years
  - 400 mg once daily for 3 days
- Children 1-2 years
  - 200 mg once daily for 3 days

TAPEWORM

Clinical features
- Usually diagnosed by the patient passing flat white segments in the stool.
- Vague abdominal pains.
- Loss of appetite and loss of weight may occur.

MANAGEMENT
If the patient has diarrhoea, wait for it to settle.

Albendazole
- Adults and children over 2 years
  - 400 mg once daily for 3 days
- Children 1-2 years
  - 200 mg once daily for 3 days

In pregnancy
Praziquantal (Biltricide)
- Adults
  - 10 mg / kg as a single dose
  - usual dose
    600 mg (1 x 600 mg tab)
  - avoid in first trimester of pregnancy

ANORECTAL CONDITIONS

SYMPTOMS OF ANORECTAL DISEASE

SEVERE ANAL PAIN

Causes

There are 5 common causes of severe anal pain

- Anal fissure
- Thrombosed pile / perianal haematoma
- Submucous abscess of the anal canal
- Perianal abscess
- Ischiorectal abscess

> **MANAGEMENT**
> - Severe anal pain is a surgical emergency and all patients need to be **REFERRED** stat
>   - even if you are not sure which of the above causes are present

SOMETHING PROTRUDING FROM THE ANUS

Causes

Non-painful
- Prolapsed, non-complicated piles
- Sentinel pile
- Rectal prolapse
- Condylomata acuminata

Painful
- Thrombosed pile
- Submucous abscess
- Anal polyp (rare)

> Treat the cause.

BLEEDING FROM THE ANUS

FRESH BLEEDING FROM THE ANUS

Causes
- Haemorrhoids (see page 124)
- Dysentery
- Anal fissure
- Trauma from enemas
- Carcinoma of the rectum

> **REFER** if you suspect carcinoma or other serious causes.

STREAKS OF BLOOD ON THE STOOL

Causes
- Anal fissure (page 123)
- Haemorrhoids (page 124)

> Treat according to the cause.

MALAENA OR CHANGED BLOOD FROM THE ANUS

Causes
- Malaena stools are black, tar-like and offensive.
- The causes for this are usually severe disease in the upper bowel or colon eg.
  - carcinoma
  - peptic ulcer disease

> *Usually the causes of malaena are serious and will need* **REFERRAL.**

ITCHING ANUS

This is called pruritis ani.

Causes
The most common cause is poor hygiene but it may be secondary to a discharge.
- Perianal fistula
- Candida or Trichomonas vaginal discharge in females
- Pinworm
- Gonorrhoea or Chlamydia in homosexuals
- Eczema
- Repeated, frequent use of anal suppositories eg. bismuth
- Contact dermatitis from soaps used for washing the anus
- Diabetes must always be considered
- Haemorrhoids

Clinical features
- There may be excoriation (abrasion) of theperianal skin due to scratching the severe itch

Treat the cause.

DISCHARGE NEAR THE ANUS

Causes
- The most common cause for this is a perianal fistula
- Prolapsed piles may give a chronic mucoid discharge
- Pilonidal sinus or abscess
- Any other causes of ulcers (see below)

Treat the probable cause.

ULCERS AROUND THE ANUS

Causes
- The most common cause for this is sexually transmitted infections eg.
    - herpes simplex
    - chancroid
- Other causes of ulcers may also have to be considered eg.
    - after trauma
    - bed sores
    - chronic diarrhoea causing excoriation (HIV/AIDS)

Treat the cause.

PAINFUL NATAL CLEFT

Causes
- Pilonidal sinus or pilonidal abscess
- Other skin diseases such as candidiasis
- Herpes simplex ulceration

- Treat the cause
- For details of pilonidal sinus, see page 126

CHANGE OF BOWEL HABIT

This means the onset of unusual, recurrent diarrhoea or constipation, or alternating diarrhoea and constipation.

Causes
- The most important cause to exclude is carcinoma of the colon
- Often these patients will also be abusing laxatives
- Chronic constipation followed by overflow diarrhoea

All patients must be **REFERRED** if they have a true change of bowel habit, to investigate for carcinoma

MASS FELT ON PR EXAMINATION

Causes
- Intramucosal mass
    - this must be assumed to be due to a carcinoma of the rectum
- In children a rare cause is an anal polyp
- A foreign body may also occur in:
    - younger children
    - mentally retarded children.

Differential diagnosis
- In warmer areas, amoebiasis may feel like a mass on rectal examination.

MANAGEMENT
REFER
- Older patients, as a carcinoma of the bowel must be excluded as soon as possible.
- Children, as a mass in the rectum is usually serious

ABUSE OF LAXATIVES AND ENEMAS

Generally this is a symptom of excessive preoccupation with bowel function and ignorance regarding the normal frequency of passage of stools.

MANAGEMENT
- The patient should be advised on:
    - correct diet
    - the need for roughage in the diet eg. bran, fruit, vegetables and dried fruit.
- The use of laxatives and enemas should be discouraged
- The patient must be carefully examined to exclude
    - signs of bowel obstruction eg. abdominal distention
    - cancer eg. weight loss, a mass on PR or occult blood in the stool
- If any of these are present, **REFER** for investigation

AN APPROACH TO THE PHYSICAL EXAMINATION

- Usually the patient is examined in the "left lateral" position
    - but proper localisation of the pathology is often difficult in this position (except in very thin patients)
  Once it has been determined that there is pathology present, (eg. an abscess), turn the patient into the dorsal or lithotomy type of position
    - both legs held up
    - knees flexed (bent)
    - a male patient may have to hold his own scrotum up out of the way
- It may be embarrassing to the patient, but it is easier for a correct diagnosis to be made
- The natal cleft is separated and abnormalities are looked for eg.
    - pilonidal sinus
    - fistula
    - anal fissure
- The patient is then asked to strain (push) down

Rectal examination (per rectum PR)
- It is important to warn the patient of the intended procedure
- The index finger (of the right hand) is rested for a few seconds on the anus and then the finger is introduced, pointing towards the umbilicus.
- A systematic examination is performed, feeling in turn anteriorly, posteriorly and laterally.
- Normally in the female, the cervix of the uterus is felt anteriorly.
- In the male, the prostate is palpated anteriorly
    - this should be firm but not hard
- Feel specifically for
    - any hard masses in the rectum
    - any ulcer
- Examine the glove for blood or discharge

ANORECTAL DISEASES

ANAL FISSURE

Clinical features
- The pain is very severe when passing a stool
- Bleeding on passing a stool
- There is usually a history of constipation
- It may follow diarrhoea (laxative abuse)
- There is a small crack or ulcer just inside the anal margin
    - this may be seen when the edges of the anus are gently pulled apart by the examiner's fingers (as the patient presses down as if passing a stool)
- The ulcer is usually in the midline posteriorly, but may be anterior, especially in females
- It is often seen together with
    - a sentinel pile (an area of hypertrophied skin at the outer end of the fissure)
    - external haemorrhoids (piles) which may obscure the fissure
- PR is very painful or impossible as the anal sphincter is in spasm

MANAGEMENT
- If it is the first episode and / or the symptoms are mild, treat as follows:
    - local anaesthetic gel / cream applied before and after each bowel action (eg. lidocaine, amethocaine)
    - laxatives eg. Senokot 2 nocte high fibre diet
    - avoid chronic use of laxatives
- **REFER** if:
    - there is severe pain
    - the anus is very tight (PR not possible)
    - it is **not** the first episode
    - not responding to the above treatment

SUBMUCOUS ABSCESS OF THE ANAL CANAL

Clinical features
- This is often very difficult to diagnose
- Painful mass protruding from the anus
- This abscess starts inside the anal margin
- The patient may be pyrexial
- PR very painful or impossible

- **REFER** stat for an incision and drainage (I&D)
- Surgery needs to be done on the same day to avoid deterioration.

PERIANAL ABSCESS

Caused by bacteria spreading through the wall of the anus into the perianal soft tissues.

Clinical features
- Initially tender indurated area immediately next to the anus
- Later soft swelling
- May be pyrexial
- PR painful, but possible

- **REFER** stat for an incision and drainage (I&D)
- Surgery needs to be done on the same day to avoid deterioration
---

ISCHIORECTAL ABSCESS

Clinical features
- These patients are usually ill and toxic
- It is more common in people with lowered resistance eg.
    - diabetics
    - alcoholics
- Pain on sitting
- May have a high temperature
- Tender induration 2-3 cms away from the anus (hard area).
- No fluctuation, unless the disease has been present for some time.
- PR is possible, but tender, because the main inflammation is lateral to the anus.

- **REFER** stat for an incision and drainage (I&D)
- *This is a surgical emergency*
- *Do not wait for fluctuation*

HAEMORRHOIDS

These are varicose veins of the ano-rectum and there are two types formed by two different groups of veins.

- "Internal" haemorrhoids caused by superior haemorrhoidal venous plexus varicosities
    - these are situated proximal to the anal sphincters and are submucosal.
- "External" haemorrhoids are varicosities of the inferior haemorrhoidal venous plexus under the skin on the edge of the anus.
- Both are common and are caused by increased hydrostatic pressure in the portal veins from:
    - pregnancy
    - straining at stool
    - cirrhosis of the liver
- The diagnosis is suspected on the history of:
    - prolapse (protrusion)
    - anal pain which is worse on defecation
    - or bleeding.

INTERNAL HAEMORRHOIDS

- Patient may complain of:
    - bright, red blood at the end of defaecation
    - blood splattering or dripping into the pan
    - blood present on the toilet paper, often as mild, fresh, red streaks, after wiping the anus.
- In an older patient **a diagnosis of an underlying carcinoma must be considered**.
- It is important to realise that uncomplicated haemorrhoids are usually painless.
- "Painful piles" means that:
    - the haemorrhoids have prolapsed through the anus
    - may have further complicated to become thrombosed or have become eroded and infected
    - or there is some unrelated cause for the pain e.g. anal fissure

There are four categories of internal haemorrhoids:
- **First degree** - varicosities inside the ano-rectum that never protrude, but which may bleed.
- **Second degree** - varicosities that may occasionally protrude but reduce spontaneously.
- **Third degree** - varicosities that protrude and need to be pushed back manually.
- **Fourth degree** - protruding varicosities that cannot be pushed back inside:
    - these haemorrhoids are the most likely to cause trouble i.e. strangulation with mucosal ulceration and infection.
- Haemorrhoids are not a common problem in children
    - other conditions causing protrusion such as rectal prolapse and anal polyp must be considered.

EXTERNAL HAEMORRHOIDS

- They cause pain of varying degrees of severity.
- Venule may rupture and cause a perianal haematoma (very painful)
    - tender, blue, dome-shaped swelling at the edge of the anus
    - may have spasm of the anal sphincter (PR examination is very painful or impossible).

MANAGEMENT

- Give reassurance:
    - many patients with mild symptoms, eg. occasional, pruritis or blood on the paper, will want to know the cause.
    - they want reassurance that it is nothing serious, such as cancer.
- The treatment is usually conservative, and improvement usually takes place within five days ("five day disease").
- Cold packs
- Stool softeners eg. Senokot 2 nocte or lactulose 10-20 ml 1-2 x daily.
- Bismuth ointment applied 2-3 x daily or suppositories
    - insert one 2 x daily
- Local anaesthetic gel if the piles are very painful
    - apply before and after each bowel action.
- Zinc and castor oil ointment can be used to relieve pruritis.
- Conservative (non-surgical) management is usually enough in most cases (first degree to third degree).
- Treat external haemorrhoids in the same way.
- Patient may need surgery for fourth degree haemorrhoids
    - this is because there is often strangulation of the veins
    - followed by thrombosis or mucosal erosion and possible infection.
- Give advice about diet and lifestyle:
    - high fibre diet
    - avoid chronic use of laxatives
    - avoid straining at stool

REFER patients with:
- Fourth degree haemorrhoids
- Milder degrees of prolapse with intermittent bleeding for treatment by rubber-banding / injection of sclerosing solution
- External thrombosed haemorrhoids / perianal haematoma if large, very painful or if not responding to conservative management
    - for possible incision, extraction of the clot and suturing/compression of the incised area

RECTAL PROLAPSE

Causes
- Malnutrition
- Chronic constipation
- Chronic diarrhoea
- Laxative abuse
- During delivery
- Worm infestation in children

Clinical features
- This happens when the rectum protrudes from the anus
- It occurs in children and adults
- In children it is associated with straining

Differential diagnosis
- In infants and children, an intussusception may look like a rectal prolapse

MANAGEMENT
- In children, treat for worm infestation (see page 119)
- When diagnosed, it must be reduced by gentle finger pressure
    - teach the parents how to do this
- Strap the buttocks together for a few hours
- **REFER** if it recurs

CONDYLOMATA ACUMINATA

Clinical features
- These are the same as genital warts, and may also occur around the anus.
- They are cauliflower-like masses
- These surround the anus
- They do not actually protrude from the anus
- They may cause itching or a mucoid discharge
- If traumatised, they may bleed slightly and become infected

See management of condylomata acuminata under Sexually Transmitted Infections page 176.

FISTULA IN ANO (PERIANAL FISTULA)

Causes
- This is a track lined by granulation tissue, extending from the anal canal or rectum, to the skin around the anus.
- It results from:
    - spontaneous bursting of an abscess
    - inadequate drainage of an abscess in the past.

Clinical features
- There is a chronic discharge from an opening near the anus
- The patient may complain of recurrent soiling of the underclothes with pus and / or faeces.
- A small elevation of granulation tissue with a bead of discharge is seen close to the anus.
- On PR, the internal opening may sometimes be felt as a nodule or detected in the mucosa.

MANAGEMENT
- **REFER** as the fistula tract needs to be excised
    - the resulting cavity must be left to close up slowly from the bottom of the cavity upwards
- Irrigation of the wound will need to be carried out a few times every day for about 2 weeks.
- The patient needs to informed about this **before REFERRAL** for surgery, so that they do not expect to come out of theatre with a neat row of stitches.

PILONIDAL SINUS

Clinical features
- A hair grows into the natal cleft skin and forms a sinus
- It is a condition usually found in hairy people
- There is discharge from the sinus, pain, or a tender swelling
- On separating the natal cleft, a small pit may be seen in the midline of the cleft, or to one side of it.

> **REFER** for operation when convenient.

PILONIDAL ABSCESS

Clinical features
- There is a painful swelling at the upper end of the natal cleft
- PR examination is normal

> **REFER** for incision and drainage.

ENDOCRINE SYSTEM

DIABETES MELLITUS

THE DIAGNOSIS OF DIABETES MELLITUS

TYPE 1 DIABETES MELLITUS

Clinical features
- Duration of syptoms: usually weeks
- Type 1 usually presents in children and young adults
- The patient often presents in coma or pre-coma
- There will be a history of weight loss - the patient is usually thin
- Polyuria
- Polydipsia
- Malaise
- Fatigue
- Polyphagia with weight loss
- Difficulty with waking in the morning
- Recurrent infection eg. boils, UTI, vulvovaginitis
- Type 1 may be brought on by a preceding viral infection
- Severe abdominal pain is sometimes the only symptom
- Severe dehydration, tachycardia, hypotension, deep sighing respiration (due to acidosis)

Differential diagnosis
- Acute abdomen
- Severe infections (pneumonia)

TYPE 2 DIABETES MELLITUS

Clinical features
- May be similar to the above
- The patient is usually overweight or even obese
- It usually presents in middle-aged patients
- There are often only mild non-specific symptoms eg. monilial vaginitis, visual impairment
- The patient may be totally asymptomatic diagnosed only by urine testing (should be done routinely)
- The patient may present with symptoms due to the complications of diabetes eg. infections, neuropathy, diabetic foot

Diagnosis
Diagnose diabetes if:
- The patient has symptoms of diabetes plus the random blood glucose (RBG) is 11.1 mmol / L or higher.
- The fasting blood glucose (FBG) is 7 mmol / L or higher.
- **OR** following 75 g oral glucose load, the 2 hour blood glucose level is 11.1 mmol / L or higher.

NB. There must be at least 2 positive tests done on seperate days for an **asymptomatic patient** to be diagnosed eg one abnormal FBG and one abnormal RBG.

This is especially important if there is an infective illness present.

Patients can only be considered to be fasting if they have not eaten for 8 hours (only water is allowed).
- In most cases these are patients who have not had breakfast following an overnight fast.
- In some cases they are patients who have had an early breakfast and nothing to eat after that
    - they are then seen at the clinic in the afternoon between 14h00 and 16h00.

SHORT-TERM COMPLICATIONS

HYPOGLYCAEMIA

This is a blood glucose below 4 mmol / L with symptoms in a known diabetic.

Causes
- The patient not eating regular meals
- The patient eating too little carbohydrates
- Too much exercise
- Too much treatment either insulin or oral agents
- Alcohol
- Prolonged vomiting (unable to eat)

Clinical features
- Sympathetic stimulation
    - hunger
    - shaking
    - trembling
    - sweating
    - palpitations
- Neurorological symptoms
    - headache
    - dizziness
    - tiredness
    - irritability
    - inability to concentrate
    - behavioural changes eg. children become "naughty"
    - confusion
    - convulsions in children
    - slurred speech
- Finally patient becomes unconscious

MANAGEMENT
*Diabetics should know the signs of hypoglycaemia and **always** have sugar with them. eg. in the form of sweets.*

Mild symptomatic hypoglycaemia
- Give glucose water to drink (4 level teaspoons of glucose (20 g) in 200 ml water).

If no obvious cause (eg. having missed a meal)
For patients on insulin therapy
- Reduce the appropriate insulin dose by 4 units
    - eg. patient on a biphasic insulin 2 x daily and the hypoglycaemia occurs during the day
    - then reduce the morning dose.

For patients on oral hypoglycaemic agents
- Reduce the sulphonylurea dose by at least 2 steps or stop the medicine depending on the severity of the hypoglycaemia.
- The metformin dose usually does not require reduction at the same time.

Severe hypoglycaemia / hypoglycaemic coma
Children
- Dextrose 10% IV, 2-5 ml / kg rapidly
    - 10% solution (dilute 1 part dextrose 50% to 4 parts water for injection)
- After dextrose bolus commence dextrose 5-10% infusion 3-5 ml / kg / hour

Adults
- Open an IV line with
    - 10% dextrose water
    - give thiamine 100 mg IVI immediately in patients at risk of thiamine deficiency eg. alcoholics or malnourished.
- Followed by a bolus of 10% dextrose water 5 ml / kg given rapidly
- If blood glucose remains less than 4 mmol / L
    - give a second IV bolus of 5 mg / kg
- Maintain with 5-10% dextrose solution until blood glucose stablised
- Once the patient is conscious, ensure he / she has something to eat.
- **REFER.**

HYPERGLYCAEMIA

Causes
- Too little treatment ie. oral agents or insulin
- Ineffective action of drugs ie. oral agents
- Incorrect diet or patient not keeping to the diet
- Patient is taking sugar
- Infections, especially urinary and chest
- Psychological stress
- Alcohol

Clinical features
Early features
- Very thirsty patient
    - a normal person should not have to drink more than 3 litres a day
- Nocturia - a normal person should not pass urine more than twice a night
- A great feeling of weakness
- Drowsiness and difficulty in waking in the morning
- Blurring of vision
- Pruritis vulvae or balanitis

Later features
- Drowsiness or varying degrees of loss of consciousness
- Abdominal pain and vomiting
- Dehydration
- Acidotic breathing
- Acetone (fruity) smell on breath
- Sugar (4 plus) in urine, with or without ketones

Note. The patient should be asked about these symptoms (especially the first two) at every visit.

MANAGEMENT
Less severe hyperglycaemia
- See Medicine protocol, page 135.

Pre-coma / severe hyperglycaemia
- **REFER** stat.
- Treat as for hyperglycaemic coma (see below)
    - but IV therapy to run at a slower rate
    - first litre to run in over 1-2 hours.
- Do not give any insulin.

Hyperglycaemic coma
- **REFER** stat.
- Start IV therapy
    - 1 litre normal saline over the first ½ - 1 hour
- Over the next 1-2 hours continue with 1 litre normal saline
    - if the transfer to hospital is delayed, continue with 1 litre every 3-4 hours depending on clinical response.
- If transfer to hospital is delayed by more than 2 hours
    - give insulin short acting, IMI, 0.1 units / kg as a bolus
    - when giving insulin IMI do not use an insulin needle

▼ **Note to doctor**
If hospital transfer is delayed
- Do an ECG to exclude hypo-kalaemia
    - then administer 5 u regular insulin (Actrapid) IVI stat
    - this procedure can be repeated hourly.
- If the ECG shows hypo-kalaemia ie. a flat T wave, prominent U wave and ST depression
    - withhold insulin
    - add 20 mmol KCL (1 amp) into the next vacolitre of saline and not into the bulb ▲

INFECTIONS

Infections are more common in uncontrolled diabetics.

Infections include
- Fungal infections such as Candida vulvovaginitis and balanitis
- Also more dangerous deep fungal infections
- TB - check poorly controlled diabetics for TB regularly
- Staphylococcal skin infections ie. boils
- Urinary tract infections
    - diabetes makes a person more likely to get pyelonephritis.

MANAGEMENT
- Treat bacterial infection seriously with an antibiotic and carefully follow up.
- The antibiotic used for skin and soft tissue infections should provide anti-staphylococcal cover e.g. flucloxacillin
- **REFER** if:
    - patient does not respond to an antibiotic
    - there is an increase in blood glucose as this often needs to be controlled with insulin.

LONG-TERM COMPLICATIONS

RETINOPATHY

This is a major cause of blindness.

MANAGEMENT
- This can now be prevented by laser therapy if performed early.
- **REFER** for fundoscopy to diagnose early reversible retinal changes in the following cases
    - *any* visual disturbance or decreased visual acuity
    - poorly controlled patients eg. where adherence is poor
    - new diabetics.
- Follow up **REFERRAL** once a year if possible
    - especially if poorly controlled or adherence is poor.

CATARACTS

MANAGEMENT
REFER for surgical removal if:
- It causes severe vision problems ie. visual acuity in both eyes 6 / 24 or less.
- It is affecting the patient's work.

DIABETIC NEPHROPATHY

Proteinuria is the most important indicator of diabetic kidney disease.

MANAGEMENT
- Any patient with proteinuria 1+ or more should have blood sent for serum creatinine and eGFR
    - **or** calculate the patient's creatinine clearance from the serum creatinine result (see page 150)
- Once the diagnosis is confirmed
    - prescribe an ACE-inhibitor in low dosage and titrate up until the maximum dose is reached, if tolerated
    - the ideal target is PCR <0.03g/mmol
    - **REFER** to specialist if eGFR/ creatinine clearance <60 ml/min
- Treat hypertension if present.
- Provide and promote other kidney and cardiovascular protection measures:
    - smoking cessation
    - aspirin therapy (if existing atherosclerotic cardiovascular disease)
    - lipid-lowering therapy

HYPERTENSION

There is increased incidence and increased severity of hypertension in diabetes.

- Hypertension must be treated with antihypertensive medicines (see page 77).
- Goal BP for all ages is <140/90 mm Hg.

DIABETIC NEUROPATHY

Peripheral (symmetrical) neuropathy
Proteinuria is the most important indicator of diabetic kidney disease.
There is "glove and stocking" sensory loss in the feet and legs causing:
- pain (worse at night)
- cramps
- paresthesia

Autonomic nerve damage
- This causes:
    - postural hypotension
    - diarrhoea or constipation
    - impotence
    - urinary retention
    - unprovoked sweating
      eg. after meals

Mononeuropathy
- There is single nerve involvement eg. radial nerve (wrist drop).
- It may involve cranial nerves eg. III and VI (double vision).

Carpal tunnel syndrome
- This is nerve entrapment.

> **REFER** if it has not been investigated.

▼ Note to doctor
Painful neuropathy
- Start with simple analgesics first.
- If response to these is poor, a tricyclic antidepressant eg. amitriptyline can be added
    - start with 25 mg at night
    - increase by 25 mg at monthly intervals to a maximum of 75 mg at night.
- Alternatively use carbamazepine
    - start with 100 mg 2 x daily
    - increasing by 200 mg / day at weekly intervals according to response
    - maximum 400 mg 12 hourly ▲

VASCULAR

- Arterial disease is common in uncontrolled diabetes
    - ie. coronary, cerebral and peripheral vascular disease
- This causes increased risk of
    - myocardial infarctions
    - cerebro vascular accidents
    - ulcers of the foot
    - kidney disease

> ### MANAGEMENT
> **REFER** if:
> - It has not been investigated.
> - It is getting worse.
>
> See pages 90-92 for management.

DIABETIC FOOT

Ulcers develop at the tips of the toes and the plantar surfaces of the metatarsal heads and are often preceded by callus formation. The ulcers can become secondarily infected.

Causes
A combination of:
- Vascular disease
- Neuropathy
- Infection

- It is very important to check the feet of diabetics as regularly as possible.

> ### MANAGEMENT
> - Relieve pressure: Non-weight bearing is essential
> - Frequent removal of excess keratin by a podiatrist to allow efficient drainage of the lesion
> - Cleanse with normal saline and apply non-adherent dressing
> - Co-amoxiclav 875/125 mg, oral, 12 hourly for 10 days
>
> **REFERRAL**
> **Urgent** if the ulcer is associated with:
> - cellulitis
> - severe hyperglycaemia
> - abscess
> - discolouration of surrounding skin
>
> **Non urgent**
> - Ulcers not responding to adequate treatment
>
> ### Advice for diabetics to prevent foot disease
> - Do not use tobacco of any type
>   - ie. do not smoke.
> - Do not apply any external heat
>   - eg. do not sit too close to a fire or use hot water bottles.
> - Do not use water in the bath which is too hot
>   - test that it is not too hot with your elbow or the back of your hand.
> - Do not walk barefoot as you can easily cut or injure your foot.
> - Do not wear bad shoes
>   - shoes with nails or wrinkled lining
>   - shoes which are too tight
>   - they can cause wounds and abscesses which will be difficult to heal.
> - Buy square-toed shoes or round-toed shoes, a half size larger than usual.
> - Do not wear tight socks or tight stockings as they block the circulation.
> - Do not perform "Home Surgery"
>   - do not cut any corns or callouses
>   - be very careful in cutting the toe nails
>   - if you are having difficulty, it is best to go to the chiropodist.
> - Do not ignore any signs of infection of the feet
>   - go to the clinic straight away.

MANAGEMENT OF DIABETES MELLITUS

GOALS OF TREATMENT
- To give the patient a feeling of health
    - physically
    - psychologically
- Acceptable glucose control. Aim for:
    - a fasting blood glucose of 6-8 mmol / L
    - a random blood glucose of below 10 mmol / L
    - glycated haemoglobin (HbA1c) 6-7.5%
- No glycosuria if possible
- Normal blood pressure, and body weight
- Prevention, early diagnosis and management of complications
- To continually educate the patient on all aspects of his condition
- Absence of hypoglycaemia

PATIENT EDUCATION
This should be started at the first visit. You should continue to re-educate the patient at every visit.

Education about diabetes
- Explain, in simple terms, that diabetes is a life-long condition that can be controlled
    - he / she must regularly attend the clinic or doctor for the rest of his / her life.
- The patient is to be given a diabetic bracelet with instructions that it should never be removed, and be replaced immediately if broken or worn.
- If the blood glucose is poorly controlled, the patient must test his blood sugar daily at home
    - the method of testing blood sugar must be shown to the patient
    - he must keep a record to show to the clinic sister / doctor every month
    - the test must be done before breakfast one day and before supper the next day, to test for control throughout the 24 hours.
- He should be warned about possible complications and advised how to recognise these early on
    - report these immediately to the clinic.
- Tell him about the danger of infection.
- He must report to the clinic immediately if he has any of the following:
    - febrile illness
    - symptoms of a urinary tract infection
    - skin infections or septic wounds, especially of the feet
    - chronic cough.
- At every visit you should check if the patient is taking his drugs correctly
    - you must also make sure he understands his condition.
- He should be praised if he has done well. He should be given advice if he has made mistakes.
- He should *never* be made to feel that he is an invalid.
- He should be encouraged to live a life that is as normal as possible.
- Explain about hyperglycaemia and hypoglycaemia.

Hyperglycaemia education
- Warn about causes and symptoms (see page 130)
- Advise that if he becomes symptomatic, to continue the usual treatment doses and to report to the clinic / hospital immediately.
- Advise that if the urine sugar stays high, he must report to the clinic / hospital as soon as possible.

Hypoglycaemia education
- Warn about causes and clinical features (see pages 129-130).
- Advise the patient always to keep some sugar near him, like sweets, cold-drinks etc. to take if symptoms should occur.
- If symptoms persist or recur frequently, he must report to the clinic.
- Instruct the patient to take regular meals and to eat
    - immediately after taking an oral hypoglycaemic drug
    - 30 minutes after insulin injection.
- Advise the patient not to do any tiring exercise
    - if unavoidable he should eat extra food before doing the exercise.

Dietary education
All patients whether obese, normal weight or underweight must be given dietary advice.
- Check at every visit whether or not the diet is being followed.
- Stress the importance of diet at each visit.

Suggested food guide for patients

Foods to be avoided
- **Sugar and foods containing sugar** such as sweets, cold drinks, colas, lemonades, ginger beer, cakes, buns and scones (unless baked with whole wheat flour), vet koek, pastries, jam, honey, syrup, condensed milk, puddings, jelly, custard, canned fruit, stewed fruit, fruit juices, e.g. Liquifruit, orange squash.

Vegetables
- Eat a variety of vegetables - several portions daily
- One portion a dark green vegetable e.g. spinach, broccoli, green beans and peas
- One dark yellow/orange vegetable e.g. carrots, pumpkin and butternut
- Other highly nutritious vegetables include morogo, cabbage, potatoes, sweet potatoes, lentils, gem squash, tomatoes, beetroot, cucumber, avocado pear.
- You may eat as much vegetables as you want.
- Potatoes to be cooked in their skins
- Eat vegetables raw or cook them in a little water for a short time.

Porridge
- Eat products with high fibre content e.g. rough maize, sorghum (Maltabela) meal, rough/rolled oats, whole wheat cereal. Eat these in moderate or small amounts only.
- Avoid commercial breakfast cereals e.g. cornflakes, Rice crispies.

Mealies
- Eat whole mealies or rough stamp mealies (Samp).

Bread
- Eat only whole wheat or brown bread and only a few slices a day.

Other grains
- Eat brown rice or whole wheat semolina pasta

Meat
- Remove excess fat; do not fry, only grill, braai or roast; avoid gravies.

Dairy
- Full cream milk and milk products and eggs can be consumed. If there is evidence of a lipid disorder recommend low fat products.

Fats and oils
- Reduce unhealthy oils such as hard margarine. Use healthy types of fat e.g. butter, avocado pear, olive oil, canola oil.

Fruit
- Eat unpeeled if possible and uncooked.
- Eat only one fruit (fresh) at a time.

Salt
- Salt restriction may help to control blood pressure
- Remove the salt from the table.
- Avoid foods containing a lot of salt such as potato crisps and other salty snacks, salty biscuits, tinned soup and tinned vegetables, tomato sauce, Worcester sauce, marmite and other bread spreads.

Alcohol
- All alcohol including beer breaks down to sugar in the body and may cause hyperglycaemia.

Lifestyle education
- Encourage regular exercise, if possible every day, eg. walking or gardening.
- Advise patient on the care of the feet and the cutting of toe nails (see notes page 132 on foot care)
    - supply advice hand-out.
- Advise patient on the care of wounds.
- Find out if it is difficult for the patient to get time off from work to come for treatment
    - where necessary supply them with a "letter to the employer"
    - for an example of this letter see page 80.

TYPE 2 DIABETES MELLITUS

Urine testing
- Test urine for glucose, ketones, protein, leucocytes and nitrites.
- Test urine at the first visit, then annually
- Test urine if the patient:
    - has symptoms or signs of a UTI
    - is ill with no known cause

Blood Glucose testing
- Finger-prick blood glucose at every visit and HbA1c testing at 3-6 month intervals in patients not meeting treatment goals.
- Blood glucose should ideally be monitored at home in all patients on 2 or more daily doses of insulin
- *A fasting blood glucose of between 5 and 7 mmol / L is ideal:*
    - *but aim for at least less than 8 mmol / L*
- *A random blood glucose between 6 and 8 mmol / L is ideal*
    - *but aim for at least less than 10 mmol / L*
- If the blood glucose is high this may be due to
    - not taking his treatment that morning
    - **and** having had breakfast
- If the blood glucose is low this may be due to
    - having taken the treatment that morning
    - **and** having missed breakfast
- An HbA1c of less than 7% is ideal
    - but aim for at least less than 8%

Note:
- Finger-prick glucose testing at each scheduled visit cannot be relied on to give accurate information regarding control or adherence in the longer term.
- HbA1c testing provides a reliable method of assessing control and adherence over the previous few months
    - this should be done annually or 3-6 monthly in patients not meeting treatment goals.

Weight and diet control
- Weigh the patient and compare weight with the previous weight and the ideal body weight
    - write down the difference in weight, *either gain or loss on the card and tell the patient what it is*
    - ideal body weight (IBW) can be easily worked out from the adult patient's height
    - IBW = height in metres without the 1 before the decimal eg. 1,75 m = 75 kg
    - normal weight = from 10% below IBW to 10% above IBW.
- Check at every visit whether the diet is being followed
    - encourage the patient to continue with his diet whether or not there is control.
- If he has not been keeping to his diet and treatment
    - try to find out the reason
    - advise and try to help eg. by making appointments at a better time for him
    - give the patient a letter to the employer
    - re-educate the patient on the importance of drug treatment and non-drug treatment
    - warn the patient of the dangers of not following the advice on diet and treatment
    - do not increase the dosage of treatment except in certain special cases eg. infections.
- Abdominal circumference measurement
    - target less than 80 cm in women and 94 cm in men

Complications
- Ask about complications especially
    - hyper / hypoglycaemia
    - infections eg. UTI, septic wounds, boils
    - pruritis vulvae
    - problems with vision
    - foot problems
- Examine patients for complications especially
    - hypertension
    - foot infections
    - skin infections
    - tuberculosis
    - pruritis vulvae
    - peripheral vascular disease
    - eye complications

■ MEDICINE PROTOCOL

INDICATIONS FOR REFERRAL

- Glycosuria combined with ketonuria (greater than 1+)
- Blood glucose (BG) 25 mmol / L or greater
- If there is any dehydration or acidosis (deep sighing respiration)
- Any change in consciousness or mental confusion
- The patient on the maximum dosage of oral therapy with BG 15-25 mmol / L
- Hypoglycaemia (see page 129)
- Chronic cough or weight loss to exclude tuberculosis
- Any fever where you cannot find or adequately treat the cause
- Pregnancy or if considering becoming pregnant
- Badly septic wound or ulcer
- Young diabetics (less than 40 years), especially if they
    - are under 30 years of age
    - are thin
    - have severe symptoms
- If possible all patients should be **REFERRED** annually for fundoscopy to exclude a diabetic retinopathy (see page 131)
    - once their blood glucose is controlled
    - or has stabilized
    - or at any time when they develop visual problems

MEDICINE DETAILS

Biquanides

- Action
    - increases tissue sensitivity to insulin
    - induces a mild degree of anorexia
- Contraindications
    - uncontrolled heart failure
    - kidney impairment, i.e. eGFR <30 ml / minute
    - severe hepatic impairment

Metformin
To be taken with meals to reduce adverse effects
- 500 and 850 mg tabs
    - starting dose 500 mg daily
    - increase to 500 mg 2 x daily
    - increase to 850 mg 2 x daily
    - maximum dose 850 mg 3 x daily

Sulphonylureas

- Action
    - stimulate insulin release from the pancreas
- Contraindications
    - pregnancy
    - kidney impairment, i.e. eGFR <60 ml / minute
    - severe hepatic impairment

Glimeperide
To be taken with or before breakfast
- 1 mg tabs
    - starting dose 1 mg daily
    - increase by 1 mg increments at monthly intervals according to response
    - maximum dose 4 mg daily

Glibenclamide
To be taken half an hour before meals
- 5 mg tabs
    - starting dose 2,5-5 mg daily (5 mg if blood glucose 17 mmol / L or greater)
    - increase by 5 mg daily at each step
    - maximum dose 10 mg morning and 5 mg evening
    - avoid in the elderly (>65 years)

BLOOD GLUCOSE MANAGEMENT

All patients are managed according to their blood glucose (BG) readings.
The readings below refer to either the fasting or the random blood glucose level, unless one or the other is specifically stated

Blood glucose (BG) 25 mmol / L or greater

- **REFER** stat
- *This may be a hyperglycaemic or keto-acidotic emergency.*
- See hyperglycaemia management (page 130)

BG 10 - 25 mmol / L
Patient on no treatment

- Lifestyle modification and appropriate diet
- Prescribe
    - metformin 500-850 mg daily
- Check patient after 4 weeks.
- For the further management follow Diagram A (page 138).

Patient already on treatment

- Provided the adherence has been good
    - increase the dose by one step
    - for the further management follow Diagram A (page 138).

Defaulters

- Manage as before, provided the treatment was correct.
- Thereafter follow Diagram A (page 138).

BG 8 - 10 mmol / L

- Fasting - increase the dose of treatment by one step if the blood glucose has been at this level for 3 monthly visits in a row
- Random - continue with the same treatment

BG 6 - 8 mmol / L

- Fasting - carry on with the same treatment.
- Random - see page 136, when to reduce drug therapy

BG 4 - 6 mmol / L

- Reduce the dosage of tablets by one step.
    - if the patient is on both a sulphonylurea and metformin, reduce the dose of the sulphonylurea by one step.

BG 4 mmol / L or less

- If symptomatic start treatment for hypoglycaemia (see page 130).
- It will be necessary to stop or reduce drug therapy depending on the severity of the hypoglycaemia.
- If the patient is on a sulphonylurea stop the medicine or reduce the dose by at least 2 steps.
- If this is due to taking treatment without eating, warn the patient about this danger.

When to reduce drug therapy
- If the blood glucose remains controlled for 3 months in a row, try to reduce the dosage of the drugs by one step beginning with the sulphonylurea.
- If this is successful, then keep on reducing the dosage every 3 months.
- It may even be possible to eventually stop all the drugs.
- If however the blood glucose rises, it may be necessary to increase the dosage again, if adherence has been good.

MONITORING
At every visit
- Finger-prick blood glucose
- Weight
- Blood pressure

Baseline
- BMI for cardiovascular risk assessment
- Abdominal circumference (target less than 88 cm in women and 102 cm in men).
- Comprehensive foot examination.
- Urine dipstix for protein.
- If dipstix negative and the patient is not on an ACE-inhibitor, send urine for albumin-creatinine ratio (ACR)
    - if abnormal (>3 mg / mmol), prescribe an ACE-inhibitor
- **Note:** If the dipstix is positive 1+ or more, in the absence of infection, heart failure or menstruation
    - confirm within 2 months
    - diagnose nephropathy (see page 131)
- Serum creatinine concentration and calculate creatinine clearance (doctor or PHCN) unless a laboratory estimated eGFR has been done
    - **REFER** to doctor if eGFR <60 ml / min
- Serum lipids (**fasting** triglycerides, total cholesterol and LDL cholesterol)
    - **REFER** to specialist if total cholesterol >7.5 mmol/l or LDL cholesterol >5 mmol/l or triglycerides >10 mmol/l.
- Eye examination to look for retinopathy
    - **REFER** to an ophthalmologist as soon as the patient's condition has stabilised.

Annually
- Foot examination
- Urine dipstix for protein.
- If dipstix negative, send urine for albumin-creatinine ratio (unless the patient is already on an ACE-inhibitor)
    - if abnormal (>3 mg / mmol), prescribe an ACE-inhibitor
- **Note:** If the dipstix is positive 1+ or more, in the absence of infection, heart failure or menstruation
    - confirm within 2 months
    - diagnose nephropathy (see page 131)
- Serum creatinine concentration and eGFR or calculate creatinine clearance (doctor or PHCN).
- Serum lipids (**fasting** triglycerides, total cholesterol and LDL cholesterol) if never previously done.
- Serum potassium concentration, if on an ACE-inhibitor or eGFR <30 ml / min.
- HbA1c in patients who meet treatment goals (3-6 monthly in patients whose therapy has changed until stable).
- Eye examination
    - **REFER** patients who are not already receiving eye-care by an ophthalmologist to check for retinopathy
- **REFER** patient to diabetes nurse educator and/or dietician annually or whenever needed.

TYPE 1 AND TYPE 2 DIABETICS REQUIRING INSULIN
- These patients are usually seen first by a doctor or at a diabetic clinic if there is one available.
- Once their condition has been stabilised they can be treated by the nurse clinician.
- If problems arise with blood glucose control they can be referred back to the doctor or diabetic clinic.

Types of insulin
- **Short acting insulins (SA)**
    - Actrapid HM
    - Humulin R
- **Intermediate acting insulins (IA)**
    - Humulin N
    - Protaphane HM
- **Biphasic insulins (combination SA + IA)**
    - Actraphane HM
    - Humulin 30 / 70

Preparations include
- 10 ml vials
- Cartridges for pen injection devices
- Disposable syringes (penset)

Note.
- All insulins are in the concentration of 100 units / ml
- Pen injection devices are generally reserved for
    - patients with poor vision
    - pregnant women

Insulin therapy
Diabetes mellitus type I
- All patients should be referred at diagnosis of drug therapy to begin and be stalilised.
- If the patient is severely symptomatic, and referral to hospital is delayed by more than 2 hours:
    - give stat dose of Actrapid insulin
    - 0.1 units / kg IMI
    - when giving insulin IM, do not use an insulin needle

Diabetes mellitus type 2
- Insulin is indicated when the patient is uncontrolled on the maximum oral therapy.
- Insulin therapy should be started under the supervision of a doctor.
- Educate patients on the following:
    - how to draw up the correct amount of insulin
    - injection technique
    - the areas for insulin injection (either thigh or abdomen) and rotation of injection sites
    - recognition and treatment of acute complications ie. hypoglycaemia and hyperglycaemia.

- Patients must ensure that they take regular meals.

For Insulin Protocol for Type 2 diabetes patients, see page 139.

Other management

To prevent long-term complications of diabetes:
- Statin therapy should be added to lifestyle therapy, regardless of baseline lipid levels, for Type 2 diabetic patients who:
    - are older than 40 years of age or have had diabetes for longer than 10 years
    - have existing cardiovascular disease
    - have chronic kidney disease (eGFR <60 ml / minute)
- Give simvastatin, orally, 10 mg at night.
- If the LDL-cholesterol remains >3 mmol/L, a higher dose may be required
    - **REFER** patient to specialist.
- Use aspirin therapy in Type 1 or Type 2 diabetic patients with a history of cardiovascular disease, i.e.:
    - ischaemic heart disease
    - peripheral vascular disease
    - previous thrombotic stroke
- Give aspirin, oral, 75-100 mg daily.

NB Avoid aspirin in patients with uncontrolled blood pressure, especially if the BP is greater than 160/100.

REFERRAL

Urgent
- Dehydration
- Keto-acidosis / acidotic breathing
- Hyperglycaemia >25 mmoi / L
- Ketonuria >1+
- Serious infections eg. pyelonephritis
- Gangrene
- Sudden deterioration of vision
- Nausea, vomiting and abdominal pain

Non-urgent
- Pregnancy
- Uncontrolled on maximum oral therapy
- Peripheral neuropathy
- Peripheral vascular disease

▼ **Note to doctor**

Guidelines for changing insulin doses

Reducing insulin doses
- Reduce the dose of the insulin most active at that time by 4 units.

Patients on a biphasic insulin twice-daily
- Time of hypoglycaemia
    - during the day, reduce morning dose
    - at night, reduce evening dose.
- Erratic meal times and content may be the cause of hypoglycaemia
    - correct these causes if possible before adjusting insulin doses.

Increasing insulin doses
- Increase only one insulin dose at a time.
- Doses should be increased gradually, not more than 4 units weekly.

Patients on a biphasic insulin twice-daily
- Time of hyperglycaemia
    - during the day, increase morning dose
    - at night, increase evening dose

- *Defaulters*
- Re-start on previous dose of insulin.
- If severely symptomatic:
    - give stat dose of Actrapid insulin
    - 0.1 units / kg IMI

Criteria for clinic doctors for admission to hospital for hyperglycaemia

- The main criteria for admission should **not** be the degree of hyperglycaemia
- Much more important are factors such as:
    - dehydration
    - acidosis
    - presence of ketones on the breath or in urine >1+
    - associated severe infection
    - a patient sleepy or obtunded (dull mental state) in any way ▲

DIAGRAM A

PROTOCOL FOR TYPE 2 DIABETES PATIENTS

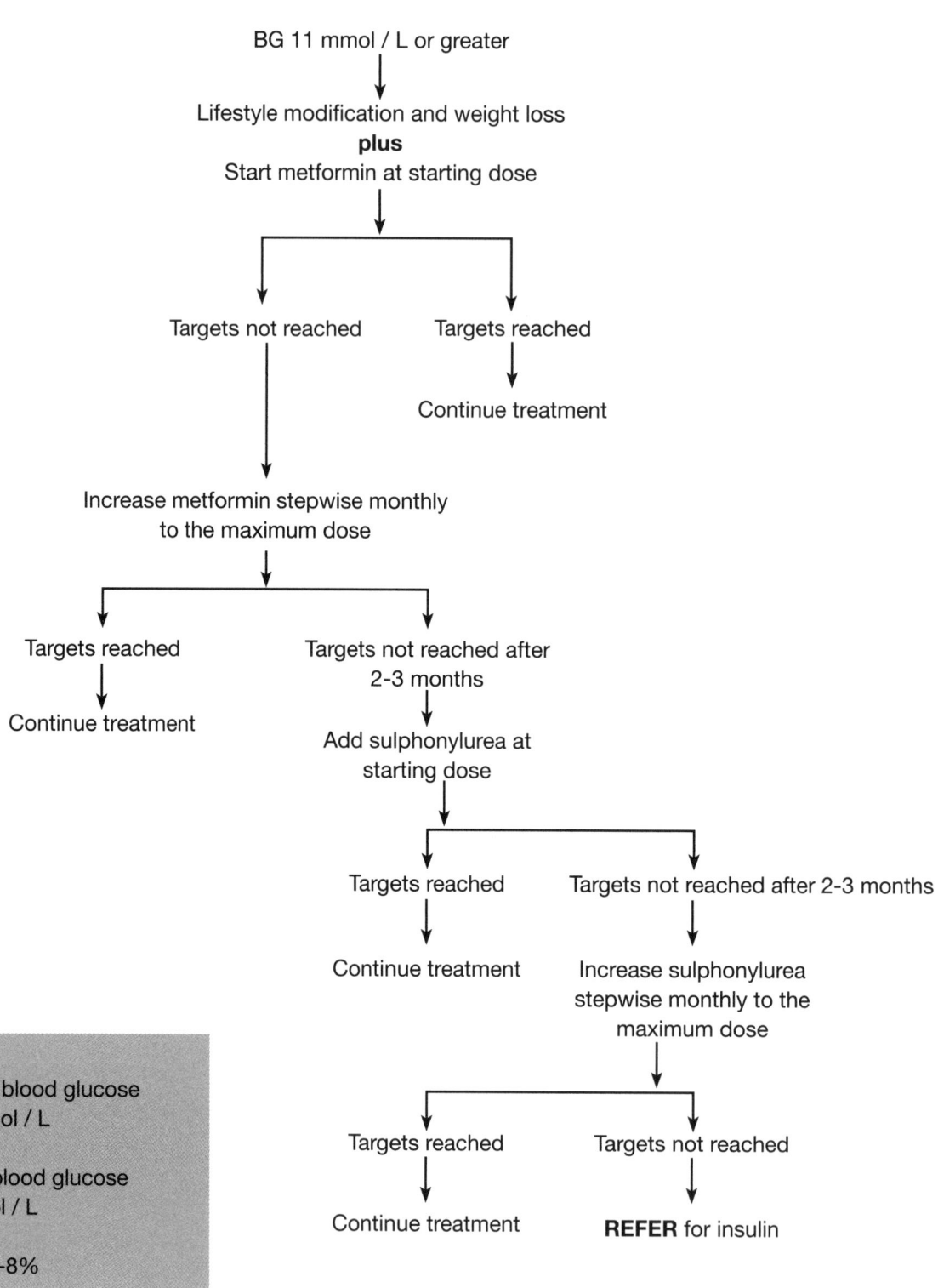

DIAGRAM B

INSULIN PROTOCOL FOR TYPE 2 DIABETES PATIENTS

Insulin as supplementation

STEP 1
- Use a basal intermediate acting insulin, eg. Protophane, Humulin N

Starting dose	Increment	Maximum daily dose
• 10 units in the evening at bedtime but not after 22h00	• Increase to 15 units if 10 units not effective	20 units

At initiation of basal insulin therapy, the sulphonylurea may be discontinued, but metformin therapy must be **maintained.**

STEP 2 (if above not effective)
- Use biphasic insulin eg. Actraphane, Humulin 30/70

Starting dose	Increment	Maximum total daily dose
Total daily dose 15 units: • 2/3 total daily dose 30 minutes before breakfast (10 units) • 1/3 total daily dose 30 minutes before supper (5 units)	4 units monthly: • First increment is added to the morning dose • Second increment is added to the evening dose • Subsequent increment to follow same pattern.	• **REFER** if total daily dose exceeds 75 units OR if more than 1 unit / kg total daily dose is needed

At initiation of biphasic insulin therapy, metformin must be continued, but sulphonylurea therapy should be **stopped.**

THYROID GLAND

THYROID GLAND PROBLEMS

HYPO-THYROIDISM

Causes
- Congenital (usually gene mutations)
- Thyroiditis
- Post-thyroidectomy
- Post-radio-active iodine for thyrotoxicosis
- Pituitary / hypothalamic malfunction
- Medicines
    - iodine excess eg. amiodarone
    - lithium
    - antithyroid drugs for Grave's disease

Clinical features
- The onset is gradual and often mistaken for ageing alone or for depression
    - **it is difficult to diagnose**
    - **it is often missed.**
- It mainly affects middle-aged females
- The symptoms are a result of decreased metabolism, with slowing of mental and physical activity
- The symptoms are often vague, multiple and chronic
- There is sensitivity to cold
- Menorrhagia (later oligomenorrhoea and amenorrhoea)
- Loss of appetite
- Constipation
- Weight gain (moderate)
- Tiredness/weakness
- Forgetfulness
- Tingling in the fingers - carpal tunnel syndrome
- Face puffy
- Stiff, aching muscles
- Dry skin which flakes easily on rubbing
- Hair becomes dry and tends to fall out
- Thinning of the outer halves of eyebrows
- Slow pulse rate (bradycardia)
- Speech is slow and slightly hoarse
- Low temperature
- Later, myxoedema results
    - dull, expressionless face
    - sparse hair
    - peri-orbital puffiness
    - large tongue
    - pale, cool skin which feels rough and like dough.
- Delayed relaxation of tendon reflexes ("hung up" reflexes)
- Pericardial effusion or other serious cavity effusions

MANAGEMENT
REFER
- If hypo-thyroidism is suspected
- Patients with a thyroidectomy scar who are not taking thyroid replacement hormones regularly, to check the thyroid levels.

▼ Note to doctor
- Check TSH concentration
- If elevated, check T4 concentration
- If TSH is elevated and T4 is low, diagnose hypothyroidism ▲

HYPERTHYROIDISM
(HYPERFUNCTION OF THE THYROID GLAND)

Causes
- Most common cause is abnormal thyroid stimulator as in Graves's disease.
- Other common causes are associated with autonomous hyperfunction within the gland, such as toxic single nodules or multinodular goitre.
- Sub-acute thyroiditis.
- Excess secretion of thyroid stimulating hormone (TSH) by pituitary tumour.

Clinical features
- The symptoms are a result of overproduction of T3 and T4
- It is more common in females
- Age 20-60 years
- There may or may not be a clinically detectable goitre
- There is weight loss, although there is **increased** appetite
    - the differential diagnosis includes diabetes mellitus.
- Preference for cold weather, sweating, heat intolerance
- Mood changes eg. irritability, patient cries easily, emotional
- Palpitations with or without symptoms of heart failure
- Nervousness
- Increased frequency of bowel actions/diarrhoea
- Polyuria
- Menorrhagia or amenorrhoea - reduced fertility
- Hyperactive (restless)
- Rapid speech
- Anxious
- Looks thin or wasted
- Tachycardia
- Arrhythmias eg. atrial fibrillation, ectopic beats
- Bounding pulse, high pulse pressure
- Fine tremors of the fingers
- Warm, sweaty hands
- Skin warm, moist and soft
- Muscle weakness
- Hyperreflexia
- Muscle wasting (proximal myopathy)
- Retraction of the upper eyelids
    - the patient appears to stare.

- Lid lag
    - the upper lid moves slower than the eye, as the patient looks down
    - as a result the white upper sclera will be obvious (as the patient looks down).
- Infrequent blinking
- Hair is fine and silky
- Failure to wrinkle the brow on upward gaze
- Onycholysis
- In addition in Grave's disease
    - exophthalmos (proptosis)
    - clubbing of the fingers
    - pretibial myxoedema (thyroid dermopathy of the shins)

MANAGEMENT
- **REFER**
- If delay in **REFERRAL** is expected, prescribe propranolol 40 mg 3 x daily
    - **or** atenolol 50 mg daily

▼ **Note to doctor**
- Check TSH and FT4 concentrations
- If TSH suppressed and T4 normal, request FT3
- If TSH is suppressed and FT4 or FT3 is elevated, diagnose hyperthyroidism ▲

GOITRE (ENLARGED THYROID GLAND)

Clinical features
- There is an anterior neck swelling on one or both sides of the mid-line.
- It moves upwards on swallowing.
- The swelling may be smooth and diffuse, e.g. Graves's disease or nodular (single nodule or multinodular).

MANAGEMENT
- **REFER** unless previously investigated.
- If excessive sympathetic symptoms, e.g. palpitations, give:
    - propranolol 40 mg 3 x daily
    - **or**
    - atenolol 50 mg daily

THYROIDITIS

Mainly viral or auto-immune in origin. The common forms can be associated at one time or another with an euthyroid, thyrotoxic or hypothyroid state.

SUBACUTE THYROIDITIS (DE QUERVAIN'S THYROIDITIS)

Clinical features
- Characterised by pain over the thyroid or pain referred to the lower jaw or ear.
- The gland is tender and nodular and the ESR is raised.
- The toxic phase lasts up to 3 months.

MANAGEMENT
- **REFER** unless previously investigated.
- If excessive sympathetic symptoms, e.g. palpitations, give:
    - propranolol 40 mg 3 x daily
    - **or**
    - atenolol 50 mg daily

SINGLE THYROID NODULE

Clinical features
- A single swelling in some part of the thyroid gland
- Rest of the gland normal
- May cause features of thyrotoxicosis

MANAGEMENT
- **REFER** for investigation as there is a possibility of it being malignant.
- If excessive sympathetic symptoms, e.g. palpitations, give:
    - propranolol 40 mg 3 x daily
    - **or**
    - atenolol 50 mg daily

THYROGLOSSAL CYST

A thyroglossal cyst may be confused with a goitre.

Clinical features
- It is a fluid-filled swelling which occurs in the remains of the thyroglossal duct.
- The thyroglossal duct is an embryonic structure which usually disappears by birth.
- It is a midline swelling.
- It moves upwards
    - on swallowing
    - when the tongue is stuck out.

REFER.

Kidney and Urological Disorders

UROLOGICAL PROBLEMS

UROLOGICAL SYMPTOMS

HAEMATURIA

Causes

Blood visible with the naked eye (macroscopic haematuria)
- Blood appearing uniformly mixed with the urine is from the kidney, ureters or bladder
- Blood appearing at the beginning of micturition
    - suggests anterior urethral or prostatic causes
- Blood appearing at the end of micturition
    - suggests the posterior urethra or bladder causes
    - it is particularly due to bilharzia
- Dark smoky urine is due to slow bleeding in the kidney eg. glomerulonephritis
- Fresh red blood in the urine is usually due to bladder disease, especially
    - bilharzia (haematuria at the end of voiding)
    - tumours
    - infection
    - stones
- Red urine which is not positive for blood on dipstix may be due to
    - beetroot
    - drugs and food colourants
    - porphyria

Blood detected on dipstix only (microscopic haematuria)

This may be due to
- Febrile illness
- Acute glomerulonephritis (AGN)
- Alcohol
- TB
- Tumours
- Trauma
- Contamination eg. menstruation
- Bleeding disorders
- Bacterial endocarditis

Other macroscopic appearances of urine

Turbid
- Consider proteinuria or infection (pyuria)
- Examine and diagnose further

Orange / red / green / blue
- Consider bilirubin, urobilin, drugs (anti-tuberculous: rifampicin), laxatives and "blood cleaning" tablets
- Examine and diagnose further

Cloudy
- Consider urates and phosphates
- This is usually normal and needs no further treatment

> **MANAGEMENT**
> - Treat the cause if you are able to, e.g. UTI
> - **REFER**
>   - all cases not associated with bilharzia or UTI
>   - any patient not responding to specific drug treatment
>   - if there is haematuria after trauma, as there might be serious underlying kidney damage with only mild haematuria

▼ **Investigation of haematuria**
- Urine microscopy for red blood cell morphology and casts
    - dysmorphic appearance of the RBCs or the presence of casts is due to kidney / glomerular disease
    - isomorphic normal-shaped RBCs may indicate a urological condition, e.g. renal calculi, prostatic disease, urinary tract tumours or menstrual contamination
- **REFER** patients with non-glomerular bleeding and those with glomerular bleeding who have reduced eGFR or proteinuria. ▲

RETENTION OF URINE

Causes
- Enlarged prostate (in males)
    - a common cause
    - particularly in the elderly
- Stricture of the urethra
- Infections
- Pregnancy
- Post delivery
- Ectopic pregnancy
- Tumours
- Brain and spinal cord disease
- Phimosis and paraphimosis

Clinical features
- Difficulty or inability to pass urine
- A poor stream of urine and dribbling (dripping) after voiding
- Pain in the lower abdomen
- Palpable bladder present

MANAGEMENT
- Treat the cause if you are able to.
- **REFER** if:
    - you are unsure
    - you suspect a serious cause
- If the patient is distressed, catheterize to relieve distension of the bladder and record the volume of urine
    - the catheter can be left in to provide relief during transport

INCONTINENCE OF URINE

Causes
- This may be due to generalised debility or confusion
- Exclude local causes eg.
    - urinary tract infection
    - neurological disorders
    - bladder prolapse

MANAGEMENT
- **REFER** unless the patient has been previously investigated
- If no treatable cause for the incontinence is found, teach the patient or family the care of whatever drainage method is being used eg. catheter
- Consider the following
    - physiotherapy for muscle weakness problems
    - occupational therapy for assistance with equipment
    - home nursing if necessary

POLYURIA

This is the excretion of increased quantities of urine.

Causes
- Diabetes mellitus
- Drugs such as diuretics
- Recovery from heart failure
- Acute kidney failure (recovery phase)
- Increased or excessive fluid intake
- Chronic kidney failure

REFER if
- You are not able to make a diagnosis
- You cannot treat the cause

BURNING ON MICTURITION (BOM)

Causes

In children
This is an unusual complaint in children.
- It is vital to exclude a urinary tract infection by testing the urine for leucocytes and nitrites with a dipstix
- More common causes are
    - phimosis or balanitis in boys due to trauma
    - wet nappies or soap powders used
    - vaginitis in girls
    - sexual abuse must always be excluded as a cause
    - vaginal foreign bodies

In men
- Urethritis is the most common cause and must be considered and treated even if there is no evidence of discharge on history or examination
    - Chlamydia is common and seldom gives a purulent urethral discharge
- If there is no evidence of a urethritis, you should look for prostatitis (see page 170)
- Balanitis is common in diabetes
    - particularly due to Candida
- Urinary tract infection (think of diabetes)
- Urinary stones
- Bilharzia
- Tumours
- Applications to the genitalia to prevent or treat sexually transmitted infections eg. Dettol, Vaseline

In women
- Urinary tract infections are common and must be checked for with a dipstix on a "clean catch" specimen (see below)
- It may be due to vaginitis or cervicitis
    - it is important to do an adequate gynaecological history and examination to exclude serious causes eg. carcinoma of the cervix
- Pregnancy must always be considered
- Bladder tumours
- Bilharzia
- The patient may say she has BOM to alert the clinician to another underlying problem eg. infertility

How to collect a "clean catch" specimen
- The vulva should be wiped / washed with Savlon or chlorhexidine
- After this the urine is obtained "midstream", ie. in the middle of micturition (voiding)

UROLOGICAL DISEASES

PROSTATE

PROSTATITIS

See section on Sexually Transmitted Infections page 170 for a discussion and management of prostatitis.

BENIGN PROSTATIC HYPERPLASIA (PROSTATISM)

Clinical features

- Some enlargement of the prostate occurring with advancing age is natural, but this may become symptomatic and will require treatment
- This occurs in men over 45 years of age
- They may complain of prostatism
    - difficulty and delay in starting micturition
    - poor urinary stream
    - difficulty in clearing all the urine, with dribbling after having finished urinating
- Nocturia
- Frequency
- They may present with
    - features of a urinary tract infection
    - urinary retention
- Prostatic examination reveals a firm enlarged prostate
- It is important to feel for hard nodules on PR which might suggest a carcinoma of the prostate

MANAGEMENT
REFER if
- you are unsure about the prostate size
- the prostate is very large
- there are nodules or you suspect a carcinoma
- there is significant difficulty in micturition
- If there is a moderate size prostate on PR and symptoms are not severe and recur now and again
    - advise patient that surgery may be needed if it gets worse
    - avoid a lot of fluid at night
- Treatment of any associated urinary tract infection may help to relieve symptoms.
- It is important to screen all patients for prostate cancer whether this is suspected or not
    - take blood for PSA (prostate specific antigen).

▼ **Note to doctor**
- Interpretation of PSA results
    - normal <4ng/ml
    suspicious
    - over 50 years > 4 ng/ml
    - over 60 years >5ng/ml
    - over 70 years >7ng/ml
    dangerous
    - >10ng/ml - all ages
- Suspicious results **REFER** for biopsy.
- Over 75 years don't **REFER** for biopsy ▲

PROSTATIC CANCER (CARCINOMA)

This is a common and serious cancer in men which is often advanced at the time of diagnosis.

Clinical features

- Prostatism uncommon
- Urinary incontinence
- Haematuria
- Erectile dysfunction
- It may present with
    - features of a UTI
    - chronic lower backache (spinal metastases) or pelvic pain
- The prostate gland is hard and often nodular
- There are general features suggesting chronic illness such as pallor, wasting and tiredness

MANAGEMENT
REFER if
- **Any** nodules are felt in the prostate on rectal examination
- You suspect a carcinoma

BLADDER

CYSTITIS

Clinical features

- The diagnosis of a urinary tract infection is confirmed if the urine is found to have nitrites **and** leucocytes
- You can suspect an infection if there are typical symptoms and signs of acute cystitis
    - dysuria
    - frequency of micturition
    - urgency of micturition
    - supra-pubic pain and tenderness
    - sometimes the urine is grossly blood-stained (haemorrhagic cystitis)
    - the urine shows leucocytes or nitrites, blood and protein
- It is important to note that some patients, especially diabetics, often do not complain of the typical symptoms of cystitis
  eg. burning on micturition (BOM) and frequency
    - *therefore if attention is not paid to the urine findings, the diagnosis may be easily missed*

Dipstix test (Multistix etc)
- The nitrites and leucocytes should be read after two minutes
    - they may become falsely positive if read later
- In patients who present with the typical symptoms and signs, but urine findings are negative, the diagnosis should only be made once other causes have been excluded eg.
    - vulvitis
    - salpingitis
    - urethritis

See management of UTI on page 151.

BILHARZIA (SCHISTOSOMIASIS)

Clinical features

- Terminal haematuria, especially if a patient is from a known bilharzia area ie.
    - N. Province, Mpumalanga, KwaZulu-Natal, Eastern Cape
    - any other African country eg. Swaziland, Mozambique, Zimbabwe
- "Swimmer's itch" (itchy skin)
- The diagnosis should be confirmed by
    - finding bilharzial ova in the urine or faeces
- *Asymptomatic infection* means there are no symptoms and the disease is discovered by chance
- *Symptomatic infection* means that the patient has symptoms of bilharzia infection
- Blood tests are not helpful in diagnosis of bilharzial cystitis as they do not show the difference between present and previous infection

MANAGEMENT

Endemic areas
- Treatment should be given to all patients even if microscopy cannot be done

Non-endemic areas
- Treatment should be given only if eggs of S haematobium or S mansoni are found in the urine or faeces
- Treatment of symptomatic cases is important as early lesions are reversible and curable
- Treatment in pregnancy should preferably be delayed until after delivery
- Praziquantel (Biltricide) is excreted in breast milk. If the mother can safely do so, she should
  - refrain from breast feeding on the day of treatment and the next 2 days
  - be instructed to express breast milk and throw it away
  - feed the baby on powdered milk or cow's milk with a cup and spoon
  - be encouraged to begin breast feeding again on the fourth day

Medicine management
- Praziquantel (Biltricide) is very effective for both S. haematobium and S. mansoni.
- Tablet 600 mg with 4 equal segments (each segment 150 mg)
  - give 40 mg / kg body mass in a single oral dose
  - the average adult dose is 4 x 600 mg tabs
- Side effects of praziquantel are few
  - may cause temporary drowsiness and dizziness

All treated cases should be advised on how to avoid re-infection.

Follow up
- Patients should be examined for the presence of living eggs 3 and 6 months after treatment (urine microscopy)
- Re-treatment is necessary if egg excretion has not decreased greatly

Prevention
- Prevent infestation of snails by providing latrines
- Provide a safe water supply for home use and recreation
- Health education
- Snail destruction
- Wear protective clothing when working in water
- Avoid slow-flowing water
- Avoid areas with a lot of vegetation in the water
- Ideally collect water
  - in the cooler time of the day at sunrise
  - near fast-flowing water
  - from areas of sandy beach
- Boil all water before use.
- Try to touch the water as little as possible.
- Avoid swimming in rivers and dams.
- Do not urinate or pass stools near water used for drinking, bathing or washing.

KIDNEY

PYELONEPHRITIS

Infection of the kidney parenchyma

Clinical features
- Pain in one or both loins, radiating to the supra-pubic area
- Fever and sometimes rigors
- Headache, malaise, vomiting
- Abdominal pain
- There may be symptoms of associated cystitis eg.
  - dysuria
  - frequency
  - supra-pubic tenderness
- The urine is often turbid, offensive and shows proteinuria, haematuria, leucocytes and nitrites on L Combu 9 testing
- Renal angle tenderness is often confused with fibrositis of the back muscles. It is only of value as a sign of pyelonephritis if the tenderness is
  - very obvious
  - usually unilateral
  - associated with other reliable symptoms and signs of pyelonephritis
- A better test is tenderness over the kidney on direct palpation from the front through the anterior abdominal wall.

MANAGEMENT
Outpatient therapy is only indicated for women of reproductive age, who do not have any of the danger signs - see referral criteria below.
- All other patients should be **REFERRED**.
- Give ciprofloxacin, orally, 500 mg 12 hourly for 7-10 days.

If severely ill
- Before **REFERRAL**, set up an IV drip of normal saline.
- Give a single dose of ceftriaxone
  - children 80 mg / kg IMI or IVI stat
  - adults 1g IMI or IVI stat

Referral criteria
- Acute pyelonephritis with danger signs:
  - vomiting
  - features of sepsis, eg. tachypnoea, tachycardia, hypotension, confusion
  - diabetes
- Acute pyelonephritis in:
  - pregnant women
  - women beyond reproductive age
  - men
- Children over 3 months who appear ill
- Children less than 3 months of age with any UTI

POST STREPTOCOCCAL GLOMERULONEPHRITIS (PSGN)

Causes
- Post streptococcal glomerulonephritis (PSGN) follows infection with a Beta-haemolytic Streptococcus
- There is an immune response to the Streptococcus aimed at destroying the invading bacterium
  - unfortunately, the immune response also destroys glomerular tissue resulting in PSGN

Clinical features

- There may be malaise, headache, anorexia, low grade fever
- Many children have a very mild asymptomatic illness
- Of those who have clinical illness, most recover rapidly
- A few will develop complications of chronic glomerulonephritis or nephrotic syndrome
- Haematuria is essential for diagnosis
    - it may be macroscopic or microscopic
    - it is usually dark and smoky if macroscopic (seen with the eye)
    - it is rare for the urine to be grossly blood-stained
- There is proteinuria usually of a mild degree and in the same proportions as the haematuria
- It is more common in boys
- It is common in the 4-15 year age group
    - very rare before 2 years
    - most common between 7-10 years
- It occurs 1-3 weeks after a streptococcal throat infection or impetigo
    - the initial infection is usually an impetigo, often associated with scabies
    - the streptococcal infection may still be present
- Prompt and adequate treatment of the strep throat (or impetigo) is not always a safeguard against glomerulonephritis
- Recurrences are very uncommon

In more severe cases

- There is decreased urine output (oliguria)
- Occasionally no urine at all (anuria)
- Oedema
    - peri-orbital
    - worse in the morning
    - may have dependent oedema (severe cases)
    - severe oedema is not usually seen
- Heart failure as shown by all the usual symptoms and signs
- Hypertension may be severe and sudden in onset
- Hypertensive encephalopathy
    - due to a severe rise in blood pressure
    - characterised by headache, restlessness, vomiting, blurring of vision and convulsions

Note. A paediatric BP cuff may be needed to measure the BP correctly in smaller children

MANAGEMENT
REFER if:
- There is macroscopic haematuria
- There is oedema
- There is hypertension
- You suspect heart failure or encephalopathy

Immediate management before REFERRAL
General measures
- Stop all fluid intake if patient does not pass urine
    - do **not** put up a drip.
- Give oxygen and nurse in semi-Fowler's position if dyspnoeic.

Medicine management
- If hypertension is present:
    - <6 years >120 mm Hg systolic BP or 90 mm Hg diastolic BP
    - >6 years >130 mm Hg systolic BP or 95 mm Hg diastolic BP

Give nifedipine, oral 0,25-0,5 mg / kg sublingually, as a single dose. Withdraw contents of 5 mg capsule with a 1 ml syringe
- 10-25 kg, give 2,5 mg
- 25-50 kg, give 5 mg
- over 50 kg, give 10 mg

- If there is respiratory distress, give furosemide as an initial bolus dose
    - in children 2 mg / kg IVI (do **not** put up a drip)

If there is blood on the dipstix only
- Test urine for nitrites and leucocytes to exclude infection
- Give penicillin VK for 10 days in a dose appropriate for age
- Ask the child to return if the symptoms get worse
- Restrict
    - fluid intake
    - salt
- Carbohydrates should be given liberally (plenty)

NEPHROTIC SYNDROME

This is mainly an immune-complex disease.

Causes
- Diabetic nephropathy
- Secondary to infections, especially AIDS
- This can be due to a variety of glomerular diseases including PSGN

Clinical features
- Oedema - severe, generalised
- There may also be ascites and pleural effusions
- Marked proteinuria with less haematuria

REFER to hospital.

RENAL CALCULI (KIDNEY STONES)

Clinical features
- A sudden onset of loin pain
- It is intensely painful
- Spasmodic
- The pain radiates down to the groin and scrotum / perineum
- It may be associated with nausea and vomiting
- There is haematuria
    - gross
    - **or** on urine dipstix

- **REFER**
- Give analgesia
    - morphine 10-15 mg IMI stat

ACUTE KIDNEY FAILURE

Causes
- Dehydration and fluid loss
- Toxins
- Urinary tract obstruction

Clinical features
- Oliguria or anuria
- Nausea and vomiting
- Confusion
- Hiccups
- Heavy haematuria and / or proteinuria

> - **REFER to hospital stat if you suspect it.**
> - If not dehydrated or shocked, stop all fluids.
> - If dehydrated or shocked, commence normal saline IV.

CHRONIC KIDNEY DISEASE

Clinical features
- Many patients with this problem are not diagnosed because the signs and symptoms may be mild and easily missed
    - suspect it particularly in diabetics and hypertensives
- Hypertension
- Anaemia
- Tiredness
- Weakness
- Weight loss
- Chronic hiccups
- Diarrhoea
- Oedema
- Proteinuria
- There may be nocturia and polyuria due to inability to concentrate urine.
- Later oliguria and anuria.

Investigations
- Any patient with proteinuria of 1+ or more in the absence of infection, heart failure or menstruation should have urine sent for spot PCR (protein-creatinine ratio).
- If the PCR >0.1 g / mmol
    - send blood for serum creatinine concentration and eGFR
    - or calculate the patient's creatinine clearance (doctor or PHCN)

> ### MANAGEMENT
> **Proteinuria**
> - Start with low dosage of an ACE-inhibitor and titrate up, for example:
>   - enalapril 5 mg 12 hourly
>   - increase to 10 mg 12 hourly
>   - then increase to 20 mg 12 hourly or until the proteinuria disappears
>
> **Diabetes mellitus**
> - When eGFR <60 ml / min:
>   - stop sulphonylurea
>   - reduce dose of metformin by 50%
> - Insulin is the preferred medicine to control blood glucose in patients with eGFR <30 ml / min
>
> **Hypertension**
> - Treat if present (see page 76).
>
> **REFER**
> - Patients with eGFR below 60 ml / min.
> - No resolution of proteinuria with ACE-inhibitor therapy.

> - If there is deterioration in the patient's condition, e.g.
>   - dehydration
>   - confusion
>   - evidence of acute infection
> - Uncontrolled hypertension / heart failure

▼ **Note to doctor**
Creatinine clearance calculation (for use in adults)
Males
$$CrCl\ (ml/min) = \frac{(140 - age) \times weight\ (kg)}{plasma\ Cr\ (micromol/L)}$$

Females
$$CrCL\ (ml/min) = \frac{(140 - age) \times weight\ (kg) \times 0.85}{plasma\ Cr\ (micromol/L)}$$ ▲

NB Ideal bodyweight should be used if the patient is clinically obese or underweight.

URINARY TRACT INFECTIONS (UTI)

Uncomplicated cystitis
- This occurs in non-pregnant women of reproductive age.

Complicated cystitis
- This occurs in all others including children, men, pregnant and post-menopausal women and diabetic patients.

UTI IN WOMEN

Causes
- Women often develop infection of the bladder, particularly
    - during pregnancy
    - as a result of trauma during delivery

Other contributing factors are
- The proximity of the external urethral meatus (EUM) to the vaginal introitus
- The shortness of the female urethra
- Patients with infections of the cervix and vagina develop a discharge and, as a result, tend to wear some occluding material to collect the discharge, such as a pad
    - this means that the urethra is bathed in infected material
- Trauma during intercourse
- The infection ascends up the urethra causing a urethritis
    - infection of the bladder (cystitis)
- The cystitis may ascend further and cause an infection in the renal parenchyma (pyelonephritis)

Clinical features
See pages 147 and 149.
A common problem is how to decide whether the symptoms in women are due to a urinary tract infection, a vaginitis or a cervicitis.

- Diagnosis of urinary tract infection is confirmed if the dipstix test records the presence of nitrites and leucocytes
    - leucocytes with no nitrites may be due to contamination with pus from a vaginitis or cervicitis (this may cause symptoms similar to a urinary tract infection)
    - presence of blood or protein in the urine is **not** diagnostic of a urinary tract infection.

- On vaginal examination, palpation of the bladder through the anterior fornix frequently causes pain
    - this is more acute on bimanual examination when the bladder is compressed
- Speculum examination may reveal whether a vaginitis or cervicitis is present (though the presence of either does not exclude a urinary tract infection)

Urine specimen
- A urine specimen for MC&S should ideally reach the laboratory within 30 minutes to obtain accurate results.
- Refrigerate specimen if delay of more than 1 hour is expected before urine reaches the laboratory.
- It should be a clean catch specimen.
- If this is not possible it may be more reliable and cost effective to send the patient to the hospital for collection of the urine specimen.

MANAGEMENT IN ADULTS

- Treat as a urinary infection if:
    - urine positive for both leucocytes and nitrites
    - urine positive for nitrites or leucocytes with symptoms of UTI
    - systemic signs and symptoms
- Urine with leucocytes only:
    - check the patient for other sources of leucocytes eg urethritis, prostatitis, vaginitis, cervicitis
    - if unsure, do a dipstix on a midstream urine
    - a quick and effective way is to give the patient a dipstix to dip into the urine in the middle of passing urine
- **REFER** for investigation if no cause for the leucocytes is found as it may be due to less obvious causes eg TB.

Referral criteria
- No response to treatment
- Relapse (i.e. recurrence of infection within 3 weeks of completing treatment)
- Recurrent UTI
    - more than 3 times in a woman
    - more than once in a man
    - within a 1 year period
- Patients with acute pyelonephritis with any of the danger signs (see page 148).
- Pyelonephritis in pregnant women, women beyond reproductive age, diabetic patients, and in men.

General measures
- Encourage high fluid intake
- Promote personal hygiene (females)
- Send urine for MC&S in complicated or recurrent UTIs
- All patients to return in 3 days if not improved
- Patients with complicated or recurrent UTI to return after 1 week to check the urine & MC&S results.

Medicine management
- Uncomplicated cystitis (18 years and older)
    - nitrofurantoin 100 mg 4 x daily for 7 days
- Pregnant / breastfeeding women and adolescents
    - nitrofurantoin 100 mg 4 x daily for 7 days
- Complicated cystitis (including men, post-menopausal women and diabetics)
    - ciprofloxacin 500 mg 2 x daily for 7 days (Dr initiated)
- Acute pyelonephritis in non-pregnant women of reproductive age who do not have any of the danger signs
    - see referral criteria page 148
    - give ciprofloxacin 500 mg 2 x daily for 7-10 days (Dr initiated)

Cystitis not responding to treatment
- Features which suggest this are:
    - the patient still has symptoms
    - urine still has evidence of leucocytes, or nitrites and possibly protein and blood.
- **REFER** or manage according to the MC&S results.

UTI IN CHILDREN

Clinical features
- This problem is very often missed because young children seldom complain of urinary symptoms
- UTI is more common in undernourished children
- Urinary tract infections should be suspected in any child with
    - nausea, vomiting, anorexia, diarrhoea
    - abdominal pain
    - fever, particularly if no other cause can be found
    - weight loss and failure to thrive
    - any urinary symptoms or enuresis
    - vague symptoms or malaise
- There are seldom any signs to be found on clinical examination
- The diagnosis is made on examining the child's urine
- Urine testing will often show urinary tract infections which are not even suspected clinically
- Other abnormalities such as haematuria due to unsuspected sexual abuse may also be found

Urine specimen

How to obtain a urine specimen in a child
- The easiest method in girls is for her to sit facing backwards on a toilet seat
    - this ensures wide abduction of the hips
    - the first few millilitres of urine is passed directly into the toilet and a midstream sample then caught
- Boys may simply pass urine in the normal manner into a container
    - where possible ensure that the foreskin is pulled back
- In younger children apply a urine bag as a first screening test

Urine specimen results
- If there are no leucocytes or nitrites, it is unlikely that the child has a UTI.
- If leucocytes and nitrites are found, the child definitely does have a UTI.
- Leucocytes together with other typical symptoms and / or signs of a UTI are also diagnostic
    - this is because the nitrite test is falsely negative when there is frequent bladder emptying (as occurs in young infants)
- If only leucocytes are found and there are no other symptoms or signs of a UTI, this may be due to contamination from the vulva, foreskin or faeces.
- Often, if the vulva is recleaned and a second specimen is tested
    - it will be found to be clear
    - if leucocytes are still found, a UTI should be suspected

MANAGEMENT

REFER
- All children under 3 months of age
- All children over 3 months who appear ill
- All children for renal tract investigation after completion of treatment
- No response to treatment
- Recurrent UTI in children for assessment and consideration of prophylaxis

Medicine management
- Co-amoxyclav 3 x daily for 7 days
    - 3-6 months 4 ml (125 / 31.2 mg / 5 ml)
    - 6-12 months 6 ml (125 / 31.2 mg / 5 ml)
    - 12-18 months 8 ml (125 / 31.2 mg / 5 ml)
    - 18 months-3 years 5 ml (250 / 62.5 mg / 5 ml)
    - 3-5 years 6 ml (250 / 62.5 mg / 5 ml)
    - 5-7 years 7.5 ml (250 / 62.5 mg / 5 ml)
    - 7-11 years 10 ml (250 / 62.5 mg / 5 ml)
- Send urine for MC&S.
- Child to return after 1 week to check the urine and MC&S result.

RECURRENT UTI

MANAGEMENT

General measures
- Women should empty their bladders as soon as possible after intercourse.
- Identify and **REFER** elderly patients with hormone-deficient atrophic vulvo-vaginitis.
- Patients with impaired bladder emptying need urological or gynaecological examination to establish the cause.

REFERRAL
Recurrent UTI if:
- more than 3 x in a women
- more than 1 x in a man
- within a 1 year period

PHIMOSIS AND CIRCUMCISION

IN ADULTS

For management see page 176.

IN CHILDREN

- It is important to realise that the foreskin is normally attached to the glans of the penis for several months after birth
- Parents often try to retract the foreskin to clean the glans, and are worried that it is not retracting "normally"

MANAGEMENT

- Parents should be advised that trying to retract the foreskin too early will result in damage and bleeding under the foreskin and later scarring and adhesions
- Parents who wish to have a baby boy circumcised should be advised
    - that it is a potentially dangerous operation
    - to only have it done by experienced people

ENURESIS

This is urinary incontinence occurring after the chronological or mental age of 5 years.

Primary
Children who have never achieved continence.

Secondary
- Children who maintain continence for at least one year, only to lose it at some point after that.
- More linked to emotional, behavioural problems and psychosocial stress (age 5-7 and adolescents are high risk).

Differential diagnosis
- Genito-urinary pathology – structural or neurological
- Infections, e.g. obstructive uropathy, cystitis, spina bifida

MANAGEMENT

General measures
- Medical cause to be ruled out.
- Behavioural treatment should be attempted first
    - record keeping
    - star chart
    - restrict fluids before sleep
    - nighttime awakenings to urinate (30 minutes to 3 hours after sleep onset)
- Retention control training

Medicine management
REFER for:
- Imipramine, used if the problem is resistant to behaviour therapy
    - however tolerance develops after 6 weeks
- Desmopression
    - wetting resumes once medication is discontinued
    - combination with behavioural methods works better

SEXUALLY TRANSMITTED INFECTIONS

HIV AND AIDS

HIV AND AIDS IN ADULTS

Human immuno-deficiency virus (HIV) enters lymphocytes and replicates. This leads to progressive destruction of the immune system, until the person becomes unable to fight infection and develops AIDS.

Primary HIV infection (seroconversion illness)
A non-specific illness which is common when HIV infection first occurs and is characterised by:
- Fever
- Lymphadenopathy
- Pharyngitis
- Erythematous, maculopapular rash
- Small, orogenital ulcers
- Myalgias or arthralgias

Illness lasts an average of 2 weeks. During its course the HIV Elisa test changes from negative to positive. There is complete recovery.

Persistent generalised lymphadenopathy
- There are enlarged lymph nodes >1 cm diameter (>0.5 cm diameter in children).
- Involves at least 2 non-adjacent sites other than inguinal nodes.

WHO STAGING FOR HIV AND AIDS IN ADULTS (MODIFIED)

CLINICAL STAGE I
- Asymptomatic
- Persistent generalised lymphadenopathy

CLINICAL STAGE II
- Moderate and unexplained weight loss (<10% of presumed or measured body weight)
- Recurrent upper respiratory tract infections (such as sinusitis, otitis media, pharyngitis)
- Mucocutaneous manifestations which include herpes zoster; recurrent mouth ulcers; papular pruritic eruptions; angular cheilitis; seborrhoeic dermatitis; fungal finger nail infections.

CLINICAL STAGE III
Conditions where a presumptive diagnosis can be made on the basis of clinical signs or simple investigations
- Unexplained persistent fever (intermittent or constant for longer than one month)
- Unexplained chronic diarrhoea for longer than one month
- Severe weight loss (>10% of presumed or measured body weight)
- Persistent oral candidiasis
- Oral hairy leukoplakia
- Pulmonary and lymph node TB,
- Recurrent severe pneumonia
- Acute necrotising ulcerative gingivitis or periodontitis

Conditions where confirmatory diagnostic testing is necessary
- Unexplained anaemia (<8g%), and or neutropenia (<500/ul) and or thrombocytopenia (<50 000/ul) for more than one month

CLINICAL STAGE IV
Conditions where a presumptive diagnosis can be made on the basis of clinical signs or simple investigations
- HIV wasting syndrome (weight loss of more than 10% of body weight plus either unexplained chronic diarrhoea or unexplained fever persisting for more than one month)
- Extrapulmonary tuberculosis
- Pneumocystis pneumonia
- Recurrent severe bacterial infections excluding pneumonia
- Chronic herpes simplex infection (orolabial, genital or anorectal > 1 month)
- Candidiasis of the oesophagus, larynx or bronchi
- Kaposi's sarcoma
- HIV encephalopathy (AIDS dementia)

Conditions where confirmatory diagnostic testing is necessary
- Extrapulmonary cryptococcosis including meningitis
- Disseminated non-tuberculous mycobacteria infection
- Cryptosporidiosis
- Isosporiasis
- Cytomegalovirus (CMV) infection (retinitis or of an organ other than liver, spleen or lymph nodes)
- Any disseminated mycosis e.g. histoplasmosis
- Lymphoma (cerebral or B cell non-Hodgkin)
- Invasive cervical carcinoma
- Central nervous system toxoplasmosis

HIV TESTING

Indications for offering the test:
Offer the HIV test to anyone you see in your consulting room in the clinic. All patients should know their status.
- People at risk
    - people with STIs
    - multiple partners
    - partner of person with HIV

- Physical findings suggestive of HIV infection
    - unexplained weight loss
    - unexplained chronic diarrhoea, fever
    - person with active TB
    - generalised lymphadenopathy
    - herpes zoster
    - oral thrush, oral hairy leukoplakia
    - folliculitis, prurigo
    - unexplained peripheral neuropathy
    - unexplained dementia
    - severe seborrhoeic eczema
    - Kaposi's sarcoma

MAKING THE DIAGNOSIS

- Adequate pre- and post-test counselling must be provided.
- Ensure patient confidentiality.

- HIV in adults must be confirmed with:
  - a second rapid test using a kit from a different manufacturer
- There is a window period of up to 3 months in which antibodies are not detected by blood tests
  - this is the time period between becoming infected and the appearance of antibodies, which are detectable by blood tests.

ADVICE ON HEALTH MAINTENANCE

- Counsel patients on preventive methods of reducing the spread of the disease:
  - use condoms during sexual intercourse
  - seek early treatment for sexually transmitted infections
  - advise on safe handling of blood spills e.g. cuts, epistaxis.
- Promote selective and family disclosure.
- Give reproductive counselling.
- Advise patients to:
  - stop smoking
  - limit alcohol intake
  - brush teeth well and see a dentist yearly
  - go for annual PAP smears.
- Consider circumcision as it is found to reduce risk of infection.

PROPHYLAXIS

Prophylaxis for opportunistic infections in adults

- Primary prophylaxis with co-trimoxazole prevents many infections e.g.
  - Pneumocystis jiroveci pneumonia
  - toxoplasmosis
  - bacterial pneumonia
  - Salmonella bacteraemia
  - Isosporiasis (a cause of chronic diarrhoea in HIV)

INDICATIONS FOR COTRIMOXAZOLE PROPHYLAXIS

- WHO Clinical Stage III or IV for HIV disease
- CD4 count less than 200
- TB co-infection

Note: In active pulmonary or extra-pulmonary TB infection, primary prophylaxis for other opportunistic infections should only begin after 1 month of intensive phase treatment has been completed.

MANAGEMENT
- Give co-trimoxazole 2 tabs (160/800) daily
  - **or** Dapsone 100 mg daily can be used where there is mild hypersensitivity to co-trimoxazole.
- Prophylaxis may be discontinued if the CD4 count increases to more than 200 cells on antiretroviral therapy for at least 6 months and the patient is well on ART.
  Note: Minor side effects e.g. nausea, mild itchy rashes should not be accepted as a reason to stop co-trimoxazole prophylaxis.
- **REFER** if severe or dangerous side effects are present e.g. fever, blistering rash, Stevens-Johnson syndrome.

TB PREVENTION THERAPY (IPT)

Patients with HIV infection are more susceptible to TB infection than HIV-negative individuals.

- It is essential to rule out active TB before IPT is given.
- Do not start IPT if the patient has any of the following:
  - active cough
  - night sweats
  - fever
  - weight loss

MANAGEMENT
- Start IPT together with ARVs:
- Isoniazid, oral, 300 mg daily for 12 months
And
- Pyridoxine, oral, 25 mg daily for 12 months.
- Monitor for development of active TB, and for side effects e.g. nausea, vomiting, yellow eyes, pain in the right upper quadrant of the abdomen.
- Patients should be followed up monthly for the first 3 months.

IPT in pregnant patients:
- CD4 > 100: defer IPT until after delivery
- CD4 < 100: exclude active TB with symptom screen, then give IPT.
- Evidence further suggests that IPT may reduce mortality amongst those tested TST-positive.

OPPORTUNISTIC INFECTIONS (ADULTS)

CHEST INFECTIONS

PNEUMONIA

This is a common opportunistic infection in both early and advanced symptomatic HIV disease. The disease is often more widespread with multilobar and bilateral disease being common.

Clinical features
- Generally similar to those in non-immunocompromised patients. But the classical signs of consolidation e.g. bronchial breathing and percussion dullness are often absent in advanced HIV infection.

Investigations
Chest X-ray
- To assess extent of the pneumonia
- To check for evidence of possible associated TB e.g. basal or midzone infiltrate, fibrocavitation, mediastinal nodes
- To look for other concomitant disease e.g. pericardial disease, lymphoma, disseminated Kaposi's sarcoma.

Other investigations
- Send sputum for Xpert MTB/RIF.
- CD4 count
  - this should preferably not be checked until the patient has fully recovered from the pneumonia.

MANAGEMENT

Indications for **REFERRAL** to hospital:
2 or more of the following:
- Confusion or decreased level of consciousness
- BP <90/60
- Respiratory rate ≥30 per minute
- Pulse rate >140 per minute
- Age >65 years
- Dehydration

Also **REFER** patients with pneumonia who are unlikely to comply with treatment.

Medicine treatment
- Give co-amoxiclav 875 / 125 mg 2 x daily for 5 days.
- In penicillin-allergic patients
    - moxifloxacin 400 mg daily for 5 days
- If no response in 48 hours, **REFER** to hospital.

PNEUMOCYSTIS PNEUMONIA

This is an AIDS-defining illness (CD4 count usually below 200). Causative organism: Pneumocystis jiroveci.

Clinical features
- Dry cough for weeks
- Dyspnoea made worse by movement or exercise
- Fever
- Night sweats
- Tachypnoea which is often marked
- Tachycardia
- Cyanosis on exertion
- Often a clear chest

Investigations
Chest X-ray
- May be normal in the early stages.
- May show bilateral interstitial infiltrate beginning in the perihilar regions
    - later a ground glass pattern (alveolar consolidation) may show.

MANAGEMENT
- Patients usually require specialist management, especially if severe
    - **REFER**.
- Less severe and specialist referral facilities are not readily available
    - give co-trimoxazole (single strength) 1 tab per 4 kg of body weight divided into 4 doses/day
    - review after 5 days
    - if a good response after 5 days, continue until 21 days of treatment have been completed.

Prophylaxis
This should be commenced after completing the course of treatment i.e. co-trimoxazole 2 tabs daily. Continue indefinitely or until the CD4 count increases to more than 200 on ARV treatment.

TUBERCULOSIS

HIV infection has become the most important risk factor for the development of active tuberculosis.

Clinical features
Pulmonary tuberculosis should be suspected if:
- Cough for >2 weeks with or without haemoptysis
- Weight loss
- Fever
- Night sweats
- Fatigue
- History of contact with active TB case

Investigations
Chest examination
- In early HIV infection the typical apical chest signs of bronchial breathing and crepitations may be heard.
- In advanced HIV disease these chest signs are more often present in the middle and lower regions
    - however chest signs are often absent.
- Fever and tachycardia are also common features in advanced HIV disease.

Making the diagnosis of TB
Every effort should be made to establish a microbiological diagnosis:
- Sputum smear microscopy in HIV/AIDS patients with TB are often negative because there is less cavitation as a result of decreased cell-mediated immunity
    - molecular techniques are more sensitive.
- If sputum is available, send a specimen for Xpert MTB/RIF.
- If the GeneXpert is negative and there is still suspicion of PTB, send a second specimen for bacteriological culture.

Chest X-ray
In patients with early HIV infection the X-ray features of TB look like those in patients without HIV infection. These are:
- Patchy consolidation especially in the upper lobes or apical segments of the lower lobes, often with cavitation.
- Fibrosis and volume loss and calcified foci which are features of healing.

In patients with advanced HIV infection atypical X-ray features are present which include:
- Lower zone infiltrate
- Consolidation, especially of the left lower lobe which may be mistaken for pneumonia.
- Features of extra-pulmonary tuberculosis which include pleural effusion, enlargement of hilar and mediastinal lymph nodes, pericardial effusion.
- Miliary tuberculosis with 1-2 mm nodules distributed evenly throughout the lung fields.

Other investigations
- Other options for investigation may be tried either immediately or if the first sputum specimens are negative e.g. aspiration of pleural fluid, lymph node FNA biopsy
    - the result of pleural aspiration may be considered positive if either the ADA level and/or fluid protein is greater than 30 and microscopy shows a lymphocyte predominance.
- Bactec TB culture of blood (if available) can be useful:
    - in patients with PUO or a pericardial effusion
    - where sputum microbiological investigation has failed.

MANAGEMENT
- Treatment of TB is the same irrespective of HIV status.
- You need to follow the most recent SA Tuberculosis Control Programme Practical Guidelines of the Department of Health.

THE MOUTH

ORAL CANDIDIASIS

Clinical features
- Pseudomembranous - white curd-like patches usually on the palate or buccal mucosa (especially behind the back molar teeth).
- Erythematous - punctate red spots or red areas.
- Hyperplastic - white plaque-like areas on the tongue that cannot be scraped off.
- Angular chelitis - fissures on the corners of the mouth that lie horizontal.

See ENT page 46

OESOPHAGEAL CANDIDIASIS

Clinical features
- Odynophagia – pain on swallowing over weeks
- Retrosternal chest pain especially when swallowing
- Oral thrush usually, but not always, present

Fluconazole tabs 200 mg daily for 14 days prescribed by a doctor.

ACUTE NECROTISING ULCERATIVE GINGIVITIS

This may be an early indicator of HIV disease.

Clinical features
- Acutely painful bleeding gums
- Halitosis
- Greyish membrane (slough) on gum margin especially between teeth (interdental papillae)
- Involvement of one tooth or many teeth

- **REFER** to dentist.
- Give chlorhexidine mouthwash.
- Give paracetamol for pain.

DIARRHOEA

ACUTE DIARRHOEA

- This is usually self-limiting and is managed by fluid replacement.
- **REFER** diarrhoea with complications.

ACUTE INFLAMMATORY DIARRHOEA (DYSENTERY)

A diarrhoea stool with blood or mucus is usually due to bacteria.

Causes
Main bacterial causes are:
- Shigella
- Salmonella
- Campylobacter
- E. coli

MANAGEMENT
- Fluid replacement with oral rehydration solution (in a cup of lukewarm water)
    - give IV fluid if the patient is vomiting or is severely dehydrated
- Give ciprofloxacin 500 mg 2 x daily for 3 days
    - children 15 mg/kg/dose 2 x daily for 3 days
- **REFER** if there is no improvement after 3 days.

CHRONIC DIARRHOEA

This means diarrhoea lasting for more than 2 weeks. The majority of cases may be HIV related.

Causes
Cryptosporidia; Microsporidia; Isospora belli

MANAGEMENT
- Send stools for ova, cysts and parasites
    - special stains are needed to identify Cryptosporidium, Isospora and Microsporidia.
- Prevent dehydration using Oral Rehydration Solution (ORS) or Sugar Salt Solution (SSS) - see page 108.
- Give loperamide (adults only) 2 mg (1 tab) as required after each loose stool (max 12 mg in 24 hours)
    - do not give loperamide in suspected dysentery
- Commence ART
    - if the patient is wasted (Stage IV)
    - if the stool is positive for Cryptosporidium or Isospora

Diet
- Children
    - if breastfeeding, give more frequent, longer feeds
    - if replacement feeding, replace milk with fermented milk products e.g. amasi or yoghurt
- Adults
    - carbohydrates: rice, maize, potatoes
    - fruit: apples, bananas, carrots
    - after 2-3 days a full general diet may be eaten

REFER patients where Isospora has been found in the stools.

▼**Note to doctor**
- Isospora responds to high doses of cotrimoxazole.
- Cryptosporidium and microsporidium do not usually respond to treatment.
- For Isospora give cotrimoxazole single strength 4 tabs 12 hourly for 10 days, then 2 tabs daily thereafter. ▲

SKIN / HAIR CONDITIONS

SEBORRHOEIC DERMATITIS

Clinical features
- Extremely common
- Main sites involved:
    - scalp, especially hair margin
    - face - eyebrows, nasolabial folds, moustache area
    - upper outer arms, central chest and upper back
    - intertriginous - inframammary, axillae, groin, scrotal, behind ears
- Erythema and scaling, sometimes acute and weeping
- Scalp greasiness
- Hyperpigmentation (hypopigmentation in children) especially in skin folds
- In severe cases most of the body surface may be covered.

> See the Skin pages 260-261

FOLLICULITIS

Clinical features
- Itchy follicular pustules with red borders or urticarial lesions

> - Give flucloxacillin 500 mg 4 x daily for 5 days
>   - or erythromycin 500 mg 3 x daily for 5 days.
> - Also chlorphenamine 4 mg 2-3 x daily.

PAPULAR PRURITIC ERUPTION

Hypersensitivity response to insect bites

Clinical features
- Common
- Very itchy
- Small erythematous papules often with scratched out centres that heal forming hyperpigmented spots with pale centres
- Frequent recurrences

> - Hydrocortisone 1% cream apply 2 x daily for 7 days only
> - Chlorphenamine 4 mg 2 x daily

SCABIES

Clinical features
- May be very florid.
- Papular eruptions usually found on finger webs, wrists, forearms, small of back that are itchy at night
    - new lesions can be found in the morning
- Eruptions can be extensive and crusting looking like seborrhoeic dermatitis - then called Norwegian scabies.

> ### MANAGEMENT
> - Give benzyl benzoate (Ascabiol)
>   - apply nightly x 3 nights.
> - If poor response to benzyl benzoate, use permethrin 5% lotion and repeat after 1 week.

HAIR ABNORMALITIES

Clinical features
- Lustreless (no shine)
- Straightening
- Diffuse alopecia
- Premature greying

VIRAL INFECTIONS

HERPES SIMPLEX CHRONIC MUCOCUTANEOUS ULCERATION

Clinical features
- Painful ulcers involving the skin around the anogenital area or occurring in the mouth in patients with advanced HIV infection.
- Ulcers persist for weeks and are very painful
    - may be small and grouped
    - may be confluent and larger, with a polycyclic edge.

> ### MANAGEMENT
> - Recommend salt water mouthwash (½ teaspoon salt in a cup of lukewarm water)
>   - gargle for one minute 2 x daily.
> - Give acyclovir 400 mg 3 x daily for 7 days.
> - Give paracetamol 2 tabs 3 x daily when needed.

HERPES ZOSTER

- This is common at all stages of HIV infection.
    - it can recur.
    - it may be the first clinical evidence of HIV infection.
- Unilateral vesicular rash following one or more dermatomes. Even in HIV, this rash usually extends from the midline anteriorly to the spine posteriorly.
- The extent and severity of the condition is often in accordance with the degree of immunosuppression.

Clinical features of herpes zoster in HIV disease
- Increased severity of pain both with the acute rash and in post-herpetic neuralgia
- Recurrent episodes
- Multidermatomal involvement
- Increased scarring and staining

> ### MANAGEMENT
> - If fresh vesicles are present:
>   - oral acyclovir 800 mg 5 x daily for 7 days
> - If secondary bacterial infection is present (uncommon)
>   - give flucloxacillin 500 mg 4 x daily for 7 days
>
> **Pain relief**
> - Paracetamol 2 tabs 3-4 x daily for 7-10 days
> - **Plus REFER** for
>   - amitriptyline 25 mg at night
>   - increasing by 25 mg every 2 weeks to maximum of 75 mg at night
>   - **and** if severe pain tramadol 50 mg 4 x daily for 5 days

Post-herpetic neuralgia and prolonged pain
- Amitriptyline as above
- **Plus** if pain not controlled **REFER** for:
    - tramadol 50 mg 4 x daily
    - may be increased to a maximum of 100 mg 4 x daily

REFER
- Involvement of the eye

MOLLUSCUM CONTAGIOSUM

Clinical features
- Dome-shaped papules with central umbilication
- May be widespread in severe immunosuppression

- Individual lesions should be treated separately
- Apply iodine solution (tincture of iodine BP) to the central core using an applicator.

DRUG REACTIONS

Drug reactions are more common in HIV disease, especially to co-trimoxazole, carbamazepine, griseofulvin and some anti-TB drugs.

Clinical features
- Most often erythematous papular or maculo-papular rash often with pruritis.
- May present with:
    - urticaria
    - erythema multiforme (target lesions)
    - Stevens-Johnson syndrome (involving mucous membrane of eyes, mouth and genitalia)
    - toxic epidermal necrolysis (large blisters which burst leaving denuded skin)

MANAGEMENT
- Stop the offending drug.
- Give chlorphenamine 4 mg 3 x daily.
- **REFER** Stevens-Johnson syndrome
    - toxic epidermal necrolysis

KAPOSI'S SARCOMA
(AIDS-DEFINING)

Cause
- Human herpes virus type 8

Clinical features
- Red-brown-purple-black plaques or nodules
    - well or ill-defined.
- The presence of >5 skin lesions suggests organ involvement.
- Can cause lymph node enlargement and may be associated with local oedema.
- Common sites are the hard palate adjacent to the second molar teeth, medial third of the lower eyelid, tip of the nose, the limbs and the penis.
- Can involve the chest
    - CXR findings can resemble PTB.

MANAGEMENT
Lesions are treated if symptomatic or if there is severe cosmetic disfigurement.

REFER for treatment:
- Painful or oedematous limbs (lymphatic obstruction)
- Possible lung involvement
- To dentist for oral lesions
    - that interfere with chewing or swallowing
    - or cause pain or bleeding
- Localised area causing problems e.g. ulceration or infection

LYMPHADENOPATHY

Clinical features
- Glands >1 cm size (adults) and > 0.5 cm size (children)
    - they can be symmetrical or asymmetrical.
- Present in 2 or more sites (excluding inguinal nodes)
    - bilateral glands count as 1 site.
- It often involves epitrochlear nodes.

Causes
Other causes include TB, lymphoma, Mycobacterium avium complex (MAC), local sepsis, syphilis and Kaposi's sarcoma.

Investigations
If TB is suspected, it is advisable to do a chest X-ray as lymphadenopathy may accompany pulmonary TB.

MANAGEMENT
REFER for fine needle aspiration to identify TB or malignancy if:
- unilateral or one dominant node
- rapidly enlarging
- matted glands
- tender
- mediastinal adenopathy on chest X-ray

NEUROLOGICAL PROBLEMS

HEADACHE

This is a potentially serious symptom in HIV and AIDS.

Causes
- Tuberculous meningitis
- Cryptococcal meningitis

MANAGEMENT
- **REFER** patients with headache for investigation if:
    - new severe headache, associated with systemic symptoms or neurological signs
    - clinically significant chronic headache
    - severe headache associated with neck stiffness, fever, vomiting, altered level of consciousness
    - focal localising signs
    - new onset seizures

HIV ENCEPHALOPATHY

This includes cognitive, motor and behavioural dysfunction:
- Early
    - difficulty concentrating
    - motor slowing
    - memory loss
- Late
    - personal neglect
    - mutism
    - paraplegia

All patients should be **REFERRED** for full investigation.

PAINFUL PERIPHERAL NEUROPATHY

Causes
- HIV itself
- ARV therapy i.e. NRTIs, especially stavudine
- INH therapy i.e. TB therapy or INH prophylaxis
- Alcohol abuse

Clinical features
- Burning, tingling or numbness of feet and/or lower legs
- Glove and stocking distribution (bilaterally equal)
- Absent ankle jerks

MANAGEMENT
Mild to moderate pain
- Paracetamol 1g 3 x daily when necessary.
- **REFER** to doctor for amitriptyline 25-75 mg nocte.
- If no doctor available give
    - carbamazepine 100 mg 2-3 x daily for 1 week (not in patients on ARVs)
    - increasing to 200 mg 2-3 x daily if no response

Patients on INH therapy
- Pyridoxine 25-50 mg 1-3 x daily
    - maximum 100 mg daily in patients on ARV therapy

Alcohol abuse
- Thiamine 100 mg daily

Patients on ARVs
- Substitute stavudine with tenofovir **only** if the patient is virologically suppressed.

Severe pain
- **Add** tramadol 50 mg 4 x daily (Dr initiated)
- **REFER**

GUILLAIN-BARRE SYNDROME

Clinical features
- Often presents early in HIV infection.
- Reflexes are notably absent or decreased.
- There is acute onset muscular weakness and mild distal sensory loss.
- Symmetrical ascending weakness usually begins in the legs and progresses to the arms.
- It may involve respiratory muscles affecting breathing.
- There is usually a satisfactory outcome.

REFER to hospital.

CRYPTOCOCCAL MENINGITIS

Clinical features
- Patients may present with a severe headache, neck stiffness, photophobia, fever, vomiting, clouding of consciousness, and focal signs and seizures.
- Often headache is the only sign.

REFER to hospital.

HIV AND AIDS IN CHILDREN

Infants are infected with HIV during pregnancy, birth or breastfeeding.
- In 25% of them the virus replicates rapidly and the child presents with signs of infection in the first year of life.
- Many children present with symptoms between the first and fifth year of life.
- Approximately 5-10% remain asymptomatic until 8 years of age.

WHO STAGING FOR HIV AND AIDS IN CHILDREN (MODIFIED)

CLINICAL STAGE I
- Asymptomatic
- Generalised lymphadenopathy

CLINICAL STAGE II
- Hepatosplenomegaly
- Seborrhoeic dermatitis
- Persistent parotid enlargement
- Papular pruritic eruptions (PPE)
- Recurrent or chronic upper RTIs (OM, otorrhoea, sinusitis)
- Angular chelitis
- Extensive molluscum contagiosum
- Recurrent oral ulcerations
- Herpes zoster

CLINICAL STAGE III
- Failure to thrive (between the 3rd percentile and 60% of expected weight)
- Unexplained persistent diarrhoea (>2 weeks)
- Oral candidiasis (after the first 6 weeks of life)
- Unexplained persistent fever (>1 month)
- Recurrent severe presumed bacterial pneumonia
- Symptomatic lymphoid interstitial pneumonitis
- Pulmonary or lymph node TB
- Chronic lung disease eg. bronchiectasis

CLINICAL STAGE IV

- Severe failure to thrive (<60% expected body weight)
- Pneumocytis pneumonia
- HIV encephalopathy
- Candidiasis (oesophageal, bronchial or pulmonary)
- Extrapulmonary TB
- Chronic herpes simplex infection (orolabial or cutaneous) of more than 1 month's duration
- Recurrent severe bacterial infection eg meningitis, bone or joint infection but excluding pneumonia
- Extrapulmonary cryptococcosis including meningitis

MAKING THE DIAGNOSIS

Children less than 18 months of age
- A positive antibody test in the child may reflect maternal antibody rather than infection in the child.
- Virological testing using DNA PCR (polymerase chain reaction) is the test of choice.

When to test (HIV PCR)
- At birth.
- Repeat at 10 week visit.
- Repeat at 18 week visit only if:
  - the child received NVP for 12 weeks (the mother received < 4 weeks of ART in pregnancy)
  - the child received dual therapy (due to maternal virological failure)
- At any time when clinical signs indicate possible HIV infection.
- 6 weeks after breastfeeding has stopped.
- Always confirm with a second HIV PCR test if the first test is positive.

Children over 18 months of age
- Two HIV antibody tests are performed
  - 2 rapid tests using kits from different manufacturers and a different blood specimen.

When to test (HIV rapid test)
- At 18 months of age if the exposed infant has not been shown to be HIV-infected.
- If the child is still breastfed, 6 weeks after stopping breastfeeding.
- Clinical features suggest HIV infection.

PROPHYLAXIS OF OPPORTUNISTIC INFECTIONS

- Primary prophylaxis with cotrimoxazole prevents many infections e.g. pneumocystis pneumonia, toxoplasmosis, bacterial pneumonia.
- Indications are:
  - all HIV-exposed or infected infants starting from 6 weeks of age
  - any child 1-5 years with CD4 <25%
  - any child >5 years of age with CD4 <350

Age	Co-trimoxazole daily dose
6 weeks - 6 months	2.5 ml
6 months - 3 years	5 ml
3 - 10 years	10 ml or 1 tab
10 - 14 years	2 tabs

Discontinutation:
- Child is HIV uninfected and has not been breastfed for at least 6 weeks
- HIV-infected child >1 year of age with evidence of immune reconstitution
  - 1–5 years: CD4 count >25%
  - >5 years: CD4 count >350 on 2 tests 3–6 months apart

OPPORTUNISTIC INFECTIONS (CHILDREN)

TREATMENT OF OPPORTUNISTIC INFECTIONS IN CHILDREN

Diarrhoea
Assess severity of dehydration using the standard treatment Guidelines of the Department of Health.

> Manage according to the hydration classification.

Tuberculosis
- TB should be considered earlier in non-resolving pneumonia.
- Tuberculin tests are often not reliable and a negative test does not exclude TB.

> Manage children with TB according to the National TB guidelines.

Pneumonia
- Consider clinic management if:
  - respiratory rate is less than 50 breaths/min in infants 2-12 months old
  - less than 40 breaths/minute 1-5 years old
  - there is no cyanosis
  - the child is tolerating oral feeds/fluids

Pneumocystis pneumonia
- Suspect a PCP (PJP) infection if the child:
- Is less than 12 months old
- Has severe tachypnoea
- Is dyspnoeic and restless
- Has cyanosis
- Has few crepitations relative to the degree of dyspnoea

> - They usually require hospital management.
> - PCP prophylaxis should continue after discharge as per guidelines.

Lymphoid interstitial pneumonia (LIP)
- This is a slowly progressive interstitial lung disease of unknown aetiology.

Consider LIP when:
- The child is older than 2 years
- There is slowly progressive hypoxia and exertion fatique
- There is digital clubbing
- Parotid glands are enlarged
- Associated recurrent bacterial respiratory infections are a feature.
- Chest X-ray shows bilateral reticulonodular infiltrates and mediastinal lymphadenopathy.

MANAGEMENT
- **REFER** to hospital for confirmation of the diagnosis.
- Steroid treatment is indicated for hypoxic children.
- Children started on steroids should also be given PCP prophylaxis for as long as they are on steroid therapy.
- Follow up and maintenance treatment at a clinic.

ANTIRETROVIRAL THERAPY (ART) IN ADULTS

GOALS OF ART

The primary goal of ART is to decrease HIV-related morbidity and mortality.

- The patient should experience fewer HIV-related illnesses.
- The patient's CD4 count should rise and remain above the baseline count.
- The patient's viral load should become undetectable (<50 copies / ml), and remain undetectable on ARV therapy.

The secondary goal is to decrease the incidence of HIV through:
- An increase in voluntary testing and counselling with more people then knowing their status and practising safer sex.
- Reducing transmission in couples where one partner is positive and one negative.
- Reducing the risks of HIV transmission from mother to child.

ART INITIATION

Eligibility for ART
- **All HIV-positive persons, irrespective of CD4 count or WHO clinical stage.**

Timing of ART initiation
- In general, ART should be started as soon as the patient is ready within 2 weeks of CD4 count result availability
- ART should be initiated *immediately* in pregnancy and during breastfeeding.
- Unless contraindicated, ART should be initiated within 1 week in the following cases:
    - CD4 count <200 (except TB patients and cryptococcal meningitis)
    - WHO Clinical Stage IV (except TB meningitis and cryptococcal meningitis)

TB patients
- In TB patients with CD4 count >50, ART should be deferred until 8 weeks after initiating TB treatment
    - this reduces the risk of deterioration due to the immune reconstitution inflammatory syndrome (IRIS).
- In TB patients with CD4 counts <50 (except TB meningitis), start ART within 2 weeks after starting TB therapy.
- In patients with TB meningitis (irrespective of CD4 count), ART should be deferred until 8 weeks after initiating TB treatment.

Cryptococcal meningitis
- In patients with cryptococcal meningitis, ART should be deferred until 6 weeks after starting antifungal treatment.

RECOMMENDED REGIMENS

FIRST-LINE REGIMEN (REGIMEN 1)

All new patients including pregnant women
- Tenofovir (TDF) 300 mg at night

WITH
- Emtricitabine (FTC) 200 mg at night

AND
- Efavirenz (EFV) 600 mg at night

OR
- A fixed dose combination of the above (FDC) taken at night is preferred.

Special considerations
- In patients with significant psychiatric co-morbidity or where the neuro-psychiatric toxicity of EFV may impair daily functioning (e.g. shift workers), use dolutegravir (DTG) or nevirapine instead of EFV
- **Note:** Avoid NVP in women with a CD4 count >250, and men with a CD4 count >400 when initiating ART due to increased risk of rash-associated hepatitis.
- Avoid dolutegravir in women of reproductive age unless they have been sterilized or are on relaible contraception i.e. IUD
- Tenovofir is contraindicated in patients with kidney disease (creatinine clearance <50) or who are on nephrotoxic medication, e.g. aminoglycoside
    - use abacavir (ABC) instead of TDF
    - a fixed dose combination of ABC and 3TC (600/300 mg) taken together with EFV 600 mg at night, is preferred.
- Weight of 25-40 kg: Use a fixed dose combination of TDF and FTC (300/200 mg) taken together with EFV 400 mg at night.

At initial diagnosis of HIV	
CD4 count and WHO clinical staging	• Baseline assessment to assess eligibility for fast-tracking
Screen for pregnancy	• For immediate initiation if pregnant
Screen for TB symptoms	• To identify TB/HIV co-infected
Do creatinine	• To detect kidney insufficiency
Do TPAB/RPR	• To detect syphilis
Do ALT: if NVP required	• To exclude liver disease

SECOND-LINE REGIMEN (REGIMEN 2)

Second-Line Regimen	
Failing on a TDF- or ABC-based first-line regimen	• Zidovudine (AZT) 300 mg 12 hourly **WITH** • Lamivudine (3TC) 150 mg 12 hourly **AND** • Lopinavir + ritonavir (LPV/r) 400/100 mg 12 hourly **OR** • A fixed dose combination of AZT and 3TC (300 / 150 mg) 12 hourly + LPV/r 12 hourly is preferred
Exceptions	
Hb <7.0 g/dL or neutrophil count <0.75	• Use TDF or ABC instead of AZT
Note: In patients who are hepatitis B surface antigen positive:	• Do not stop TDF as this may cause a severe flare up of hepatitis B • Use a combination of TDF and FTC (300/200 mg) daily and add AZT + LPV/r 12 hourly.
Dyslipidaemia or diarrhoea associated with LPV/r	• Switch LPV/r to ATV/r
Anaemia and kidney failure	• Use ABC

Routine monitoring for adults with HIV

On ART	
CD4 at 1 year on ART	• To monitor immune response to ART
VL at 6 months, 1 year and then every 12 months	• To identify treatment failures and problems with adherence
If on TDF, do creatinine at 3 and 6 months, 1 year and then every 12 months	• To identify TDF toxicity
If on AZT, do FBC at 1, 2, 3 and 6 months	• To identify AZT toxicity
If on LPV/r, do fasting cholesterol and trigiycerides at 3 months	• To identify LPV/r toxicity

Viral load monitoring	
Viral load level	**Recommended response**
<50 copies/ml Lower than detectable limit	• 2 monthly viral load monitoring
50-1000 copies/ml Detectable but <1000 copies / ml	• Assess adherence carefully • Repeat viral load in 6 months, and manage accordingly
>1000 copies/ml	• Give intense adherence support • Repeat viral load in 2 months, and check HBV status • If viral load confirmed >1000, switch to second-line therapy

At routine follow-up visits for those opting to defer ART	
Screen for TB symptoms	• To identify TB/HIV coinfection
Repeat CD4 count every 6 months	• To determine eligibility for OI prophylexis
Offer advice on secondary prevention of HIV	• To prevent HIV transmission and reinfection
Treatment failure with Regimen 2	
Failing second-line for >1 year and good adherence documented	• **REFER** for specialist opinion • Genotype antiretroviral resistance testing must be done • The regimen will be determined by an expert committee

Interrupted ART
- Recommence previous regimen and do VL
- Repeat VL in 2 months. Target is greater than the 1 log (10 fold) decrease

IMMUNE RECONSTITUTION INFLAMMATORY SYNDROME (IRIS)

Clinical deterioration after starting ART

This is due to the improving immune system interacting with organisms that have already infected the body. There are 2 forms:

- Unmasking: this occurs when a previously unsuspected condition becomes clinically evident.
- Paradoxical: this occurs when a known condition on appropriate treatment becomes worse.

IRIS most commonly occurs in association with opportunistic infections such as TB, MAC, cryptococcal infection, CMV and hepatitis B or C.

Clinical features
- IRIS usually presents during the first 6 weeks after starting ART.
- IRIS caused by MTB is the most common clinical presentation and may present with:
  - fever
  - lymphadenopathy
  - worsening of the original tuberculous lesion and/or
  - development of other TB manifestations, such as miliary TB or pleural effusion

PROPHYLAXIS OF OPPORTUNISTIC INFECTIONS

- Co-trimoxazole prophylaxis must be continued in all patients on antiretroviral treatment until the CD4 count is >200 cells/mm^3 for at least 6 months and the patient is well on ART.
  - recommence if the CD4 count drops to <200 cells/mm^3 or if regimen failure.
- Patients who have had cryptococcal meningitis must continue taking fluconazole prophylaxis until the CD4 count is >200 cells/mm^3.

CONCOMITANT TUBERCULOSIS

- HIV-positive TB patients qualify for lifelong ART, regardless of their CD4 count.
- TB patients with a CD4 count >50 should complete 2 months of TB therapy before commencing ARVs.
- Patients with a CD4 count of <50 need to be fast-tracked and ART initiated within 2 weeks
    - however make sure the patient is tolerating TB treatment and symptoms are improving before commencing ARVs
- In patients with TB meningitis (irrespective of CD4 count), ART should be deferred until 8 weeks after initiating TB treatment.
- Patients on lopinavir / ritonavir should have their dose doubled slowly over 2 weeks (to 800/200 twice a day)
    - monitor ALT monthly

PREVENTION OF MOTHER-TO-CHILD TRANSMISSION

For the woman

1st antenatal visit	
All women to be counselled and tested for HIV, unless known positive	• HIV-positive women to be initiated on a fixed dose combination (FDC) of TDF, FTC and EFV same day • Send blood for creatinine and CD4
Currently on lifelong ART	• Continue the current ART regimen • Check VL same day if the woman has been on ART >3 months
2nd antenatal visit (1 week later)	
Creatinine < 85	• Continue FDC
Creatinine > 85 (TDF contraindicated)	• Stop FDC • **REFER** urgently to Dr - initiation of alternative triple regimen (usually ABC, 3TC, EFV) - Investigation and management of kidney disease
Viral load monitoring	
Women newly initiated on ART	• First viral load will be done 3 months after ART initiation
Woman already on ART > 3 months	• VL to be repeated on the day of pregnancy confirmation
Viral load lower than detectable level	• Continue on current ART regimen • Repeat VL 6-monthly throughout pregnancy and breastfeeding; return to annual VL monitoring only once she has stopped breastfeeding
Viral load < 1000 copies/ml	• Assess adherence carefully • Continue on current ART regimen, provide adherence counselling support • Repeat VL **within** 6 months, if suppressed continue with 6-monthly VL testing.
Viral load > 1000 copies/ml	• Provide adherence counselling, **repeat VL in 1 month**. • If second VL result is undetectable or has shown a reduction in VL of 1 log (10-fold) or greater, continue with the existing regimen. • If the viral load is unchanged or has not shown a 1log reduction or has increased, the woman should be switched to second-line therapy urgently.

For the HIV-exposed infant

Low risk	
Situation	Infant prophylaxis
Mother on lifelong ART **OR** Mother started ART more than 4 weeks prior to delivery **AND** viral load <1000 copies/ml	• NVP at birth and then daily for 6 weeks • Do HIV PCR at birth • Repeat HIV PCR at 10 weeks • If birth or 10-week PCR is positive: • Stop NVP, start infant ART and cotrimoxazole prophylaxis • Encourage and support exclusive breastfeeding
High risk	
Mother started ART less than 4 weeks prior to delivery **OR** Mother diagnosed at birth or within 72 hours of delivery	• NVP at birth and then daily for 12 weeks • Do HIV PCR at birth • Repeat HIV PCR at 10 weeks • Repeat HIV PCR at 18 weeks • If birth, 10- or 18-week PCR is positive: Stop NVP, start infant ART and cotrimoxazole prophylaxis • Encourage and support exclusive breastfeeding
Mother failing 1st line and initiated on 2nd line **AND** Viral load < 1000 copies/ml	• > 4 weeks before delivery - AZT + NVP for 6 weeks • < 4 weeks before delivery - AZT for 6 weeks + NVP for 12 weeks • Do HIV PCR at birth • Repeat HIV PCR at 10 weeks • Repeat HIV PCR at 18 weeks if on NVP prophylaxis for 12 weeks • If birth, 10- or 18-week PCR is positive: Stop NVP, start infant ART and cotrimoxazole prophylaxis • Encourage and support exclusive breastfeeding
Mother failing 2nd line	• Refer for specialised management

NB. If infants test HIV PCR positive at any stage, initiate ART immediately and send confirmatory HIV PCR test.

Unknown risk	
Abandoned or orphaned baby with unknown maternal HIV status	• Do immediate Rapid HIV test • If positive: - Give NVP daily for 6 weeks - Do HIV PCR and repeat at 10 weeks If negative: - no prophylaxis

ANTIRETROVIRAL THERAPY (ART)
IN CHILDREN

GOALS OF ART

The goal of antiretroviral therapy in children is to increase survival and decrease HIV related morbidity and mortality.

- The child's CD4 percentage should rise and remain above the baseline percentage.
- The child's viral load should become undetectable (<400 copies/ml)
    - it should remain undetectable on ART.
- In some children the best achievable goal may be:
    - a suppressed though detectable viral load
    - with sustained elevation in CD4 percentage
    - absence of intercurrent and/or opportunistic infection

ELIGIBILITY FOR ART

Eligible to start ART
- **All HIV positive children irrespective of CD4 count or clinical stage.**
- If no medical contraindication, ART should be initiated within 1 week in the following cases:
    - Children <1 year of age
    - WHO Clinical Stage IV
    - MDR or XDR-TB
    - CD4 count < 200 or <15%

Social criteria
There must be at least one identifiable caregiver who is able to supervise the child and/or administer medication.

RECOMMENDED REGIMENS

First-Line Regimen	
> 3 months-3 years **OR** Older children < 10 kg	• ABC + 3TC + LPV/r
> 3 years and > 10 kg	• ABC + 3TC + EFV
Adolescents >15 years and >40 kg	• TDF + FTC + EFV

Adjustment of previous First-Line Regimens	
Changing first line children regimen to adult treatment, if >15 years and > 40 kg	If viral load suppressed and on: • ABC + 3TC + EFV - change to TDF + FTC + EFV • ABC + 3TC + LPV/r - change to • TDF + FTC + EFV

Second-Line Regimen	
The most common cause of treatment failure is poor adherence. Adherence has to be addressed before switching to 2nd line therapy. Do not change regimens or move to 2nd line without clear guidance from a practitioner experienced in child ARV medicine.	
Failed first line NNRTI based regimen (consult with a specialist before changing) Failed ABC + 3TC + EFV	• AZT + 3TC + LPV/r
Failed first line protease inhibitor-based regimen Failed ABC + 3TC + LPV/r	Referral to a specialist

Routine monitoring for children with HIV

At initial diagnosis of HIV	
Hb or FBC	• If <8g/dl, **REFER** to doctor
CD4 count and percentage	• Baseline assessment - do not wait for CD4 result to start ART
Cholesterol + triglyceride (if on a PI-based regimen)	• Baseline assessment
ALT (if jaundiced or on TB treatment)	• To detect liver dysfunction
On ART	
Height, weight and head circumference (<2 years)	• To monitor growth and development
CD4: 1 year on ART, and then every 12 months	• To monitor response to ART
VL: At 6 months and 1 year on ART, then annually	• To monitor viral response to ART
If on AZT: Hb or FBC at 1, 2, 3 months and then annually	• To identify AZT-related anaemia
If on a PI-based regimen: cholesterol + triglyceride at 1 year and then 12-monthly	• To monitor for PI-related metabolic side effects

CONCOMITANT TUBERCULOSIS

- If TB treatment started first, commence ART if ALT is normal.
    - within 2 weeks if CD4 < 50
    - after 8 weeks if CD4 > 50
- If the child is to be initiated on or is already taking lopinavir / ritonavir
    - add extra ritonavir to boost the dose (1:1).
- If the child is on an EFV-containing regimen, there should be no change to the ARVs.

POST-EXPOSURE HIV PROPHYLAXIS

Exposure to infectious material from HIV sero-positive individuals including blood, saliva, semen and vaginal secretions.

HIGH-RISK INJURIES

Needlestick injury

The risk increases when:
- The injury is deep.
- It involves a hollow needle.
- The source patient is more infectious, e.g.
  - terminal AIDS
  - seroconversion illness
  - patient known to have a high viral load

Sexual violation injury

- High risk is defined as:
  - pre-pubertal children
  - genital or anal laceration
  - anal receptive exposure

MANAGEMENT
General measures

Needlestick injury

- Squeeze the needlestick site so that bleeding occurs.
- Wash the site with soap and running water.
- Apply a povidone-iodine wound dressing.

Exposure through eye or mouth

- Flush out very well with water.

TESTING THE SOURCE PATIENT

- Give counselling and get the patient's informed consent for testing.
- The following blood tests must be done:
  - Rapid HIV test (unless known HIV positive)
  - HIV Elisa test
  - Hepatitis B surface antigen (HBsAg)
  - Hepatitis C antibody (HCAb) (if occupational exposure)
  - Treponema pallidum antibody (TPAB) and RPR (if sexual offender)

TESTING THE EXPOSED HEALTH WORKER / SEXUAL OFFENCE VICTIM

- Counselling must be provided before an exposed health worker/sexual offence victim is tested for infection.
- Baseline tests are required to prove seroconversion for compensation later.
- The following blood tests must be done:
  - Rapid HIV test (unless known HIV positive)
    PLUS
  - HIV Elisa test (unless known HIV positive
  - Repeat HIV Elisa at 6 weeks and 4 months (to check for seroconversion).
  - Hepatitis B surface antibody (HBsAb).
  - Hepatitis B surface antigen (HBsAg) at 4 months (to check for seroconversion).
  - Serum creatinine if TDF part of PEP
  - FBC if AZT part of PEP
- The following blood tests must be done only if the source patient was positive:
  Occupational exposure:
  - Hepatitis C antibody (HCAb).
  - Hepatitis C PCR after 6 weeks if HCAb was negative.
  Sexual offence victim:
  - Treponema pallidum antibody (TPAB) and RPR and repeat after 4 months if RPR was negative (to check for seroconversion).

MANAGEMENT
Medicine treatment

- Initiate post-exposure prophylaxis (PEP) immediately after the injury and within 72 hours
  - do not wait for the test results on the source patient and health worker.
- With very high-risk exposures, treatment may be considered beyond 72 hours
  - but not beyond 7 days
- PEP is not indicated:
  - for victims / health workers who are HIV infected (they may need prophylaxis if the source patient has a resistant strain and is on a different regimen - these cases must be discussed with HIV expert).
  - when the source patient is HIV negative unless there are features suggesting seroconversion illness.
- Test for HIV infection at the time of exposure and then at 6 weeks and 4 months.

- Tenofovir 300 mg daily for 4 weeks
and
- Emtricitabine 200 mg daily for 4 weeks
and
- Atazanavir/ritonavir 300 / 100 mg daily for 4 weeks

If tenofovir is contraindicated or if source patient is known to be failing a tenofovir-based regimen, replace tenofovir and emtricitabine with:
- Zidovudine 300 mg 12 hourly for 4 weeks
and
- Lamivudine 150 mg 12 hourly for 4 weeks

PEP following hepatitis B exposure

Source patient HBsAg positive or HBsAg unknown

<u>Health care worker unvaccinated or vaccinated and HBsAb titre < 10 units / ml</u>
Refer to the nearest district hospital for:
- hepatitis B immunoglobulin (HBIG), IM, 500 units
- hepatitis B vaccination

<u>Health care worker vaccinated and HB5Ab titre ≥ 10 units / ml</u>
- no treatment required.

OTHER SEXUALLY TRANSMITTED INFECTIONS

It is important to take a good sexual history and undertake a thorough examination. The history should include questions concerning symptoms, sexual orientation, the possibility of pregnancy, antibiotic allergy and recent travel.

QUALITY CARE FOR PEOPLE WITH STIs

Provide information, education and counselling
- Inform patients about STIs i.e. how they are transmitted, the symptoms, signs and complications.
- Explain that STIs increase the risk of getting HIV disease

The full treatment must be completed
- Emphasize that the full treatment must be completed to prevent complications.
- Emphasize the importance of sexual abstinence until cured.

Counsel on safe sex
- Have a non-judgemental attitude
- Help patients make changes in their attitudes, behaviours and lives
- Provide the patient with a choice of ways to reduce the risk of acquiring another STI, including HIV
    - reduce the number of sexual partners
    - have protected sex by using condoms
    - seek prompt treatment for STIs
- Promote circumcision

Promote the use of condoms
- Demonstrate how to use a condom
- Supply condoms freely

Contacts must be managed
- Counsel on the importance of treating all sexual partners and on ways in which to inform them.
- Provide letters that must be given to the partners

URETHRITIS

Causes
- Gonorrhoea
- Non-gonococcal urethritis
- Mixed gonococcal and non-gonococcal urethritis

GONORRHOEA

Cause
- The causative organism is *Neisseria gonorrhoeae*
    - incubation period is 1-10 days

Clinical features
In males
- It presents as dysuria and a purulent urethral discharge which may become tinged with blood.
- It is however occasionally asymptomatic
- Rectal infection is common in homosexuals
- If untreated, the condition may become chronic and progress to involve the:
    - prostate
    - epididymis
    - peri-urethral glands.
- Urethral stricture is a late complication of untreated or inadequately treated urethritis.

In females
- The primary site of infection is the endocervix, but the urethra and Bartholin's glands may also become infected.
- It is usually asymptomatic
- However, there may be dysuria and a vaginal discharge seen to be arising from the cervical os.
- This discharge may cause soreness (not itchiness)
- If untreated, the condition may progress to involve the uterus and tubes causing acute or chronic salpingitis.

In both sexes
- Gonorrhoea may complicate systemically with dissemination via the blood stream.
- It is then associated with intermittent fever, arthralgia, tenosynovitis or arthritis
    - particularly of the knees, ankles, wrists
    - often involves several joints
- Other complications include conjunctivitis, iritis and endocarditis.

In neonates
- It can cause conjunctivitis with:
    - a profuse purulent discharge
    - oedema of the lids and they may be stuck together
    - severe chemosis.
- Incubation period 1-10 days
- If untreated, serious visual loss may occur as a result of:
    - corneal ulceration
    - panophthalmitis (infection of the whole eye).
- For treatment see ophthalmia neonatorum page 238.

NON-GONOCOCCAL URETHRITIS

A urethritis where gonococci cannot be demonstrated by microscopy or culture.

Causes
- The most common cause for this is Chlamydia trachomatis (types D-K)
    - incubation period 7-21 days
- Less common causes are:
    - ureaplasma urealyticum
    - mycoplasma genitalium

Clinical features
- Symptoms are often mild with a mild urethral discharge
    - they can be more severe with
      a profuse discharge

- Many patients, both male and female, are symptom-free.

In males
- It can spread to involve the epididymis
- It can cause infertility

In females
- It can spread to involve the fallopian tubes causing salpingitis and sterility.

In neonates
- It can cause conjunctivitis with:
    - a watery or purulent discharge
    - swelling of the eyelids.
- Incubation period 5-12 days
- It can also cause an afebrile pneumonia

SYNDROMIC MANAGEMENT OF URETHRITIS
- Confirm discharge
- Consider treating a person with burning on micturition without a discharge
    - this should be done if there is a significant risk of the person having acquired an STI **and** provided urinalysis result does not indicate a urinary tract infection

Medicine management
- Ceftriaxone 250 mg IM as a single dose
- **Plus** azithromycin 1 g as a single oral dose.
- **Add** metronidazole 2 g as a single oral dose if the sexual partner has an abnormal vaginal discharge.

Female contacts
- Treat the same as the male partner.

Penicillin-allergic patients
- People who are penicillin allergic may also react to cephalosporins.
- If there is severe penicillin allergy i.e. angioedema, anaphylactic shock or bronchospasm:
    - omit ceftriaxone / cefixime
    - increase azithromycin dose to 2 g as a single oral dose

If symptoms persist
- Re-examine the patient and confirm that the discharge is coming from the EUM.
- Ask whether the sexual partner has been treated
    - if not, establish whether the patient had unprotected sexual intercourse with the partner since the previous treatment
- If the above is considered to be the cause:
    - repeat the above treatment and re-emphasise the importance of treating the partner
- If the above cannot explain the lack of response
    - suspect resistant gonococcal infection

Suspected treatment failure
- Ceftriaxone 1 g IM as a single dose (Dr initiated)
- **Plus** azithromycin 2 g as a single oral dose
- **Plus** (if not previously given) metronidazole 2 g as a single oral dose

Suspected 1g treatment failure
- **REFER** within 7 days for further investigation and management

EPIDIDYMO-ORCHITIS

Clinical features
- Painful swollen testis
- Very tender
- Often redness of the scrotal wall
- Associated urethral discharge which is commonly, but not always, present
- Exclude trauma or torsion of the testis as a possible cause

SYNDROMIC MANAGEMENT OF EPIDIDYMO-ORCHITIS
- Give ceftriaxone 250 mg IMI stat
- **Plus** azithromycin 1 g as a single oral dose
- Give a scrotal support if the patient has severe pain or give ibuprofen, oral, 400 mg 3 x daily for 5 days

Penicillin-allergic patients
- If there is severe penicillin-allergy, i.e. angioedema, anaphylactic shock, bronchospasm:
    - azithromycin, oral, 2 g as a single dose
    - review after 7 days or earlier if necessary.

If no response
- It is important to exclude other possible causes of testicular swelling, e.g. testicular tumour tortion or TB
    - **REFER**.

BALANITIS

Causes
- Candidiasis (thrush)
- Secondary to genital ulceration eg. chancroid, chancre herpes genitalis (see genital ulceration below)
- Secondary to urethral discharge (treat for urethritis as above)
- Fusospirochaetosis (see page 174)
- Allergic reaction to washing powder or fabric softener

GENITAL CANDIDIASIS

Causes
- Caused by a yeast, Candida albicans

Clinical features
- It is often found in association with:
    - diabetes mellitus
    - HIV disease/AIDS
    - the use of broad spectrum antibiotics.
- Slight to severe redness of the glans and prepuce
- Surface covered with adherent (sticky), streaky or curd-like white patches.
- Sometimes fissuring of the skin at the preputial opening.

- Wash head of penis with soap and water.
- Imidazole cream e.g. clotrimazole to be applied 2 x daily.

SECONDARY TO GENITAL ULCERATON

- Confirm swollen prepuce and a discharge coming out from under the prepuce.
- Commonly associated with phimosis (inability to retract the foreskin).

> For management see under syndromic management for genital ulcers page 173.

PROSTATITIS

Clinical features

There may be any of the following features associated with urethritis or cystitis (nitrites, bacteruria) in males.
- Perineal pain
- Pain on defaecation
- Lower abdominal pain
- Low back pain
- Rectal examination reveals a tender, enlarged prostate

> **MANAGEMENT**
>
> **REFER** if symptoms are severe.
>
> *If it is secondary to cystitis:*
> - Give ciprofloxacin 500 mg 2 x daily for 14 days.
>
> *If it is secondary to urethritis:*
> - Ceftriaxone 250 mg IM stat.
> - **Plus** azithromycin 1 g as a single oral dose

GENITAL ULCERATION

General considerations
- All treatment for ulcers must include treatment for syphilis (primary chancre) because it is not clinically possible to exclude the presence of syphilis in any genital ulcer.
- The only exception is a recurrence of herpes genitalis ulceration (see page 172).

SYPHILIS

A common sexually transmitted infection caused by a spirochaete (Treponema pallidum).

- It is usually spread by sexual contact but can be transmitted from skin, mucosal lesions or in fluids (saliva, blood).
- The spirochaete crosses the placenta to the foetus
- It is capable of infecting any organ of the body
- It is possible to become re-infected after treatment ie. there is little immunity.

Syphilis can be divided into a number of stages:
Early syphilis
- Primary
- Secondary
- Early latent

Late syphilis
- Late latent
- Tertiary

PRIMARY SYPHILIS

Clinical features

The chancre
- The typical lesion is the chancre which appears at the site of inoculation 9-90 days following exposure.
- It usually occurs on the genitals but may be found on the lips, in the mouth, at the anus or on the cervix.
- It is seen rarely on the breast or on a finger
- It arises as a papule or erosion and develops into a painless, round or oval ulcer which is:
    - superficial
    - or raised
    - often indurated.
- The ulcer surface is smooth and covered with serous fluid
- Although usually single, there can be multiple lesions in about 20% of cases.
- "Kissing chancres" may result from auto-inoculation
- Secondary infection of chancres is uncommon
- There is associated *bilateral lymphadenopathy* and the glands are felt to be moderately enlarged, discrete, rubbery and non-tender
    - suppuration of these glands is very uncommon
- Healing occurs without treatment usually in 3-8 weeks
- The RPR blood test becomes positive 4-6 weeks following exposure.

In females
- Chancres are not as typical and are easily missed
- There may be marked oedema of the labia

In males
- There may be marked oedema of the prepuce

> See management of all genital ulcers (page 173).

SECONDARY SYPHILIS

Clinical features
- The interval between the appearance of the primary chancre and the onset of secondary syphilis is 6-8 weeks.
- In about a third of patients the primary lesion is still evident when the secondary manifestations occur.
- *It is highly infectious*
- The lesions may last from hours to months

Presentations
- Skin, hair and mucosal lesions
- There may also be a constitutional upset
- Lesions affecting the brain, kidney, liver, hair, eye and heart are rare.

Skin lesions
- These are usually found together with generalised lymphadenopathy
- They are usually macular, papular or papulo-squamous (scaly papules)
- However they may be:
    - pustular
    - follicular
    - **or** a combination of any of these types.
- Typically non-itchy
- The lesions are bilaterally symmetrical, involving the neck, trunk and inner aspects of the arms and thighs.
- The condition must be suspected if the palms and soles are involved.
- Annular lesions which look like ringworm may be seen, particularly around the mouth and neck.

Mucous membrane lesions
- There is a diffuse redness (eg. in the pharynx)
- Ulcers and papules of the lips, mouth and throat
- Mucous patches may be seen on the genitalia and in the mouth
    - they are rounded and have a grey-white base surrounded by a red areola
    - they may coalesce (come together) to form serpiginous lesions between them, called "snail track ulcers"
- Commonly seen are the *condylomata lata* around the anus and vulva
    - they are papular lesions which enlarge to form broad, moist, pink or grey-white, flat-topped plaques which may become eroded.

Note. Blood tests are always positive in secondary syphilis.

MANAGEMENT

Doxycycline 100 mg 2 x daily for 14 days
In pregnancy:
- Give benzathine penicillin 2,4 million units IMI stat.
- Blood tests e.g. TPAB / RPR are not indicated unless difficulty is experienced in making a definite diagnosis in a patient presenting with a rash.
- Contacts to be treated the same as patients.

If penicillin-allergic and pregnant
- **REFER** for confirmation of a new syphilis infection and penicillin desensitisation

LATENT SYPHILIS

This is the clinically inactive stage of syphilis occurring between the secondary and tertiary stages.
- It may be divided into early latent and late latent syphilis
- It is diagnosed by blood tests TPAB / RPR

MANAGEMENT

Doxycycline 100 mg 2 x daily for 28 days
In pregnancy:
- Give benzathine penicillin 2,4 million units IMI stat and repeat at weekly intervals x 2, i.e. a total of 7,2 million units
- For contacts in pregnancy:
    - Doxycycline 100 mg 2 x daily for 28 days
- If a patient defaults in having any injection for more than 3 days, he/she should be re-treated fully with 3 injections
    - in such cases the importance of adherence must be strongly re-emphasised.
- Repeat TPAB / RPR after 6 weeks in pregnancy to exclude reinfection
    - see page 339

If penicillin-allergic and pregnant
- **REFER** to hospital for penicillin desensitisation

After 6 months
- If titre shows a four-fold or greater reduction, discharge the patient
- If titre shows less than a four-fold reduction,
    - retreat with doxycycline 100 mg 2 x daily for 14 days
- Note: if the original titre was less than 1:8, further reduction may not occur (serofast).

TERTIARY SYPHILIS

This may develop at any time after secondary syphilis.
- It is uncommon
- It may never develop

Clinical features
The following lesions are found.

Gummas
- These are areas that have become hard, in which the centre breaks down.
- They are found in the skin and long bones

CVS
- Aortic aneurysm and aortic valve incompetence
- Coronary ostial stenosis (causing angina)

CNS
- Meningitis
- Tabes dorsalis
- General paralysis of the insane (GPI)

- *Tertiary syphilis is very difficult to treat*
- *All suspected cases must be **REFERRED** for inpatient treatment*

CONGENITAL SYPHILIS

An infected pregnant woman may
- Abort after the 4th month
- Give birth to a macerated stillbirth
- Give birth to a baby with congenital syphilis with:
    - bullous skin eruptions (syphilitic pemphigus)
    - serous or sero-sanguinous nasal discharge (snuffles).
- Give birth to a baby who develops stigmata later eg.
    - Hutchinson's teeth (notched incisors)
    - deafness
    - bone deformities

MANAGEMENT

Pregnant women should be treated with the penicillin regime appropriate for the stage of syphilis diagnosed.
- Provided the penicillin treatment had been completed more than *4 weeks* prior to delivery, there is little risk to the infant.
- Therefore, it is not necessary for these babies to be notified

Notification

Notification is indicated in the following situations
- Untreated mothers
- Inadequately treated mothers or where the course of penicillin treatment was completed less than 4 weeks prior to delivery.

Examination of baby

Any infant must be examined at birth for evidence of congenital syphilis if the mother
- had a positive RPR blood test
- had other evidence of syphilis in pregnancy (regardless of treatment)
- was unbooked

- If clinical evidence of congenital syphilis is found, the infant must be **REFERRED** to hospital for full evaluation (including CSF examination) and treatment.
- If **NO** evidence of congenital syphilis is found, the infant must be given benzathine penicillin 300,000 u (1 ml) IM as a single dose if the mother:
    - was not treated
    - has received <3 doses of benzathine penicillin
    - delivers within 4 weeks of completing treatment

NB Treat the mother and partner, unless this has already been done.

Follow up

- For those infants not treated at birth, the 6 week follow up visit is an important time to check for congenital syphilis
    - this is because in the majority of infants, physical signs do not appear until 2-8 weeks after birth

GENITAL HERPES (HERPES GENITALIS)

Causes

- A venereal disease caused by Herpes simplex virus type 2
- Incubation period varies from 2-20 days
    - but is usually about 1 week

Clinical features

- Recurrent attacks are common
- There is usually something that sets off the attacks eg.:
    - menses
    - stress
    - intercourse.
- Usually a few days before the rash appears, the patient has symptoms (a prodrome) of itching or burning associated with a localised reddish patch.
- Later groups of vesicles appear
- Lesions may fuse
- Rupture of these vesicles results in the formation of painful, small superficial ulcerations or erosions.
- There is sometimes an associated lymphadenopathy
- The glands are painful, discrete and usually small
- Herpes should be suspected if the patient gives a history of repeated sores or blisters recurring at the same time.

MANAGEMENT

There is no specific curative therapy for herpes genitalis. Treatment is aimed at reducing the duration and severity of episodes.

Patient advice

The patient should be told that:
- The disease often has repeated episodes.
- The disease cannot be cured, and treatment can only lessen symptoms.
- Each episode is self-limiting and will usually clear up spontaneously in 10-14 days.
- The area must be kept as clean and dry as possible to avoid secondary infection and to speed up healing.

Medicine management

See page 173 - Magangement of all genital ulcers.
- if only blisters are present, treat with acyclovir alone
- **Note**: acyclovir is less beneficial if it is started after 48-72 hours following onset of symptoms

- At subsequent visits for recurrences, it is not necessary to repeat the benzathine penicillin
    - treat with acyclovir only
- If secondary bacterial infection is present (uncommon), give ciprofloxacin 500 mg 2 x daily for 5 days
- The patient should abstain from sexual intercourse or use condoms from the onset of the prodrome (itching or burning over a localised area) until the lesions have completely healed - usually 10-14 days.
- Encourage VCT for HIV disease.
- Contacts are to be examined for evidence of genital ulceration
    - if lesions are found, treat as above
    - if lesions are not found, no treatment is required (recommend VCT for HIV disease)

Other management

In pregnancy

- Pregnant women with a history of genital herpes should be carefully monitored during their pregnancy for evidence of active disease.
- If they should have an active infection during labour, a Caesarean section can be done to avoid neonatal infection, which can cause encephalitis and possible death.

CHANCROID

This is a soft genital sore caused by Haemophilus ducreyi.

Clinical features

- It presents 1-9 days following intercourse with an affected partner
- It can occur anywhere on the genitalia
- It may also be found at the anus or on the cervix
- It appears as a painful ulcer with a distinctive red margin
- It is soft to the touch, extends deeply, with a raised irregular edge
- It has a base which is covered by a purulent, dirty exudate and bleeds easily
- There may be single or multiple ulcers
- "Kissing" lesions may result from auto-inoculation

- Lymphadenopathy is variable
    - they are often unilateral but may be bilateral
    - frequently the glands are tender
    - they may become matted with overlying erythema
    - they may suppurate forming draining sinuses

> **MANAGEMENT**
> - Give syndromic management for genital ulceration (see Syndrome Protocol opposite).
> - Patients with matted, hot, tender inguinal glands (pre-suppuration) are to return after 5-7 days if they have not improved.
> - Fluctuant inguinal gland abscesses must be aspirated, not incised
>   - see Management of buboes below

LYMPHOGRANULOMA VENEREUM (LGV)

Causes
- Caused by *Chlamydia trachomatis* serotypes L1, L2 and L3
- Incubation period is usually about 3 weeks

Clinical features
- It is less common in major centres of South Africa.
- Relatively common in Swaziland and adjoining areas of Mpumalanga and KwaZulu-Natal, Transkei, Lesotho
- It begins as a single, small, painless ulcer (< 5 mm in diameter)
- Lesion heals early and is seldom seen
- It drains to the lymph nodes which causes unilateral or bilateral tender lymphadenopathy
    - often both the inguinal and femoral nodes are involved giving a groove in between ("groove sign")
- The glands fuse, soften and form multiple draining sinuses
    - these cause extensive scarring

> **MANAGEMENT OF BUBOES**
> **Matted, tender lymph glands or abscess (bubo)**
> (All cases whether ulcer present or not)
> - Give syndromic management for LGV and chancroid
>   - azithromycin 1 g, as a single oral dose and repeat weekly for 2 weeks
> - **REFER** fluctuant lymph glands for aspiration.

MANAGEMENT OF ALL GENITAL ULCERS

> **MANAGEMENT**
> *Because it is not clinically possible to exclude the presence of syphilis in any genital ulcer, all treatment for ulcers must include treatment for syphilis (primary chancre). The only exception is a recurrence of herpes genitalis ulceration (see page 172).*
>
> **Medicine management**
> - Doxycycline 100 mg 2 x daily for 14 days
>
> In pregnant / lactating women:
> - Give benzathine penicillin 2,4 million units IMI stat
>
> **Plus**
> - Acyclovir 400 mg 3 x daily for 7 days
> - Encourage VCT (voluntary counselling and testing) for HIV disease.
>
> **Penicillin-allergic patients**
>
> *Penicillin-allergic men and non-pregnant women:*
> - Doxycycline, oral, 100 mg 2 x daily for 14 days
>
> **Plus**
> - Acyclovir 400 mg 3 x daily for 7 days
>
> *Penicillin-allergic pregnant / breastfeeding women:*
> - **REFER** for confirmation of a new syphilis infection and penicillin desensitisation

SYNDROMIC PROTOCOL FOR GENITAL ULCERATION

Patient complains of genital sore
- Take history and examine
- Genital ulcer present?

Yes:
Genital ulcer management (see above)
- Counsel on adherence and risk reduction
- Promote and provide condoms
- Contact management
- Review in 1 week

No:
- Counsel
- Educate
- Promote and provide condoms

Ulcer healed or improving?

No:
- Azithromycin 1 g as a single oral dose.
- If no response in 48 hours, **REFER**.

Yes:
Discharge patient

FUSOSPIROCHAETOSIS

Clinical features
- This occurs under the foreskin in uncircumcised males
- It presents as a profuse, offensive, rapidly-drying, watery discharge
- It is often associated with irregular map-like areas of superficial ulceration or erosion of the prepuce or glans of the penis

> **MANAGEMENT**
> - Give benzathine penicillin 2,4 million units IMI stat (to cover for primary chancre)
>
> *Penicillin-allergic patients*
>   - doxycycline 100 mg 2 x daily for 14 days (to cover for primary chancre)

MATTED TENDER LYMPH GLANDS OR ABCESS AND GENITAL ULCER

> - See management of buboes page 173

GENITAL ULCER AND URETHRITIS

> **MANAGEMENT**
> - Ceftriaxone 250 mg IM as a single dose.
> - **Plus** azithromycin 1 g as a single oral dose.
> - **Plus** (if sexual partner has an abnormal vaginal discharge)
>   - metronidazole 2 g as a single oral dose
> - Acyclovir 400 mg 3 x daily for 7 days
> - Review after 7 days

GENITAL ULCER AND SCROTAL SWELLING

> **MANAGEMENT**
> Give the following:
> - Ceftriaxone, IM, 250 mg as a single dose
>   - **plus** azithromycin 1 g as a single oral dose
> - Acyclovir 400 mg 3 x daily for 7 days
> - Ask patient to return after 7 days if not improved.

VAGINAL DISCHARGES

Sexually transmitted causes
- Vaginal infections
- Cervical infections
- Pelvic inflammatory disease - see upper genital tract diseases page 197

VAGINAL INFECTIONS

TRICHOMONAS INFECTION
This is often contracted during sexual intercourse and is usually a sexually transmitted infection.

Clinical features
In females
- Incubation period of 5-28 days
- A sudden onset of a smelly, frothy vaginal discharge varying from cream to green in colour.
- It often begins with the menses.
- There is vulvar erythema, itchiness and vaginal tenderness which may lead to dyspareunia.

In males
- Often asymptomatic.
- It may cause a mild urethritis that only lasts a short time.
- It may cause prostatitis.

> For management see under syndromic management for vaginal discharge (see opposite).

BACTERIAL VAGINOSIS

Causes
- *Gardnerella vaginalis* together with certain anaerobic bacteria

Clinical features
- There is a grey-white vaginal discharge that sticks to the walls
- It may be profuse
- It has a typical fishy odour
- It is not associated with:
  - pruritis
  - dysuria
  - dyspareunia.

> For management see under syndromic management for vaginal discharge (see opposite).

GENITAL CANDIDIASIS

Causes
- Caused by a yeast, *Candida albicans*

Clinical features
- It is often found together with other conditions
    - pregnancy
    - AIDS
    - diabetes mellitus
    - use of oral contraceptives or broad spectrum antibiotics
- There is vulval irritation and vaginal discharge
- The vulva and vaginal wall are often reddened
- The discharge
    - may be scanty or profuse
    - is thick, curd-like and white
    - sticks to the vaginal wall

- Clotrimazole 500 mg pessary
    - insert at night as a single oral dose
- **Or** clotrimazole 200 mg pessary nightly for 3 nights

CERVICAL INFECTIONS

Causes
- Gonococcal infection
- Non-gonococcal infection

GONOCOCCAL AND NON-GONOCOCCAL INFECTION

Clinical features
- Seen on speculum examination as a mucopurulent discharge coming out of the cervical os.
- A red granular cervical erosion is diagnostic of chlamydial cervicitis.

SYNDROMIC MANAGEMENT OF VAGINAL DISCHARGE

Not sexually active within the last 3 months
Vulval or vaginal itchiness and vulva scratched/inflamed and/or curd-like discharge:
- Clotrimazole vaginal pessary 500 mg as a single dose to insert nocte.

If prominent vulval symptoms:
- Clotrimazole cream 1% applied to vulva 2 x daily for 7 days.

If no vulval or vaginal itchiness and no curd-like discharge:
- Metronidazole, oral, 2 g as a single dose.

Sexually active within the last 3 months or a contact of male urethritis syndrome

No lower abdominal pain:
- Ceftriaxone 250 mg IM as a single dose

Plus
- azithromycin 1 g as a single oral dose

Plus
- metronidazole 2 g as a single oral dose.

Lower abdominal pain:
- Do abdominal and PV examination
- Do speculum examination whenever possible

Pain on moving the cervix/lower abdominal tenderness:
- Ceftriaxone 250 mg IM as a single dose

Plus
- azithromycin 1 g as a single oral dose

Plus
- metronidazole 400 mg 2 x daily for 7 days

If vulva red/scratched and/or curd-like discharge:
- Clotrimazole vaginal pessary 500 mg as a single dose to insert nocte.

REFER if any of the following are present:
- abdominal guarding and/or rebound tenderness
- abdominal mass
- fever > 38 degrees C
- abnormal vaginal bleeding
- recent delivery, TOP or miscarriage

If severely ill patient (before referral):
- Ceftriaxone, IV or IM, 1 g as a single dose

Plus
- Metronidazole, oral, 400 mg as a single dose

No pain on moving the cervix and no lower abdominal tenderness:
Treat as above under heading "No lower abdominal pain"

Male contacts and pregnant women
Treat as above under heading "No lower abdominal pain"

GENITAL ULCER AND VAGINAL DISCHARGE

MANAGEMENT

No pain on moving the cervix and no lower abdominal pain
- Ceftriaxone IM 250 mg stat
- **Plus** azithromycin 1 g as a single oral dose
- **Plus** metronidazole 2 g as a single oral dose
- **Plus** acyclovir 400 mg 3 x daily for 7 days

Pain on moving the cervix / lower abdominal pain
- Ceftriaxone 250 mg IMI stat
- **Plus** azithromycin 1 g as a single oral dose
- **Plus** metronidazole 400 mg 2 x daily for 7 days
- **Plus** acyclovir 400 mg 3 x daily for 7 days

GENITAL WARTS
(CONDYLOMATA ACUMINATA)

Causes
- Caused by the Human papilloma virus (HPV)

Clinical features
- They can be especially numerous in pregnancy
- They begin as small, pointed projections which grow upwards and become pedunculated (on stalks).
- These growths multiply and usually form clusters which will finally give the lesions a cauliflower appearance.
- They grow quickly in warm, moist areas
- Because of the collection of purulent material in the clefts, they:
    - become offensive
    - appear as pale, greyish growths.
- Perianal and rectal warts
    - may occur as a result of perineal spread in women
    - are commonly found in homosexual men
- Warts can be soft or hard

Differential diagnosis
Condylomata lata which are due to secondary syphilis.
- These warts are low flat-topped, painless and moist
- There are usually other features of secondary syphilis
    - generalised rash
    - generalised lymphadenopathy
    - a history of a recent painless ulcer

Carcinoma of the vulva
- A history of a chronic growth with no response to treatment
- The growths are very offensive or ulcerating

MANAGEMENT
In most cases, warts resolve without treatment after 2 years in non-immunocompromised patients
- In pregnancy there is no treatment
- Patients to return 6 months after delivery for treatment by which time the majority will have regressed
- **REFER** all patients with:
    - hard hyper-keratinised warts
    - warts larger than 1 cm in size
    - intra-vaginal, cervical or urethral meatal warts
- **REFER** females to gynaecologists and males to surgeons for cryotherapy, cauterisation or excision.

NB.
- *The use of condoms may also be helpful in preventing repeat infections*
- The patient should be warned that there is strong evidence that this virus predisposes the woman to several carcinomas of the genital tract, especially **carcinoma of the cervix.**
- Therefore, all women who have condylomata acuminata (or whose contacts have had them) should be advised to have **annual PAP smears** until at least the age of 50 years.

Medicine treatment
Podophyllin 20 % in Tinct. Benz Co, topical.
- Apply at weekly intervals to lesions by a healthcare professional until lesions disappear.
- Apply petroleum jelly to surrounding skin for protection.
- Wash the solution off after 4 hours.
- Contraindicated in pregnancy.

REFERRAL
Extensive or recurrent anogenital warts.

MOLLUSCUM CONTAGIOSUM

Clinical features
- Dome-shaped papules with central depression (umbilication)
- The number varies from occasional lesions to large crops scattered across the genital area, including the pubis.
- Other sites which may be affected are the perineum and inner thighs.

MANAGEMENT
- Usually no treatment is necessary unless requested by patient.
- Individual lesions have to be treated separately.
    - apply tincture of iodine to the central core of each lesion using an applicator.

PARAPHIMOSIS

Causes
This is caused by a mild phimosis (narrowing of the opening of the foreskin) which gets caught behind the glans of the penis during erection.

Clinical features
- The tight foreskin constricts the penis and causes severe oedema and pain
- Severely swollen glans (end) of the penis
- In early cases there is no ulceration
- In late cases ulceration occurs secondary to exposure of the mucous membrane

---

- Attempt to reduce the paraphimosis by gentle pressure
- **REFER** if not successful

▼ **Note to doctor**
- Anaesthetise the penis with local anaesthetic (without epinephrine)
- Use 14 cc 1% lignocaine for an adult
- Inject 3 cc at the dorsum of the base of the shaft of the penis, with needle touching on hard penile tissue
- Infiltrate the rest of the local in a triangle around the base of the shaft of the penis, at the level of the junction of penile and scrotal skin.

NB. Do not do it halfway along the shaft, as the pressure of the local can cause ischaemia.

- Once the local anaesthetic is working (about 10 minutes) attempt to pull foreskin over by squeezing and pulling the foreskin forward.
- In rare cases, a dorsal slit is necessary
    - make a 1 cm incision along the tightest point of constriction, dividing the superficial fibres
- Check after 2 weeks
    - if there is a residual phimosis, **REFER** for circumcision
    - before **REFERRAL** inform patient that circumcision does not prevent STIs ▲

Female Reproductive System

GYNAECOLOGICAL SYMPTOMS

COMMON CAUSES

LOWER ABDOMINAL PAIN

There are many causes of lower abdominal pain in a woman. It helps to look at the four organs that are the main cause of pain.

- Bowel disease. Nearly half of lower abdominal pain is considered to be due to spastic colon.
- Disorders of the renal system e.g. urinary tract infection
- Pain from the muscles of the abdomen e.g. after severe exertion or coughing
- Gynaecological disease

COMMON GYNAECOLOGICAL CAUSES

■ PRE-PUBERTY AND PUBERTY

Pain in this age group is virtually never gynaecological.
Possible gynaecological causes are:
- Is there a history or suggestion of sexual abuse and / or vaginal discharge?
    - this suggests the possibility of infection of the genital tract or urinary tract infection.
- Is there accompanying abdominal swelling or a mass?
    - rarely there may be an ovarian swelling or tumour.
    - think pregnancy in the older pubertal group, even if they have not had a period.

■ REPRODUCTIVE AGE GROUP

Cyclical pain (coming every month)
Physiological
- Related to menses - primary dysmenorrhoea
- Mid-cycle ovulation and related functional cysts
    - usually unilateral and may be accompanied by a marked mucous physiological discharge.

Pathological
Related to menses:
- Uterine eg. fibroids, secondary to an IUCD
    - usually a colicky type of pain.
- Endometriosis
    - bowel symptoms are often exacerbated during menses
- Chronic pelvic inflammatory disease
    - if this becomes severe, pain may be continuous but made worse by menses.

Non cyclical
Pregnancy-related - associated with vaginal bleeding
- Abortions
- Ectopic
- Pseudocyesis with dysmenorrhoea, after a variable period of amenorrhoea

Pregnancy-related - NOT associated with vaginal bleeding
Genital tract origin:
- Uterine
    - round ligament tenderness, usually only from about 20 weeks. The ligament can invariably be palpated as the only tender area on the lateral side of the uterus.
    - red degeneration of a fibroid. This can cause severe pain. Often the patient will know that she has a fibroid, or the fibroid can be felt as a distinct tender mass, or masses of variable size on the uterus. The uterus will usually be large for dates.
- Ovarian
    - an ovarian cyst may complicate during pregnancy
    - early pregnancy always has a corpus luteum of pregnancy that maintains the early pregnancy
    - if this ruptures or bleeds, it may be associated with pain and bleeding and may lead to abortion.

Non-genital tract origin
- These occur coincidentally during pregnancy eg. UTI, appendicitis, cholecystitis, typhoid.

Not related to pregnancy
Associated with infection
- Endometritis and cervicitis
    - usually minor suprapubic pain and no fever
    - often discharge with minor urinary symptoms
    - there may be post-coital or abnormal bleeding.
- Infection of the upper genital tract (PID)
    - usually more severe pain and constitutional symptoms of infection
    - extent of the pain and severity varies with the stage of infection
    - often associated with dyspareunia.
- Secondary to vulval infections causing suprapubic or inguinal pain associated with the disease or tender lymphadenopathy eg.
    - herpes
    - infected vulval tumours or ulcers
    - lower limb infection.

Neoplasm or cysts
- Ovarian
    - complications of an ovarian cyst ie. rupture, torsion or haemorrhage; this is usually unilateral and may be associated with bleeding.
    - neoplasia; abdominal swelling usually precedes pain.
- Uterine and cervical
    - neoplasia
    - usually presents with abnormal bleeding and/or discharge, and/or dyspareunia.

NON-GYNAECOLOGICAL CAUSES

Urinary
- Cystitis
  - severe dysuria usually more marked than the lower abdominal pain.
- Pyelonephritis
  - usually poorly localised abdominal pain and constitutional symptoms of infection
- Renal colic

Gastrointestinal
- Appendicitis
- Colic followed by gastroenteritis
- Constipation
- Other GIT disease eg.
  - diverticulitis
  - intestinal obstruction.

Musculoskeletal
- Hernias
- Trauma
- Pain referred from the spine or hip
- Secondary to exertion
  - the pain will be associated with movement
  - there may be a precipitating cause.
- Psoas abscess

Anxiety
There can be anxiety about the following:
- Sexually transmitted infections especially HIV
- Cancer
- Infertility
- An unwanted pregnancy
- Sexual problems

■ POST MENOPAUSAL

- Lower abdominal pain in this age group is rarely gynaecological.
  - **Note** the section on non-gynaecological causes of pain (see above).
- **NB.** urinary tract infections are common in elderly, oestrogen-deficient women.

CLINICAL FEATURES

The history is most important. Features suggesting a gynaecological cause are:
- Pain coming in cycles
- Associated features such as abnormal bleeding, vaginal discharge, dyspareunia, dysuria, changed pain with menses.

On examination
- Examination checks the patient's general condition looking for pyrexia, pallor or shock.
- Abdominal examination checks for:
  - rebound tenderness suggesting peritonitis
  - the maximal site of the pain
  - any masses.

Note:
- Vaginal examination is of great value even if the patient is bleeding. It should only be avoided where a placenta praevia is suspected.
- Tumours of the cervix may be easily palpable on digital, vaginal examination, as are prolapsed fibroids.

VAGINAL DISCHARGE

The patient may be able to give a valuable opinion about whether the discharge is normal or not.
Physiological discharges vary during the month.

Causes of abnormal discharge
- Carcinoma of the cervix or uterus (older women)
- Reactions to soaps, washing powders, fabric softeners, deodorants and antiseptics
  - chemicals that may cause a reaction are Dettol, Savlon, Jeyes Fluid - these may cause thrush.
- Vaginitis
- Cervical infections
- Endometritis
- Genital ulceration
- Foreign body
- Sexual abuse in children (see page 193)

Clinical features of abnormal discharge
- Often smells bad
- May cause burning or itching
- May look different
- May be increased in amount

See sexually transmitted infections page 174.

PAIN WITH MENSES (DYSMENORRHOEA)

Dysmenorrhoea may be primary or secondary.

PRIMARY (NORMAL) DYSMENORRHOEA

Clinical features
- This is a normal (physiological) body reaction. Each woman learns to know her own normal pattern of pain.
- The pain is often worse when the periods become regular
  - it is increased when ovulation starts after menarche because the ovulation releases more prostaglandins
  - primary dysmenorrhoea suggests that ovulation is taking place.
- The pain is worse for the first 2 days, and similar to cramp.
- There may be dull backache and lower abdominal pain before the period starts.
- The pain responds to anti-prostaglandins such as ibuprofen.
- It commonly occurs in young women.
- Pain and bleeding may change after the woman has given birth.

MANAGEMENT
General measures
- Patients are advised about the nature of the condition and encouraged to carry on with their normal everyday activities.

- Advice to young women to fall pregnant to improve this condition is wrong and dangerous. Pregnancy may not stop the dysmenorrhoea but may result in:
    - unwanted pregnancies
    - sexually transmitted infection
    - difficult relationships with future partners
    - marital problems

Medicine management
- Give an anti-inflammatory drug
    - ibuprofen 400 mg
      3 x daily for 2-3 days
    - **or** diclofenac 25 mg
      3 x daily for 2-3 days.
- Oral contraceptive pills can greatly help relieve symptoms
- If the pain is severe
    - **add** combined oral contraceptive tablets e.g. Nordette 1 tab daily
    - review after 3 months

SECONDARY DYSMENORRHOEA

Secondary dysmenorrhoea is not normal. It is often a warning of an underlying gynacological disorder.

Common causes
- Pelvic inflammatory disease
- Endometriosis
- Fibroids
- Other masses or tumours

Clinical features
In secondary dysmenorrhoea there is a change in the nature of the period pain. The woman knowing her normal menstrual pattern is often best able to decide if it is different.
- It may occur earlier than usual starting before menstruation. It may:
    - be more severe
    - last longer
    - be a different type of pain
    - or radiate more to other areas.
- There are often other associated gynaecological symptoms e.g. dysparunia, menorrhagia, abnormal bleeding.

NB. It is important to look for pathological causes. Do an abdominal and vaginal examination and speculum to look for possible causes.

MANAGEMENT
- Treat for pelvic infection if you suspect it (see page 197)
- Give an NSAID
    - eg. ibuprofen 400 mg 3 x daily for 2-3 days
- If pain is severe or if no response and if pregnancy is not planned
    - give combined oral contraceptive e.g. Nordette 1 tablet daily for 3 months
- **REFER** if:
    - there is uncertainty about the diagnosis
    - you suspect a serious cause
    - there is no response to the above treatment

AMENORRHOEA

PRIMARY AMENORRHOEA

Causes
- It is quite possible for puberty to be delayed up to the age of 18 years
    - however, secondary sexual characteristics should be present.
- Ask about a familial tendency to late puberty.

A useful way to decide on the possible cause is to check:
- If there is any regular menstrual like pain (cyclical pain)
- If there is the development of normal secondary sexual characteristics of enlarged breasts, axillary and pubic hair.

If these are not present, the problem may be in the pituitary, uterus or ovaries such as a congenital abnormality.
If the pain is regular and there are secondary sexual characteristics, the hormonal system is probably working.

The causes to look for then are:
- An unsuspected pregnancy
- Hidden menstruation (cryptomenorrhoea) caused by an imperforate hymen, a vaginal septum or another congenital abnormality
    - this will cause severe dysmenorrhoea
    - on examination the intact hymen may be seen bulging with a blue colour
    - there may be a palpable abdominal mass if the uterus is distended with blood.

The other important cause for delayed menarche is any chronic illness, such as heart disease, tuberculosis and anorexia nervosa. This often shows itself with weight loss or other symptoms.

MANAGEMENT
If there is any suspicion of pregnancy check:
- by palpating the abdomen
- by doing a pregnancy test

REFER if:
- The genitalia are abnormal.
- The patient has not menstruated by 16 years of age.
- The patient is 14 or older with no secondary sexual characteristics.
- The patient is having cyclical pain but there are no visible menses.
- You suspect any serious medical cause.

SECONDARY AMENORRHOEA

This is when the woman has previously been having normal menses and now stops menstruating.

Causes
- The first diagnosis to look for should always be **pregnancy**. Quite often the patient will actually come wanting to confirm if she is pregnant or not
    - if she has not been pregnant before, she may not know the symptoms.
- A common cause is when a patient is desperately wanting a baby (psuedocyesis) and misses her period because of her anxiety.

Other causes

Normal causes for no menstruation
- Breast feeding
    - the menses may only start 6 months or more after delivery.
- Post-abortion or termination of pregnancy
- Menopause with:
    - hot flushes
    - change in menstrual pattern recently.
- Excessive exercising as may occur in athletes.

Due to medication (iatrogenic)
This is an important cause. Often patients do not understand the possible effects of contraceptives.
- Depo injections such as Depo-Medrol may cause prolonged amenorrhoea.
- Prolonged use of oral contraception may also cause amenorrhoea.
- Treatment for other diseases, such as depression or hypertension.
- Gynaecological treatment or surgery, such as hysterectomy

Emotional stress
This may be due to many causes such as:
- Family problems particularly changes in a relationship or death in the family.
- Work-related, particularly unemployment.
- Personal trauma such as a motor vehicle accident, assault or criminal episode.
- Travel or moving house.

Chronic or severe medical illness
Usually this will give other symptoms. An important symptom is significant weight loss in the last month.
Important diseases are:
- Tuberculosis
- HIV/AIDS
- Diabetes, heart disease, chronic lung or kidney disease
- Alcohol and drug abuse
- Malnutrition
- Carcinoma, especially if under treatment with radiotherapy or anti-cancer drugs

Endocrine causes
- Occasionally a tumour of the pituitary gland may affect the gynaecological hormones
    - a symptom that may suggest this is the recent onset of breast milk secretion
    - some medication may do this, but profuse breast milk secretion suggests a prolactinoma tumour.
- Thyroid disease is easily missed. This usually shows itself as:
    - weight change
    - recent onset of discomfort with hot or cold weather.

MANAGEMENT
- Check for pregnancy
- Many patients will respond well to an honest discussion about the probable cause, especially if it is related to contraception.
- Patients sometimes worry that the lack of menstruation will cause the "bad blood" to be retained
    - it may help to explain that not menstruating helps the body retain iron
    - this in turn helps increase resistance.
- Good treatment of a disease may result in a normal menstrual pattern returning.
- If a disease is suspected, it should be treated or the patient **REFERRED** for investigation.

▼ Note to doctor
* If the patient requests help in having a menstrual cycle:
    - reassure
    - if no obvious cause is found and the pregnancy test is negative, she can be given medroxyprogesterone (Provera) 10 mg daily for 10 days.
- If the endometrium has been prepared by oestrogen
    - the progesterone will cause a withdrawal bleed 5-7 days after conclusion of the treatment
    - if there is no withdrawal bleed, it suggests there is not enough oestrogen
    - this may be due to causes arising from the hypothalamus and pituitary to the ovaries
    - give an oral contraceptive (oestrogen, progesterone combination) tablet eg. Nordette, Triphasil for 1 month
    - if there is no withdrawal bleed after use of these drugs, it suggests there is significant disease
    - **REFER** for investigation. ▲

MENOPAUSE

Menopause means the permanent cessation of normal menses at the end of the reproductive age group. The average age of menopause is 52 with a wide variation. Menopause is usually defined as occurring after 6 months of amenorrhoea at this age group. It is associated with a massive rise in FSH and a decrease of oestrogen.

Climacteric is the time around menopause which may be associated with a gradual loss of regular cycle of periods, and is associated with the following symptoms.

Clinical features
- Hot flushes
- Psychological upsets
    - difficulty with sleeping
    - irritability
    - tiredness
    - headache
    - anxiety and nervousness.
- The vaginal epithelium is sensitive to oestrogen withdrawal causing:
    - senile atrophic vaginitis (common)
    - dyspareunia
    - more frequent urinary tract infections.
- Bowel symptoms
    - increased constipation
    - abdominal distension
    - flatulence
- Because of re-absorption of calcium, bones become more fragile and fractures may occur more easily.

MANAGEMENT
Advice and reassurance
- Often a careful discussion about what happens in menopause will help the patient to deal with many of the symptoms.
- Explain what menopause is and that it is a normal process.

REFER any patient with:

- Early onset of menopause before 40 years
- Increased bleeding or bleeding between periods around the climacteric as this is an important symptom of carcinoma of the cervix or uterus
- Any post menopausal bleeding.

If symptoms are severe at the time of menopause
Analyse the major problems:
- If there are debilitating hot flushes and no contraindications to oestrogens, then start oral oestrogen therapy
    - **plus** progesterone if uterus is intact.
- If vaginal and or urinary symptoms are dominant, give one course of vaginal oestrogen cream.
- If there is a history of osteoporosis, or osteoporosis-induced fracture, start hormonal therapy (HT).

Oestrogen therapy
Important contraindications to oestrogen therapy
- History of deep vein thrombosis or pulmonary embolus
- Coronary artery disease
- Stroke
- Oestrogen-dependent tumours of the breast or endometrium
- Women >60 years of age
- Acute liver disease

NB. If oestrogens are contraindicated, treat the problem with:
- Antidepressants
- Specific anti-osteoporosis therapy
- B blockers for hot flushes

▼ **Note to doctor**
If the uterus is still present, the patient must not be given oestrogen alone. She should be given sequentially opposed or continuous combined therapy. Sequentially opposed preparations are preferred for women who are still menstruating (or have recently stopped) and will result in regular menstrual periods.

Sequentially opposed therapy
- Give at least 10 days of a progestogen a month in addition to the oestrogen.
- The progestogen causes the endometrium to slough and for menstruation to occur.
- This removes abnormal cells and prevents carcinoma of the uterus developing.
- Give conjugated oestrogens (Premarin), oral, 0.3-0.625 mg daily for the first 11 days followed by the addition of medroxyprogesterone acetate 5-10 mg daily for the next 10 days
    - followed by no therapy for the last 7 days
    - **or** oestradiol valerate 1-2 mg daily for the first 11 days followed by the addition of cyproterone acetate 1 mg daily for the next 10 days
    - followed by no therapy for the last 7 days

Continuous combined therapy
- Continuous combined preparations are often preferred if the woman had her last menstrual period over a year ago.
- Give conjugated oestrogen, oral, 0.3-0.625 mg daily

plus
- Medroxyprogesterone acetate 2.5-5 mg daily

or
- Oestradiol valerate 1 mg daily

plus
- Norethisterone acetate 0.5-1 mg daily

If the uterus is absent (post-hysterectomy)
- Patient can be offered oestrogen only
    - oestradiol valerate 1-2 mg daily
    - **or** conjugated oestrogens 0.3-0.625 mg daily
- Try to start on the lowest possible dose of oestrogen.

- Try to wean the patient from oestrogen after a maximum of 5 years
    - there is an increased risk of breast cancer after 5 years of therapy and even more after 10 years.
- Vaginal oestrogen is useful in the management of atrophic vaginitis. However the oestrogen will stimulate the lining of the uterus if given over a prolonged period.
- All patients on oestrogen therapy should have their breasts checked regularly
    - they should ideally have a mammogram once a year.
- The need to continue HT should be reviewed annually. ▲

CHANGES IN MENSTRUAL BLEEDING

- The normal cycle and bleeding pattern is unique to each person. The patient will usually know her regular pattern and be able to say in what way it has changed.
- The normal time between periods varies from 22-36 days
    - the time between periods must be counted from the 1st day to the 1st day.
- It may help to ask the woman to write down her menstrual bleeding for one or several months to get a more objective idea of the amount and type of abnormal bleeding.
- In the time before the menopause (pre-menopause) the bleeding may become lighter, then heavier, and decrease at the end.
- Because the patient knows her menstrual pattern best, she may be able to guide the clinician to possible causes to explore further on history and examination.

ABNORMAL UTERINE BLEEDING

INCREASED MENSTRUATION (MENORRHAGIA)

Menorrhagia is when cyclical, regular menstruation is increased, either in amount or duration or both.

Clinical features
- Pallor
- Large clots
- "Flooding" resulting in the blood soiling her clothes, running down her legs, needing increased sanitary protection.
- There may be associated increased dysmenorrhoea.
- The bleeding may be affecting work or social activity.

Causes
- Chronic pelvic infection
- Fibroids or gynaecological tumours
- Anovulatory cycles (where an ovum is not produced) leading to prolonged unopposed oestrogen stimulation of the endometrium
    - early periods following puberty
    - after childbirth or abortion

- pre-menopause
- stress such as death of a loved one, or physical or psychological trauma
- Endocrine disease e.g. hypothyroidism
- Iatrogenic
  - intra-uterine contraceptive device
  - following tubal ligation
- Bleeding disorders e.g. thrombocytopaenia, leukemia

INTER-MENSTRUAL BLEEDING

This is irregular spotting or bleeding occurring between the normal menstrual periods.

Causes
- Use of hormonal contraceptives, especially depo injections
- Anovulation due to poor follicular development and function, as well as low cyclic oestrogen levels
- Tumours e.g. carcinoma cervix or body of the uterus
- Abortion
- Breastfeeding
- Cervical polyps
- Polycystic ovarian syndrome
- Hyperprolatinaemia

DYSFUNCTIONAL UTERINE BLEEDING (DUB)

This is abnormal uterine bleeding that is not due to an organic cause of the genital tract or systemic condition. It may present as menorrhagia, inter-menstrual bleeding or an irregular cycle.

Causes
- Breakthrough bleeding in patients on hormonal contraceptives.
- Anovulatory cycles

MANAGEMENT OF ABNORMAL UTERINE BLEEDING

- Try to find the cause and treat accordingly
  - **Note:** It is most important to do a vaginal examination (and speculum if available), to look for possible causes such as carcinoma of the cervix.
- **Note:** it is most important to do a **vaginal examination**. Even if a speculum is not available, carcinoma of the cervix may be felt on vaginal examination as a rough irregular hard cervix. There may also be a particularly offensive discharge that may smell of decaying tissue.
  - if there is any suspicion of carcinoma, do a PAP test if possible
  - or **REFER** to exclude malignancy.
- Treat for salpingitis if you suspect it.
- **REFER** if:
  - organic disease is present which you are not able to treat e.g. fibroids
  - the heavy bleeding is around the menopause or after the menopause

---

- the bleeding is severe
- she is severely pale
- she has symptoms or signs of heart failure as a result of the blood loss
- you are unsure of the cause, and she is not responding to clinic treatment
- you suspect a serious cause

▼ **Note to doctor**
For menorrhagia associated with chronic salpingitis:
- Give combined contraceptive pill e.g. Nordette 1 tablet daily for 3 months
- It is helpful to give ibuprofen if there is associated dysmenorrhoea
  - 400 mg 3 x daily with or after food for 2-3 days
- If an IUCD is present, consider requesting its removal.
- Treat the patient with STI syndromic treatment

For excessively heavy anovulatory dysfunctional bleeding:
- Give norethisterone, oral, 5 mg 4 hourly (5 x daily) for 24-48 hours.
- Tranexamic acid (Cyclokapron) can be given instead of norethisterone; this works by stabilising platelet clots that are only present in the early part of the menses.
  - Cyclokapron should therefore only be given for the first 4 days of the period
  - 1 g 4 x daily

- Thereafter continue with a combined oral contraceptive, e.g. Nordette 1 tablet 3 x daily for 7 days, omitting placebos in the pack
  - then 1 tablet daily including placebos for 6 months, to restore cyclicity

For moderate anovulatory dysfunctional bleeding:
- combined oral contraceptive e.g. Nordette 1 tablet daily for 3 months

For progesterone breakthrough bleeding due to a very thin endometrium, e.g:
  - perimenopausal women
  - chronic Depo-provera usage
  - subdermal implants
  - long-term COC usage
- Treat with conjugated oestrogens 0.625 mg daily for 21 days with the addition of medroxyprogesterone 10 mg daily from day 11 to day 21
  - use for 3-6 cycles

If bleeding not controlled:
REFER for specialist investigation. ▲

DECREASED MENSTRUATION (OLIGOMENORRHOEA)

If the bleeding is still in a regular pattern and cycle, it suggests a less serious cause. If the bleeding is irregular, it is important to look for serious causes, particularly carcinoma of the cervix.

Causes
If the time between periods is longer (>35 days) but still cyclical, common causes are:
- Polycystic ovarian syndrome
- Contraception with depo injection
- Pre-menopause (anovulatory cycles)

- Explain the reason and reassure.
- **REFER** if a serious cause is suspected, e.g. polycystic ovarian syndrome

POST-MENOPAUSAL BLEEDING

Vaginal bleeding in a woman who has reached menopause is often the earliest and only sign of carcinoma of the uterus.

Other causes of bleeding
- Vaginal or cervical infection or trauma

> **REFER** unless a treatable cause is obvious.

POST-COITAL OR CONTACT BLEEDING

This means bleeding after sexual intercourse. It is often a symptom of serious disease, especially in a woman over the age of 30.

Causes
- A common and dangerous cause is carcinoma of the cervix
- Carcinoma of the uterus
- Infection associated with an intra-uterine contraceptive device
- Infection of the cervix
- Polyps of the uterus

> **MANAGEMENT**
> - Do a vaginal examination.
> - The patient must have a PAP smear to exclude carcinoma.
> - Treat the cause if possible.
>
> **REFER** if:
> - There are no PAP smear facilities.
> - You suspect carcinoma of the uterus or cervix.

PRE-MENSTRUAL TENSION SYNDROME (PMT)

These are changes affecting the woman's body as a result of hormonal changes during the menstrual cycle.

Clinical features
- The symptoms are usually worse before or during menstruation.
- Features suggesting that the cause is hormonal are if the symptoms occur in cyclical pattern associated with menses, and disappear afterwards.
- Keeping a calendar of when the symptoms occur and their relation to the menstrual cycle may help the patient and clinician decide on the possible cause of the symptoms.

Neurological
- Headaches may occur before, during or after menstruation.
- Migraines may be precipitated.
- Epilepsy may be worse at certain times during the cycle.
- Irritability and depression
    - the hormonal changes do not cause these problems but make underlying depression or stress worse.

Abdomen
The woman may notice:
- Constipation or diarrhoea
- Abdominal bloating and distension
    - this may be due to making an underlying irritable bowel syndrome worse.

Breast
- There may be distension and tenderness.

Oedema of parts of the body
- This may affect different parts such as fingers or ankles.

> **MANAGEMENT**
> - Do a physical examination to look for any underlying causes.
> - Depression is common and may make pre-menstrual symptoms worse.
> - Reassurance and explanation often helps.
> - Treat any possible underlying problem.
> - Bloating may be helped by eating less gas-producing foods such as beans or cabbage.
>
> **REFER** if:
> - Symptoms are significantly affecting her life
> - You suspect a more severe underlying condition eg. depression.

DIFFICULTY WITH SEXUAL INTERCOURSE

DYSPAREUNIA (PAIN ON INTERCOURSE)

This is when there is pain on intercourse and not just difficulty or discomfort. It is often a symptom of underlying gynaecological disease.
There are two main types of pain:

■ SUPERFICIAL DYSPAREUNIA

Pain may occur superficially in the vulva or vagina at the beginning of penetration.

Causes
- Infections
    - herpes
    - candida
    - genital ulcers
    - Bartholin's abscess

- Fear causing spasm of the muscles around the vulva and vagina (vaginismus). This may be due to:
  - previous painful intercourse
  - rape or sexual abuse
  - fear of a sexually transmitted infection or AIDS
  - fear of pregnancy
- Congenital abnormality eg. a very thick hymen
- Vulval disease such as carcinoma or previous scarring

■ PAIN WITH DEEP PENETRATION (DEEP DYSPAREUNIA)

If this occurs often or always on intercourse, it suggests more serious gynaecological disease.

Causes
Causes of frequent or constant pain are:
- Salpingitis
- Endometriosis
- Carcinoma of the cervix or uterus
- Disease of the ovary
- Tumours such as fibroids
- Bladder infection or disease

MANAGEMENT
- It is important to take a good history and examination to find the possible causes of the pain. If the pain is due to disease, there will usually be other gynaecological symptoms such as
  - secondary dysmenorrhoea
  - menstrual change
  - changed vaginal discharge.
- Treat if it is likely to be due to salpingitis.
- **REFER** if there is no response or if you suspect a serious cause.

LOSS OF INTEREST IN INTERCOURSE (DECREASED LIBIDO)

- Loss of interest eg. poor relationship with her partner or struggling to satisfy her partner
- All of the causes of dysparunia as on pages 185-186
- Fertility problem
- Women who have had a termination of pregnancy may have residual fears and guilt for many years.
- Medical problems such as orthopaedic problems, diabetes, heart disease, asthma, epilepsy
- Mental illness eg. depression
- Severe stress, either mental or physical.

MANAGEMENT
- It is important to do a thorough history and gynaecological examination to look for possible physical causes.
- Treat the underlying condition as far as possible
  - **REFERRAL** may be necessary for psychological or marriage counselling.
- It may help to explain basic aspects of anatomy and physiology.

SORES OR ULCERS OF THE GENITALIA

Ulcers may be difficult to see, especially in the vagina.

Single ulcers suggest
- Syphilis
- Chancroid
- Lymphogranuloma venereum
- Granuloma inguinale
- Carcinoma of the vulva

Multiple ulcers suggest
- Herpes genitalis
- Multiple chancroids
- Secondary syphilis with condylomata lata

Differential diagnosis
The patient may call the lesion a sore or an ulcer, but it may be a painful area due to other causes such as:
- Infection of the hair follicles of the pubic area (folliculitis). This may be due to:
  - irritation of the vulva or vagina due to applications such as Zambuck, Savlon, Dettol.
  - it is more common in patients with HIV disease.
- Diseases of the skin e.g. eczema

MANAGEMENT
- Do a careful and thorough examination.
- Treat the cause if possible.
- For sexually transmitted infection management, see page 173.

INFERTILITY

Infertility can cause great emotional distress to a couple and may seriously damage a marriage.

It is useful to find out if this is:
- Primary infertility ie. the patient has never been pregnant.
- Secondary infertility where there has been previous pregnancies but now there is a period of involuntary infertility.

The patient may not be absolutely sure of the answer:
- They may have had an incident, when younger, of irregular menstrual bleeding which they thought was a pregnancy but it was just an irregular cycle.
- They may have had an abortion which they do not want to tell you about.

Examination of the cervix will confirm whether there has been a previous pregnancy, as any pregnancy or abortion will cause dilation of the cervix. This will:
- Result in tearing of the cervix
- Be visible on speculum examination as a lacerated cervix.

Specific causes in women
60% of cases of infertility are due to a problem in the female partner.
- The most common cause is tubal disease i.e. pelvic inflammatory disease.

- the woman may not even be aware that she has salpingitis, especially if the organism was chlamydia.
- Endometriosis possibly due to the direct effects of tubal adhesions.
- Anovulation due to:
  - poor hypothalamic or pituitary function (low FSH, LH and oestradiol)
  - polycystic ovarian syndrome (irregular cycles and hyperandrogenism)
  - poor ovarian function (low oestradiol with increased FSH)
- Uterine or cervical abnormalities, e.g. cervical stenosis
- Congenital abnormalities

Specific causes in men
40% of cases of infertility are due to a problem in the male partner.
- Primary testicular failure
  - low sperm count and sperm abnormalities
- Previous episodes of STIs causing epididymo-orchitis
- Impotence
- Retrograde ejaculation
- Alcohol and drug abuse

MANAGEMENT
- Sadly, infertility is often difficult to treat. However showing concern and genuine interest and attempting to find the cause may bring help and relief to the couple.
- Look for possible treatable causes from the history and examination of both partners. This will involve a full history and examination of them both.

The following advice can be given to patients to help them get pregnant:
- The couple should try to have daily intercourse at the time of ovulation and for several days afterwards.
- Show the patient how to work out the optimum (best) time for intercourse
  - ie. at ovulation, 14 days before her next expected period.
- She may also be able to assess anovulation by:
  - taking her temperature daily (it goes up after ovulation)
  - noting changes in her discharge (the discharge is thinner and more profuse).
- She may have symptoms of ovulation (mittelschmertz)
  - sudden lower abdominal pain
  - feeling faint.
- During intercourse it may help if:
  - the woman avoids getting up immediately after intercourse
  - the man does not withdraw his penis immediately after intercourse, to allow as much sperm as possible to drain into the vagina.
- The man should be advised about ways of ensuring maximum sperm amounts. He should avoid:
  - excessive intercourse
  - wearing tight underpants
  - having very hot baths

- excessive alcohol and drugs.

REFERRAL
- Many hospitals have stopped investigating infertility due to staff and cost constraints.
- Usually both partners need to be tested for HIV
  - the male partner will need to be investigated for causes of male infertility as well.
- It would be advisable to find out about local hospital protocols for the investigation of infertility. If the patient can afford the high costs, private hospitals offer sophisticated investigation and management of infertility problems.

"SOMETHING COMING DOWN" OR "FALLING OUT"

Causes
- This is usually due to prolapse of the uterus.
- Cystitis may give similar symptoms.

Clinical features
- Low back pain or a dragging feeling
- Difficulty with defecation that is relieved by pressure on the perineum
- Urinary incontinence
- On examination:
  - the uterus and cervix may be seen prolapsing
  - a swelling may be seen in the upper or lower wall of the vagina due to prolapse of the bladder or rectum.

MANAGEMENT
- If the prolapse is mild:
  - reassure her
  - encourage weight loss
  - avoid straining when passing stool ie. treat for constipation
  - teach her pelvic floor exercises to strengthen the muscles of the perineum.
- **REFER**
  - if the prolapse is marked
  - if the symptoms are causing concern.

URINARY INCONTINENCE

This is a common problem, but patients are often too embarrassed to complain of it unless asked directly.
It is very embarrassing socially, as the person may wet her clothes or the chair.

STRESS OR URGE INCONTINENCE

- Stress incontinence may occur with any increased intra-abdominal pressure eg. coughing, laughing, sneezing.
- With urge incontinence the patient may feel the need to pass urine but not be able to stop herself urinating until getting to the toilet.

Causes
- Poor pelvic muscles usually due to trauma during childbirth.

Clinical features
- On examination:
  - prolapse of the bladder may be seen
  - the patient might leak urine when asked to cough or strain.

> **MANAGEMENT**
> - If associated with a urinary tract infection, treatment of the infection may relieve the problem.
> - Physiotherapy
> - **REFER** for other causes.

CONTINUOUS INCONTINENCE

This may be due to overflow incontinence when the bladder remains full and leaks urine all the time. It may also be due to total incontinence when the urine drains all the time and the bladder remains empty.

Causes
- Vesico-vaginal fistula
- Carcinoma of the cervix
- Spinal cord damage or other neurological disease

Clinical features
- The history of a continuous leak of urine without the need to ever pass urine.
- With overflow incontinence a distended bladder may be palpated supra-pubically.
- On examination of the vulva, a trickle of urine may be seen.

> **MANAGEMENT**
> - **REFER** when convenient unless it is an acute obstruction.
> - If there is chronic obstruction to urine flow with a full bladder and overflow incontinence
>   - it is safer to **REFER** the patient to be catheterised in a hospital so that the urine loss can be monitored.

LOWER GENITAL TRACT DISEASES

INFECTIONS OF THE VULVA

FURUNCULOSIS

These are infections in and around the hair follicles.

Causes
- Shaving of the pubic hair
- Poor personal hygiene
- Pubic lice and scabies
- Secondary to eczema

Clinical features
- Papules, pustules and crusted lesions.
- Regional lymph glands are not generally greatly enlarged unless the infection is severe.
- Commonly more than one furuncle is present at a time.
- Care must be taken not to confuse these with sexually transmitted ulcers.

> **MANAGEMENT**
> - Give flucloxacillin 250-500 mg 4 x daily for 5 days.
> - If the patient is penicillin-allergic, use azithromycin 500 mg daily for 3 days.
> - Chlorhexidine solution or Betadine is given for local swabbing.

INTERTRIGO

Intertrigo is a condition that occurs in areas where sweat and sebum collect ie. where large areas of skin are in close contact.

Clinical features
- It occurs under large pendulous breasts, under "aprons" of fat in the abdomen and between the thighs and buttocks.
- In the vulval area the condition may be made worse when a vaginal discharge is present.
- The constant friction of the skin in these places gives rise to shiny, often offensive areas
    - these occasionally show signs of secondary infection due to thrush and other organisms.
- The condition is uncomfortable for the patient, particularly in hot weather.

> **MANAGEMENT**
> - Advise the patient to wash frequently with water and to dry well.
> - Treat any associated vaginal discharge.
> - Advise patients to lose weight.
> - Aqueous cream may sooth the affected area.
>
> **Contraindications**
> - Toilet powders become sodden and form a paste that make the condition worse
> - Oils and ointments
> - Soaps and antiseptics such as Savlon

GENITAL HERPES

These are clusters of small blisters that break down to become small superficial ulcers. These may coalesce (come together) and are very painful.

> For details and management see Sexually Transmitted Infections (page 172).

GENITAL WARTS (CONDYLOMATA ACUMINATA)

> For details and management see Sexually Transmitted Infections (page 176).

SWELLINGS OF THE LABIA

BARTHOLIN'S ABSCESS

Causes
- The most common cause is gonorrhoea.

Clinical features
- The patient complains of severe pain in the labium, which will make walking and intercourse difficult.
- An obvious swelling is visible in the posterior third of one of the labia majora.
- The abscess bulges inwards, sometimes hiding the urethra.

- On palpation the swelling:
  - is very tense
  - has shiny, reddened skin covering it
  - is extremely tender.
- The patient looks miserable and may be pyrexial.
- If untreated this may become a Bartholin's cyst.

MANAGEMENT
- This requires incision and drainage under general anaesthetic.
- Also treat for gonorrhoea (see syndromic management of urethritis page 169).

BARTHOLIN'S CYST

Clinical features
- The cyst is quite easily seen and felt in one of the labia majora.
- It is the size of a small plum.
- On palpation it is:
  - tense
  - painless

If the patient wishes to have it removed, **REFER** her for surgery.

SEBACEOUS CYST

Clinical features
- These may occur in or around the labia.

REFER.

VAGINAL DISCHARGE

- There is **normally** a physiological discharge from the vagina
  - however infections of the vagina are common.
- Many women tolerate markedly abnormal discharges
  - due to lack of money or time to seek medical assistance
  - because they do not think the discharge is serious.
- Vaginal discharges are commonly associated with infections of the cervix.
- An important defence mechanism of the vagina is the presence of acid-forming bacteria
  - these break down glycogen in the epithelial cells of the vagina to form acid
  - a high glycogen content is directly related to a high oestrogen level
  - women are therefore more vulnerable before puberty, after menopause and at the time of menstruation.

Causes
- Often a vaginal infection is caused by a mixed group of organisms, and it is seldom possible to be sure of the exact cause
- Sexually transmitted infections
- Post-delivery or after trauma eg. episiotomy
- Sexual abuse must be kept in mind in a young girl with an abnormal vaginal discharge
- Foreign bodies especially in children or mentally abnormal patients
- Disease of the cervix, e.g. cervicitis, carcinoma
- Pedunculated fibroids in the cervical canal, or cervical polyps, may cause an increase in seemingly normal vaginal secretion.
- Due to applications and allergies:
  - deodorants
  - contraceptive applications
  - soap powders especially in underclothing
  - vaginal douches to try to prevent infection or pregnancy. Often these are too strong eg. Dettol, and may result in a severe chemical reaction

MANAGEMENT
- Always do a vaginal examination even if the woman is bleeding as it may be possible to feel an abnormal cervix.
- If possible do a speculum examination as this often shows the cause of the problem, especially during pregnancy.
- Carcinoma of the cervix may have no obvious visible abnormality on the cervix
  - always do a PAP smear unless she has had one in the last 12 months
  - encourage her to have regular PAP smears
- In the clinic situation it is not possible to identify the specific organism causing the discharge.
- It is always a good policy when dealing with vulval infections to advise the patient:
  - to wear cotton panties
  - to wash frequently, using soap and water
  - about the importance of proper drying
  - to avoid bath oils and foams
  - to stop using Dettol, Savlon, etc.

Medicine management
Sexually active within the last 3 months or partner has MUS (male urethritis syndrome):
- Ceftriaxone 250 mg IM as a single dose
  - **plus** azithromycin 1g as a single oral dose
  - **plus** metronidazole 2 g as a single oral dose
- Bring contacts for treatment

Not sexually active within the last 3 months:
If curd-like vaginal discharge:
- Clotrimazole vaginal pessary 500 mg inserted as a single dose at night

If valvul itchiness/excoriation:
- Clotrimazole topical cream to apply 2 x daily for 7 days

If no valvul irritation and no curd-like discharge
- Metronidazole 2 g as a single oral dose

VULVO-VAGINITIS

This is commonly caused by the candida albicans fungus (thrush) and is a distressing condition.

Causes
- Diabetes
- Pregnancy
- Malnutrition (especially in alcoholics)
- Patients who have been taking broadspectrum antibiotics
- Psychological stress
- Oral contraceptive use
- If severe or persistent, consider AIDS
- Wearing of tight panties, especially nylon, which causes the vulva to remain too moist

Clinical features
- It causes severe itchiness and burning in the vulva and around the introitus.
- It may cause superficial and deep dysparunia.
- The typical vaginal discharge is thick, white and cottage cheese-like in consistency.
- The lesions on the vaginal wall look like splashes of white paint
    - if rubbed off, they leave a raw, bleeding area.

MANAGEMENT
- Find the cause and treat eg. diabetes.
- Give clotrimazole 500 mg pessary
    - insert high into the vagina as a single night-time dose.
- Imidazole cream eg. clotrimazole cream to apply to vulva 3 x daily.
- Apply a weak vinegar solution (2 tablespoons/30 ml of white vinegar in a litre of mildly warm water) 2 x daily by douche or washing
    - this helps to destroy the fungus by acidifying the vagina.

BACTERIAL VAGINOSIS

- This is strongly suggested if the patient complains that she noticed a discharge with a fishy odour after intercourse, or the fishy odour is detected on vaginal examination.
- Medical staff should be careful about sniffing vaginal discharges as this may lead to infection with organisms from the vagina.

- Metronidazole 2 g as a single oral dose.
- Avoid in the first trimester of pregnancy.

TRICHOMONAS VAGINITIS

Clinical features
- The main complaint is of a frothy or bubbly, yellow or green-coloured, watery, vaginal discharge.

DISEASES OF THE CERVIX

CERVICITIS

Clinical features
- A persistent vaginal discharge, usually white or grey
- Dull low backache
- On vaginal examination the cervix may be:
    - enlarged
    - irregular
    - eroded.
- Speculum examination is essential in making a proper diagnosis of cervicitis.
- Only the cervix has cells that make mucus. Any vaginal discharge with mucus means that part of the discharge is coming from the cervix.

NB. Any cervical lesion should be viewed as likely to be a carcinoma.

Differential diagnosis
Ectopy (ectropion) of the cervix
- This is the appearance of normal endo-cervical mucosa at the cervical os.
- It is a normal finding in the following conditions:
    - pregnancy
    - puberty
    - while taking the contraceptive pill

MANAGEMENT
- A PAP smear should be done, unless the patient has had one within the last 12 months.
- If a PAP is done when severe infection is present, it is difficult for the laboratory to diagnose. It is advisable to:
    - treat the infection first
    - bring the patient back for a PAP smear when the infection has cleared.
- Infections of the cervix are difficult to treat successfully by medical means mainly because of:
    - the mixed nature of infecting organisms present in the region
    - the nature of the cervical mucosa that creates crypts that store organisms
    - possible recurrent infection by the partner if not treated.

No treatment is required unless the patient is observed to have a yellow, mucoid (mucopurulent) discharge from the external os.

If there is a mucopurulent discharge and you suspect infection, treat as follows:
- Advise to abstain from sexual intercourse until treatment is completed.
- Bring contacts for treatment.
- Give ceftriaxone 250 mg IM stat
    - **plus** azithromycin 1 g as a single oral dose
    - **plus** metronidazole 2 g as a single oral dose.
- **REFER** if there is an inadequate response

CARCINOMA OF THE CERVIX

In South Africa this is one of the most common cancers in women. The important thing to remember is that it can be cured if detected at an early (pre-malignant) stage.

Risk factors
- Promiscuity (having many sexual partners)
- First coitus at a young age
- Pregnancy at an early age
- High parity
- Uncircumcised partners

Causes
- Certain subtypes of the human papilloma virus may cause carcinoma of the cervix.
- Herpes simplex type 2 may also contribute.

Clinical features
In the early stages there are no clinical features. In the later stage may there be:
- Dysparunia
- Post-coital bleeding
- Offensive vaginal discharge
- Cervical lesions visible on speculum examination:
    - as a growth
    - as an ulceration.
- There may be irregularity of the cervix on vaginal examination.

MANAGEMENT
- Encourage women to have regular PAP tests:
    - at the age of 30 and every 10 years after that
    - every year if she or her partner has had condylomata accuminata.
- If there is a suspicion of a cervical lesion, the patient should have a PAP smear.
- Follow the guidelines to further management given in the PAP report from the laboratory.
- If there is an obvious cervical tumour, **REFER.**

TRAUMA

RAPE

- Victims of alleged rape should be dealt with sympathetically and with dignity.
- Make sure the consultation is as private as possible, and that the patient is not exposed unnecessarily.
- Obtain as full a history as possible
    - the history taken by a nurse clinician may give more information than given to the doctors
    - this may especially be so with language or cultural differences.

History
A general history should include:
- Date and time of alleged offence
- Number of people who raped her
- Details of the alleged rapist
- Details of any physical violence or trauma to her
- If she scratched the man
- If the intercourse was vaginal, anal or oral, and whether a condom was used
- Whether she has changed clothes, washed or passed urine since the incident
- Other diseases that may be important eg. HIV

Take a full gynaecological history
- Age of menarche
- Number of pregnancies
- What contraception she is using
- Last menstrual period
- Date of last consenting intercourse and whether condoms were used

Examination
- Mental state
- Give detailed description of bruises, lacerations etc.
- In children if there is blood in the urine, it suggests there was recent damage to the genitals

Gynaecological
- This should be done only by the person doing the medico-legal report.
- The nurse clinician should take care not to interfere with the vagina in any way, unless emergency treatment is needed.

MANAGEMENT

REFER the following patients:
- To the medico-legal clinic:
  - any person who alleges he/she was raped
  - even if at present the patient does not want to make a case, the patient may change his/her mind later.
- To the hospital for immediate treatment if there is evidence of serious injury to a child or adult.

General measures
- If victim wants to open a case, the Family Violence, Child Protection an Sexual Offences Unit (FCS) must be summoned.
- It is the patient's choice to have immediate HIV testing
- If the patient declines, give a 3-day starter pack of PEP and encourage the patient to reconsider testing within those 3 days
- No further PEP will be given in the case of continued refusal of HIV testing

Medicine management
The patient should receive all the necessary medicines at the medico-legal clinic. However, if there is likely to be a delay or difficulty in getting to the medico-legal clinic, treatment should be started immediately.

Adults and adolescents over 14 years of age:
- Emergency contraception (if not on contraception and it is within 72 hours of the event):
  - levonorgestrel 1.5 mg as a single oral dose
- Antibiotics to prevent sexually transmitted infections:
  - ceftriaxone 250 mg IM as a single dose
  - **plus** azithromycin 1 g as a single oral dose
  - **plus** metronidazole 2 g as a single oral dose.
- PEP should not be given to a previously infected HIV person as it may lead to the development of viral resistance.

PEP treatment
- If the patient presents within 72 hours of the event, PEP should be offered:
  - fixed dose combination of tenofovir (TDF) 300 mg daily
  - **and** emtricitabine (FTC) 200 mg daily (Truvada)
  - **and** atazanavir/ritonavir (ATV/r) 300/100 mg daily for 28 days

- If tenofovir is contraindicated or if the source patient is known to be failing a tenofovir-based regimen, replace tenofovir and emtricitabine with:
  - fixed dose combination of zidovudine 300 mg 12 hourly
  - **and** lamivudine 150 mg 12 hourly (Lamzid)
  - for 28 days

Follow-up support
- Discuss issues relating to stress management at subsequent visits
- Refer where appropriate to:
  - Psychologist, social worker, local organisations that may be able to assist, e.g. POWA

CHILD ABUSE

SUSPECTED SEXUAL ABUSE

- This is a growing problem.
- The majority of cases are girls, but a small number of boys are sexually abused.
- All ages are affected.
- The abuser is often a man close to the family, often a member of the family.
- Abduction and rape by a stranger can also occur.

■ WHEN TO SUSPECT SEXUAL ABUSE

Common presentations
- History of rape
- Brought by a family member or teacher because of a suspicion of interference
- Vaginal discharge or bleeding
- Soreness of introitus / vagina
- Abnormal vaginal discharge
- Genital warts or ulcers

The child presents with another problem
- Urinary problems
  - unexplained haematuria
  - leucocytes in urine
  - a urinary tract infection
  - dysuria
- Abdominal pain (look for evidence of genital infection)
- Fever
- Evidence of psychological disturbance eg.
  - enuresis (bedwetting)
  - encopresis (inappropriate passing of faeces)
  - sexually advanced behaviour
- Any neglected child

History
- It is important to decide who is the best person to take the history eg. doctor, PHC sister, social worker.
- The more people involved, the more stressful it will be for the child and escort.
- Generally the child will give an honest history
  - this may be strongly denied by the escort if they are feeling defensive about the information.
- If the history is given spontaneously, get all the possible details:
  - ask who is responsible, when, where, how often (these details are important)
  - ask questions carefully and non-threateningly
  - do not push them further than they want to go as they are often frightened.
- The escort may also be concerned about the implications of this information for the family, so be sensitive to the escort's needs as well.
- Ask the escort and the child what is worrying them most at the moment
  - escorts are often worried about pregnancy, STIs, AIDS.
- Explore the social, psychological and medical history as needed.

Examination

- Get consent from the parent or escort to examine the child.
- This is a threatening examination so make contact with the child first and gain her/his confidence.
- If the child is old enough, explain:
  - what you are going to do
  - that you will be gentle.
- Ensure privacy during the examination.
- Identify who should be present during examination:
  - escort
  - nurse assistant if appropriate
- It is helpful not to undress the child completely
  - let the child keep his/her top on while examining genitalia.
- Put mother/escort at the head of the child to reassure her/him.
- The child may be examined in a number of positions:
  - left lateral
  - supine
  - on mother's lap, allowing legs to flop open.
- If necessary, let the child expose her own genitalia so that she feels she is able to control the examination
  - put gentle pressure on inner aspect of the labia and dilate the vagina. This helps you to see the hymen better.
  - it is sometimes useful to view the hymen when the child is in kneeling position with the buttocks pointing upward. Gravity pulls the other tissues of the vulva down and allows the hymen to be seen better.
- Check urine for blood or leucocytes. If there is blood in the urine it may be due to:
  - recent genital trauma
  - other trauma to the area
  - infection in the area
- Examine the genitalia and check the hymen for tears
  - it is often difficult to decide if there has been any damage to the hymen.
- Look for scars or damage to the fourchette or fossa navicularis.
- Look for thickening of the edge of the hymen.
- Do not forget to check the anus for sores, reflex dilatation, loss of tone that may be due to:
  - penetration
  - enema abuse
- Examine the rest of the child for evidence of trauma.
- Record details of physical examination on the clinic record card and make a duplicate (using carbon paper if available).

Differential diagnosis

- Children are often brought because a relative is worried about abuse.
- Careful history and examination may demonstrate that it is not abuse but a vulvo-vaginitis which is common before puberty.

Common causes

- Contact dermatitis due to applications to the genitalia
  - antiseptics such as Dettol are common causes.
- Irritation from panties especially nylon that may be made worse by the use of strong washing soaps or "Stay Soft".
- Self-exploration or masturbation
- Worms from the anus going into the vagina.

MANAGEMENT
General measures

- **REFER** any child if there is any suspicion of abuse for further medico-legal assessment to:
  - police child abuse unit (FCS)
  - local medico-legal services
- Cases must be opened in all cases of suspected or alleged rape/sexual abuse in children
- The patient and her family should be **REFERRED** to a social worker or psychologist by the medico-legal services for counselling.
- If badly injured, the child needs **REFERRAL** to hospital.

Legal requirements

NB. It is a legal requirement to notify child abuse, including sexual abuse, even if you only suspect it.

- Notify the most appropriate authorities eg. special police units for child abuse.
- To protect yourself keep a copy of the clinical notes and draw pictures of what you found, for later evidence.
- The case should be entered into the clinic child abuse register and the notification forms should be filled in if available.

Safety of the child

- If the child is in danger and cannot return home safely, he or she may need to admitted to hospital.
- The child must be seen by a doctor first.
- The social worker must be contacted so she can arrange a more permanent place of safety.
- In addition, a retention order may be needed if the relatives refuse.

Medicine management

- The patient should receive all the necessary medicines at the medico-legal clinic.
- However if there is likely to be a delay or difficulty in getting to the medico-legal clinic, treatment should be started immediately

Adolescents over 14 years:

- See management of adult victims of rape (page 193)

Children
- **REFER**
- Ceftriaxone IM 50 mg/kg/dose (max 250 mg) as a single dose

Plus
- Metronidazole as a single oral dose
  - 1-3 years: 500 mg (12.5 ml)
  - 3-7 years: 600-800 mg (15-20 ml)
  - 7-11 years: 1g (5 x 200 mg tabs)
  - 11-15 years: 1.6 g (4 x 400 mg tabs)

Plus
- Azithromycin as a singe oral dose
  - 1-3 years: 120 mg (3 ml syrup)
  - 3–5 years: 160mg (4 ml syrup)
  - 5-7 years: 200 mg (5 ml syrup)
  - 7-11 years: 250 mg
  - 11-15 years: 500 mg

HIV prophylaxis (PEP: Post-Exposure Prophylaxis)
- Obtain consent for HIV testing before initiating PEP.
- If the child presents within 72 hours of the event, and is HIV uninfected or HIV status is unknown, PEP should be offered
    - AZT, oral, 12 hourly for 28 days; maximum 300 mg/dose
    - 6-9 months   9 ml solution
    - 9 months-3 years   12 ml solution
    - 3-6 years   15 ml solution
    - 6-8 years   2 x 100 mg caps
    - > 8 years   1 x 300 mg cap

  AND
    - 3TC 4 mg / kg / dose oral 12 hourly for 28 days

  AND
    - lopinavir/ritonavir, oral, 12 hourly for 28 days
    - 6-12 months   1.5 ml solution
    - 1-3 years   2 ml solution
    - 3-6 years   2.5 ml
    - 6-8 years   2 x 100/25 tabs
    - 8-12 years   3 x 100/25 tabs
    - maximum 400/100 mg/dose

If you are sure it is just a pre-pubertal vulvo-vaginitis and not abuse:
- Clotrimazole cream to apply around the introitus
    - this may help prevent the parents from applying home solutions such as toothpaste and Zambuck etc.
- Application of a weak white vinegar solution (30 ml in a litre of water) 2 x daily by washing around the genitalia.
- **Plus** metronidazole as a single oral dose (see opposite)

OTHER FORMS OF CHILD ABUSE

- Manage in a similar manner as for sexual abuse.
- Treat injuries.
- Keep records as for sexual abuse.

UPPER GENITAL TRACT DISEASES

DISEASES OF THE UTERUS

FIBROIDS OF THE UTERUS

Clinical features
- Menorrhagia that may cause severe anaemia
  - this is often the presenting complaint.
- Pain due to:
  - degeneration of a fibroid
  - dysmennorrhoea
  - infection of the fibroid
  - prolapse of a fibroid causing severe colicky pains and a vaginal discharge
  - dysparunia
- Mass
  - in the abdomen
  - this may be palpable on vaginal examination.
- Pressure symptoms
  - urinary frequency due to an anterior fibroid
  - urinary retention secondary to upward displacement of the bladder and stretching of the urethra
  - rarely constipation
  - venous congestion and pedal oedema
  - sacral plexus pressure causing backache and neurological symptoms in the legs
- Infertility
  - due to tubal obstruction
  - deforming of the endometrium due to the masses protruding

Differential diagnosis
- Pregnancy (this may occur in a patient with a fibroid uterus)
- Full bladder
- Ovarian tumours
- Hydrosalpinx and other swelling of the fallopian tubes
- Red degeneration in a fibroid may present as an acute abdomen
  - consider all the causes of acute abdomen
- Carcinoma of the uterus

MANAGEMENT
If asymptomatic
- Reassure the patient and advise her that:
  - the fibroids will get smaller after menopause
  - they seldom become malignant.
- Supply her with iron and folic acid if there is associated menorrhagia, as many women are iron-deficient from their diet and previous pregnancies.
- She must come back if she starts getting symptoms.

If symptomatic
- Treat for infection, pain and anaemia.
- Advise her that the only therapy is surgery
  - hysterectomy is often the only safe treatment especially for large or multiple fibroids
  - if she wants to keep her uterus and only wants to have myomectomy, warn her that this may not guarantee fertility and that there are dangers with the operation.
- There is no point in referring her until she is prepared to consider surgery
  - encourage her to discuss this possibility with her relatives
  - then to return when she is prepared to have surgery.

ENDOMETRITIS

Causes
- Commonly postpartum, either after a full-term delivery or an abortion
- After the insertion of an intra-uterine contraceptive device (IUCD)
- Tuberculosis
- Septic (criminal) abortion

Clinical features
- Lower abdominal pain, general malaise, headache, and offensive, profuse vaginal discharge
- If severe, the patient may look ill and toxic, and have a high fever.
- There may be tenderness of the uterus on palpation.
- If there are retained products of conception:
  - the uterus may be sub-involuted (not fully contracted)
  - the cervical os may be open.

MANAGEMENT
If severe, postpartem, or if you suspect a criminal abortion:
- Put up a drip.
- **REFER** stat.
- Give ceftriaxone 1 g IVI stat.
  - **and** metronidazole 400 mg orally stat if there is likely to be any delay in admission.

SALPINGITIS / PELVIC INFLAMMATORY DISEASE (PID)

ACUTE SALPINGITIS

Clinical features
- Gradual onset of lower abdominal pain, usually sub-umbilically.
- It may be felt in the iliac fossa or generally over the whole lower abdomen.
- She will complain of fever, general malaise and headache.
- She usually has urinary symptoms.
- Vaginal discharge is also a common presenting symptom.

If severe
- The patient has difficulty walking and usually enters the consulting room bent over and holding her abdomen.
- The patient is ill.
- The temperature is high.
- Pulse rate is rapid and thready.
- Respiration tends to be shallow and panting.
- She is restless while on her back
    - these patients prefer to lie on their sides with thighs flexed on the abdomen
- There will be limitation of movement of the abdomen with distension, severe tenderness, guarding and rebound, especially in the lower abdomen.

PV examination
- If the patient is severely ill, vaginal examination will cause such severe pain that it is both pointless and cruel.
- In less severe illness, vaginal examination will show the features of inflammation of the pelvic peritoneum:
    - tenderness of the fornices
    - there may be fullness in the posterior fornix suggestive of a tubo-ovarian abscess
    - movement of the cervix will be tender (cervical motion tenderness)

Stage	Manifestations
Stage 1	Cervical motion tenderness and/or uterine tenderness and / or adnexal tenderness
Stage 2	As per Stage 1, plus pelvic peritonitis
Stage 3	As per Stage 2, plus tubo-ovarian abscess
Stage 4	Generalised peritonitis due to ruptured tubo-ovarian abscess

Differential diagnosis
- *The most important differential diagnosis is an ectopic pregnancy. Acute pelvic inflammatory disease without a fever should be assessed as an ectopic pregnancy until proved otherwise.*
- It may be difficult to be sure of the diagnosis, especially if it is a chronic, bleeding ectopic, which may have clinical features very similar to a mild salpingitis.

Features that suggest an ectopic pregnancy
- Sudden onset of pain at the beginning
- Previous ectopic pregnancy
- Pain radiating to the right shoulder
- History of fainting associated with the pain
- Pallor on examination
- Mild or no pyrexia
- Distended "doughy" abdomen, not quite as tender as in salpingitis
- Positive pregnancy test

MANAGEMENT
All patients with stages 2-4 must be hospitalised for parental antibiotic treatment.

Medicine management (Stage 1)
- Ceftriaxone 250 mg IMI stat
- **Plus** azithromycin 1 g orally stat
- **Plus** metronidazole 400 mg 2 x daily for 7 days
- Ibuprofen 400 mg 3 x daily for 2-3 days taken after meals
- Any patient with an IUCD must be considered for:
    - possible removal of the IUCD
    - a change of contraception.

Patient advice
- She must be advised to:
    - abstain from intercourse until her treatment is completed
    - tell her partner to come for treatment as well
    - consider using condoms for more protection.
- Warn the patient that this infection may:
    - make future pregnancies more difficult
    - increase the possibility of ectopic pregnancy.
- She should come back in 2-3 days if there is no adequate response

REFER if:
- Suspicion of an ectopic
- Any doubt about the diagnosis
- High temperature (above 39°)
- Ill patient
- Patient not taking adequate fluids orally
- Pallor
- Any symptoms or signs of pelvic peritonitis such as:
    - severe guarding
    - rebound tenderness on percussion
    - tenderness on palpation of the umbilicus
- There has been no adequate improvement after 48 hours or the patient's condition deteriorates on treatment.

Before REFERRAL:
- Put up a drip.
- Give analgesics eg. ibuprofen 400 mg orally stat.
- Give ceftriaxone 1 g IM stat.

Plus
- Metronidazole 400 mg orally stat.

CHRONIC SALPINGITIS

Clinical features
- Lower abdominal pain
- Vaginal discharge
- Urinary symptoms
- Congestive dysmenorrhoea
- Deep dysparunia
- Secondary infertility
- Menorrhagia may occur
- The only positive findings on abdominal examination are tenderness with slight guarding of the areas above the inguinal ligaments
- Rebound tenderness is not present
- The cervix is relatively immobile and there is mild tenderness in attempting to move it from side to side and up and down (cervical excitation tenderness - CET)

- The uterus may be found out of position
  - usually displaced to one or other side or retroverted and fixed
  - mobility may be limited
  - it may be bulky and tender on movement
- In some patients swellings in the adnexae may be felt.

Differential diagnosis
The most important diagnosis is a chronic ectopic pregnancy as mentioned above.

MANAGEMENT
- *If the pain is quite severe, it suggests she is having an acute attack as well as the chronic salpingitis*
  - give the medicines used for an acute attack.
- *Chronic salpingitis can be very resistant to treatment.*
- **REFER** if the patient is having 3 or more attacks of salpingitis in a year:
  - chronic salpingitis can cripple a woman's life with severe dysmenorrhoea and lower abdominal pain
  - surgery such as hysterectomy may be the only way to effectively relieve chronic pain and discomfort
  - physiotherapy may be helpful.

ADNEXAL SWELLING ON PV EXAMINATION

Causes
- It is seldom easy to be sure what is causing the mass.
- This may be due to masses in the fallopian tubes or ovaries.
- Carcinoma of the ovary is an important cause.

REFER if there is any doubt about the diagnosis as a carcinoma of the ovary must be excluded.

PELVIC ABSCESS

Clinical features
- There will be a history of a recent attack of salpingitis.
- On examination the patient will be ill with a fever and tenderness in the lower abdomen.
- The typical vaginal findings are a soft, extremely tender, fluctuant mass, felt in the Pouch of Douglas, through the posterior fornix.

MANAGEMENT
- **REFER** stat.
- If there is any delay give:
  - ceftriaxone 1 g IVI or IMI
  - analgesics as required.

ENDOMETRIOSIS

This is the presence and proliferation of endometrial tissue outside the uterine cavity, usually within the pelvis.

Clinical features
- Dysmenorrhoea
- Dysparunia
- Chronic pelvic pain
- Infertility

Diagnosis
Made by laparoscopy

MANAGEMENT
REFER:
- If you suspect it
- Women with chronic pelvic pain
- Women with endometriosis who wish to conceive

Symptom recurrence is common following cessation of treatment.

MISCARRIAGE (ABORTION)

DIAGNOSIS

A miscarriage should be suspected if the patient has the following:
- Vaginal bleeding with a history of amenorrhoea or symptoms / signs of pregnancy.
- **Or** if the woman herself suspects that she is pregnant and then has:
    - sudden onset of colicky lower abdominal pain, similar to labour pain
    - vaginal bleeding, especially if there are clots.
- The patient may have seen foetal parts
    - she may describe it as having passed "something like meat".
- The findings of a dilated cervix or products of conception are diagnostic of a miscarriage.

Differential diagnosis
- If the cervix is closed, other conditions must be considered eg.
    - a heavy menstrual period after a delayed or missed period. If she desperately wants a child, she may interpret this as a miscarriage to satisfy her need to be pregnant.
    - other causes of vaginal bleeding such as cervical carcinoma.

MANAGEMENT
Note: In any woman with PV bleeding, unless she is more than 20 weeks pregnant, it is important to do a **vaginal examination** to exclude a carcinoma of the cervix as the cause of the bleed.
- Put up a drip.
- **REFER.**

TYPES OF MISCARRIAGE

THREATENED MISCARRIAGE

Clinical features
- History of amenorrhoea or clinical evidence of pregnancy
- Usually no lower abdominal pain
    - if present, usually mild
- Vaginal bleeding (mild)
- Speculum examination will reveal blood coming through the cervical os
- Cervical os closed

MANAGEMENT
- The patient should be asked to rest in bed as much as possible.
- She should not have sexual intercourse until she is sure the bleeding has settled.
- If the pain and bleeding settle, she should continue with normal antenatal clinic attendance.
- She should be advised to come immediately if the bleeding or pain becomes more severe.

REFER patients for sonar at hospital to establish the diagnosis if the pain or bleeding is getting worse, even though the cervix is closed,.

INEVITABLE MISCARRIAGE

Clinical features
- Any dilatation of the cervix
- Any prolapse of foetal parts
- More severe pain
- Mild or moderate vaginal bleeding

- Give oxytocin 20 units IV in 1 litre normal saline and infuse at 125 ml / hour (2 ml / minute).
- **REFER.**

INCOMPLETE MISCARRIAGE

This is when some parts of the placenta are retained in the uterus. Most pregnancies that abort at less than 12 weeks gestation are incomplete. Many later miscarriages are also incomplete.

Clinical features
- Usually last menstrual period less than 12 weeks previously
- A history of having passed products of conception
- Heavy vaginal bleeding often with clots
- Bulky uterus < 12 weeks in size
- An open cervix
- Cramping pain persists

MANAGEMENT
- The only way to manage the problem is dilation and curettage (D&C) to remove the retained products.
    - this may be life saving as the vaginal bleeding can be severe and continuous.

Before REFERRAL:
- Remove any products of conception from the cervix.
- Give oxytocin 20 units IV in 1 litre Ringers lactate or normal saline and infused at 125 ml / hour.

COMPLETE MISCARRIAGE

This is when all the products of conception are passed. It occurs generally in a pregnancy of more than 12 weeks gestation.

Clinical features
- The full products of abortion may have been seen
    - by the patient
    - or by the clinician
- There will be minimal vaginal bleeding or it will have stopped.
- The cervix may be closed.
- The uterus will be well contracted.
- No more cramping pain will be felt.
- After 18 weeks gestation, the placenta can be checked for completeness.

> **MANAGEMENT**
> - Reassurance
> - Help the mother and father with grief process at the loss of the child.
> - **REFER** for confirmation
>   - if the woman is Rh negative for anti-D immunoglobulin to prevent Rh incompatibility in the next pregnancy
>   - see Maternity page 343
> - **REFER** if the patient is having recurrent miscarriages (after recovery from this one)
>   - she should report to the clinic for **REFERRAL** the next time she misses her second period.

LEGAL MISCARRIAGE

Women may now have terminations of pregnancy if they wish. It is illegal to attempt to prevent or obstruct a woman from having a termination of pregnancy.

Primary care clinician's role
- To confirm that the woman is definitely pregnant
- To estimate the duration of pregnancy
- To form good relationships so that women will report unwanted pregnancies before 12 weeks
    - this makes termination much easier
    - access to termination after 12 weeks is more limited
    - termination is more traumatic to the mother and child after 12 weeks.
- To help the woman clarify her reasons for the termination
    - often the initial decision to terminate is an emotional one, which may be a response to pressure from the father of the child or from other family members.
    - the more clearly the woman has worked through her emotions and come to terms with the decisions, the less likely she is to suffer from post-miscarriage complications such as depression.
- To warn her that it is a traumatic procedure and that there may be psychological effects later of guilt or depression
    - these may only surface 10 years or more after the episode.
- To advise her to grieve the loss of the child before and after the termination
    - it sometimes helps to name the unborn child.
- To look carefully at all the options available for dealing with the unwanted pregnancy such as:
    - keeping the child
    - adoption
- To help her to plan ways of preventing a repeated unwanted pregnancy
    - discuss ways of safe sex.
- To ask her who she thinks can help her
    - family
    - friends
    - religious organisation
    - clinic, social worker or psychologist
    - support groups or NGOs that specialise in helping women with unwanted pregnancies.
- To follow up the woman after the termination for any medical, psychological or spiritual complications.

> **MANAGEMENT**
> - If the gestation is less than 12 weeks, **REFER** to local health facilities with the necessary equipment and staff.
> - **REFER** to hospital if:
>   - the gestation is over 12 weeks
>   - less than 12 weeks but with complications of heart disease or previous Caesarean section.

UNSAFE (SEPTIC) MISCARRIAGE

Septic miscarriage still occurs mainly because of lack of access to legal abortion facilities.

Clinical features
- She may present with other unrelated symptoms eg. fever or headache.
- The woman may be very ill.
- On examination:
    - a high fever and rigors
    - tachypnoea and tachycardia
    - pallor
    - low blood pressure
    - abdomen usually shows tenderness and guarding
    - offensive vaginal discharge and products of conception may be present
    - there may be evidence of trauma to the cervix on speculum examination.
    - uterus is palpable abdominally (> 12 weeks in size)
- Delay in the diagnosis of this condition may result in:
    - severe complications
    - death of the patient.

> **MANAGEMENT**
> - Resuscitate the patient.
> - Put up a drip.
> - Ceftriaxone IV 1 g stat.
> **AND**
> - Metronidazole, 400 mg orally stat
> - Warn the patient that an operation may be necessary. If the patient is less than 18 years, get consent, if possible
>   - the patient or relatives should be advised that she may need a hysterectomy if the sepsis is severe
>   - this could save her life.

ECTOPIC PREGNANCY

ACUTE ECTOPIC PREGNANCY

Clinical features
- The history and findings are usually quite typical.
- The patient says that she has missed one or two periods and suspects pregnancy.
- Usually while busy with daily duties she develops a severe, sharp, stabbing type of pain
    - in one of the iliac fossae
    - severe enough in many cases to cause her to collapse and lose consciousness.
- On recovering from this, she finds that the pain is no longer present
    - she may have continued with what she was doing.
- Shortly after this she begins to feel dizzy and weak and may faint again.
- Pain felt in right shoulder tip, due to blood under the diaphragm, is strongly suggestive of an ectopic pregnancy.
- The clinical findings will vary according to the stage at which the patient is seen.
- The patient is often restless and anxious but may not complain of pain.
- Abdominal examination shows:
    - marked discomfort on moving the abdomen
    - moderate or mild lower abdominal distension
    - guarding is often not marked
    - the "feel" of the abdomen is quite typical - like "kneading bread dough"
    - rebound tenderness is quite violent and this test must be done gently eg. by gentle percussion or palpation of the umbilicus.
- On vaginal examination:
    - extreme tenderness is felt when the cervix is touched
    - PV bleeding that may be mild
- Urine pregnancy test is usually positive:

> **MANAGEMENT**
> - **REFER** stat.
> - Set up an IV drip using a large bore Jelco because she may need a lot of fluid quickly to maintain her blood pressure
>   - normal saline
>   - run the drip fast to maintain a systolic BP of 80-90 mm Hg, as the shock is often severe and is made worse by the trip to hospital (see shock page 271).

CHRONIC ECTOPIC PREGNANCY

Clinical features
- The patient will often say that she has missed one or two periods, or she thinks she is pregnant, but the pregnancy "does not feel normal".
- The patient often gives a history of repeated attacks of pain
    - sharp and stabbing in nature
    - in one of the iliac fossae.
- She eventually comes to the clinic because of a persistent dull, aching pain in the lower abdomen, which is not relieved by any medication.
- She may also have a reddish-brown, infrequent vaginal discharge.
- The signs and symptoms of pregnancy have lessened.
- The abdomen:
    - moves freely with respiration
    - is hard on palpation, due to voluntary guarding and some rigidity.
- Rebound tenderness is present.
- On PV:
    - cervical excitation tenderness is present
    - a mass may be palpated in an adnexal region, which is hard, irregular and tender.
- Urine pregnancy test is usually positive:

> **REFER** if you suspect it.

POST-PREGNANCY COMPLICATIONS

For routine postnatal care and other common postnatal problems, see the Puerperium in the Maternity section, page 351.

PUERPERAL SEPSIS

Puerperal sepsis is a dangerous, infective condition

Causes
The following conditions predispose to infection
- A dead foetus with membranes ruptured
- Prolonged rupture of membranes prior to delivery
- Instrumental delivery (forceps)
- Assisted delivery (internal version for transverse lie)
- Breech delivery
- Retained products
- Manual removal of the placenta, performed without due care to strict aseptic techniques
- Prolonged labour
- Too many PV examinations or unsterile techniques

Clinical features
- Fever
- Malaise
- Headache
- Painful lower abdomen
- Temperature is high, pulse rate fast, respiration fast and shallow
- Palpation of the abdomen reveals a soft tender mass which
    - arises out of the pelvis
    - is the large, tender, infected uterus
- Rebound tenderness, guarding, rigidity are frequently present
- A profuse, offensive, vaginal discharge - reddish brown in colour
- The history of a recent delivery plus the above findings are sufficient to make an assessment as to how to manage the patient
- It may be confused with a septic episiotomy, or the two conditions may occur together
- If you suspect retained products, do a vaginal examination to exclude an open cervix

MANAGEMENT
- If the condition is mild give:
    - co-amoxyclav 875 / 125 mg 2 x daily for 5 days
- Care of the newborn baby must also be taken into consideration in your decision about management
- **REFER** if:
    - there is any doubt about the care at home
    - the mother is ill
    - you suspect retained products
    - the cervix is open

PERINEAL LACERATIONS AND EPISIOTOMIES

A common problem is sepsis in a sutured episiotomy or a gaping perineal laceration.

Clinical features
- Septic wound
- Purulent discharge
- Localised tenderness
- No abdominal tenderness

MANAGEMENT

With mild sepsis
- The septic lacerations are swabbed
- All visible suture material is removed from the wound if possible
- Give chlorhexidine in water, Savlon or Betadine to make a swabbing solution
    - do not use chlorhexidine in alcohol as it burns
- Advise how and when to swab the area
- It is necessary to keep the wound as clean and dry as possible

More severe sepsis
- If the patient has systemic signs or symptoms eg. fever, tachycardia, treat as above
- Give co-amoxyclav 875 / 125 mg 2 x daily for 5 days
- Generally these wounds heal well because of the good blood supply in the area

Third-degree tears
- These usually have the elements of a second degree tear plus laceration of the rectal sphincter and / or the rectal mucosa
- It is however possible for the rectal sphincter to be torn with minimal damage to the perineum
- It is essential that these tears be repaired as soon as possible after the placenta is delivered
- If there is undue delay before such a repair is undertaken, the chances of a breakdown of the wound increase proportionally with each hour of the delay ie.
    - the longer the delay the greater the chance of wound sepsis and breakdown
    - and the greater the chance of formation of a recto-vaginal fistula

Indications for REFERRAL or secondary suture are
- Wounds not responding to treatment
- Very large wounds needing secondary suturing, when the sepsis has completely cleared at 6 weeks

BREAST CONDITIONS

CRACKED NIPPLES

- In normal sucking, the baby takes the whole nipple into its mouth and bites on the areola behind the nipple as this is where the milk is pooled
- Moderate pressure here results in an efficient release of milk
- However, the baby cannot get access to the areola area if:
    - the breasts are over distended
    - the nipples are retracted
- The baby instead applies pressure on the nipples
- This results in a vicious cycle of
    - an increasing distension of the breast because the milk is not being drained
    - an increasingly hungry and frustrated baby who traumatises the nipple further
    - an increasingly distressed and desperate mother
    - cracked nipples and subsequent spread of infection into the breast, full of retained milk
    - breast abscesses
- A natural response to cracked nipples, is for the mother to take the baby off the breast and to bottle feed
- *This is a serious step to take, because breast milk is vital for the health of the baby*
- *Disease and death may be the end result, particularly in areas where people are poor*

Causes
Common errors causing over-distension of the breast are:

- Supplementing with powdered milk or water, due to fear that the breast milk is inadequate
- Schedule feeding eg. only feeding every 2 hours, or every 4 hours
    - demand feeding is the best method.
- Not breast feeding adequately at night eg. due to the baby being separated from the mother
- Mother starting work and being forced to use another method of feeding
- Bottle feeding and dummies which decrease the emptying of the breast

Clinical features
- The mother complains of severe pain in the nipple
- This may be associated with cracks and bleeding

MANAGEMENT
Breast feeding advice
Advise the patient about good breast feeding practices.

- Demand feeding
- Have the baby at the bedside or sleep with the baby
- Do not supplement with water, other milks or foods
    - for the first 4 months
    - and ideally for the first 6 months if the baby's growth is adequate
    - this has the added benefit of lessening the development of allergy in the baby
- Avoid introducing a bottle as
    - this decreases the amount of time the baby spends sucking the breast
    - the baby begins to prefer the bottle as it is easier to suck

- Keep the breasts soft
    - the best breast pump is the baby
    - if the baby is not able to do this, then the mother should express constantly, until the breasts are soft

Mechanism of breast feeding
- Explain the mechanism to the mother so that she will understand how to do it properly
- During a feed the breast supplies 3 types of milk rather like a 3 course meal
    - the first milk is high in fluid and low in protein and nutrition (the soup course)
    - the middle milk is high in protein and nutrition (the main course)
    - the end milk is high in sugar which satisfies the baby and he stops feeding (the dessert)
- Giving each breast for only a short time during each feed may result in malnutrition, as the baby only receives the first milk (the soup course) from each breast all the time
- Adequate emptying of one breast makes sure the baby gets all 3 types of milk
- The breast which is not being used may become engorged
    - this soon settles spontaneously
    - no treatment is needed apart from reassurance

Inverted and cracked nipples
- When inverted nipples are present, nipple shields can be provided
- If the pain is so severe that the mother cannot breast feed, advise and encourage her to
    - express the breasts
    - feed the expressed breast milk (EBM) to the baby by means of a cup and spoon, and *not* a bottle. Bottles, even though well sterilised, may result in chest, ear and gastrointestinal infections
- A barrier ointment will help healing, eg. Zinc and Castor oil

Working mothers
- Working mothers should be encouraged to
    - express the breasts before going to work
    - leave the EBM to be given by cup and spoon while she is away
- It will help if she can
    - take the child to work with her
    - or possibly come home to feed during tea or lunch times
- She should breast feed as much as possible when she is at home, especially at night

Note.
- There is no current evidence that preparation of the nipple during pregnancy with spirits etc. has *any* positive effect of "toughening up" the nipple
- Often it results in damaging the nipple and making it more vulnerable to infection
- All that should be done during pregnancy is
    - normal hygiene
    - washing with water and a bland soap

ENGORGED BREASTS

Causes
- Poor feeding practices as above
- A still-birth or a very sick child who cannot suck
- Production of a large amount of milk

Clinical features
- Breasts are engorged during the first 2-3 days after birth (which is normal)
- Dilated and enlarged veins are seen on the surface of the breasts
- Congested overlying skin
- On palpation they are very tense, hard and knotty, and extremely painful
- **Tail of Spence** (under the arm) can become engorged

MANAGEMENT
Advice and reassurance
- The best machine to empty the breasts and keep them soft is the baby!
- Alternatively use manual expression or a breast pump to keep the breasts soft
- Encourage frequent feeding
- Advise on how to feed the baby
- Advise the mother to wear a good supporting brassiere
- If the cause is inverted or small nipples, supply a nipple shield
- Use of warm water applied to the breasts helps to express the milk and ease the pain, eg. using a hot towel or warm water in a bath
- For tail of Spence use a rolled-up towel under the arm while feeding
- To reduce the amount of milk production until the feeding pattern is established, reduce fluid intake while engorgement is present
- The pain is helped by giving paracetamol 2 tabs 3 x daily for 3 days

After a neonatal death
- When a neonatal death or a fresh still-birth occurs, it is necessary to avoid breast engorgement if possible, before it becomes a problem by
    - fluid restriction
    - breast binders
    - diuretics are effective in most instances
    - analgesics
    - high doses of pyridoxine and Vitamin B Co may also assist in suppressing lactation

MASTITIS

Generally this occurs in women who are breast feeding.

Causes
- If mastitis occurs in non-breast feeding women, carcinoma of the breast *must* be excluded as a cause
- Other causes include
    - trauma
    - blood-spread infections

Clinical features
- The patient has a temperature which is often high
- She complains of malaise and looks ill
- The infection ascends from the nipple
- The affected breast may show a reddened area over the site of the infection which is hot and tender to touch
- There may be a purulent discharge from the nipple

Differential diagnosis
- It is often difficult to decide whether this is only a mastitis, or whether there is an abscess
- Breast abscesses are difficult to diagnose because fluctuation may occur late or not at all
- Generally our patients present late and therefore are more likely to have an abscess than a mastitis
- For features of an abscess see below

MANAGEMENT
- Give flucloxacillin 500 mg 4 x daily for 5-10 days
    - **or** azithromycin 500 mg daily for 3 days if penicillin-allergic
- Analgesics - paracetamol 2 tabs 3 x daily as required
- Encourage the patient to continue with breast feeding, but if she cannot do so
    - take the baby off the breast and show her how to express all the milk to avoid stagnation in the ducts
    - she should feed this milk to the baby by cup and spoon
    - try and avoid bottle feeding if at all possible
- If there is any doubt, it is better to assume that it is an abscess
    - it may help to confirm the diagnosis by trying to aspirate the area of maximum tenderness with a syringe and large needle
    - if this yields pus, the patient should be **REFERRED**
- The patient should come back in 24-48 hours if not improved.

BREAST ABSCESS

Causes
- A breast abscess results from failure of treatment of acute mastitis because
    - the patient has received insufficient therapy
    - treatment was begun too late
- The generalised infection becomes localised as a result of the body defences
    - it then becomes encapsulated to form an abscess

Clinical features
- Severe pain, for at least 2 days duration
- Throbbing pain, severe enough to affect sleep
- Localised tenderness
- There may be pus coming out of the nipple
- The patient looks ill, has a high temperature and a rapid pulse
- On examining the affected breast a red, localised area is seen which can be situated anywhere in the breast
- On palpation this area is relatively fixed and tender
- Fluctuation is *not* a feature until very late in the disease
- The axillary glands may be tender and enlarged, if the outer quadrants are involved

MANAGEMENT
- Advise about breast feeding methods to prevent mastitis and breast abscesses
- **REFER** for incision and drainage, if there is any suspicion of an abscess

BREAST LUMPS IN PREGNANCY

Causes
- This is usually a galactocoele which is due to trapped milk in a duct
- Fibroadenoma, also called a lactating adenoma
- Engorged tail of Spence in lactation (see opposite)

REFER all breast lumps.

BLOOD-STAINED NIPPLE DISCHARGE (DURING PREGNANCY OR POST PARTUM)

MANAGEMENT
- This may not need treatment
- The baby may suckle the breast without any harm
- **REFERRAL** is only necessary if the blood-stained discharge
    - persists for >72 hours
    - appears when the mother is not breast feeding
    - is only coming from one duct
    - there is an associated palpable breast lump

CONTRACEPTION

METHODS OF CONTRACEPTION

Sometimes during a routine consultation, you will become aware that the patient has a problem with contraception, even though it may not have been the patient's presenting problem. This can provide a very valuable opportunity for assisting the patient.

A common example is seeing a teenager who is sexually active, but has not yet considered contraception or the effects of her sexual practices.

Factors you should take into consideration when advising a patient on contraceptive practice are that

- There is an increasing incidence of potentially life-threatening, viral, sexually transmitted infections eg.
    - Hepatitis B
    - Papilloma virus
    - the AIDS virus (HIV)
- Correct contraceptive methods may be a significant factor in improving the patient's relationship with her partner as it may remove fears and anxieties about
    - pregnancy
    - infections

INTRA-UTERINE CONTRACEPTIVE DEVICES (IUCDs)

- The IUCD is a highly effective safe long-term contraceptive method.
- It is not contra-indicated in HIV infection and may be the most suitable contraceptive for women on ART.

Advantages
- Provides long-term protection i.e. 5 years
- Fertility returns on removal of IUCD
- Women in whom adherence is likely to be a problem, e.g. mental retardation.
- Women taking medicine that can interfere with hormonal contraception, e.g. anticonvulsants.
- Women with medical contraindications to pregnancy, e.g. kidney or heart disease.

Disadvantages
- Some discomfort or cramping following insertion of IUCD

Contraindications
- Menorrhagia or unexplained uterine bleeding
- A bleeding tendency or in patients using anticoagulants
- Valvular heart disease
- Active pelvic inflammatory disease
- Purulent cervicitis
- Previous history of ectopic pregnancy
- Small uterus (less than 5 cm)
- Distorted uterine cavity as a result of
    - fibroids
    - a congenital abnormality
- Fixed retroversion of the uterus
- Cervical stenosis
- Carcinoma of the cervix / uterus
- Repeated expulsions

▼ **Note to clinic doctor**
Missing IUCD
- A routine abdominal X-ray only shows whether the IUCD is in the pelvis or not. It does not show whether it is definitely in the uterus or not
- The best way to locate a missing IUCD is to insert a sterile probe into the uterus first and then X-ray ▲

CONDOMS

- Condoms are effective as barrier contraceptives and in preventing transmission of sexually transmitted infections, if used correctly
- Failures do occur as a result of the condom breaking or coming off too soon

---

MANAGEMENT
- Patients must be warned that they are not absolutely safe
    - in preventing STIs
    - as contraception
- Patients who choose to use this method must be given careful instruction as to how
    - to apply the condom correctly
    - to hold the base of the condom on withdrawal to prevent any spilling of semen after intercourse

---

SUBDERMAL IMPLANTS

- The subdermal implant is a very effective long-term contraceptive method.

Advantages
- It provides long-term protection, i.e. 3-5 years.
- Fertility returns on removal of the implant.
- Can be used in women >35 years who:
    - are obese
    - smoke
    - have diabetes or hypertension
    - a history of venous thromboembolism

Disadvantages
- Frequent bleeding irregularities
- Implant must be inserted or removed by a trained healthcare professional
- Insertion of the implant may result in local pain and bruising

Contraindications
- Patients who have active liver disease
- Unexplained uterine bleeding
- Patients on long-term medicines that induce the metabolism of progestins including efavirenz, rifampicin, phenytoin, carbamazepine and phenobarbital

MANAGEMENT
- For pain after insertion:
  - ibuprofen 400 mg 3 x daily for 5 days
- **REFER** if:
  - heavy or prolonged bleeding despite treatment with combined oral contraceptive
  - infection at insertion site inadequately responding to initial antibiotic treatment.
  - failure to locate an implant (in the arm) by palpation

INJECTABLE CONTRACEPTIVES

- Injectable contraceptives are private and effective with a very low failure rate.
- They do not protect the patient against infections.

Advantages
- Once injected, the patient is protected for
  - 12 weeks with medroxyprogesterone acetate (Depo-provera)
  - 8 weeks with norethisterone enanthate (Nur-Isterate)
- The action does not depend on patient adherence.
- They can be used post-partum
- Can be used in women >35 years who:
  - are obese
  - smoke
  - have diabetes or hypertension
  - a history of venous thromboembolism
- Interactions with other medicines do not lower contraceptive effect.

Disadvantages
- A delay in return of fertility of up to 1-2 years (average 6-9 months) after the last injection
  - patients should be advised about this
- Possible prolonged amenorrhoea
- Possible heavy or prolonged menstrual bleeding
- Weight gain in some women

Indications
- They may be used in women in whom oestrogen-containing contraceptives are contra-indicated
- They can be used for post-partum contraception and during lactation but should not be used within 48 hours of childbirth

Contraindications
Absolute contraindications
- Patients who have liver dysfunction
- Unexplained uterine bleeding
- Malignancy of the breast or genital tract

Relative contraindications
- Any woman planning pregnancy within a year
- Previous depression

Heavy or prolonged bleeding
- Women should be advised to report if they bleed for more than 10 days

▼ **Note to doctor**
- Give combined oral contraception for 21 days (omit inactive pills)
- If unacceptable bleeding recurs, treatment may be repeated for 2 or 3 cycles
- **REFER** if:
  - heavy bleeding despite treatment with combined oral contraceptive ▲

COMBINED ORAL CONTRACEPTIVES (COC)

- Recommended for highly motivated women where reliable adherence is more likely.
- Does not prevent sexually transmitted infections including HIV.

Advantages
Patients with any of the following may benefit from the use of OCs:
- Dysmenorrhoea
- Menorrhagia and dysfunctional uterine bleeding
- Premenstrual tension syndrome
- Fertility returns 1–3 months on discontinuing the COC
- Endometriosis
- Benign breast conditions
- Polycystic ovary syndrome
- Long-term protection against ovarian, endometrial carcinoma
- Improves bone mineral density

Disadvantages
- Interactions with other medicines can lower contraceptive effect
- Avoid in women over 35 years of age who smoke >15 cigarettes/day or have risk factors for cardiovascular disease

Contraindications
- Unexplained vaginal bleeding
- Less than 4 weeks after delivery
- Hypertension
- Myocardial infarction
- Angina pectoris
- A history of thrombo-embolism, arterial or venous
- Stroke
- Heart valve lesions
- Uncontrolled diabetes
- Active or recent liver disease
- Gall stones
- Migraine sufferers
- Malignant melanoma
- Psychosis
- Breast carcinoma
- Carcinoma of the cervix or uterus
- Psychosis or severe depression
- Systemic lupus erythematosus
- Kidney disease
- Porphyria
- Prolonged confinement to bed
- Proposed major surgical operation
- Leg immobilisation after a fracture

Breast feeding
- Delay initiation of contraception until 6 months post-partum

Medicines decreasing the action of oral contraception
These are mainly liver enzyme-inducing agents
- Anti-epileptic medicines
    - phenytoin (Epanutin)
    - phenobarbitone
    - carbamazepine (Tegretol)
- Antituberculous
    - rifampicin
- Antiretrovirals
    - efavirenz
    - lopinavir / ritonavir
    - nevirapine

Antibiotics
- Possible lowering of contraceptive effect and a condom should be used for the duration of that menstrual cycle as well.

Laxatives
- Very loose stools may cause malabsorption of oral contraceptives.

Medicines affected by oral contraception
- Oral contraceptives may lower the effect of some medicines, e.g. lamotrigine, by their effect of increasing the action of liver enzymes which metabolise medicines.
- Asthmatic women on oral contraceptives may need to have their theophylline dose reduced to avoid toxicity.

TYPES OF ORAL CONTRACEPTIVES

■ COMBINED CONTRACEPTIVES

These contain a synthetic oestrogen and progestogen

Monophasic preparations

Nordette
Content
- 21 tablets 30 mcg ethinyloestradiol (EE)
- 150 mcg levonorgestrel (LG)
- 7 tablets placebo - this is a low dose for general use

Ovral
Content
- 21 tablets 50 mcg ethinyloestradiol
- 500 mcg norgestrel
- 7 tablets placebo - this is a high dose of hormones

Indications
- For post-coital contraception
- Up to 72 hours after rape

Triphasic preparations
These copy the physiological cycle more closely

Triphasil
Content
- 6 tabs 30 mcg ethinyloestradiol (EE) and 50 mcg levonorgestrel (LG)
- 5 tabs 40 mcg EE and 75 mcg LG
- 10 tabs with 30 mcg EE and 125 mcg LG
- 7 tablets placebo

■ PROGESTOGEN ONLY PILLS

Microval
Content
- 30 mcg levonorgestrel

Advantages
- Fertility returns immediately on discontinuing the tablet
- Can be used post-partum

Disadvantages
- Less reliable than combined oral contraceptive
- Frequent bleeding irregularities
- Should be taken at the same time every day - if taken more than 3 hours late and unprotected intercourse has occurred in the past 5 days
    - give emergency contraception
- Interactions with other medicines can lessen contraceptive effect

Indications
- Can be used post partum
- Can be used in women >35 years who:
    - are obese
    - smoke
    - have diabetes or hypertension
    - a history of venous thromboembolism

Contraindications
- Abnormal uterine bleeding
- Myocardial infarction or stroke
- Liver disease
- Cancer of the breast or genital tract

STERILISATION

- This is a free service if organised through family planning clinics
- The use of sterilisation should be considered in those cases where a patient must under no circumstances become pregnant eg.
    - medical conditions which will be made much worse by pregnancy and may even result in the death of the patient during pregnancy eg. severe heart disease
    - very high chance of a severe genetic disorder or a history of previous seriously abnormal children
    - serious mental disease
    - seriously retarded patients
- In women over the age of 35 there is
    - an increasing tendency not to use oral contraceptives
    - a world wide increase in the use of sterilisation for couples in this age group, (particularly when their families are complete)
- Even if the couple are young, sterilisation may be the method of choice, and they should be allowed to consider this method if it is suitable.

MANAGEMENT

Sterilisation of the male (vasectomy)
- This is a simple, safe out-patient procedure with few complications or side effects
- It should be encouraged whenever possible instead of sterilisation of the female
- The man must be warned that he will still be fertile for 3 months after the operation and should take precautions during this time
- He must be reassured that it has no effect on potency

- It may actually improve the sexual relationship with his partner as there will be freedom from fear of conception
- Neither sterilisation nor circumcision prevent sexually transmitted infections

Sterilisation of the female (tubal ligation)
- When sterilisation is considered by the couple, it must be made quite clear to them that it is usually irreversible in the female partner (when properly performed)
- This is more dangerous than sterilisation of the male
- Sterilisation is extremely difficult in a woman who is very obese. Alternative methods may be safer
  - sterilisation of her male partner
  - Depo-provera

Legal requirements
- Because sterilisation is considered by law to be a mutilating operation performed on healthy tissue, care must be taken to comply with all legal requirements
- Any woman who is mentally normal, may sign consent for sterilisation herself, without needing her husband's signature
- Mentally subnormal women need to be certified as such by a specialist psychiatrist, and a certificate obtained from the Minister of Health
  - **REFER** to a hospital where these facilities are available

SPECIAL SITUATIONS

POST-COITAL CONTRACEPTION

MANAGEMENT
To prevent conception after unprotected intercourse eg. rape or where there has been a problem with contraception

- Give levonorgestrel 1.5 mg as a single oral dose, no later than 5 days after intercourse
  - this should be used in emergencies only. Repeat the dose if the woman vomits within 2 hours
- **Or** insert an IUD within 5 days.

SPOTTING (BREAKTHROUGH BLEEDS)

This suggests that there is an incorrect dosage of either the oestrogen or the progesterone component of the contraceptive.

The patient needs more oestrogen if:
- The breakthrough bleeding occurs in the first half of the cycle
- The woman complains of
  - vaginal dryness
  - decreased libido

The patient needs more progesterone if:
- The break-through bleeding occurs in the second half of the cycle
- The woman may complain of:
  - acne-like skin problems
  - premenstrual tension syndrome

- Allow a 3-month trial on the pill
- If the bleeding persists, **REFER**

WHEN TO USE AN ADDITIONAL CONTRACEPTIVE METHOD

Use an additional contraception method if:
- The woman has had to take a course of antibiotics while on contraceptives
- There has been spotting or break-through bleeding
- There has been diarrhoea or vomiting

- An additional method of contraception should be added for at least 2 weeks, or until the next menstrual period
- Advise to use condoms during this period

CONTRACEPTION IN HYPERTENSION

MANAGEMENT
- The preferred hormonal contraceptive for hypertensive patients is injectable progestogen-only contraceptive or the IUD
- Barrier methods

CONTRACEPTION IN DIABETES

MANAGEMENT
- Combined oral contraceptive pills should be used with caution due to lipid side effects.
- The preferred hormonal contraceptive for diabetics is the IUD or injectable progestogen-only contraceptive

CONTRACEPTION FOR EPILEPTICS

MANAGEMENT
- Anti-epileptic medicine such as phenytoin, phenobarb and carbamazepine are enzyme-inducing and interfere with hormonal contraceptives
  - the preferred contraceptive is the IUD
- If she has completed her family, discuss the possibility of sterilisation for her husband or herself
- If she is mentally subnormal and her family do not want her to get pregnant, **REFER** to arrange sterilisation under the Act
  - see opposite Sterilisation management and legal requirements

NERVOUS SYSTEM

EPILEPSY

ASSESSMENT OF SEIZURES

*Epilepsy is a disorder of the brain, which shows itself by **repeated unprovoked seizures** (fits).*

- Epilepsy cannot be diagnosed on **one** fit alone.
- A seizure (fit) is the result of an abnormal sudden discharge of cerebral neurones, rather like an electrical short circuit.
- This "short circuit" may affect:
    - only a part of the brain (partial seizure)
    - parts of the brain in progressive stages (Jacksonian epilepsy)
    - all of the brain simultaneously (generalised seizure)
- For a full assessment of a patient with seizures, you need
    - a careful history
    - a physical examination
    - relevant investigations

STEP 1 - DECIDE IF THE PATIENT IS HAVING TRUE SEIZURES

If an eye witness to the event is present at the interview, try to obtain an accurate picture of what occurred. If possible ask the witness to demonstrate the episode.

Features suggesting a true seizure:
- Jerking movements or stiffness. Ask whether this involved the whole body or part/s of the body
- Deviation of the eyes
- Tongue biting or incontinence
- Post ictal (post-fit) confusion, drowsiness or complaints about a headache
- Abnormal behaviour before, during or after the fit.

If there were none of these, it would more likely suggest a syncopal attack.

■ SYNCOPE (FAINTING) WHICH MAY BE CONFUSED WITH SEIZURES

Clinical features
- The loss of consciousness in syncope is produced by inadequate blood circulation to the brain.
- Syncope may occur in response to
    - strong emotional stimuli eg. the sight of blood
    - standing for long periods
    - standing up after sitting
    - after an episode of gastroenteritis
    - after severe physical exercise eg. long distance running
- Syncope usually starts gradually with a feeling of faintness, greying out of vision, nausea, sweating, pallor, followed by falling and unconsciousness
    - the body is limp (flaccid)
    - there is no rigidity (increased tone) in the muscles
    - there is no twitching

Some important causes of syncope
Cardiac arrhythmias and disease
- There will often be a history of:
    - previous heart disease or symptoms of heart disease
    - use of beta-blocker drugs.
- There may also be a history of palpitations.
- There may be clinical signs such as abnormal blood pressure, irregular pulse, murmurs and bradycardia.

Transient ischaemic attacks (TIAs)
- These are due to some interruption in the blood flow to a part of the brain and may be due to:
    - emboli
    - atheroma
- They produce transient, localised, neurological signs and symptoms eg.
    - blurring of vision in one eye
    - weakness and numbness of part of the face or of a limb
- There is often **no** loss of consciousness.
- The attacks last for a short time and then the symptoms and signs disappear in less than 24 hrs.
- If the ischaemia is severe, it may go on to become a stroke, with permanent damage to that part of the brain affected.

Hypoglycaemia
- This is common in alcoholics especially after a bout of heavy drinking.
- **Note.** Hypoglycemia may present as a true seizure also.

Simulated attacks (hysteria)
- These "attacks" often occur before an audience but it may be difficult to tell the difference between true epilepsy and hysteria.
- Be cautious of making the diagnosis of hysteria, unless you can be fairly certain there is no genuine disease causing the attacks (see page 225).

STEP 2 - CLASSIFY THE TYPE OF SEIZURE

The clinical description of the seizure will affect decisions about the patient's treatment and his working situation.

- The description from a witness is important.
- Patients with epilepsy, who have an aura or warning, may be able to prepare for the fit, eg.
    - if walking down stairs, they will be able to sit down
    - if they are driving, or using dangerous machinery, they will be able to stop
    - if they are in a street, they could ask a passerby to stay with them during the fit
- Patients with generalised epilepsy, without warning symptoms, are at a disadvantage, because they cannot take precautions
    - the fit comes totally unexpectedly.
- Primary generalised fits are usually not associated with any treatable cause, and investigations are usually negative.
- Partial fits have an 80% chance of being associated with some definite disease eg. tumour or cyst
    - therefore patients with partial epilepsy should **always** be investigated.

■ PARTIAL SEIZURES

- These are seizures which may or may not go on to become generalised.
- The usual cause of this type of fit is some localised disease or damage (focus) in the brain.
- It is associated with some warning sign, as the damaged portion discharges first, before spreading to other parts of the brain.

Note. There may or may not be loss or change of consciousness in partial seizures.

Simple partial seizures
Cause motor, sensory, autonomic or psychic symptoms without altered consciousness
- Motor eg. limb-jerking on one side of the body
- Sensory eg. numbness in an arm
- Autonomic eg. unpleasant smell or taste
- Psychic eg. sense of fear, auditory or visual hallucinations

Complex-partial seizures (temporal lobe epilepsy)
- As above but is followed by a period of impairment of consciousness (they do not fall)
- During the seizure automatism may occur
    - uttering noises and words, chewing and lip smacking, walking aimlessly
- When the seizure ends the individual is amnesic for events which took place during the seizure.

Epilepsy partialis continuans
- This is a partial seizure where a part of the body may have jerking movements continuously but the patient is fully conscious.

Jacksonian epilepsy
- This is a partial seizure which arises in the motor cortex of the brain.
- Jerking starts in a part of a limb, then spreads up the limb and may then progress to involve one whole side of the body
    - but it does not cause loss of consciousness or become generalised.

Todd's paralysis
- Following a seizure patients may experience a localised paresis for up to 24 hours, and then it clears.

Partial seizures which become generalised seizures
- These are generalised (grand mal) seizures that are preceded by any kind of aura.
- Examples of auras:
    - unpleasant smell - temporal lobe focus
    - visual disturbance - occipital lobe focus
- On investigation with electro-encephalogram (EEG), a focus or starting point can be found.

■ GENERALISED SEIZURES

Primary generalised seizures
- These are seizures where there is no warning beforehand ie.
    - no focal signs
    - or the aura is very short
- There is loss of consciousness at the onset.
- Some of these seizure types are hereditary, which suggests a biochemical mechanism.

Absence seizures (petit mal)
- Occur mainly in children.
- Start with sudden arrest of speech and movement.
- Patients stare unresponsively ahead.
- There may be eye blinking, lip smacking and fidgetting.
- Duration is 4-6 seconds with no post-ictal confusion.
- Attacks may occur daily.

Febrile convulsions
- This is a form of generalised seizure accompanied in susceptible children by a high fever.
- It occurs in the 6-month to 5-year-old-age group.
- The seizure occurs during the rising phase of the temperature curve (ie. during the first day).

MANAGEMENT OF FEBRILE CONVULSIONS
- **REFER** if it is the first episode or if you cannot exclude a possible meningitis.
- Antipyretic agents should only be considered in children with fever who appear distressed, for symptomatic relief
    - they do not prevent febrile convulsions
- It is necessary to treat the cause of the fever (e.g. meningitis, systemic infections)
- Tepid sponging is not recommended for the treatment of fever
    - children with fever should not be undressed or over-wrapped

---

STEP 3 - DETERMINE THE PRECIPITATING FACTORS OF THE SEIZURE

The following factors are not themselves the cause of the fits, but will precipitate a fit in someone who is vulnerable to them, ie. someone who is already an epileptic.

- It is important to discuss these factors with the patient.
- Examples of precipitating factors are
    - stress of any kind, physical or mental
    - lack of sleep
    - alcohol
    - hypoglycaemia
    - pyrexia
    - TV / strobe light
    - computers

MANAGEMENT OF EPILEPSY

NB. Exclude hypoglycaemia.

Management of a generalised seizure
- Turn the patient on his side
- Loosen tight clothing or collars
- Remove any dangerous objects near the patient
- Do not put anything between the teeth or try to press on the tongue
- Put something under the patient's head
- Watch the patient so as to be able to record the type and duration of the seizure
- **REFER** unless the patient is a known epileptic

GENERAL MANAGEMENT
Discuss the following with the epileptic patient:
- The diagnosis of epilepsy
- The possible cause of the epilepsy
- The possible precipitating factors
- The complications of epilepsy
- The medicines and their side effects, and how to deal with these side effects
- The necessity for good adherence
- The aims of treatment, and the limitations of treatment, ie. that it:
    - ***cannot cure*** epilepsy
    - can only control the fits and then only if the treatment is taken correctly
- The effects of the seizures and of the treatment on the person's lifestyle, social situation, and on the family.
- The fact that if the tablets are stopped suddenly, worse fits may occur.

- The best lifestyle to adopt in order to prevent further seizures, and to be able to enjoy as normal a life as possible.

Seizure diary
- Patients should keep a diary of the number of fits they have had.
- They should also record what happened before the fit, so as to try and assess what possible precipitating factors there may have been.
- The aims of the diary are to:
  - involve the patients in their own care
  - try to discover any preventable precipitating factors
  - assess the degree of control of the fits
  - detect any side effects of the drugs.
- It is essential to ask the patient about his seizure diary if you have asked him to keep one
  - the information can be of great value
  - it will show the patient that you are genuinely interested in his condition and that it is worth his effort in keeping the diary.

Medicine interaction vigilance
- Other medicines may affect the blood level of anti-epileptic drugs, and vice-versa.
- Oral contraceptives, sub-dermal implants, warfarin and ARVs may be less effective.
- Progestogen only injectable contraceptives or IUDs are preferred.

Lifestyle education
- The patient should try to lead as *normal* a life as possible.
- Work should be encouraged.
- Disability grants should not be encouraged. It is important for epileptics to take a normal role in society
  - however, these grants may be a great help to a family struggling to cope with a severely handicapped epileptic with mental retardation or other sequelae
  - **REFER** the family to the social workers if you think they will benefit.
- Patients should not be discouraged from marrying and having a family
  - if genetic counselling is requested, they should be **REFERRED**.
- Normal sports and exercise should be encouraged if at all possible, especially for children. However
  - swimming must be supervised
  - contact sports should be avoided eg. boxing, karate, rugby.
- Driving and other dangerous occupations need to be assessed individually
  - they need to be discussed with the patient and his employer if possible
  - all concerned should be aware of the possible problems.

  Note. *Uncontrolled epileptics should **not** drive. Patients may resume driving if fit-free for 2 years on treatment. They should be discouraged from driving public transport vehicles.*
- Alcohol should be stopped because it:
  - causes liver enzyme induction which then causes metabolism of the anti-epileptic drugs to be speeded up, decreasing concentration
  - lowers the threshold for seizures.
- Good patterns of regular meals, recreation and exercise to relieve stress and regular sleeping patterns should be encouraged.
  - this may help considerably in lessening fits
  - patients should also be counselled and helped to learn to deal with stress and anxieties before they affect the epilepsy

The first visit
- **REFER** if:
  - this is the first fit even if you are unsure whether the fits are genuine or not
  - this is a repeat fit **and** the patient has never had the fits investigated
  - there has been no previous therapy
  - the patient is not sure about his / her drugs

Subsequent visits
- If the patient is fit free, then continue with previous therapy.
- Check that the patient understands his / her disease and the management.
- Find out if there are any serious side effects from the anti-epileptic treatment.
- Check that the patient's family, social and work environment are satisfactory.
- Check that drug adherence is satisfactory.
- Check the seizure diary if the patient has kept one.
- If there have been fits, and the problem is not one of adherence or alcohol abuse
  - then increase dosage by one step
  - drug levels can be used to check whether patient is receiving enough medication.

MEDICINE MANAGEMENT
Also see Pharmacopoeia pages 383, 389 and 396.

The goal of treatment is to *completely* stop all fits, provided this can be achieved without too many side effects from the medicines.

- Usually this is best achieved with the use of only **one** medicine, and **not** with mixed therapy.
- If the fits are not controlled in patients taking dosages within the maintenance range, then blood levels of the medicines should be obtained if possible.

Medicine choice
- The clinic doctor or hospital will start the treatment with a medicine effective for the type of seizure diagnosed.

Adults
- The medicine of choice for most adult patients is either carbamazepine or lamotrigine.
  - Carbamazepine should preferably be avoided in pregnant women and is contraindicated in HIV-infected patients on ART
- Lamotrigine is the preferred medicine for HIV-infected adults on ART and in pregnant women.
- Valproate is strongly contraindicated in pregnancy and should not be initiated in women of child-bearing potential

Children
- Carbamazepine or valproate is the best choice.
- Carbamazepine may exacerbate myoclonic seizures and absence seizures
- Phenobarbitone is used only in children under 6 months of age
  - it should be avoided in older children as it causes sedation and interferes with concentration (school work)
- Valproate is the preferred medicine for HIV infected children

Carbamazepine
Adults
- Start treatment with:
  - 100 mg 12 hourly for 1 week
  - then 200 mg 12 hourly
- If seizures are not controlled, increase by 200 mg / day at 2-weekly intervals up to a maximum of 1 200 mg / day
  - in 2-3 evenly spaced divided doses.
- Once a dose of 400 mg 12 hourly or 15 mg / kg / day has been reached, any further increases should be guided by blood level estimations
  - the maintenance range is usually 600-1 200 mg / day in divided doses
  - encourage patients to take doses as close to the scheduled time as possible.

Children
Initial dose:
- Syrup (100 mg/5ml)   5 mg/kg/day, given in divided doses, 8 hourly.
- Tablets (200 mg)   5 mg/kg/day, given in divided doses, 12 hourly.
- Depending on response to treatment, increase slowly by 5 mg/kg/day, if necessary, at 2 weekly intervals to a maximum of 20 mg/kg/day or 1 g/day.

Lamotrigine
Adults
- Initially 25 mg daily for 2 weeks
  - then 50 mg daily for 2 weeks
- Thereafter increase by up to 50 mg / day every 2 weeks according to response up to a maximum of 200 mg daily.
- Usual maintenance dose 100-200 mg / day as a single dose or 2 divided doses.
- The dose of lamotrigine will need to be doubled when patients on ART are changed to lopinavir / ritonavir.

Phenytoin
- This is not usually the drug of first choice because of its side effects. These include:
  - skin thickening, gum hypertrophy, hirsutism, acne
  - long-term therapy can cause folate deficiency
- An overdose may cause fits. The signs of overdose may be:
  - ataxia, nystagmus, tremor, speech disturbance

Adults
- Usual daily dose 300 mg at night.
- All doses above 300 mg / day are potentially toxic and should be monitored carefully, both clinically and by drug levels.

Valproate (Epilim CR)
Adults
- Initially 300 mg 12 hourly
  - increase by 200 mg / day at 2 weekly or monthly intervals until control is achieved
- Usual dosage range 1-2 g / day in 2 divided doses
- Contraindicated in women of childbearing age and in HIV infected patients on zidovudine

Children (males only)
- Initially 5 mg / kg 12 hourly increasing according to response
- Maximum dose 15 mg / kg 12 hourly

Achieving a steady plasma level
- To get to the right plasma level of the medicine usually takes several days (5 times the drug's half life) eg.
  - phenytoin has a half life of 24 hours, therefore it will take 5 days to reach a steady blood level
  - carbamazepine has a half life of 25-65 hours for a single dose and 8-29 hours with chronic use and will take 2-5 days to reach steady state.
- After reaching a steady blood level, the medicine level gradually begins to drop after several months.
- This is because the liver becomes more efficient in metabolising the medicine, due to improvement in the liver enzyme medicine breakdown system.
- As a result, the patient may begin to fit again after some months of good control, and an increase in dosage is required.
- Drug blood levels may be helpful after some months of initiating treatment to assess whether increased dosage is necessary.

Changing medicines
NB: HIV-infected individuals on ARVs
Adults
- Lamotrigine is preferred because of fewer medicine interactions.
- When switching to lamotrigine
  - commence treatment as outlined above
  - discontinue the other anticonvulsant after 28 days
- The dose of lamotrigine will need to be doubled when patients on ART are changed to lopinavir / ritonavir.

Poorly controlled epilepsy
Ask the patient or family member or care-giver about the following:
- Adherence with medicine therapy.
- If non-adherence has been established, ask for reasons contributing to non-adherence and offer guidance.
- Use of other medicines which may cause drug interactions
- Substance abuse or traditional medicine use.
- Alcohol abuse.

If one or more of the above are present, address the problem/s but leave anticonvulsant therapy unchanged (unless dose adjustment is necessary because of a drug interaction).

Fit-free on treatment for two years
- If patients have been free of fits for more than 2 years, then you should discuss with them and / or their family whether they would like to try and stop treatment.
- There is always the danger of a breakthrough fit, with its possible embarrassment socially or at work
  - some patients may rather choose to continue with treatment for life than take the chance of having a fit
  - some patients are keen to come off treatment.
- Decrease the dose **gradually** by one step a month
  - it should take 3-4 months to wean patients off their medicines.

Epilepsy control during pregnancy

- During pregnancy one third of epileptic patients improve, one third stay the same and one third get worse.
- *Avoid changing epileptic drugs during pregnancy.*
- These patients should be **REFERRED** if there are any problems.
- It may be necessary to increase the dose.

REFERRAL
- Increased number of seizures
- Patients who have been seizure-free for 2 years, to review therapy
- Pregnancy
- Development of neurological signs and symptoms
- Symptoms of toxicity, e.g. ataxia, tremor, nystagmus

STATUS EPILEPTICUS

Status epilepticus means repeated generalised fits, with no regaining of consciousness between each fit.

This is a medical emergency.

Effects of status epilepticus
- Cardiorespiratory dysfunction
- Hyperthermia
- Metabolic derangements
- Decreased respiration resulting in anoxia to the brain
- Increased acidosis due to
  - poor respiration
  - excessive muscle exercise
- Damage to the neurones and progressive brain damage
- Eventual exhaustion and death due to anoxia and acidosis

Causes
- Not taking treatment correctly
- Hypoglycaemia
- Overdosage of anti-epileptic drugs
- Alcohol excess
- Other brain diseases eg. meningitis

MANAGEMENT
General measures
- Call for the doctor if available.
- Do not allow the patient to injure him- or herself but avoid excessive restraint.
- Place patient on his or her side.
- Ensure the airway is open by:
  - extending the neck
  - removing any obstructions to respiration.
- Administer high-flow oxygen.
- Check the blood glucose.
- If blood glucose is low.
  - Establish an IV line (10% dextrose solution)
  - Administer 2-5 ml/kg rapidly
- Do not push a spatula or spoon into the patient's mouth
  - the patient will not choke on his / her tongue but he / she may choke on a tooth broken off when trying to put in the spatula or spoon.

Medicine management
Children < 12 years of age
- Midazolam, buccal, 0.5 mg / kg / dose
  - use midazolam for injection 5 mg in 1 ml
  - draw up the required volume in a 5 ml syringe
  - administer into the buccal cavity, between gum and cheek on the dependent side
- Dose:
  - 6 months-1 year   0.8 ml
  - 1-3 years   1 ml
  - 3-5 years   1.5 ml
  - > 5 years   2 ml
- May be repeated after 5-10 minutes if convulsions continue

Note:
- Buccal midazolam should not be used in infants <6 months of age

OR
- Midazolam, IM
- Child >13 kg: midazolam, IM 5 mg
- Repeat after 5-10 minutes if still fitting

OR
- Diazepam, intra-rectal
  - use diazepam for injection 10 mg in 2 ml
  - draw up the required volume in a 2 ml syringe
  - remove the needle, then inject the barrel of the syringe into the rectum
  - Inject the contents
  - remove the syringe while at the same time holding buttocks together to prevent leakage
- Dose 0.5 mg / kg / dose
  - 6 months-1 year   2.5 mg (0.5 ml)
  - 1-5 years   5 mg (1 ml)
  - 5-8 years   7.5 mg (1.5 ml)
  - 8-14 years   10 mg (2 ml)
- May be repeated after 10 minutes if convulsions continue.

Uncontrolled seizures (doctor only)
- Give phenobarbitone tablets, oral, crushed by nasogastric tube at a loading dose of 20 mg/kg as a single dose
- Maximum dose: 210 mg (7 x 30 mg tablets)

Adults
- Midazolam, 10 mg, IM, as a single dose
- May be repeated after 5-10 minutes if still fitting

OR
- Diazepam, intravenous
    - this is very effective but if given too fast it can easily cause respiratory arrest.
- Dose 0.1 mg / kg
    - give 2 mg per minute to a maximum of 10 mg
- Do not add to the vacolitre.
- Diazepam must not be mixed with other medicines or solutions.
- Repeat the dose if necessary after 5-10 minutes
    - maximum dose of 20 mg within 1 hour

OR
- Midazolam, buccal, 10 mg using the parenteral formulation
- Repeat after 5-10 minutes if still fitting
- If no response after 2 doses of midazolam or 2 doses of diazepam and if the seizure has lasted more than 20-30 minutes, **REFER** urgently to hospital.

NEUROLOGICAL PROBLEMS

HEADACHE

The reaction of both the patient and medical attendant to a headache is the fear that the cause is serious disease of the brain.

However, the great majority of headaches are not due to a serious cause.

*Headaches are not a common symptom in **children** and must be taken seriously, as it is more often associated with serious disease than it is in adults.*

- Important clues helping to establish the real cause of the headache are obtained from the patient's history.
- Allow and encourage the patient to speak and explain:
    - their feelings about the headache
    - what they associate with the cause of the headache.
- A thorough history and general and neurological examination is essential to detect any other symptoms or signs which may point to a more serious cause, eg.
    - meningitis
    - brain tumour
    - illness elsewhere in the body

Clinical features

Features suggesting a serious cause

- Headaches getting progressively worse over some months
- Headaches waking a patient at night
- A headache that is worse in the morning and improves during the day, which may suggest increased intracranial pressure.
- Any associated neurological symptoms, especially if they are:
    - of recent onset
    - progressive.
- Other signs of systemic illness eg. weight loss, chronic cough, fever, pallor etc.
- A person with chronic headaches who notices a definite change in the pattern of the headache.
- Recent onset of a severe headache, especially if it is the first episode.
- Dull, aching, deep pain

Features suggesting less serious causes (eg. stress)

- Headaches occur every day
- The patient has been having them for months or years
- Triggers of the headache eg. food, stress, weather

Headache diary

Record details of each headache

- Which day
- What time of the day
- Which part of the head is involved
- How long it lasted
- Possible causes at the time
    - eg. stress, foods, exercise or rest
- At work or at home
- Activities before or at the time of the headache
- Drugs at the time eg. contraceptives, over-the-counter medications
- Menstrual pattern in women
- What makes the headache better or worse

ACUTE HEADACHES

Causes

Generalised headaches

- Meningitis
    - acute, bilateral with drowsiness and neck stiffness
    - cryptococcal
    - tuberculosis
- Systemic infections eg. measles, pneumonia, typhoid, malaria, tick bite fever
- Urinary tract infections
- Gastrointestinal disease
- Poisoning eg. glue-sniffing, insecticides
- Prescribed drugs, analgesics
- Carbon monoxide poisoning
    - there will be a history of having slept in a room with a burning fire, with no openings for free air entry
- Epilepsy (post-ictal)
- Stress eg. school, family or work problems
- Hypoglycaemia
- Post traumatic
- Dental disease
- Cerebro vascular accident
- Tumour
- Osteo-arthritis of neck or other neck problems
- Subarachnoid haemorrhage (acute single episode)

Localised or unilateral headaches

- Tumour
- Brain abscess
- Migraine (acute headache, recurrent attacks)
- Cluster headache (acute headache, recurrent attacks)
- Ear disease
- Eye disease
- Dental disease
- Sinusitis in older children and adults
- Giant cell arteritis

MANAGEMENT

REFER if
- No obvious treatable cause is found
- The headache has not improved with your treatment
- You suspect a serious cause

CHRONIC / RECURRENT HEADACHES

Chronic or recurrent headaches are a common complaint in adults.

The majority are not due to serious illness and are due to stress and anxiety, but serious causes must be excluded.

Other possible causes

Increased intracranial pressure

- May be due to a brain tumour or chronic meningitis such as tuberculosis, cryptococcosis or a subdural haematoma.

- The features will be a headache which is:
  - occurring every day
  - relieved on sitting, worse on lying down
  - worse by coughing or bending forward
  - getting progressively worse
  - most noted in the morning
  - relieved during the day
  - associated with nausea and vomiting.
- Physical examination may reveal localising signs eg. neck stiffness, cranial nerve abnormalities, papilloedema
- If you suspect this, **REFER** stat

Cysticercosis of the brain
- This is being recognised increasingly as a cause of chronic headache and neurological disease, especially fits.
- There are no specific features except for:
  - a chronic headache
  - the fact that the person comes from an area where meat is eaten without adequate abattoir facilities.

Chronic diseases
- Chronic renal disease
- Early kidney failure
- A good history and thorough examination should detect these causes.

Analgesic abuse
- This occurs particularly in middle-aged women
- Initially they have recurrent headaches due to tension
- They begin to take over-the-counter analgesics regularly
- Headaches start to recur (especially between doses) which in turn causes the patient to take more analgesics
  - a vicious cycle develops
- If you suspect this, ask how long a bottle of analgesics or pack of headache powders is lasting them
  - if they are using more than a bottle or pack per week, they are suffering from analgesic abuse
- This is an increasingly common cause of kidney failure
  - **REFER** if evidence of kidney damage
- Counsel the patient very strongly against this dangerous practice and **REFER** to a substance abuse clinic if necessary.

Hypertension
- Commonly thought by the patient to be a cause of headache
- However headaches only occur with a very high diastolic pressure.
- Many of the headaches that hypertensive patients complain of, are due to other causes.

Other causes
- Some of the causes mentioned under "acute headaches" (see page 219) may also result in a chronic or recurrent headache.

STROKE / CEREBRO VASCULAR ACCIDENT (CVA)

ACUTE STROKE

Most strokes are ischaemic (thrombosis or embolism), while others may be caused by cerebral haemorrhage.

Clinical features
- Usually when relatives bring in a patient whom they suspect has suffered a stroke, the diagnosis is obvious from the clear neurological damage already present:
  - weakness and/or loss of sensation on one side of the body including possible facial weakness on the same side
  - difficulty in speaking or understanding (dysphasia or aphasia) when the dominant hemisphere is involved
  - impairment of gait or stance
  - sometimes visual loss or disturbance
- Stroke symptoms and signs which resolve within 24 hours suggest a transient ischaemic attack (TIA) due to an embolus or thrombosis.
- Check for clinical features of possible underlying conditions that may have led to the stroke e.g.
  - diabetes
  - myocardial infarction

MANAGEMENT
REFER
- All acute strokes
- Patients who may have suffered a TIA to try to prevent a full-blown stroke or to exclude myocardial infarction

Emergency treatment
- If the patient is conscious
  - give aspirin 300 mg as a single oral dose
- If the blood pressure is elevated, control should be done gradually
  - dropping a high blood pressure too swiftly can make the brain damage caused by the stroke worse
  - avoid antihypertensive therapy before **REFERRAL**

Note. Patients with "old strokes" that have been present for several months or who have been treated in the past and have not fully recovered, will only need **REFERRAL** if they are deteriorating. Otherwise they should be treated at the clinic.

OLD STROKES

MANAGEMENT
General measures
- A major aim of management is to restore and maintain as much brain and body function as possible.
- Ideally this will allow the patient to return to normal function at home and at work.
- This requires hard work and co-operation from the family, the patient and the assistance of a full health team.

Physiotherapy
- This is vital to strengthen and to maintain nerve and muscle function.

Occupational therapy
- To help the patient adapt the remaining function to the work and home situation.

Speech therapists
- If there is a speech or swallowing problem

Domiciliary (home) nursing services
- If available or needed

Medicine management
- Patients should take aspirin 75-100 mg daily for the rest of their lives, if the cause of CVA was thrombosis / embolus.
- For patients with thrombatic stroke, for secondary prevention, irrespective of the LDL cholesterol level
    - give simvastatin, oral, 40 mg nocte (10mg nocte for patients on amlodipine)
- Blood pressure should be controlled

SUB-ARACHNOID HAEMORRHAGE

Clinical features
- The headache is of sudden onset and is unbearable
- The patient may describe it as being "hit by a bolt of lightning"
- These headaches may be recurrent becoming more severe
- Commonly there are associated signs of meningism eg.
    - neck stiffness
    - positive Kernig's test
- There may be other neurological signs and symptoms
- May affect adults in any age group
- The blood pressure is usually elevated

REFER for investigation if you suspect a sub-arachnoid haemorrhage.

MENINGITIS

Clinical features
Young babies
- The signs of meningeal irritation are often absent
- Failure to suck, vomiting and fever are important symptoms of meningitis
    - though a normal temperature does not exclude the possibility of meningitis
- Neck stiffness is a late sign
- Possible signs are:
    - fullness or loss of pulsation of the fontanelle
    - high pitched cry
    - irritability or lethargy
    - convulsions or any symptoms that suggest fitting, eg. jerking of the eyes, twitching of the limbs
- Petechial rash suggests meningococcal septicaemia

Older children and adults
The symptoms and signs in older children become more definite and more like those in adults
- Headache
- Photophobia
- Impaired level of consciousness
- Vomiting
- Neck stiffness
    - *this must be properly done, trying to get the chin onto the chest*
    - children or adults with meningitis may only show stiffness and pain when the neck is fully flexed (terminal neck stiffness)
- Convulsions
- Pyrexia
- Other signs of meningeal irritation eg.
    - Kernig's test: pain and resistance on passive knee extension when hips fully flexed
    - Brudzinski test: hips flex on bending head forward
- Other neurological signs may be present eg. cranial nerve lesions
- Petechial rash, if a meningococcal septicaemia is present

Note. In patients with lowered resistance (eg. diabetics, AIDS, the elderly), the symptoms and signs may be much less obvious.

MANAGEMENT
- If there is **any** possibility of meningitis, it is obligatory and vital to **REFER** for a lumbar puncture stat
    - this is the only way of confirming the diagnosis
- *If meningitis is strongly suspected or if any danger signs are present e.g. depressed level of consciousness, purpura:*
    - *give immediate antibiotic therapy (ceftriaxone IMI or IVI)*
    - *neonates, infants and children 80 mg / kg stat (see pharmacopoeia)*
    - *adults 2 g stat*
    - ***this should be given before REFERRAL***

Prophylaxis of meningococcal meningitis
In cases of confirmed meningococcal infection, the following close contacts should receive prophylaxis:
- Household members
- Child-care centre contacts
- Health care workers who have resuscitated patients before treatment

Medicine management
- Children < 6 years
    - ceftriaxone, IM 125 mg single dose
- Children 6-12 years
    - ciprofloxacin, oral 250 mg single dose
- Children >12 years and adults
    - ciprofloxacin, oral 500 mg single dose
- Pregnant women
    - ceftriaxone, IM, 250 mg as a single dose

TENSION HEADACHES

This is probably the most common type of headache.

Clinical features
- They tend to occur late in the day, but are often present all day.
- The headache is bilateral, usually bifrontal or occipito-nuchal, but may be felt over the entire head
    - often described as a "tight band" around the head
    - or sometimes described as throbbing
- There is often associated dizziness and /or blurring of vision
- They may persist for weeks or months
- A useful physical sign is that usually this headache is associated with spasm of the occipital muscles of the neck
    - palpation of the neck will reveal tenderness in these muscles

Differential diagnosis
- It may be difficult to decide if this is due to migraine or not
    - a history of stress, and the nature and duration of the headache may help

- An important differential diagnosis is cervical spine disease with nerve entrapment (see page 223)
    - if there is a possibility of this diagnosis, **REFER**.

Note. Physiotherapists, if available, may be able to help distinguish the two causes

- Underlying depression should be kept in mind
    - this may be detected by associated sleep disturbance, appetite and mood changes and suicidal thoughts
- It is important to exclude analgesia overuse as a cause of the headaches.

MANAGEMENT
- Try and help the patient identify the cause of the tension.
- Counsel as far as you can.
- Give simple analgesics eg. paracetamol, aspirin, ibuprofen, unless abuse of these is considered to be the cause of the headache.

REFER
- For relaxation therapy if available
- For further counselling if necessary
- If there is doubt about the diagnosis
- If not responding, for medicine therapy
    - amitriptyline 25-75 mg at night

MIGRAINE

This is a unilateral recurring headache, usually occurring with pain-free intervals and almost always provoked by the same stimuli.

CLASSICAL MIGRAINE
(MIGRAINE WITH AURA)

These are headaches associated with characteristic prodromal sensory, motor or visual symptoms (aura)

Clinical features
- There may be a family history of migraine
- It is more common in women and often occurs premenstrually
- Attacks may occur months or years apart
- The aura may take the form of visual hallucinations e.g. zigzag lines, scotomas (blind spots)
- The patient may complain of photophobia (visual intolerance to light), dizziness or tinnitus
- The patient may not tolerate loud noises (phonophobia)
    - he will want to lie in a dark, quiet place
- Headache is often accompanied by nausea and vomiting
- Less commonly one may get dramatic focal neurological features (complicated migraine)
    - numbness (paraesthesias) of body parts
    - nerve palsy
    - sensory changes
    - hemiplegia of short duration
- The patient may be able to pinpoint certain triggers to the migraine, such as:
    - many food substances (eg. red wine, chocolate, cheese)
    - contraceptive pill
    - anxiety
    - travel
    - exercise
    - hypoglycaemia
    - bright lights.

COMMON MIGRAINE
(MIGRAINE WITHOUT AURA)

Clinical features
- This is the more common type of migraine
- It differs from classical migraine in not having the aura or prodrome preceding the headache
- The symptoms are:
    - episodic severe headache
    - sometimes photophobia, phonophobia
    - nausea or vomiting
    - the headache is throbbing, fronto-temporal and often unilateral
    - it may last from hours to 1-2 days
- There may be a positive family history

MANAGEMENT
General measures
- It is important to recognise the headache as migraine
- If certain triggers to migraine are recognised, these should be avoided.
- Eliminate any food suspected of contributing to the symptoms
    - e.g. chocolate, cheese and monitor the response
- Avoid bright lights and loud noises eg. discos
- Keep to a regular sleep and eating pattern so as not to miss meals (avoid hypoglycaemia)

Medicine management
Due to gastric stasis during a migraine attack, the absorbtion of drugs may be decreased
- Medication should therefore be taken as early as possible during an attack.
- Patients should also be advised to rest for at least an hour after taking medication.

Treatment of acute migraine
- Simple analgesics, for example:
    - paracetamol or aspirin may be moderately effective.
- Non-steroidal anti-inflammatory drugs are often effective, for example:
    - ibuprofen 800 mg stat, then 400 mg 8 hourly if needed
- Morphine-like drugs may be effective, but use with caution as there is a possibility of overuse and addiction, for example:
    - tramadol
- **NB.** If nausea and vomiting are prominent, use an anti-emetic, for example:
    - metoclopramide 10 mg 3 x daily oral / IMI.

Migraine prophylaxis
If patient's attacks are very frequent, you may be concerned about the high intake of analgesic medicines. You may want to try other medicines that are used for migraine prevention (prophylaxis). These include the following:
- Antidepressants, such as amytriptyline and imipramine
    - 10-25 mg at bedtime
    - increasing every 2 weeks up to a maximum of 75 mg at bedtime
- Beta-blockers, eg:
    - propranolol 80 mg 2 x daily
- Calcium channel blockers eg:
    - flunarizine hydrochloride (Sibelium) 5-10 mg at night

- Anticonvulsants e.g. carbamazepine, valproate
- Carbamazepine dose:
  - initially 100 mg 2 x daily
  - increasing every 2 weeks according to response up to a maximum of 400 mg 12 hourly

CLUSTER HEADACHES

Clinical features
- The headache is strictly unilateral and concentrated in or around the eye.
- It may affect the cheek or temple area
- Blocked or runny nose on the same side as the headache
- Red, inflamed watery eye on the same side as the headache
- There may be a partial ptosis of the affected eye
- Usually nocturnal occurring within 1-3 hours after falling asleep
- It lasts for 15 minutes - 2 hours
- There may be more than one attack in 24 hours
- They occur in clusters
  - bouts of frequent attacks
  - can last for weeks to months
  - they then disappear for months or years
- Alcohol may bring on an attack or make an attack worse
- Specific food may rarely be the cause

Features which differentiate these headaches from migraines
- More common in males, especially middle-aged
- Not familial
- The patient is very restless, unlike with migraine
- They may even bang their heads against the wall

MANAGEMENT
General measures
- Simple measures such as rest
- Avoid alcohol

Medicine management
- Analgesics and anti-inflammatory drugs are ineffective
- To induce rapid remission:
  - prednisone 40 mg daily for 5-10 days
- **REFER** if no response to prednisone

SPACE-OCCUPYING LESION

- Infection eg. tuberculoma, toxoplasmosis, Nocardia
- Tumour either benign, malignant or haematological

Clinical features
- Headaches which occur with increasing frequency and severity
- Throbbing or non-throbbing, unilateral or bilateral
- Activity or change in position of the head may worsen pain
- Unexpected, sometimes projectile vomiting

REFER patients with headaches that are new and progressive.

CERVICAL SPINE DISEASE

This is more common in older people due to osteo-arthritis and osteoporosis.

Clinical features
- Headache, especially occipital
- Pain or paraesthesia (pins and needles) may be present
  - radiating down one or both arms (radial side)
  - may be related to movements of the neck
- Pain in the shoulders
  - it often looks exactly like fibrositis of the neck muscles
- There may be signs of weakness or specific areas of sensory loss in one or both the arms, hands or fingers (radial side).
- There may be severe limitation of neck movement or an acute torticollis.

Causes
- Post traumatic
- Osteo-arthritis
- Tuberculosis or malignancy of the cervical spine
- Osteoporosis with collapse

Differential diagnosis
- Fibrositis
  - this will not give any loss of sensation in the arms
  - the pain seldom radiates down the arms

MANAGEMENT
REFER
- If you suspect this problem
- If there is any evidence of neurological damage
- If it does not respond quickly to analgesics and rest
- Physiotherapy may be helpful
- X-ray of the cervical spine

OTHER CONDITIONS CAUSING HEADACHES

EYE DISEASE

CLOSED ANGLE GLAUCOMA

Clinical features
- Acute onset
- Nausea and vomiting
- Severe pain typically behind the orbit but need not be well localised
- Decreased visual acuity
- Coloured haloes seen around lights
- A moderately dilated pupil which does not respond to light
- Hazy cornea
- Inflamed conjunctiva pericorneally

For management see The Eye pages 239-240.

REFRACTORY ERRORS
(DIFFICULTY WITH VISION)

Clinical features
- Usually mild headache will come on gradually as the person stresses his / her eyes eg. with reading or studying.
- It can be confirmed by testing for visual acuity with a Snellen chart and a Near Vision book.
- If looking through a pin-hole improves the vision, this confirms that the patient has a refractory problem
    - eg. short-sightedness

REFER for refraction and spectacles.

MENINGEAL IRRITATION

This is usually caused by either meningitis or subarachnoid haemorrhage.

Clinical features (see also meningitis page 221)
- Severe persistent headache
- Neck stiffness
- Fever (not subachnoid haemorrhage)
- Confusion
- Vomiting (especially in children)

PAIN IN MAXILLA OR MANDIBLE

DENTAL DISEASE

Clinical features
- Dental caries may be responsible
    - this can be detected by examining the teeth
    - percussion over the affected tooth should give a pain similar to the one the patient is complaining about
- Dental abscess
    - severe throbbing pain

TEMPERO-MANDIBULAR JOINT

Pain in the tempero-mandibular joint is common.
- This occurs as a result of malocclusion of the teeth causing a crooked bite and stressing the tempero-mandibular joint during chewing.
- Direct palpation of the joint should reveal tenderness if this is the cause.

REFER.

DISEASES IN THE EAR, NOSE AND SINUSES

Clinical features
- Sinusitis is a common cause of headaches in adults and in older children (see page 36)
- Otitis media
- Mastoiditis or intracranial complicatoins of chronic ear infections

- Manage the underlying condition
- If there is doubt, **REFER**

MALARIA

Falciparum malaria is common in southern Africa.

Clinical features
- A history of recent travel to, or coming from, a malaria area
- Severe headache
- Muscle and joint pains
- High fever
- Rigors (shivering)
- Jaundice
- Enlarged liver or spleen
- Pallor

- If there is any possibility of malaria, **REFER** stat.
- See Malaria, page 367.

TICK BITE FEVER

Clinical features
- A severe generalised headache
- A history of having been in an area where ticks are common
    - ie. any rural area of southern Africa
- A septic bite on the body (eschar)
    - this may be in an area the patient cannot see eg. the back or perineum so check the whole body
    - the bite will have a black, necrotic centre
- Associated lymphadenopathy of the regional glands
- Fever and rigors
- Macular-papular red rash in some patients including the palms and soles
- Occurs usually one week after the bite occurred

- Responds well to doxycycline
    - 100 mg 2 x daily for 7 days
- **REFER** if unsure or the patient is seriously ill

POST-TRAUMATIC HEADACHE

POST-CONCUSSION HEADACHES

- These may occur for months or years even when no loss of conciousness reported.
- They are not usually associated with anatomic lesions of the brain.

SUBDURAL HAEMATOMA

Clinical features
- Patient is often elderly
- There may be a chronic headache
- History of trauma or fall or sudden movement of the head especially in the elderly or those with a bleeding disorder
- There may be a personality change
- There may be localising neurological symptoms and signs
    - unequal pupils
- There may be a fluctuating level of conciousness
- There may be spacticity and hyperreflexia

REFER if subdural haematoma suspected.

HEADACHES DUE TO MEDICINES

Causes
- Prescription medicines are a common cause eg.
    - sulphonylureas e.g. glimepiride
    - oral contraceptives
    - zidovudine (AZT), efavirenz
- Anti-inflammatory drugs (NSAIDs)
- Medicine abuse or their withdrawal must be considered
    - e.g. glue-sniffing, alcohol, dagga, Mandrax, etc.

EPILEPSY

- Headache postictal (post fits)
- Consider epilepsy if the headache is
    - recurrent
    - associated with any change in consciousness or behaviour
- Several types of epilepsy are not associated with loss of consciousness eg. temporal lobe epilepsy

See Epilepsy page 213.

HYPERTENSION

Acute or severe blood pressure elevation may induce headaches.

HYPOGLYCAEMIA

Causes
- Many people find that if they miss food or a meal they develop a headache.
- Diagnostic feature: the headache is relieved by food
- If this occurs in diabetics, their treatment should be reviewed to exclude drug-induced hypoglycaemia
    - this may be a particular problem with insulin dependent diabetics, in the early morning hours

MISCELLANEOUS

Causes
- Hormonal effects
    - this may occur as a result of hormonal effects especially in the second half of the menstrual cycle when high levels of oestrogen and progesterone cause fluid retention
    - this may affect the brain and cause headaches
- Pregnancy complications eg. pregnancy-induced hypertension
- Women with unwanted pregnancies, or women desperately wanting a child may present initially with a "headache"
    - this is just a method of seeking advice and help with their problem

REFER if you suspect a serious cause.

WEAKNESS

ON ONE SIDE OF THE BODY

Possible causes
Face only
- Cerebro vascular accident or TIA
- Cranial nerve entrapment
- Bell's palsy

Body (including face)
- The most common cause for unilateral weakness of the body is cerebro vascular accident or stroke.
- Transient ischaemic attacks are strokes caused by small emboli
    - symptoms and signs last less than 24 hours
- Hypoglycaemia may present with unilateral weakness and signs of a stroke which resolve when the glucose level is restored.
- Poliomyelitis must be kept in mind

- One-sided weakness may be the presenting complaint of a patient with depression or a psycho-social problem
  - definite neurological signs may not be found or are confusing
- Todd's paresis ie. weakness occurring after a partial seizure

> **MANAGEMENT**
> **REFER**
> - Any definite neurological deficit
> - All children with these symptoms even if there are no neurological signs on examination.
> - For counselling if found to be due to anxiety

- Guillain Barre syndrome
- Neoplastic conditions
- Thiamine deficiency

> **REFER** all patients

GENERALISED WEAKNESS

This is often the presenting complaint of patients with diseases of any of the organs, but there are also many neuromuscular disorders that one must bear in mind.

Myopathic disorders (muscle weakness)
There are many causes
- Inflammatory causes eg.
  - infections by viruses (coxsackie, HIV, influenza)
  - bacteria
  - parasites
- Endocrine (hormonal dysfunction) eg.
  - hyper- and hypothyroidism
  - Cushing's disease
- Metabolic (electrolyte) disturbances, especially hypokalaemia
- Inherited muscular dystrophies
- Drug induced / toxin induced eg.
  - alcohol, antibiotics, pethidine, steroids, chloroquine etc.

Neuromuscular junction disorders
- Such as myasthaenia gravis

Neurogenic disorders (nerve disease)
- Metabolic defects eg. porphyria etc.
- Polyneuropathies associated with:
  - diabetes mellitus
  - malnutrition
  - vitamin deficiencies (B12 and folate).
- Toxins
  - lead, mercury, chemicals
- Neuropathies associated with:
  - malignancies (carcinoma lung, breast, stomach)
  - haematological malignancies.
- Infections eg. leprosy
- Connective tissue disease
  - systemic lupus erythematosis
  - scleroderma

General diseases (non-specific weakness)
- Heart failure
- Chronic obstructive airways disease
- Anaemia
- Systemic infections
- Cirrhosis of liver
- Kidney failure
- Anxiety stress depression
- Ageing

> **MANAGEMENT**
> - Manage the cause if you are able to
> - **REFER**
>   - if you are not sure of the cause
>   - if you suspect a serious cause
>   - for physiotherapy

BELLS PALSY

This is unilateral facial muscle paralysis. Most patients recover within a few weeks or months.

Clinical features
- Unilaterally the forehead is unfurrowed.
- The eye will not close partially or completely.
- The cheek on the affected side cannot be blown out.
- The corner of the mouth drops and is unable to move sideways.
- Taste sensation may be lost unilaterally.
- Hyperacusis (painful sensitivity to loud sounds) may be present.

> **MANAGEMENT**
> - HIV testing
> - Eye pad protection of the eye during sleep.
>
> *Adults*
> - Prednisone 60 mg daily for 7 days started within 3 days of onset (doctor prescribed).
>
> *Children*
> - Prednisone 2 mg/kg daily for 7 days started within 3 days of onset (doctor prescribed).
>
> **REFER** all patients for physiotherapy if available.

AFFECTING BOTH LEGS (PARAPARESIS)

Acute myelopathy presents with a sudden onset of paraparesis with associated sensory loss. Incontinence and autonomic instability may be present.

Causes
- Inflammatory (myelitis), usually viral in origin
  - HIV infection
  - herpes zoster
- Infectious conditions, e.g. TB / bilharzial granulomas, abscesses causing external compression of the spinal cord

CHANGE IN SENSATION

ONE SIDE OF THE BODY

Causes
- Similar to the causes for weakness of one side of the body (see page 225)

REFER if you suspect genuine neurological disease.

LEGS OR ARMS (PERIPHERAL NEUROPATHY / POLYNEUROPATHIES)

Defective functioning of peripheral nerves.

Clinical features
- The condition usually starts distally and spreads proximally
- Initially tingling, burning, pins and needles in the soles of the feet or tips of the toes
- Later sensory loss over both feet
- Patients may experience difficulty in walking and an unsteady ataxic gait
- Foot drop may become apparent

Causes
- HIV disease
- Metabolic
    - diabetes mellitus, kidney failure
- Alcohol
- Infections
    - tuberculosis, syphilis, leprosy
- Vitamin deficiencies
    - B1, B6, B12, folate
- Medicines - INH, phenytoin, metronidazole
- Carcinoma
- Toxins, eg. lead, organophosphates

MANAGEMENT
Check urine for diabetes.

Alcohol abuse
- Advise patient to stop drinking and **REFER** to SANCA or Alcoholics Anonymous (AA).
- Encourage the patient to eat an adequate diet.
- Prescribe thiamine 100 mg daily

Patients on INH therapy
- Give pyridoxine 25-50 mg 3 x daily
    - maximum 100 mg daily in patients on ARV therapy

Mild to moderate pain
- Give paracetamol 1g 3 x daily when necessary
    - **Plus** amitriptyline 25-75 mg nocte (doctor initiated)
- If no doctor available give
    - carbamazepine (not in patients on ARVs)
    - 100 mg 2 x daily for 1 week
    - then 200 mg 2 x daily
    - increasing by 200 mg / day at weekly intervals according to response
    - maximum 400 mg 2 x daily

Severe pain
- Add tramadol 50 mg 4 x daily for 5 days
    - **REFER** to doctor

REFER if
- No response to treatment
- Unsteady / ataxic gait
- Foot drop
- Severe sensory loss

AFFECTING ONLY ONE AREA (MONONEUROPATHIES)

If the patient can clearly localise the area of sensory loss, and this is confirmed on examination, it suggests single nerve disease.

Causes
- Nerve entrapment syndromes eg.
    - carpal tunnel syndrome of the hand
    - entrapment of the superficial nerve of the thigh
- Diabetes
- Leprosy
- Trauma or surgery to that area
- Spinal disease eg. prolapsed intervertebral disc

REFER so as not to miss any treatable causes

PAIN RADIATING DOWN A LIMB

Causes
- Osteo-arthritis trapping the nerves coming through the spinal foramina
- Prolapsed intervertebral disc (pain radiates down radial side of arm)
- Cervical rib will give pain radiating down the ulnar side of an arm
    - when the person looks strongly in the opposite direction
    - if the neck is flexed strongly away from the area of pain
- Spinal tumours
- Diseases in other organs
    - heart disease giving pain in the left arm
    - gynaecological disease giving pain in one or both legs
- Diabetes

- Tertiary syphilis (tabes dorsalis) which classically gives shooting pain down the limb
    - this condition is rare

Clinical features
- Patients may complain of pain or pins and needles radiating down one or both limbs.
- They may have severe shooting pain down the concerned limb eg. tabes dorsalis.

> **REFER** if you suspect a serious cause.

MENTAL CONFUSION (AND CHANGE IN CONSCIOUSNESS)

This is usually a sign of severe systemic or neurological disease.

Causes

There are many causes.

D - drugs (intoxication and withdrawal)
I - infections e.g. pneumonia, meningitis
M - metabolic e.g. hypoglycaemia, organ failure
T - trauma e.g. chronic subdural haematoma
O - oxygen deprivation e.g. hypoxia, carbon monoxide poisoning
P - pre-existing neurological disease e.g. epilepsy and dementia

NB. It is **vital** to do an urgent blood glucose estimation on **any** patient of **any** age who has acute confusion, to exclude hypoglycaemia.

Acute confusion in the elderly
- This must **not** be considered to be due just to old age or senility
- Very often it is a sign of systemic illness eg.
    - urinary tract infection
    - heart failure
    - drug side effects
- Often the confusion will respond well to correct treatment of the cause.
- Subdural haemorrhage needs to be excluded

Confusion in alcoholics
- It may be due to the alcohol
- It may also be due to more serious causes eg.
    - chronic subdural haemorrhage
    - systemic infection such as meningitis, pneumonia, hypoglycaemia etc.

Emergency treatment
If the most likely cause of the delirium is a medical disorder and if very restless:
- Haloperidol, IM, 5 mg immediately

If alcoholic/ataxic:
- Thiamine IV/IM, 100 mg immediately

If the delirium is caused by seizures or substance withdrawal or if communication is difficult:
- Midazolam, IM, 7.5-15 mg immediately
    - repeat after 30-60 minutes if needed

TREMOR

Patients often do not mention tremors even if severe. They may only be observed by yourself on examination.

Causes
- Drugs, especially alcohol
- Diseases of the cerebellum, especially as a result of alcohol abuse
- Anxiety and stress
- Benign essential tremor

Parkinsonism
- This may be due to the effect of drugs, especially antipsychotics such as haloperidol.
- This may also be due to Parkinson's disease
    - this occurs in older patients
    - they often have dull, expressionless faces and dull, monotonous voices
    - they have difficulty with walking due to rigidity, and do not swing their arms
    - their writing becomes smaller and smaller
    - the tremor of the hand is described as being similar to rolling pills or a cigarette

> **MANAGEMENT**
> - **REFER** any severe tremor
> - Treat any cause you can manage eg. alcohol or anxiety
> - No need to refer if the patient has been investigated previously, unless there is deterioration

DIZZINESS AND FAINTING (SYNCOPE AND BLACKOUT)

Causes

If there is genuine loss of consciousness, serious causes must be looked for.

- Arrhythmias and heart disease
- Epilepsy
- Transient ischaemia of the brain or a full CVA
- Hypoglycaemia
    - sweating, cold extremities and forehead
- Hypertension
- Medicine side effects eg. antihypertensives, tranquillisers, antipsychotics
- Alcoholism
- Severe systemic infections
- Fever
- Gastrointestinal illness eg. gastritis, gastroenteritis
- Prolonged bed rest and getting up too quickly
- Debilitating illnesses
- Prolonged standing
- Anaemia
- Emotional causes eg. anxiety or fear
- Fainting may be precipitated by coughing, micturition or hyperventilation (this is rare)
- Ear disease causing vertigo which may be confused with dizziness
    - for the differential diagnosis of dizziness, see ENT page 20
- Hysteria
    - this occurs particularly in young women

- take care with diagnosis so you don't miss more dangerous causes
- if there is any doubt, **REFER**

Features which may help make the diagnosis of hysteria
- Some stress factor before the collapse
- Falling slowly, usually forwards or sideways
- No evidence of significant injury as result of fall eg. bruises
- Fluttering of the eyelids (rapidly blinking)
- Strong tension keeping the eyelids closed when you attempt to open the eyes
- Unusual neurological symptoms or signs
- Reflexes are not generally brisk in hysteria

MANAGEMENT
- Do a blood glucose estimation if there is any suspicion of hypoglycaemia
- Exclude disease by general examination
- If nothing abnormal is found, reassure the patient that no treatment is required
- Treat the cause if you are able to
- **REFER** if you suspect a serious cause

If you suspect hysteria
- Reassure the patient
- Often getting them to obey commands while doing the physical examination will help them to improve eg.
    - get them to breathe while auscultating their lungs
    - get them to sit up and undress etc.
- Remove them from the source of stress eg. by admission to hospital which may
    - help the problems
    - bring quicker healing and relief
- Violent methods of waking the patient up are cruel
    - eg. slapping or spraying with ethyl chloride

DEMENTIA

Progressive loss of cognitive function usually of slow onset. Initial presentation may be with mild personality and memory changes.

Common reversible causes of dementia

Metabolic:
- Hypothyroidism
- Vit B 12 deficiency
- Pellagra

Medication and drugs
- Long-term alcohol abuse
- Many medications with CNS side effects

Infections
- Neurosyphilis
- HIV dementia

General Measures
- Disclose the diagnosis to family members/primary care giver
- Explain that the condition is evolving and future planning is necessary
- Discuss home safety risks
- Ensure that the patient has a caregiver that can supervise medication taking when the patient is unable to do so him/herself.

THE EYE

PROBLEMS OF THE EYE

INDICATIONS FOR REFERRAL

Useful guidelines which usually suggest that an eye problem is serious:
- Pain or redness in *one eye only*
    - **REFER** unless you can confirm a treatable cause
- Visual acuity that has changed

REFER the following conditions on the same day:
- Complicated foreign bodies (FBs)
    - all FBs older than 36 hours (see page 241)
    - deep penetrating FBs
- Unresponsive conjunctivitis, if no improvement after 4-5 days treatment, and the patient has:
    - pain
    - poor vision
- Sudden visual loss in one or both eyes for which you cannot find an obvious treatable cause
- Trauma with any complication eg.
    - hyphaema (blood in the anterior chamber)
    - poor vision
    - laceration of cornea or sclera
- Chemical burns
- Recent proptosis of one or both eyes
- Squint of recent onset
- Retinal tear or detachment suspected
- Diplopia/double vision
- Shingles affecting the eye

Less urgent REFERRAL
- Eyelashes rubbing on the cornea (trichiasis)
- Eyelids bent into the eye (entropion)
- Eyelids bent out too much (ectropion)
- Any disorder of refraction eg. short sight, long sight etc. which will need referral to an optometrist
- Cataracts
- Slow loss of vision
- Chronic glaucoma
- Long-standing blindness
- Squints (under 2 years of age)
- Diabetics - once a year

When to REFER children
- Leucocoria (white reflex from the pupil)
    - usually due to the presence of a retinoblastoma (tumour of the retina) or cataract
- Enlargement of the eye (buphthalmos / kerato globus) due to:
    - congenital glaucoma
    - acquired glaucoma
- Hazy cornea (corneal oedema)
- Squint at **any** age if not previously investigated by an ophthalmologist
- Excessive tearing (epiphora)
    - sign of glaucoma
    - blocked tear ducts

SYMPTOMS OF EYE PROBLEMS

BILATERAL RED / PAINFUL EYES

Causes
- Viral and secondary bacterial infections
- Primary bacterial infection eg. Haemophilus, Gonococcus
- Anxiety eg. scholars having difficulty studying
- Referred pain from related structures eg.
    - sinus disease
    - nasal disease
    - intracranial disease eg. meningitis
- Trauma which has affected both eyes
- Trachoma (scratchy, gritty eyes)
- Ectropion, especially in the aged, or entropion with trichiasis
- Arc eye (due to welding without protective glasses). This is very painful and is associated with blepherospasm of the eyelids

UNILATERAL RED / PAINFUL EYE

This usually suggests serious disease.

Less serious causes
- Inflamed pinguecula (see page 238)
- Foreign body not embedded
- Infections of the eye lid such as
    - styes
    - infected meibomian cysts
- Phlyctenular conjunctivitis (see page 237)
- Referred pain from
    - local sinus infection
    - nasal disease
- Migraine giving unilateral eye pain
- Cluster headaches

Causes usually needing REFERRAL
- Any doubt as to the cause
- Trauma, unless minor
- Foreign body if embedded
- Corneal ulceration eg.
    - pneumococcal
    - herpes simplex
- Keratitis
- Uveitis
- Acute glaucoma
- Burns eg. chemical, flash

BILATERAL ITCHY EYES

Causes
- Viral infections ("pink eye")
- Allergies especially
    - "hay fever" reaction
    - eye medication
    - eye make-up
- spring catarrh (vernal conjunctivitis)
- Blepharitis

UNILATERAL ITCHY EYE

Causes
- Allergies of the eyelid eg. blepharitis
- Early conjunctivitis with signs only in one eye

DIFFICULTY WITH VISION

This usually suggests serious disease if it occurs suddenly.

Causes

Causes usually needing REFERRAL:
- Trauma - recent or previous
- Cataract
- Diabetes
- Hypertension
- Corneal damage due to infection
- Refractive errors needing referral to an optometrist
    - short sighted
    - long sighted
    - presbyopia (poor vision in the elderly)
- Increased intra-ocular pressure as in glaucoma
- Uveitis
- Trauma
- Glaucoma

Less serious causes
- Stress and anxiety, if no other eye pathology can be found
- Use of atropine drops or "over the counter" whitening drops eg. Eyegene may cause poor accommodation

Clinical features

Symptoms depend on the cause
- Frequent headaches and eye fatigue suggests
    - refractive errors
- Severe headaches with nausea suggests
    - acute glaucoma
- Black spots floating in the eye suggests
    - vitreous opacities
- Gradually diminishing vision in one or both eyes suggests
    - cataract formation or chronic glaucoma
- Bumping into objects and cannot see to the sides of the eyes suggests
    - chronic glaucoma (advanced disease)

MANAGEMENT
- Determine visual acuity accurately in both eyes.
- If the vision is diminished and there is no evidence of cataracts, previous trauma, hypertension, diabetes, etc, then check patient's vision by the pin hole test.

Pin hole test
- Make a hole in a piece of dark paper with a large pin, needle or point of a pen or pencil so that it is about 2 mm wide.
- Ask the patient to look through this hole at the Snellen chart
    - if vision improves, this suggests that the patient has a refractive error and needs glasses
    - if no improvement or it becomes worse, then it is probably due to a cataract or vitreous or retinal disease, and needs to be **REFERRED**.

▼ Note to clinic doctor

If vision does not improve through a pin hole, check for the presence of a red reflex.

Red reflex test

Procedure
- The patient looks past your head.
- The examiner stands about 60 cm away from the patient.
- With the ophthalmoscope at 0 (zero) the examiner keeps it close to his eye and then focuses the beam of light so that it falls on the pupillary area of the cornea.
- In normal individuals, you should be able to see a red or pink colour (reflex) through the pupil
    - this is the retina.

Significance of an absent red reflex
- If there is a history of trauma, the absence of a red reflex is probably due to:
    - retinal detachment
    - a vitreous haemorrhage
- Cataracts - one usually sees
    - black shadows against the red in immature cataracts
    - absence of red reflex in mature cataracts
- In a patient above the age of 50 years with no history of trauma or previous eye disease, an absent red reflex is almost sure to be due to cataract formation (especially with decreased visual acuity).
- If vision is normal in both eyes and all other structures appear normal, then give a placebo like normal saline drops.
- If the patient's vision is 6/12 or better, explain to him what is causing this decreased vision. This will later require treatment, when it begins to interfere seriously with function at home or at work
    - spectacles will not help him in this case
    - he should return when vision is seriously affected.
- In patients with vision of 6/18-6/60
    - **REFER** for treatment.

NB. Associated diabetes or hypertension should be adequately controlled before **REFERRAL** ▲

DOUBLE VISION

Causes
- Damage to the nerves controlling eye movement from intracranial disease
- Hypoglycaemia
- Anxiety
- Myasthenia gravis
- Thyroid eye disease
- Fracture of the orbit with extraocular muscle entrapment

SEEING THINGS MOVING OR FLOATING IN THE EYE ("FLOATERS")

Causes
- May be normal if minor (fleeing flies)
- Post trauma with blood inside the eye
- Vitreous opacities
- Cytomegalovirus (CMV) retinitis seen in advanced HIV disease

SUDDEN FLASHES OF LIGHT

Clinical features
- Usually in the peripheral vision. May be accompanied by the presence of floaters (black spots).
- If sudden in onset, may indicate the presence of a retinal tear that may progress to a retinal detachment.
- Retinal detachment is suspected when the patient complains of a shadow in the peripheral visual field that extends towards the centre of vision.
- This is more common in middle-aged and elderly myopic patients following blunt ocular trauma.

> It is an extremely dangerous condition and needs REFERRAL stat.

STRABISMUS / SQUINT
(CROSS-EYES)

Causes
- An important cause for sudden squinting is neurological disease.

Method of testing for squint
- Shine a light towards the eyes from an arm's length away.
- See if the light reflection is in the same area of the cornea of both eyes.

> **MANAGEMENT**
> **REFER:**
> - Any baby of more than 3 months, whose eyes are not parallel at all times when awake.
> - Any patient who suddenly develops a squint at any stage
>   - REFER stat.

EXCESSIVE LACRIMATION

Causes
- Blocked tear duct
- Any infection in the eye
- Eyelid bent outwards (ectropion) or inwards (entropion)
- Allergies
- Foreign body
- Eye make-up (also due to allergy)
- Effect of eye medication
- Anxiety and emotion (crying)
- Keratitis / corneal ulcer
- Scleritis

DRY EYE

Causes
- Decongestant eye drops
- Old age
- Systemic illnesses eg. Sjögren's disease; rheumatoid arthritis (common problem)
- Vitamin A deficiency
- Tear film deficiencies
- Facial nerve palsy (due to poor lid closure)

SWOLLEN EYELID

This more commonly affects the upper eyelid.

Causes
- Allergies of the eye lid
  - commonly due to eye make-up eg. mascara, eyeliners
- Insect bite near the eye, e.g. mosquito bite
- Infection of the eye lid
  - stye
  - meibomian abscess
  - cellulitis of the eyelid from an infection of the skin near the eyes - common in children with an insect bite
- Following any trauma around the eye
- Severe conjunctivitis, e.g. ophthalmia neonatorum

PERIORBITAL SWELLING

In severe cases swelling may involve the eyelids as well.

Causes
- Orbital cellulitis
  - in this condition there will be severe pain in the eye, and vision and eye movements will be affected
  - proptosis (protrusion of the eye)
  - there may be no obvious external source of infection
  - this is a very serious condition and may extend into the brain and cause a cavernous sinus thrombosis
  - **REFER** stat
- Sinusitis and associated osteomyelitis of a facial bone eg ethmoid bone
  - this can result in the development of an orbital cellulitis
- Trauma
- Allergies e.g. angioedema
- Cellulitis
- Kidney disease
- Thyroid disease

DROOPING EYELID (PTOSIS)

Causes
- Neurological disease, eg. invasion of nerves by carcinomas of the lung or brain
    - this **must** be considered if there is an acute onset of ptosis, and no other obvious cause can be found
    - **REFER**
- Congenital ptosis
    - **REFER** early due to risk of amblyopia (disuse blindness)
- Infection or allergy causing swelling of the eyelid
- Diseases of the muscles of the eye
- Trauma

PHOTOPHOBIA
(SENSITIVE TO BRIGHT LIGHT)

Causes
- Meningitis or other neurological diseases
- Effect of eye medication eg. over the counter eye drops
- Treatment to dilate the pupil eg. Atropine eye drops
- Anxiety
- Post traumatic paralysis of the 3rd nerve causing dilation of the pupil
- Migraine
- Acute glaucoma
- Keratitis
- Dry eye
- Uveitis

DISEASES OF THE EYE

VIRAL CONJUNCTIVITIS
("PINK EYE")

Commonly caused by adenoviral infection. It may be unilateral, but is usually bilateral.

Clinical features
- This is a highly contagious, viral infection which is spread by contact - hands, towels, face cloths
- Itchy eyes
- Sore eyes, feeling of grittiness (roughness) or burning which is often described by patients as being painful
- Photophobia
- Reddened conjunctivae that may become haemorrhagic
- Watery discharge from the eyes
- If the discharge is yellow there is secondary bacterial infection
- There may be swelling of the eyelids
- The cornea, iris and pupil are completely normal
- Normal visual acuity
- There may be preauricular lymphadenopathy
- **If unilateral watch out for:**
    - bacterial conjunctivitis
    - iritis
    - foreign body
    - trauma
    - phlyctenular conjunctivitis (see page 237)
    - keratitis
    - acute glaucoma.

MANAGEMENT
- Apply cold compresses to relieve symptoms

Adults and children 6 years and older
- Instil oxymetazoline drops
    - 1 drop 4 x daily for 5-7 days
- Paracetamol 3-4 x daily, when required
- Advise the patients:
    - not to share towels, face cloths, pillows
    - to wash their hands before and after instilling eye drops
- Contact lenses should not be worn.
- **REFER** if there is:
    - unilateral conjunctivitis for more than 1 day
    - corneal ulceration / haziness
    - pupil irregularity
    - diminished visual acuity
    - severe pain in the eye
    - poor or no response after 4-5 days
- Off work / school according to severity
    - usually 3-5 days, but symptoms can persist for 2-3 weeks.

BACTERIAL CONJUNCTIVITIS

Clinical features
- Mucopurulent discharge from one or both eyes, especially in the morning
- Sticky eyes
- Significant irritation
- Possible swelling of the eyelids
- Redness especially of the conjunctival angles

MANAGEMENT
- Advise the patient to remove crusts and discharge by cleaning the eyes with saline drops or clean warm water.
- Chloramphenicol eye ointment to be applied into the eyes 4-6 hourly for 7 days.
- Paracetamol 3-4 x daily, when required
- Advise the patients:
    - not to share towels, face cloths, pillows
    - to wash their hands before and after applying ophthalmic ointment
- Contact lenses should not be worn.
- **REFER** if there is:
    - unilateral conjunctivitis
    - corneal ulceration / haziness
    - pupil irregularity
    - diminished visual acuity
    - severe pain in the eye
    - poor or no response after 4-5 days
    - copious purulent discharge suggestive of gonococcal disease
    - neonatal conjunctivitis

▼ **Note to doctor**
Patients not responding
- Check for complications such as corneal ulceration by fluoroscein-staining of the cornea.
- Check for iritis.
- **REFER** to ophthalmologist ▲

ALLERGIC CONJUNCTIVITIS

Causes
- Allergy to pollens, grasses, animal fur etc.
- Allergy to eye medication eg. chloramphenicol
- Cosmetics, especially eye make-up

Clinical features
- There may be photophobia
- Bilateral conjunctivitis with itching, irritation and watering.
- Conjunctiva may appear normal or slightly red.
- More severe reactions may result in eyelid swelling and also conjunctival swelling due to oedema (chemosis).
- There may be associated blepharitis (inflammation of eye lid margin) if the allergy is due to applications
    - eg. eye make-up or eye medication.
- It is often associated with allergic rhinitis.

MANAGEMENT
- Remove the cause if possible
- Apply cold compresses to relieve symptoms
- Contact lenses should not be worn

Adults and children 6 years and older
- Oxymetazoline drops: instil 1 drop 4 x daily for 5-7 days.

plus
- Chlorphenamine. oral, at night for 7 days.
If no response within 7 days or if history of recurrent seasonal allergic conjunctivitis, change to:
    - sodium cromoglycate eye drops:
       instil 1 drop
    - 4 x daily (Doctor initiated)
    - use for 1-3 months

plus
- Cetirizine, oral, 10 mg once daily
    - use for 1-3 months

Children 2-6 years
- Chlorphenamine. oral, at night for 7 days
If no response within 7 days or if history of recurrent seasonal allergic conjunctivitis, change to:
    - sodium cromoglycate eye drops:
       instil 1 drop 4 x daily (Doctor initiated)
    - use for 1-3 months

plus
- Cetirizine, oral, 5 mg once daily
    - use for 1-3 months

SPRING CATARRH (VERNAL CONJUNCTIVITIS) / CHRONIC ALLERGIC CONJUNCTIVITIS

Causes
- This occurs mainly during the spring and summer months
    - September to February.
- It is common in children and teenagers
- Allergy to grass, tree pollens and other environmental allergens
- More common in children with a history of atopy eg atopic eczema

Clinical features
- Severe itching and a white discharge
- Conjunctivae commonly have a brown discolouration on the exposed parts
- Tiny silvery-white nodules at the edge of the cornea (Tranta's dots) are often seen
    - more common in black patients.
- The upper palpebral conjunctiva may have flat-topped papillae that give the conjunctiva a cobblestone appearance

MANAGEMENT
Adults and children 6 years and older
- Sodium cromoglycate eye drops: instil 1 drop 4 x daily (Doctor initiated)
    - use may be seasonal for 1-3 months or long term

plus
- Cetirizine, oral, 10 mg once daily
    - use may be seasonal (1-3 months) or long term

Children 2-6 years
- Sodium cromoglycate eye drops: instil 1 drop 4 x daily (Doctor initiated)
    - use may be seasonal for 1-3 months or long term

plus
- Cetirizine, oral, 5 mg once daily
    - use may be seasonal for 1-3 months or long term

- If the condition is severe, **REFER** to ophthalmologist for a short course of steroid eye drops (5 days)

REFER
- Persons wearing contact lenses
- Children under 2 years

▼ **Note to doctor**
- Steroid drops should be reserved for *severe* cases only and for a maximum of 5 days.
- Long-term steroid use can lead to steroid-induced glaucoma and cataracts.▲

PHLYCTENULAR CONJUNCTIVITIS

Causes
- Can be due to an allergic reaction in the eye to the presence of TB elsewhere in the body
- It is seen most commonly in children with primary tuberculosis (non-cavitatory type)
- It may also occur as a reaction to
    - Staphylococcal infection
    - seborrhoeic dermatitis

Clinical features
- Presents as a small, yellow or white nodule bordering on the corneal margin.
- There are localised inflamed blood vessels radiating away from the nodule

MANAGEMENT
- Exclude the diagnosis of tuberculosis on:
    - history
    - examination
- **Do not do a PPD test** as this condition is a hypersensitivity manifestation of primary tuberculosis
    - a PPD test may result in a severe conjunctival reaction leading to corneal ulceration and perforation.
- **REFER** for chest X-ray to establish whether or not hilar glands are present.
- If TB excluded, treat with
    - chloramphenicol eye ointment
      3 x daily for 7 days.

OPHTHALMIA NEONATORUM

Causes
It is not always easy to decide on the specific cause.
- Gonococcal infection
- Chlamydial infection

Clinical features
- Features which suggest gonococcal infection are:
  - maternal history of a purulent vaginal discharge
  - onset within 4 days of birth
  - profuse purulent discharge, often associated with severe oedema of the eyelids
- Features which suggest chlamydial infection are:
  - onset after the 4th day
  - slight watery or mildly purulent discharge
  - mildly inflamed conjunctivae
  - pneumonia
- The mother may complain that the baby's eyes are sticky

MANAGEMENT
- Pus under the eyelids is destructive.
- It can destroy the cornea and result in:
  - perforation
  - intra-ocular infection
  - blindness
- It is imperative that the pus is washed out as soon as possible.
- **REFER** for admission, to ensure adequate irrigation.

Profuse purulent discharge and/or swollen eyelids and / or corneal haziness
- Ceftriaxone 50 mg/kg IM stat
- Eye irrigation hourly until referral
- **REFER** to hospital

Eye irrigation
- Normal saline or sterile water can be used.
- Use a dropper or wet cotton-wool and wash beneath both the upper and lower eyelids.
- Cleanse immediately and then hourly until referral.

NB. *The mother should be advised that she herself is infected, and that both she and her partner need treatment.*

Mild purulent discharge, eyelids not swollen, no corneal haziness
- Ceftriaxone 50 mg/kg IM stat
- Chloramphenicol eye ointment applied 4 x daily for 7 days
- Review daily until discharge has cleared
- **REFER** if no improvement within 2 days

Sticky eyelids, no purulent discharge
- Chloramphenicol eye ointment applied 3 x daily

INFLAMED PINGUECULA

A pingueculum is a heaping-up or thickening of the conjunctiva usually medial to the cornea.

Causes
- Chronic irritation from atmospheric pollutants and sunlight

Clinical features
- It is usually pale or slightly yellow in colour.

Complications
- It may become the site of conjunctival infection.
- A pingueculum may grow over the cornea forming a pterygium which may:
  - affect the eyesight by approaching the pupillary area
  - cause drying out of the cornea by preventing it from getting wet by tears.

MANAGEMENT
No treatment is required unless:
- The lesion is overgrowing the cornea
  - **REFER** for surgery.
- It is inflamed
  - treat with chloramphenicol eye ointment 3 x daily
  - the patient should be encouraged to wear spectacles or dark glasses.

Note. Encourage the patient to wear dark glasses whenever exposed to the sun.

CORNEAL ULCERATION

Ulcers are usually due to a underlying cause such as trauma and poor nutrition:

Causes
- Traumatic, especially a foreign body
- Infective eg.
  - herpes simplex keratitis
  - pneumococcal keratitis
- Exposure keratitis eg. in an unconscious patient
- Contact lenses, especially soft contact lenses, worn for too long
- Often associated with lowered immunity and lowered nutrition (especially lack of Vitamin A). This tends to occur:
  - in alcoholics
  - in a child who is deficient in Vitamin A and has measles. This may cause such a severe corneal ulceration that it results in perforation and blindness
  - AIDS

Clinical features
- Decreased visual acuity
- Photophobia
- Lacrimation
- Unilateral pain and redness
- Conjunctival discharge
- There may be associated hypopyon (pus in the anterior chamber)
- Enlarged blood vessels in the conjunctiva next to the ulcer
- Staining the cornea with fluorescein will make the ulcer more easily visible. When examined with cobalt blue light of the ophthalmoscope, ulcer or corneal epithelial defect stains green.

Complications
- Visual impairment or blindness as a result of:
  - corneal scarring
  - intra-ocular infection
- Corneal perforation with prolapse of the iris
  - this is often missed unless you routinely check the shape of the pupil

- in perforation, the pupil will be an inverted tear-drop shape towards the area of perforation
- Secondary iritis

> **MANAGEMENT**
> - If you suspect this condition **REFER.**
> - If referral is deferred and a culture cannot be done within 12 hours:
> - Chloramphenicol 1% eye ointment applied 6 hourly
> - Pad the eye.

TYPES OF CORNEAL ULCERATION

■ HERPES SIMPLEX KERATITIS

Clinical features
- This is more common than the bacterial causes of keratitis (inflammation of the cornea).
- There may be a history or evidence of recent lip vesicles.
- One or more irregular, superficial branching (dendritic) ulcers may be seen, especially if the eye is stained with fluoroscein.
    - **OR** round dull swollen area in the central cornea (disciform keratitis)

> **REFER** to ophthalmologist for:
> - Topical acyclovir ointment
> - Possible debridement of corneal epithileum

■ PNEUMOCOCCAL KERATITIS

Clinical features
- It is a well-circumscribed, larger, central grey ulcer.
- Hypopyon (pus in the anterior chamber) is often present.

> **REFER** if you suspect it.

■ ARC EYE

This is due to exposure to excess ultra violet light.

Clinical features
- It commonly occurs in people who have been welding without adequate eye protection.
- They complain of severely painful eyes and photophobia some hours later.
- The conjunctivae are inflamed.

> **MANAGEMENT**
> - Instil tetracaine 0.5% drops immediately
> - Rest the eyes eg. use dark glasses.
> - Insert chloromycetin eye ointment 3 x daily plus tear substitutes.
> - Give analgesics.
> - Use proper tinted goggles when welding.

Note. Local anaesthetic eye drops block the eye defenses and may result in more damage. They should **never** be given to patients to take home.

UVEITIS

This is inflammation of the iris and ciliary body anteriorly and / or the choroid posteriorly.

- The most common form is idiopathic (unknown cause).
- Numerous systemic diseases can cause uveitis. Included among them are rheumatoid arthritis, sarcoidosis, tuberculosis, syphilis, Reiter's syndrome, toxoplasmosis, chlamydial infection, gonorrhoea.
- Uveitus causes photophobia, ocular pain and sometimes visual blurring.
- The physical signs include:
    - circumcorneal conjunctival inflammation
    - a small pupil which may be irregular due to the formation of posterior synechiae
    - hypopyon may be present
    - decreased visual acuity, often <6/18, especially if the choroid or retina is affected or with exudation into the vitreous cavity
- Complications include secondary glaucoma and secondary cataract.

> **REFER** to ophthalmologist immediately.

GLAUCOMA

Glaucoma involves damage to the optic nerve and visual field loss caused by an increase in intra-ocular pressure.

ACUTE CLOSED ANGLE GLAUCOMA

Clinical features
- Acute onset of extremely severe, piercing pain
- A unilateral, temporal headache, after being exposed to a period of darkness eg. cinema
- This causes:
    - dilation of the pupil
    - obstruction to the flow of intra-ocular fluid into the canal of Schlemm (drainage system)
- There is nausea and vomiting in severe cases
    - it may even be confused with an acute abdomen
- Sudden decreased visual acuity within hours
- Coloured haloes around lights (bright rings)
- It is unilateral
- There is congestion around the cornea (circumcorneal congestion)
    - cornea gives a hazy or cloudy appearance rather like steam behind a window
- The pupil is mid-dilated, oval, non-reactive
- The eye feels hard, compared with the other eye, when measured with finger palpation
    - this is not an accurate test
- Visual field loss.

> **MANAGEMENT**
> - **REFER** stat.
> - Give acetazolamide oral (Diamox) 500 mg, immediately followed by 250 mg 6 hourly.
> - If pupil is dilated, instil pilocarpine 1% drops ¼ hourly x 4 doses, starting 1 hour after giving acetazolamide.

▼ **Note to doctor**
- If a Schiotz tonometer is available, it may be used to measure the eyeball pressure, if there is any doubt about the diagnosis
- The mean normal intra-ocular pressure by Schiotz tonometer is 16,1 mm Hg (± 2,8).
- The eye should first be anaesthetised with tetracaine 0,5% ▲

OPEN ANGLE GLAUCOMA

This is an extremely common cause of blindness in people over the age of 40.

If it is diagnosed early it can be treated effectively.

Delay in diagnosis results in:
- irreversible damage to the retina
- progressive visual loss

Clinical features

It is more likely if:
- there is a family history of glaucoma
- the person has myopia or diabetes

- The disease has **few** or **no** symptoms.
- It is commonly only detected at an advanced stage.
- Bumping into objects due to loss of peripheral field vision
    - advanced disease.
- Patients are usually over 40 years old but in the black population, it may present earlier.
- Visual field changes: tunnel vision
- Glaucomatous cupping of the optic disc
    - this will only be seen by those who are skilled in examining the optic nerve with an ophthalmoscope
- Visual acuity remains normal until the intra-ocular pressure is grossly increased.
- Intraocular pressure may be raised or normal.
- As the disease is often asymmetrical, there is often a difference in pupil reactions between the two eyes.

> **MANAGEMENT**
> - If there is *any suspicion* of glaucoma the patient must be **REFERRED** for accurate testing.
> - Patients over the age of 35 years should be encouraged to have eye pressure tested routinely if possible
>   - eg. when going to opticians to buy glasses.
> - Any patient over the age of 30 with a unilateral visual acuity <6/18 should be referred for glaucoma assessment.
> - Patients who have been put onto maintenance therapy with specific drugs which decrease intra-ocular pressure such as acetazolamide (Diamox) or Timolol eye drops must:
>   - be encouraged to take their treatment regularly
>   - keep to their hospital appointments.

- Care must be taken in giving them any other medications or tablets as this might make the glaucoma worse e.g. antihistamine, amitriptylline and other tricyclic antidepressants.

EYE INJURY

CHEMICAL BURNS

This is an emergency. Chemical burns, especially alkali (eg. cement) or acids, can cause serious eye damage.

Clinical features
- Pain
- Inability to open eyes
- Blurred vision
- Blindness
- Excessive tearing

> **MANAGEMENT**
>
> *Immediate action is necessary as follows:*
> - Irrigate the eye with **large** amounts of water.
> - Try to get the patient under a tap and hold the eye lids open while the water pours continuously into the eye
>   - for at least 20 minutes
>   - for longer in a severe alkaline burn
> - It is important to remove any particles.
> - If this is very painful
>   - instil 1 drop tetracaine 1% local anaesthetic eye drops into the affected eye
>   - **or** if unavailable ordinary lignocaine, 2-3 ml
>   - then try to irrigate again.
>
> **Note.** Local anaesthetic eye drops should never be given as a TTO (the anaethetised eye cannot protect itself against damage).
>
> - After the urgent thorough irrigation, obtain a more detailed history.
> - It is important to find out exactly what splashed into the eye
>   - acid
>   - or alkali (this is far more damaging).
> - Examine the eyes and determine visual acuity
> - Adequate irrigation of the eye is vital in preventing serious damage to the eye
>   - it must be done **before REFERRAL,** to prevent ongoing damage
>   - if possible irrigate with normal saline attached to a drip set.
> - Chloramphenicol 1% eye ointment, applied stat before **REFERRAL.**

TRAUMA TO THE EYE

How to examine a traumatised eye
- When an eye is traumatised, many different parts may be damaged.
- It is vital to adequately examine all parts of the eye when assessing the severity of the injury.
- With severe trauma, the eyelids are often so swollen that examination of the eyeball is difficult.

First step
- Palpate the full circumference of the orbital margin - it should be clearly felt.
- A possible fractured orbit will be shown by:
    - acute tenderness on one particular point of the orbital margin
    - the presence of a notch in the margin on palpation
    - double vision.

Second step
If palpation of the orbit is normal, then the next step is to examine the eye itself.

If the lids are very oedematous do the following:
- Instil tetracaine 0,5% local anaesthetic eye drops into the swollen eye.
- Take 2 paper clips (Gem clips) and bend the rounded end over to make a U-shape.
- Use the clips as retractors to pull the swollen eyelids open, so that the eyeball can be seen.
- Check vision (visual acuity). If there is a difference try and establish whether:
    - it is related to this episode of trauma
    - there was a difference previously.
- Check if the cornea is clear.
- Check specifically for blood in the anterior chamber (hyphaema) as noted by a dark, fluid level in the lowest part of the anterior chamber, behind the cornea.

If there has been a fracture of one of the orbital bones, the eye muscles may get caught in the pieces.

This can be checked by testing for any double vision, or limitation in movement of the eyes in any direction.
- Get the patient to follow a sharp object eg. a pencil being moved in all 6 directions ie. up, down, horizontally to each side, and then obliquely in all directions.
- Ask the patient if there is double vision in any direction
    - this suggests muscle damage.
- Watch each of the eye's movements to note any limitation of movement.
- If you need 2 hands to hold the swollen lids open, an assistant may be needed to shine the light on the cornea and to move the pencil around.
- If there is any doubt, the patient should be brought back in 1 week to check the eye movements again.
- Nerves may also be caught in the fracture
    - this causes loss of sensation in the cheek.

Check the pupils as they are often useful in assessing intra-ocular trauma
- The pupils should be clear and perfectly circular.
- They should react well and equally to light.
- If there is any abnormality it suggest serious damage.

Red reflex test
- Check the red reflex if possible (see page 234).

MANAGEMENT
REFER if there is:
- Acute change in vision in any eye to 6/12 or less on the Snellen chart
- Lid laceration
- Laceration, perforation or diffuse damage of the cornea or sclera
- Blood in the anterior chamber (hyphema)
- Unequal, irregular or sluggish (slow reacting) pupils
- Limitation of movement of the eyes
- Visual abnormalities

Treatment at the clinic
- If there is marked photophobia or haematoma
    - give choramphenicol eye ointment to be applied 6 hourly.
- Do not use an eye pad with haematoma, lid oedema or bleeding
    - Use an eye shield only

FOREIGN BODY (FB)

If a patient complains of a foreign body, their complaint should be taken seriously.
- If the FB is translucent (can see through it), it may be missed on examination.
- It will only be seen on the cornea if the light is shone from the side
    - **or** if the cornea is stained with fluoroscein.
- The FB may be lodged under the upper eye lid
    - it is, therefore, **essential** to examine the upper conjunctiva if you suspect an FB.
- A particularly dangerous type of FB is when a flake of metal comes off a hammer, chopper or a grinding stone and is travelling at high speed when it enters the eye
    - it may penetrate deep into the eye
    - to begin with there will be no symptoms or signs
    - some time later there will be symptoms and extensive damage.
- The patient must be **REFERRED** for X-ray.

How to examine the upper conjunctiva
- It is **very important** to make sure that the patient keeps looking down **all the time.**
- Grasp the eyelashes between finger and thumb and pull downwards
    - at the same time press down on the upper eyelid with a match, the point of a pen, or a finger
    - this is held horizontally across the eyelid, to get above the cartilage in the upper eyelid.
- Flip the eyelid upwards.
- The eyelid should turn inside out (evert) and the superior fornix can now be seen.

MANAGEMENT
- If needed, only to remove the foreign body, tetracaine 1% eye drops 1 drop instilled into the affected eye
- If the foreign body is on the sclera or conjunctiva and not embedded
    - it can be removed with a corner of a piece of gauze, handkerchief, or a cotton wool bud.
- If the FB is on the cornea or embedded
    - **REFER.**
- If you cannot see the FB, but there is a clear history of injury
    - **REFER** for X-ray as this may be the only way of detecting a deep-seated, metallic FB
    - **REFER** urgently to opthalmologist.

▼ **Note to doctor**

If the foreign body is on the cornea:
- Insert a couple of drops of tetracaine 0,5% local anaesthetic into the eye
    - this can be repeated after a minute or two.

- Obtain good magnification if possible eg.
  - by wearing a Berger's Loupe
  - by using a magnifying glass
    on the auroscope
    or ophthalmoscope.
- Lie the patient down and ask him to keep both eyes open and to fix his vision on a particular spot
  - on the ceiling if lying down
    (which is easier)
  - **or** on the wall if sitting up.
- Try to remove the FB with a cotton wool bud first.
- If this fails, then usually the FB can be easily lifted out with a 25 gauge needle from the side, not from the front.
- Once the FB is out, look to see if there is a residual rust ring.
- If so, attempt to scratch it away with the needle point.
- If successful
  - insert an eye ointment
    (either tetracycline or
    Chloromycetin)
  - pad the eye.
- The eye should remain padded for about 12 hours, until the local anaesthetic has worn off. This is because an an aesthetised eye has no reflexes to protect it from dust or other FBs.
- If the rust ring cannot be removed adequately, the eye should be padded and the patient **REFERRED** within a day or two
  - it is often easier to remove the rust ring the next day ▲

HERPES ZOSTER OPHTHALMICUS

Clinical features
- Vesicular rash involving skin of forehead and periorbital.
- Rash stops abruptly at the midline.
- Ocular involvement includes conjunctivitis, kerato-uveitis and ocular cranial nerve palsies.
- High rate of HIV positivity in patients younger than 50 years presenting with this condition.
- Permanent sequelae may include chronic ocular inflammation, loss of vision, and debilitating pain.

> **MANAGEMENT**
> - Acyclovir, oral, 800 mg 5 x daily for 7 days.
> - Give oral anagesic eg. paracetamol.
> - Give antibiotic if secondarily infected.
> - For neuralgic pain:
>   - amitriptyline, oral, 25 mg at night for 1-3 months
> - **REFER** all patients for exclusion of ocular complications mentioned above.
>
> Note:
> - Patients need to be counselled that an HIV test will be one of the investigations done.

CATARACT

A cataract is an opacity of the lens of the eye. It most commonly occurs due to old age, but may occur earlier in patients with diabetes or trauma to the eye.

Clinical features
- Gradual onset of loss of vision (although more sudden following trauma).
- Absence of pain.
- Absence of red reflex: a dark shadow or complete block of the red reflex.
- A normal pupil reflex should be present.

> **REFER** to ophthalmologist for surgery; urgent referral if patient has bilateral dense cataracts.

EYE ABSCESSES

EXTERNAL HORDEOLUM (STYE)

This is an abscess of the follicle of an eyelash.

Clinical features
- It is situated at the **outer** edge of the eyelid
  - it differs from a meibomian abscess which is situated in the **body** of the eyelid.

> **MANAGEMENT**
> **Warm compresses**
> - These warm the area and encourage the pus to come to the surface.
>
> **Other management**
> - Pulling out the eyelash at the abscess can help the pus drain out.
> - Apply chloramphenicol eye ointment.
> - Apply an eye pad with 2 oblique strips of sticky tape.

MEIBOMIAN ABSCESS

This is an abscess of the meibomian gland, which is situated on the inner surface of the eyelids, beneath the cartilage plate.

Clinical features
- An acutely tender swelling in the middle of the eyelid
- There is typically a history of acute onset of pain and swelling in the last two days.

> **REFER** for incision and drainage.

CHALAZION

Clinical features
- This is similar to a meibomian abscess except there is a longer history.
- There is no pain or tenderness.
- The content is not pus but thick material.

> - **REFER** if it is worrying the patient, for possible surgery.
> - Treatment is not urgent.

THE SKIN

PROBLEMS OF THE SKIN

ASSESSMENT OF RASHES

Skin rashes

- Skin rash is a very common symptom, particularly in children.
- Rashes are often difficult to diagnose and more than one skin disease may occur in the same rash eg.
    - scabies with associated impetigo
    - contact dermatitis due to applications.
- It is useful to decide whether the rash is due to
    - local factors eg. applications
    - systemic illness of the body, that shows on the skin eg. measles.

History

- A careful history is important.
- Systemic causes will often give general symptoms
    - eg. fever and symptoms in other systems of the body.
- The patient may associate the onset with a specific incident eg.
    - the history of applications
    - new cosmetics
    - soaps
    - food

Examination of the skin

- Examination of the whole skin is important in diagnosing the rash.
- Patients will be reluctant to undress completely
    - use care and tact and ensure adequate privacy
    - cover one area of the body with a blanket, or some of the patient's clothes, while examining another area
    - try and ensure patients do not get cold, while you are examining them.
- Rashes due to applications will only be in an area where they can be easily applied eg. face, lower arms, legs, front of the chest (ie. localised).
- A generalised rash, especially if symmetrical, suggests a systemic cause.
- Remember to check the mouth for a rash that may be due to
    - a systemic illness (eg. syphilis, viral rashes)
    - drug reactions (eg. Stephens Johnson syndrome).

General examination

- It is important as well, to do a general examination to detect signs of systemic illness eg.
    - enlarged liver or spleen
    - lymphadenopathy
    - weight loss
    - pallor
    - cyanosis
    - clubbing
    - urine changes
    - pyrexia
    - chronic cough
    - jaundice
    - tachycardia
- This is particularly important, as AIDS patients may present initially with only a skin rash
- In adults and older children it is important to check the genitalia to exclude syphilis as a cause of the rash
    - secondary syphilitic rashes are common
    - they may look like many other types of rashes
- For your own protection, it is best to use gloves when examining rashes
    - which are infected
    - where you suspect syphilis or AIDS

MANAGEMENT

What to do if you are unsure of the diagnosis

REFER if:
- You suspect a serious cause
- No response to treatment
- There are systemic symptoms or signs of illness
- The rash is petechial or haemorrhagic
    - eg. meningococcal septicaemia
- If you suspect
    - a drug reaction
    - a severe allergy
    - an anaphylactic type reaction

If you do not think the cause is serious

- If none of the above conditions apply, many eczematous diseases of the skin improve by being kept moist
    - try ung emulsificans ointment (UE) which is safe
    - observe the response.
- Itchiness can often be controlled by advising the patient to cool the skin by applying wet cloths.

RASHES IN NEONATES AND INFANTS

It is very important in neonates to exclude systemic illness causing rashes.

CONGENITAL SYPHILIS

Clinical features
- Rash, of the palms and soles, particularly with peeling, must be thought to be due to congenital syphilis until proved otherwise.
- With any rash look for other signs of syphilis eg.
    - hepato-splenomegaly
    - snuffles (profuse, watery, frothy, sometimes blood-stained nasal discharge)
    - condylomata lata.
- Check the mother's syphilis blood tests and if positive whether she was treated properly.

Differential diagnosis
- Post mature infants
    - they will have peeling of the whole body and not just of the palms and soles.

MANAGEMENT
- **REFER** if you suspect a syphilitic skin rash, as these babies need to be investigated to exclude neurological syphilis
- Remember to advise the mother and her contact
    - they must be treated or re-treated as necessary.

MILIARIA (HEAT RASH)

Clinical features
- Small papulo vesicles surrounded by redness on the face and upper chest in neonates
    - these start to dry up and form crusts
- The child is otherwise well.
- There may be a history of dressing the child in too many clothes.

MANAGEMENT
- Reassurance.
- Do not overdress the child.
- Advise to avoid harmful applications eg. petroleum jelly (Vaseline).
- Give aqueous cream (ung emulsificans aquosum UEA) if the mother is anxious to have an application.

CONTACT DERMATITIS

Clinical features
- A history of application of lotions, oils (baby oils), rarely petroleum jelly (Vaseline), glycerine, "Hartman's druppels".
- Ask the patient specifically about applications of cosmetics, hair-dyes, soaps (eg. Lifebuoy, Tetmosol), disinfectants (eg. Dettol)
    - these commonly cause localised rashes.
- Distribution will be where the application has been applied
    - this is commonly on the child's face.
- The rash may be worse
    - in the morning if the application was applied at night
    - after the child gets hot and sweats.
- The rash may be inflamed and itchy with fine papules or vesicles
    - or if more chronic, scaly with hyper- or hypo-pigmentation.

MANAGEMENT
- Advise to avoid all applications unless prescribed.
- If the mother is anxious to have some medication
    - give ung emulsificans
- Prescribe steroid cream / ointment if the rash is severe.

NAPPY RASH

Causes
- Irritation from sodden and soiled nappies being left on for too long
- Use of waterproof pants to cover the nappy
- Diarrhoeal stools
- Washing powder enzymes and fabric softeners
- Secondary infection from candida (thrush)
- Other skin diseases (check other areas also)
    - psoriasis
    - seborrhoeic dermatitis

Clinical features
Irritant dermatitis
- Red patchy rash, sometimes with erosions, limited to upper thighs, pubic area and genitalia, but not the flexures (genitocrural folds and natal cleft).
- Due to irritation from moisture, urine breakdown products and faecal enzymes.

Candida dermatitis
The rash is bright red and raw.

There may be papules and pustules located away from the main area of the rash (satellite lesions).

The rash usually extends into the skin folds.

There may be evidence of thrush in the mouth.

Allergic dermatitis
Allergy to the chemicals in nappy cream, soaps or laundry detergents, perfumes. It can occur anywhere the allergen touches the skin.

MANAGEMENT
- Change soiled nappies as soon as possible.
- The use of a barrier ointment will help if it is an irritant or allergic dermatitis e.g.
    - zinc and castor oil ointment
    - white soft paraffin
- Treat candidiasis if you suspect that it is present
    - use an imidazole cream e.g. clotrimazole 2% under the barrier cream
    - in addition it may be advisable to prescribe nystatin oral suspension, 1 ml 4 x daily for 5 days
- If you suspect another skin disease e.g. seborrhoeic dermatitis treat for that condition specifically.

COMMON CHILDHOOD RASHES

PAPULAR AND MACULO-PAPULAR RASHES

STREPTOCOCCAL INFECTION (SCARLET FEVER)

Clinical features
- A diagnostic feature is a red throat and exudate on the tonsils which may be follicular or membranous.
- This however may be mild and therefore easily missed clinically.
- The rash is diffuse, finely papular and has a sandpaper feel
    - there is often skin erythema
- The rash is most intense in the axillae, groins and base of the neck, face.
- There may be an associated
    - strawberry tongue (coated tongue with red papillae protruding)
    - petechiae on the palate

Genital and perianal infections in small children
- Well-defined erythema with scaling or weeping around the anus or vaginal introitus or on the prepuce.

> **MANAGEMENT**
> - Treat for the streptococcal tonsillitis with penicillin VK 2 x daily for 10 days
>   - 1-9 years 250 mg
>   - 10 years and older 500 mg
> - Aqueous cream can be applied to the rash if the mother strongly wishes to have a skin application

RUBELLA (GERMAN MEASLES)

Clinical features
- An erythematous maculopapular rash
- The patient will tell you that it started behind the ears and spread over the face and upper body.
- There may be mild conjunctivitis and fever before the onset of the rash (prodrome).
- A diagnostic feature is significantly enlarged occipital lymph glands
    - this only occurs in 70% of patients.
- Children may normally have mildly enlarged occipital glands
    - these must not be confused with those of rubella which are much larger and more obvious.

> **MANAGEMENT**
> - Treatment is symptomatic only
> - The important management is to advise the escort to keep the child away from
>   - women who are pregnant
>   - women who are in their child-bearing age.
>
> **REFER**
> - Pregnant women with rubella.
> - Pregnant women who have been in contact with a patient with rubella.

MEASLES

Clinical features
- It looks very much like a severe upper respiratory tract infection for the first 3 days (prodrome)
    - severe conjunctivitis with photophobia
    - severe rhinitis
    - high temperature
    - ill-looking child
    - dry barking cough due to a laryngotracheo-bronchitis
- The diagnostic feature is the appearance of Koplik's spots (small white spots, the size of a pinhead)
- Koplik's spots are seen before the generalised rash appears
    - on the inner lining of the cheeks (buccal mucosa)
    - on the gums.
- The rash starts behind the ears and spreads over the face and body
    - it is a reddish rash of papules and macules which join together (become confluent)
- It is not always easy to be sure of the diagnosis
    - but it is important to always check for Koplik's spots.

> **MANAGEMENT**
> - The most important treatment is to **prevent** measles
>   - encourage mothers to have their children immunised.
> - The mothers should be encouraged to keep the child's nutrition and resistance high. This lessens
>   - the effect of measles if the child should become infected
>   - the complications and possibility of death.
> - Vitamin A has been shown to have an important effect in reducing complications
>   - encourage yellow vegetables in the diet
>   - give Vitamin A 200 000 iu orally stat (100 000 iu if child under 12 months)
> - Paracetamol may be given for a very high fever with distress.
> - Antibiotics are not to be used routinely
>   - only give if the child needs them (otitis media, bronchopneumonia).
> - It is important to **notify** the health authorities of all patients with measles.
>
> **Indications for REFERRAL**
> - All adults
> - Children <6 months of age
> - Children with lowered resistance due to
>   - HIV disease
>   - malnutrition
>   - tuberculosis
> - A very ill child
> - Serious complications of measles eg.
>   - bronchopneumonia
>   - neurological symptoms or signs eg. confusion
>   - dehydration or severe gastroenteritis
>   - stridor / croup

ALLERGIC RASH

Clinical features
- This rash will be typically itchy.
- There may be a history of the rash being associated with
    - the use of a medicine, e.g. penicillin
    - a food
- There may be a history of a previous similar episode.
- The rash may be red, itchy, papular.
- Wheals may occur (raised, itchy, circumscribed lesions larger than papules).
- There may be signs of scratching.
- There may be other features of allergy eg.
    - wheezes
    - oedema of the face.

> **MANAGEMENT**
> - Treat as for allergic reactions (see page 7) if
>   - the rash is severe
>   - the child has any systemic features eg. oedema, difficulty with breathing, wheezes, severe itching.
> - If mild, treat with an antihistaminic eg. chlorpheniramine 3 x daily for 3 days.
>   - Note: oral antihistamines are contra-indicated in children under 2 years of age
> - Aqueous cream or Calamine lotion may bring relief.
> - Advise to apply wet cloths to relieve severe itching.
> - Advise the escort about avoiding the medication in future.
> - Give the child a "medic alert" bracelet if you suspect a medicine as the cause of the rash (eg. penicillin).
> - If there is doubt about whether it is due to penicillin, a RAST blood test can help confirm the diagnosis.

SCABIES

> For clinical features and management see pages 255-256.

VESICULAR RASHES

There are many causes for a vesicular rash in children.

CHICKENPOX (VARICELLA)

It is due to the Herpes zoster virus.

Clinical features
- General malaise and fever precede the rash (prodrome).
- The rash of chickenpox has different stages, all occurring together at the same time.
- The rash starts as a papule which becomes a superficial vesicle.
- A valuable diagnostic sign of chickenpox is
    - the whole top of the vesicle collapses inwards, (rather like a baked cake which has flopped and collapsed in the middle)
    - this is called "umbilication"
    - the centre of this vesicle becomes black and crusted.
- If there is doubt about the diagnosis, it is useful to carefully search the child's body for a vesicle which has become umbilicated and scabbed
    - this will help confirm the diagnosis of chickenpox.
- Some vesicles may evolve into pustules.
- The rash of chickenpox is mainly on the trunk and face, and minimally on the lower arms and legs.
- The individual is infective until all the lesions have crusted.
- The duration of the infection is about 1 week.

> **MANAGEMENT**
> - Aspirin, or any compound containing aspirin, must **not** be used as it may cause Reye's syndrome which may cause hepatic encephalopathy and death.
> - Paracetamol may be used if the child has fever with distress.
> - Calamine lotion can be used
>   - it helps to relieve itch by cooling the skin
>   - the escort should, however, be advised that it is extremely poisonous if swallowed
> - For the itch, give chlorphenamine oral 3 x daily
>   - dosage according to age
>   - do not use in children under 2 years of age
>   - treat until the skin crusts have dropped off and the itch has subsided
> - Give acyclovir 4 x daily orally for 7 days, dosage according to age for:
>   - all severe cases
>   - immune-compromised patients
>   - adults and adolescents presenting within 24 hours of the onset of the rash
>
> **REFER**
> - Severely ill patients
> - Complications such as:
>   - pneumonia
>   - meningo-encephalitis
> - Pregnant women
> - Neonates with clinical chickenpox
> - Asymptomatic neonates whose mothers had chickenpox 7 days before or after delivery

HERPES ZOSTER

For clinical features and management see page 251-252.

NUTRITIONAL SKIN DISEASES

KWASHIORKOR

See also Gastrointestinal System page 113.

Skin lesions
- Similar to pellagra, only it occurs in both exposed and unexposed areas.
- Areas of hyper-pigmentation, peeling, hypo-pigmentation, ulceration, cracks.
- Can look similar to burns if severe.
- The buttocks and perineum are often involved in toddlers.
- The hair is sparse, straight, thin and easily pulled out.
- The hair often undergoes a colour change
    - reddish or grey.

MANAGEMENT
- **REFER** if:
    - the dermatitis is weeping
    - the child is ill.
- **REFER** stat if there are any poor prognostic signs
    - hypothermia
    - jaundice
    - severe infections
    - hepato-splenomegaly.
- Milder cases of kwashiorkor can be handled at the clinics.
- The most important aspect of the treatment is the diet (see management of malnutrition page 113).

PELLAGRA

Pellagra occurs mainly in areas where the staple food is maize.

Causes
- Deficiency of nicotinic acid, brought about by:
    - starvation
    - unbalanced diet
    - alcoholism

Clinical features
- Dermatitis - peeling dark areas with fine, irregular cracks ("crazy paving") that affect the sun-exposed parts of the skin eg.
    - back of the hands
    - neck
- The skin may ulcerate
- Dementia ie. mental changes and confusion
- Diarrhoea

MANAGEMENT
- Ordinary balanced diet.
- Give nicotinic acid (Nicotinamide) 100 mg daily orally.
- Give Vitamin B Co 1 tab 2-3 x daily.
- The skin lesions do not require specific treatment unless secondary infections are present.

SCURVY

Causes
- Due to a lack of Vitamin C in the diet

Clinical features
- Most common in alcoholics.
- There are spongy gums which bleed readily.
- Purpuric lesions occur in the skin and mucous membranes.
- Bleeding into the back of the thighs.
- The patient, especially a child, may present with a limp.

MANAGEMENT
- Oranges and green vegetables must be eaten.
- Give Vitamin C 1 tab (100 mg) 3 x daily.
- The patient recovers with this treatment in 3-4 weeks in uncomplicated cases.

BACTERIAL CONDITIONS

IMPETIGO

Causes
- Staphylococcus aureus
- Beta-haemolytic streptococcus
- Usually by both

Clinical features
- Most common in children.
- It may be contagious.
- It may follow minor trauma, eczema or scabies.
- It may start spontaneously in children with lowered resistance.
- The lesions start as superficial, thin-walled vesicles which soon rupture to exude a serous or pussy exudate
    - this dries to form honey-coloured crusts.
- The lesions enlarge and spread rapidly
    - the remains of the vesicles are usually visible around the edges of the crusts.
- Spread to other areas is common and results from scratching.
- Impetigo often starts around the nose because many people carry Staphylococci there.
- Other common sites are:
    - the scalp (often secondary to either ringworm or lice in the scalp)
    - the buttocks (usually secondary to scabies)
    - the arms and legs.
- The lesions are usually multiple.
- Enlargement of regional lymph nodes is often a feature.

MANAGEMENT

- Cephalexin or flucloxacillin 4 x daily for 5 days, dosage according to age.
- **Or** if penicillin-allergic azithromycin daily for 3 days, dosage according to age
- Polyvidone iodine (Betadine) cream or ointment
    - apply 2-3 x daily
- Larger, moist areas are dressed with Betadine solution
- Separate towels, toilet articles and clothing must be used to stop the spread of infection.
- Treat any associated cause eg. scabies.

ECTHYMA ("VELD SORES")

This is a bacterial infection of the skin.

Clinical features

- This occurs particularly in the undernourished.
- There are small, deep, crusted ulcers which may eventually heal with scarring.

For management see impetigo above.

CELLULITIS

This is a widespread skin infection affecting all the layers (epidermis, dermis and subcutaneous tissue), and it does not have clear edges.

Clinical features

- The affected area is usually warm, tender and swollen.
- There is usually lymphadenitis.
- It may cause fever and severe systemic illness.
- If in a child's limb, **osteomyelitis** must be excluded.

MANAGEMENT

Mild infection
- Give flucloxacillin or cephalexin 4 x daily for 5 days, dosage according to age
- **Or** if penicillin-allergic azithromycin daily for 3 days, dosage according to age

More severe infection
- Flucloxacillin or cephalexin 4 x daily for 10 days but review after 5 days.

Severe cases or rapid progression of erythema
- **Refer** for intravenous antibiotics
- **REFER** to surgeon
    - if the response is poor
    - if necrotising fasciitis is suspected

(necrosis, gangrene, gas in the tissues or haemorrhagic bullae).
- if the cellulitis is severe
- any child with cellulitis of a limb when associated with significant pain, swelling or loss of function

ERYSIPELAS

This is a superficial, well-demarcated skin infection due to Streptococcus pyogenes.

Clinical features

- There is spreading erythema and swelling.
- Sometimes there is blister formation on the surface.
- Common sites are the face and legs.

For management see cellulitis above.

BOIL

Clinical features

- Infection in, and around, a hair follicle
- Firm, painful, red nodules which soften in the centre to discharge pus
- It is often difficult to decide when pus is present.
- Features which suggest an abscess are
    - throbbing pain
    - pain so severe it interferes with sleep
    - inflammation of more than 48 hours
- Fluctuation if the pus is near the skin surface

- Treat as for carbuncle (see below).
- See Surgery pages 279-281 for details of other abscesses and management.

CARBUNCLE

Clinical features

- Infection of several adjacent hair follicles
- They contain multiple fistulous tracts

> **MANAGEMENT**
> - Exclude underlying precipitating factors especially
>   - diabetes
>   - other causes of immuno-suppression
>   - poor hygiene.
> - Prescribe antibiotics
>   - flucloxacillin or cephalexin 500 mg 4 x daily for 5 days
>   - **or** if penicillin-allergic azithromycin daily for 3 days.
> - Abscesses must be incised and drained.

LEPROSY

Leprosy is a slightly contagious, chronic infection caused by Mycobacterium leprae.

- Spreads by nasal droplets from cases of lepromatous leprosy
- The worst damage is to the
  - peripheral nerves
  - skin
  - mucosa of the upper respiratory tract
- Nerve damage results in loss of sensation in skin lesions
- There is sensory and motor damage in the peripheral nerve trunks which become thickened.
- Clinical changes depend on the patient's cell mediated immunity (CMI) to *Mycobacterium leprae*.

Clinical features

- Pale macules, with loss of sensation, should be suspected of being leprosy
  - they may be single
  - they are hairless
  - they may be a little raised at the edges.
  Note: any pale patch should be checked for sensation.
- Thickening of the skin of the face with increase in the depth of the folds of the skin
  - this is called leonine or lion-like because of the prominence of the skin folds.
- Loss of the lateral side of the eyebrows.
- The changes in the hands and feet may be the first notable sign of the problem. These are:
  - chronic ulcers of the fingers often looking like bad burns, with progressive shortening of the fingers
  - clawing of the fingers and toes
  - when tested for sensation, there is complete loss of sensation in the areas affected by the ulcers.
- Thickened nerves may be palpated or seen in the neck or in the arms.

Differential diagnosis

- Ringworm may look very similar but there will be normal sensation in the centre of the pale area.
- Other fungal infections eg. pityriasis versicolor.

> **MANAGEMENT**
> **REFER**
> - Any pale patch which has loss of sensation
> - If you suspect leprosy
> - For multi-drug therapy combination
>   - rifampicin
>   - dapsone
>   - clofazimine

TUBERCULOSIS

Clinical features

- Lupus vulgaris
  - appears as a thick, reddish-brown, scaly plaque
  - this often occurs on the face, nose, ears and neck.
- Scrofuloderma (lymph node abscesses) ie. "cold" abscesses
  - seen particularly in the neck as a mixture of abscesses, puckered scars and sinuses.

> - **REFER** if you suspect it.
> - The treatment is similar to that used for active pulmonary TB (see pages 66-67).

VIRAL CONDITIONS

HERPES ZOSTER

Varicella and Herpes zoster are caused by the same specific virus.

- Primary infection results in chickenpox.
- The virus may then settle in any of the peripheral or cranial nerves and may stay alive for many years.
- Reactivation of this dormant, live virus can lead to a vesicular rash in the area of skin supplied by that nerve.

Causes

In any young adult or child with herpes zoster, an underlying cause for the lesion should be considered eg.

- Emotional or physical stress
- Malnutrition
- Chronic disease
- Malignancy
- HIV infection

Clinical features

- Found mostly in adults and geriatrics.
- It appears as groups of small vesicles on erythematous areas of the skin, in a line along the distribution of a sensory nerve on **one** side of the body only.
- Characteristically this stops in the mid-line.
- It affects the intercostal nerves mainly, and often the 5th cranial (trigeminal), which supplies sensation to the face.
- The lesions clear in 2-3 weeks.
- It may be followed by severe, chronic, post-herpetic neuralgia, particularly in the elderly
  - this is very difficult to treat.
- It may be severe and affect more than one dermatome in immuno-compromised patients
  - especially HIV-positive patients.

> **MANAGEMENT**
>
> *Mild cases*
> - Calamine lotion
> - Paracetamol 2 tabs 3 x daily as required
>
> *More severe neuralgia*
> - Give paracetamol 2 tabs 3-4 x daily for 7-10 days
> - **Plus**:
>   - amitriptyline or imipramine
>   25 mg at night for 14-28 days
> - **Plus** if severe neuralgia, tramadol 50 mg 4 x daily for 5 days (Dr initiated)
> - **Plus** if fresh vesicles are present
>   - give oral acyclovir 800 mg 5 x daily for 7 days
>
> *Post-herpetic neuralgia*
> - Give paracetamol 2 tabs 3-4 x daily when needed
> - **Plus** amitriptyline or imipramine 25 mg at night, increasing if necessary by 25 mg at 2-weekly intervals to 75 mg at night
> - **Plus** if pain not controlled **REFER** for:
>   - tramadol 50 mg 4 x daily for 5 days
>   - may be increased to a maximum of 100 mg 4 x daily

HERPES SIMPLEX

Clinical features

Primary infection
- Gingivo-stomatitis and pharyngitis in infants and children which may be subclinical or severe
    - i.e. multiple intra-oral ulcerations, especially on the tongue
    - the ulcers are painful, small, shallow and covered by yellow-grey membrane

Secondary infection – herpes labialis / nasalis (fever blisters)
- Lesions are mostly on the lips or nose often in association with upper or lower respiratory tract infection.
- Clusters of vesicles (i.e. grouped) on a red base, preceded by tingling or burning sensation.
- They dry up within 2 weeks.
- There may be extensive ulceration in and around the mouth in immuno-compromised patients.

Recurrent herpes simplex
- In some individuals reactivations are common and are precipitated by:
    - fever
    - menstruation
- The virus remains alive but inactive (latent) in the dorsal nerve root ganglion of cutaneous nerves, between attacks.
- It most frequently affects the lips, penis and labia.
- Herpes simplex infection is a common cause of erythema multiforme (see page 257).

Eczema herpeticum
- Sufferers from atopic eczema are particularly susceptible.
- It may occur in immuno-suppressed patients.
- The vesicles are numerous, diffuse, not grouped and surrounded by erythema.
- Many of the vesicles are crusted.

Chronic mucocutaneous ulceration
- Occurs in patients who are severely immuno-compromised.
- Single or multiple painful ulcers with polycyclic edge.

- Most commonly seen in and around the mouth and in the perianal and genital areas.
- Lesions persist for months.

Genital herpes simplex
- See page 172 under STIs.

> **MANAGEMENT**
>
> *For gingivo-stomatitis:*
> - Paracetamol syrup for pain relief.
> - If the ulcerations are extensive, accompanied by difficulty in feeding:
>   - acyclovir 10 mg / kg / dose 3 x daily for 7 days or dosage according to age
>   - children >6 years: tetracaine 0.5% gel, applied 4 x daily
>
> *For eczema herpeticum, extensive herpes (oral-facial or genital) and chronic herpes simplex ulcers:*
> - Oral acyclovir, 400 mg 3 x daily for 7-10 days.
> - Keep the skin lesions clean and dry.

MOLLUSCUM CONTAGIOSUM

Clinical features

- In children usually acquired from family members or other children.
- The lesions occur anywhere on the body, but in children are common on the forehead and face.
- Pearly papules with central umbilication.
- May resolve spontaneously in immune-competent patients, but this may take up to 2 years.

> **MANAGEMENT**
>
> - Allow to heal spontaneously if the lesions are few in number and the patient is not immune-compromised.
> - In adults the core can be expressed manually
>   - careful disposal of the contents of the core is required as this is infectious
> - The standard treatment is to apply tincture of iodine to the central core of each lesion using an applicator.

WARTS

COMMON WARTS

Clinical features
- Usual raised nodular type.
- They are common in children.
- They spontaneously improve sooner or later.

> **MANAGEMENT**
>
> - They may be left alone to wait for improvement.
> - Salicylic acid 15-30% topical liquid application
>   - protect surrounding skin with petroleum jelly
>   - apply daily to wart and allow to dry

- occlude for 24 hours with plasters
- soften lesions by soaking in warm water and remove loosened keratin by light abrasion
- repeat process daily until the wart disappears
- **REFER** patients with extensive warts for liquid nitrogen freezing of the warts by a dermatologist.

PLANE WARTS

Clinical features
- Multiple flat-topped warts.
- They are typically found on the face, forehead, back of hands and knees.

- Salicylic acid 15-30% topical liquid application
  - apply daily until the warts disappear
- **Or REFER** to dermatologist

PLANTAR WARTS

Clinical features
- Found on the soles of the feet where, due to pressure, they are level with the surface of the skin.
- Often they are thick and hard, due to increased keratin.

MANAGEMENT
- Never excise or remove them surgically.
- Salicylic acid 15-30% topical liquid application
  - protect surrounding skin with petroleum jelly
  - apply daily to wart (see common warts above)
- **REFER** patient if no response to dermatologist for liquid nitrogen freezing of the warts.

GENITAL WARTS
(CONDYLOMATA ACUMINATA)

The major complication of these is the development of carcinoma, especially of the cervix.

Clinical features
- Raised papular lesions with the surface made up of many small filamentous projections
- The papules enlarge and join together to form plaques

Differential diagnosis
- Condylomata lata of secondary syphilis, which are broad, flat-topped, moist plaques seen in skinfold body areas

For management see Sexually Transmitted Infections page 176.

FUNGAL DISEASES

CANDIDIASIS

Clinical features

Mucosal - thrush
- Curd-like, white flecks in the mouth and throat or thick, white coating on the tongue
- Angular chelitis (fissures in the corners of the mouth)
- Vaginitis
- Balanitis

Cutaneous - Candidal intertrigo
Primary type in infancy
- Common in the neck folds
- Well-defined areas that are moist and macerated with satellite pustules away from the main eruption

Secondary type
- Often secondary contamination of seborrhoeic dermatitis
- Occurs in skin folds
  - beneath the breasts
  - axillae
  - groins
  - perineum
  - natal cleft
  - unterdigital
- Typical appearance is glazed (shiny), red, well-defined patches with peripheral white or yellow pustules and red, scaly lesions (satellite lesions) away from the main area of the rash.
- Always check the mouth and perineum for possible GIT involvement.

MANAGEMENT
Intertrigo
- Imidazole cream e.g. clotrimazole 2% cream 2 x daily for 2 weeks
- Or nystatin ointment 2 x daily for 2 weeks

Oral
- Nystatin suspension (not absorbed from the bowel) 1 ml 4 x daily for 5 days.
- Exclude diabetes mellitus
- Consider HIV, especially if severe

PITYRIASIS VERSICOLOR

Clinical features
- Common in adults in hot climates.
- Mostly found on the chest, back and neck.
- The rash is asymmetrical, of various shapes and sizes.
- The lesions are macules which are either lighter than normal skin (hypopigmented) or darker (hyperpigmented).
- The rash spreads with the formation of new macules on the periphery
    - the more central ones join together as they increase in size
- Pigmentation may take months to return to normal.
- Recurrence is common.

MANAGEMENT
- They may be left alone if mild and the patient does not specifically ask for treatment.
- Selsun shampoo
    - lather on affected areas
    - allow to dry and leave overnight before washing off
    - repeat weekly for 3 weeks

OR
- Imidazole cream eg. clotrimazole 2% cream
    - apply 2 x daily for 2 weeks.

TINEA CAPITIS

Infection from cats, dogs or humans.

Clinical features
- It affects mainly children between 5-10 years.
- It disappears spontaneously at puberty.
- There are round or patchy, bald areas with scaling.
- Also thickened, black broken-off hair stumps.

Management as for kerion below.

KERION

Clinical features
- A spongy, inflammatory and pustular area on the scalp.
- It is a reaction to a fungal, not a bacterial infection.
- Regional lymphadenopathy is frequently associated.

MANAGEMENT
- Avoid shaving the head in children.
- Give fluconazole.
    Adults:
    - 200 mg weekly for 6 weeks
    Children:
    - *6 months-3 years:* 50 mg daily
    - *3-7 years:* 100 mg daily
    - *7-11 years:* 150 mg daily
    - *>11 years:* 200 mg daily
    - as a single dose for 28 days
    - mix contents of capsule/s with unheated food or fluid

TINEA CORPORIS (RINGWORM)

Clinical features
- It is more common in children but also occurs in adults.
- It has a round, active, raised, scaly edge, with a healing centre which may be hyperpigmented.
- They can be single or multiple.
- Extensive disease is common in HIV-infected individuals.

MANAGEMENT
- Apply imidazole cream e.g. clotrimazole 2% cream 2 x daily.
- Continue for at least 2 weeks after lesions have cleared.
- Give fluconazole for 2 weeks if:
    - poor response
    - the condition is widespread

TINEA CRURIS

Clinical features
- It occurs in the groins and perineum.
- Usually occurs in males with tinea pedis.
- Red, slightly raised, scaly border.
- Affected area may show hyperpigmentation.

MANAGEMENT
- Apply topical imidazole cream e.g. clotrimazole 2% cream 2 x daily.
- Continue for at least 2 weeks after the condition has cleared.

TINEA PEDIS (ATHLETE'S FOOT)

Clinical features
- The skin between the toes becomes soft, white and moist (maceration).
- Fissures form between the toes.
- The infection may spread to the foot, especially the instep, producing itching, erythema, scaling and peeling.
- Secondary infection is common.
- It spreads by contact, including from floors.
- An allergic reaction (Id reaction) is seen as an eczematous rash on the hands, especially the sides of the fingers, during acute tinea pedis.

MANAGEMENT
- Apply imidazole cream e.g. clotrimazole 2% cream 2 x daily and continue for 2 weeks after the condition has cleared.
- Give fluconazole for 2 weeks if:
    - poor response
    - the condition is severe
- Give antibiotics if secondary infection is present.

TINEA UNGUIUM

The fungus invades the nail bed leading to hyperkeratosis and separation of the nail from the nail bed.

Clinical features
- The nails are lifted, later thickened, deformed and crumbling.
- The colour is opaque, white or discoloured.

Differential diagnosis
- Psoriasis may give a similar appearance.

> **REFER** to dermatologist only if the patient is concerned by the cosmetic appearance.

PARASITES AND INSECTS

LICE (PEDICULOSIS)

Any situation where there is a heavy concentration of people, with lack of sanitary facilities, is likely to cause an epidemic of lice.

There are three varieties of lice that attack humans.

PEDICULUS CAPITIS (HEAD LOUSE)

Clinical features
- The adult parasite crawls about the scalp.
- The females attach their ova (nits) to the side of the hair by means of a tough cement substance.
- The ova hatch out in about a week.
- The duration of life in the female is about a month.
- The parasite causes intense irritation and, as a result of scratching, secondary infections develop.

> **MANAGEMENT**
> - Apply permethrin 5% lotion
>   hair must be dry or towel-dried first
>   - comb into hair repeatedly with the fine lice comb provided ensuring that all areas of the scalp are covered completely
>   - rinse the lice comb in a white bowl filled with hot water to identify removed lice, or detach on white tissue paper
>   - keep combing with fine lice comb for half an hour while rinsing or wiping comb frequently
>   - after combing, rinse hair with lukewarm water and wash permethrin 5% lotion out with normal shampoo
>   - the procedure should be repeated every 5 days for 3 weeks
> - Give an antibiotic for secondary infection.
> - Avoid contact with eyes and broken skin or sores

PEDICULUS CORPORIS (BODY LOUSE)

Clinical features
- It lives in the patient's clothes.
- It is similar to the head louse.
- Itchy, red, inflammatory nodules may be present, especially on the trunk.

> **MANAGEMENT**
> - Benzyl benzoate 25% lotion, applied over the whole body
>   - leave on overnight and wash off the next day
>   - repeat once a week for up to 3 weeks
> - Give antibiotic for any secondary infection.
> - Regularly wash bed linen and underclothes in hot water and expose to sunlight.

PEDICULUS PUBIS (PUBIC OR CRAB LOUSE)

Pubic lice are acquired as STIs.

Clinical features
- They live in the pubic hair and nits (eggs) are found attached to pubic hair.

> **MANAGEMENT**
> - Shaving is usually unnecessary.
> - Apply benzyl benzoate lotion 25%
>   - leave on overnight and wash off the next day
>   - repeat once a week for up to 3 weeks.
> - Sexual partners must be treated.

SCABIES

Scabies is caused by a mite, Sarcoptes scabiei.

The disease is acquired from contact with infected persons, their clothing, or bed linen contaminated with the adult female mite, its eggs, larvae, or nymphs.

Clinical features
- It is especially disturbing at night.
- The female digs under the horny layer, to form a burrow, in which 40-50 eggs are laid.
- The eggs pass through various stages as larvae to become, finally, adults in about 8 days.
- The major symptom of scabies is severe itching, which occurs when the skin is warmed, especially just after going to bed.
- The itching ("lekkerkrap") is produced by the parasites burrowing into the skin.
- This leads to abrasions of the skin which may become secondarily infected.
- The diagnostic features are irregularly scattered papules and vesicles especially over
  - the sides of fingers adjacent to web spaces
  - the flexor aspects of wrists and elbows
  - the nipple area of the breasts
  - the belt and pubic area

- buttocks
- the lower legs
- Impetigo lesions are commonly present especially on the limbs and buttocks
  - this is almost always due to secondary infected scabies.
- The face and neck are seldom affected in older children.
- In infants, it may present with vesicles and pustules on the palms and soles and sometimes on the scalp.

Differential diagnosis
- Bugs, fleas or flies may produce skin disorders
- A useful diagnostic feature is that the bites occur usually in a line along the arm or leg and only in one area.

MANGEMENT
The only way to control the disease is to get rid of the parasites.
- All persons suspected of having scabies should be treated at the same time.
- For adults and children >6 years of age:
  - an emulsion containing benzyl benzoate 25% (Ascabiol) is applied to the entire body, with the exception of the face and head
  - rub in well
  - leave on for 24 hours and then wash off with soap and water
- The procedure is repeated after 24 hours or once within 5 days
- Clothing and bed linen should be changed after each application.
- All persons living in the household and likely to contract the infection should be treated at the same time
- For children <6 years:
  - permethrin 5% lotion applied over the whole body from the neck to the feet
  - leave on overnight and wash off the following morning
  - repeat treatment after 1 week
- Clothing, bed linen and towels should be washed in hot water and exposed to sunlight.

Scabies with secondary infection
- Benzyl benzoate and permethrin are is contra-indicated in septic scabies and on open wounds
- The impetigo must first be treated with a systemic antibiotic (cephalexin / flucloxacillin) plus polyvidone iodine cream.
- Once the infection has cleared, or has dried up, the above treatment can be applied.

Scabies in infants
- Advise the mother to scrub the bullae with a soft brush or wash-cloth and soap and water.
- Then apply permethrin lotion as above.

ALLERGIES

Causes
- Many different causes can be seen in different people.
- A first contact causes the person to become excessively sensitive.
- The skin disease then shows on subsequent exposure to the cause.
- It often is made worse by many other different causes.

Factors which may make the reaction worse
- Genetic defects.
- Susceptible target organ (skin and other systems).
- Allergens inhaled and ingested (swallowed).
- External exposure.
- Scratching, rubbing or itching.
- Heat, humidity
- Sweat retention
- Sudden temperature changes
- Soap, detergents
- Psychological stress
- Infection (local or systemic)

Note. Allergic reactions can occur in **all** organs and in **any** system. The skin is frequently involved in many different forms of allergy.

URTICARIA AND ANGIO-OEDEMA

URTICARIA

This is an acute, chronic or recurrent inflammatory condition.

Causes
See below under causes of angio-oedema.

Clinical features
- There are whitish, pinkish or reddish wheals due to dermal oedema.
- These are transient lesions (come for a short time and then disappear) which give rise to
  - burning
  - itching
  - stinging sensations.
- The wheals differ greatly in size and shape, and usually appear suddenly.
- Any or all parts of the body may be affected.
- In ordinary cases the lesions last for a few minutes to several hours (usually less than 24 hours)
  - they then disappear spontaneously, leaving no sign of them
  - commonly patients come the next day when the wheals have disappeared.

ANGIO-OEDEMA

Causes

In 50% or more of cases, no cause is found.

IgE-dependent (specific antigen sensitivity)
- Infections
  - streptococcal tonsillitis is common especially in children
  - viral illnesses in children
  - urinary tract infection
  - vulvo-vaginal candidiasis
  - sinusitis
- Inhaled or physical contact
  - pollens
  - animal fur
  - mould spores, fungi
- Medicines
  - penicillin
  - sulphonamides
- Dietary
  - specific foods eg. fresh fruit, shellfish, peanuts
  - additives to foods eg. colourants, flavourings,
  - preservatives
  - alcohol

- Parasites
    - intestinal worms
    - giardiasis
    - bilharzia

Non-immunological
- Medicines
    - ACE-inhibitors
    - aspirin and NSAIDs

Physical agents
- pressure, heat, cold and sunlight

Clinical features
- Swelling of the face, tongue and occasionally the larynx.
- Most common sites are the lips and periorbital.
- The oedema and swelling are in the deeper layers of the skin, including the subcutaneous tissue.
- There is diffuse swelling.
- There is no itch.
- It is found alone or in association with urticaria.

MANAGEMENT

Acute urticaria and angioedema
- Remove the cause or treat it, e.g. worm infestation, aspirin, NSAIDs, streptococcal sore throat, alcohol
- Antihistamines are useful
    - e.g. chlorphenamine 3 x daily
    - use regularly until the urticaria subsides
- Calamine lotion can be applied on the skin in urticaria.
- Applications to the skin are not helpful in angioedema.
- For severe cases, prescribe promethazine (Phenergan) 25-50 mg IM immediately.
    - **NB**: antihistamines have no role if angioedema is due to an ACE inhibitor
- Epinephrine, IM, 0.5 ml 1:1 000 into the lateral thigh immediately.
    - where angioedema is part of anaphylaxis
- Epinephrine, IV, 5 ml 1:10 000 is given for patients with laryngeal oedema (hoarseness, difficulty in breathing) or shocked/hypotensive
- For all cases of angioedema
    - hydrocortisone, IV / IM 100 mg immediately
- Observe all cases until resolution.

Chronic urticaria
- Less sedating antihistamines are preferable
    - cetirizine 10 mg daily

REFERRAL
Angioedema
- For admission for airway obstruction or anaphylaxis.
- If there is no response.

Urticaria
- For investigation if the individual lesions remain for longer than 48-72 hours.

PAPULAR URTICARIA

Lesions due to insect bites.

Clinical features
- Lesions often grouped or in a linear arrangement
    - may show a central bite mark
- Itchy red papules that may form blisters, become scratched and then heal with hyperpigmentation
- Chronic severe persistent reactions may be seen in immuno-compromised patients, e.g. HIV infection, malnutrition

---

MANAGEMENT
- Examine carefully for burrows to rule out scabies
- Oral antihistamine, e.g. chlorphenamine at night as needed
- Hydrocortisone 1%, topical, apply 2 x daily for 5 days
- Antibiotics where necessary for secondary infection
- Appropriate insect-control measures
    - the patient should use insect-repellents if possible, either topical or aerosol spray.
- **REFER** non-responsive cases

ERYTHEMA NODOSUM

This is due to the effects of the body's reaction against foreign material.

Causes
No cause may be found

Possible causes
- **S** Streptococcal tonsillitis (most common cause)
- **T** Tuberculosis (primary)
- **O** Oral contraceptives
- **P** Pregnancy

- **S** Sulphonamides and penicillin
- **I** Inflammatory bowel disease (ulcerative colitis and Crohn's disease)
- **N** Non-Hodgkins lymphoma
- **S** Sarcoidosis

Clinical features
- Mainly young adults, especially females, are affected.
- Painful, red nodules appear on the shins (seldom elsewhere).
- Nodules disappear leaving a bruise-like appearance within 6 weeks.
- They may recur after weeks or months.
- Recurring form common in children with tonsillitis.

MANAGEMENT
- Remove or treat the cause.
- Self-limiting and usually resolves itself within 3-6 weeks
- Symptomatic treatment
    - anti-inflammatory drug eg. ibuprofen 400 mg 3 x daily for 5-7 days
    - analgesics.
- Corticosteroids are contra-indicated.
- **REFER.**

ERYTHEMA MULTIFORME

Causes
- Infections
    - herpes simplex (most common cause)
    - enterovirus infection in children
    - mycoplasma infection
- Less commonly: medicines e.g. sulphonamides, penicillin, anticonvulsants
- Malignancy

Clinical features
- The eruption is acute in onset.
- Pink-red macules of varying sizes and shapes.

- The characteristic lesions are described as iris or target lesions
    - dark centre, pale and red concentric rings.
- When severe, the centre of this target lesion consists of a vesicle or a sizeable bulla.
- The main sites are:
    - extensor surfaces of limbs
    - especially hands and forearms
    - palms and soles
    - can involve mucous membranes, but not more than one surface
    - when severe the rash may be much more widespread with a large part of the body-surface being involved

---

- Remove or treat the cause.
- Self-limiting and requires no treatment.
- Usually lasts 10-14 days.

SEVERE CUTANEOUS ADVERSE DRUG REACTIONS

The most commonly associated medicines are sulphonamides, anticonvulsants, penicillin, NSAIDs

Stevens Johnson syndrome
- An acute systemic condition involving skin and mucous
- membranes (2 or more mucosal surfaces).
- This may occur together with ordinary erythema multiforme
- lesions
    - in more severe cases, there may be a vesicle or bulla in the central area of the target lesions
- There are often widespread bullae and erosions of the skin
- and mucous membranes.
- The patient is unwell and often febrile.
- The mucosa of the lips, cheeks and tongue is shed leaving a raw, red surface with bits of mucosa still sticking to it
    - similar changes can occur in the eyes and genitalia
- Mucosal involvement of this type can occur in all 3 sites with
- very little or no involvement of the skin
    - this is uncommon
- This syndrome most commonly occurs
    - as a complication of medicine therapy, especially penicillin, sulphonamides, anticonvulsants and allopurinol
    - **or** following the use of laxatives containing phenolphthalein

Toxic epidermal necrolysis (TEN)
- A more severe form of the condition and is suggested if the skin lesions cover more than 30% of the body surface area.
- There are sheets of desquamation of necrotic epidermis that look like burns.

MANAGEMENT
- Stop the offending medicine.
- **REFER**
    - all cases with systemic features
    - mucosal involvement
    - bullous rash
- Systemic corticosteroids are contraindicated.

OTHER DRUG ERUPTIONS

Causes
- Any drug should be suspected.
- The most common are sulphonamides, laxatives and "blood cleaning mixtures" which contain phenolphthalein.
- For diagnosis to be precise, take a detailed drug history
    - ask about new, recently-introduced drugs
    - ask about self-medication
    - be aware of cross-sensitisation and related drugs.

Clinical features
Drug eruptions can take the form of any type of rash eg. eczema, urticaria, vasculitic, purpura morbilliform, erythema multiforme etc.

FIXED DRUG ERUPTION

Clinical features
- Lesions can be eczematous.
- They recur on the same spot and increase in number with each successive attack.
- Typically large, round, well-circumscribed, black-coloured residual macules between attacks.
- In the acute stage they are itchy, red or even bullous.
- The time between taking the drug and getting the symptoms becomes shorter with each attack
    - later it is within minutes of ingesting the drug.

MANAGEMENT
- This depends on the nature and severity of the drug eruption.
- The majority of mild drug eruptions decrease rapidly when the drug is stopped.
- Hydrocortisone ointment
    - apply 2 x daily for 5 days.
- Antihistamines may be used to releive itch.
- Hyperpigmentation may take many months to resolve.

ECZEMA

An inflammatory skin disorder which shows itself characteristically in its acute stage by vesicle formation in the epidermis.

- The terms "eczema" and "dermatitis" are often used interchangeably for the same disease
- "Dermatitis" is also used for other unrelated diseases and should preferably be limited to eczema resulting from external contact i.e. contact dermatitis.

Causes
Many different causes can be identified: external and internal; alone or combined.

Clinical features
- Eczema may begin in infancy, and last through life
    - it may occur in infancy only
    - it may appear for the first time in adult life or old age.
- By a mechanism of auto-sensitisation, eczema lesions may spread far beyond the primary area of inflammation.
- An itch is an important symptom.

Acute eczema
- Redness and oedema
- Superficial vesicles may open to discharge a watery exudate ("weeping eczema")
- Crusting (serous fluid and cellular debris)
- Scaling
- Pustules if secondarily infected

Chronic eczema
- Lichenification (leathery feel due to thickening of the epidermis)
- Darker or lighter colour (hyper- or hypo-pigmentation)
- More obvious normal skin creases
- Papules
- Nodules
- Scaling

Secondary changes
- Infection: pustules or cellulitis
- Exfoliative dermatitis (erythroderma): diffuse, generalised redness and scaling of the skin
    - **REFER** patient for admission

ECZEMA ELICITED BY VARIOUS FACTORS

Causes

Dryness
- Also known as asteatotic eczema.
- Commonly found on the shins in elderly people.
- Also found in infants and children.

Infection
- This is infective or bacterial eczema.
- Found around any infection eg. a discharging otitis media.

Contact dermatitis
- Irritant causes either strong (acids, alkalis) or milder (detergents, washing powder, especially those containing enzymes, strong soaps)
    - trauma and drying out or excessive moisture (maceration) of the skin are contributing factors
- Allergic causes eg. nickel (jewellery), chrome (cement), resins (nail varnish), latex (rubber) gloves, formalin (in cosmetics) etc.

Venous stasis (varicose eczema)
- Found mostly above the medial malleolus of the ankle
- Tends to spread to the other leg, then to the rest of the body

Trauma
- Injuries or burns
- With or without secondary infection

Sunlight
- Photosensitive eczema
    - idiopathic
    - drug-induced eg. thiazides, phenothiazines

Sweating
- This is called dyshidrotic eczema or pomphylyx
- It may cause a vesicular eczema of the palms and soles

Systemic causes
- - infections e.g. tonsillitis
- - drugs eg penicillin

ENDOGENOUS ECZEMA

■ ATOPIC ECZEMA

- It is often associated with asthma, allergic rhinitis and urticaria.
- The serum IgE levels are raised.
- Relapses and recurrences are common.

Common associations
- Xerosis (dry skin)
- Susceptibility to infection (staphylococcus, HSV)
- Recurrent allergic conjunctivitis
- Orbital darkening
- Pityriasis alba

Clinical features

Infantile atopic eczema
- Mostly 3 months to 3 years of age
- Mainly found on the face, extensor surfaces of the limbs and the trunk
- Erythema, exudation and crusts
- Rash is itchy, irritating, especially at night

Flexural
- Older patients
- Found on
    - the backs of knees
    - fronts of elbows and wrists
    - neck and eyelids
- Chronic course and rash becomes lichenified

Nummular eczema
- Occurs in adults
- Coin-shaped discs covered with papulovesicles, and oozing and crusting may result
- Mostly on the limbs (trunk sometimes)

Follicular eczema
- In adults
- Small follicular papules
- Mainly on the limbs

Hand and foot eczema
- Children or adults
- Vesicles and bullae on sides of fingers, palms and soles
    - later redness, hyperkeratosis (thickened skin) and fissuring

Pityrlasis alba
- Rounded or irregular patches with slight scaling on the cheeks which become hypopigmented.
- It has a mild course.

■ SEBORRHOEIC DERMATITIS

- Sometimes started or made worse by infection (Staphylococcus, Streptococcus, Malassezia spp).
- Mostly reddening and scaling but sometimes acute and weeping.
- The scalp, face, presternal, axillae, groins are commonly affected.

Clinical features

Infantile type
- Soon after birth to about 6 months
- Distribution: face, scalp ("cradle-cap"), groins, axillae, behind ears, but the rash may generalise
- Sometimes moist and infected

Adult type
- Involves mainly the scalp, face, upper trunk
- Scalp
    - diffuse or localised around hair margin
    - dry or greasy scaling
- Face
    - central areas of the face (forehead, eyebrows, eyelid margins, nasolabial folds, upper lip)
    - pinnae (within and behind)
- Presternal

Intertriginous eczema
- Involves skin-folds of the axillae, groins, scrotum, sub-mammary and gluteal cleft
- Scaling and erythema
- In severe cases there may be oedema, scaling and weeping, particularly in the scrotal and gluteal regions.
- More severe forms may cause a widespread, generalised dermatitis with hyper- and hypo-pigmented patches and plaques.

MANAGEMENT

General principles of treatment
- Explain the disease to the patient or parent.
- Treat eczema actively, otherwise it spreads to the rest of the skin.
- Remove causes or aggravating factors such as contact allergens.
- Treat infection if present
  - treat skin infections
  - treat any systemic infections e.g. sore throat.
- Avoid use of soap on affected areas
- use aqueous cream instead.

Atopic eczema
- Infantile atopic eczema
- Avoid topical steroids if condition is mild.
- Use ung emulsificans (UE) instead.
- Explanation and reassurance is necessary.
- Avoid skin contact with rough or woollen clothes.
- Avoid overheating by blankets at night.

Acute moist or weeping eczema
- Saline dressings, applied daily or twice daily.
  - saline can be made at home i.e. 1 cup of water,
  - ½ teaspoon of salt
- Avoid use of soap on affected areas.
- Hydrocortisone 1% cream, applied 2 x daily, until improved.
  - Topical steroid should be applied to both moist and dry inflamed areas.
- If infection is present (yellow pustules that crust):
  - flucloxacillin or cephalexin 4 x daily for 5 days
  - dosage according to age
- If penicillin-allergic:
  - adults and children: azithromycin daily for 3 days.
- If there is a good response:
  - maintain treatment with emulsifying ointment (UE)
  - applied 2 x daily.
- For itching:
  - chlorphenamine may be given 3 x daily or, in mild cases, only at night to avoid sedation.

Dry eczema
- Hydrocortisone 1% ointment, applied 2 x daily for 7 days or until improved.
- If there is a good response:
  - maintain treatment with UE ointment thereafter.
- If there is a poor response or more severe eczema:
  - **REFER** for betamethasone 0.1% ointment (more potent topical steroid) applied once daily for 7 days
  - **do not** apply to face, neck and flexures.
- If there is a good response:
  - wean to hydrocortisone 1% ointment applied twice a week.
- In chronic eczema moisturising creams and ointments should continue permanently as maintenance even if the dermatitis is controlled.

- For itching not controlled with topical treatment:
- chlorphenamine may be given 3 x daily or, in mild cases, only at night (to avoid sedation).
- For long-term use in adults and school-going children and for day-time itching:
- cetirizine, oral, 10 mg once daily (5 mg once daily in children 2-6 years of age).

REFERRAL
- No improvement in 2 weeks
- Severe eczema (after initiating treatment)

Seborrhoeic dermatitis
- Cradle cap
  - use aqueous cream to remove scalp scales.
- Use Selsun shampoo for scalp itching, scalp scaling and dandruff
  - apply by lathering on scalp
  - rinse off after 10 minutes.
  - apply weekly until improved and every second week thereafter to maintain control
- Hydrocortisone 1% cream / ointment applied 2 x daily until improved
  - then once or twice weekly for maintenance as needed.

Severe dermatitis
- betamethasone 0.1% ointment applied once daily for 7 days (Doctor initiated)
- **do not** apply to face, neck and flexures

Pityriasis alba
- Direct sunlight exposure should be avoided.

MISCELLANEOUS CONDITIONS

PITYRIASIS ROSEA

A common disease of unknown cause, probably due to human herpes virus infection (HHV-7).

Clinical features
- Occurs mostly in spring and autumn
- Most common in young adults but any age may be affected
- The rash involves the trunk, neck and proximal parts of the extremities ("vest and pants")
- In severe cases it may extend to the face, arms and forearms
  - but this is uncommon
- Generalised rash usually preceded by one (rarely 2 or 3) larger, oval, slightly scaly areas called "herald patch"
  - commonly found in the scapular area or lower abdomen
  - often mistakenly diagnosed as ringworm because of its peripheral scaling
- Within 1-2 weeks, a widespread rash starts to appear
- The rash has 2 parts which vary in size
  - pink papules
  - oval macules, which are slightly scaly towards the edge of the lesions
- The lesions on the thorax are characteristically parallel to the long axes of the ribs ("Christmas tree" distribution).
- Those on the abdomen and lumbar areas form roughly transverse lines (across).
- The itch is usually mild, with few or no constitutional disturbances.
- It is self-limiting within about 4-8 weeks but may persist for longer.
- Occasionally the eruption is limited to the sun-spared areas of the axillae or groins

Differential diagnosis
- Seborrhoeic dermatitis
- Secondary syphilis (always examine the genitalia)
- Psoriasis

> **MANAGEMENT**
> - Symptomatic
>   - aqueous cream
>   - antihistamine eg. chlorphenamine or cetirizine given at night for 4-8 weeks
> - Reassurance is most important

LICHEN PLANUS

Causes
Unknown

Clinical features
- Most cases subside within 3 months to 2 years but may relapse.
- Typical lesions are shiny, flat-topped, angulated papules characteristically violet in colour.
- Commonly seen on anterior wrists, lips, penis, legs and mucous membranes.
- Itching is mild to severe.
- Healing is accompanied by greyish, hyperpigmentation (which eventually disappears).
- May become hypertrophic and warty, especially on shins.
- Mouth lesions in some cases
    - white, lacy network especially on buccal mucosa

> - Strong topical corticosteroids.
> - **REFER** to dermatologist.

PSORIASIS

An inflammatory condition of the skin and joints of unknown aetiology.

Causes
- Genetic predisposition
- Provoking and relieving factors
    - a streptococcal infection may bring on the guttate form
    - endocrine – tends to improve with pregnancy
    - psychogenic – stress often makes psoriasis worse

Clinical features
- It starts at any age, mostly 20-40 years.
- It is persistent, variable, unpredictable.
- It improves and gets worse on its own.
- Typical lesions (plaques) are well-circumscribed, slightly raised, red or pink areas of skin covered with silvery scales.
- Chronic plaques occur, especially on the knees, elbows, sacrum and scalp, where the scale
    - is thick
    - sticks to the underlying skin
    - is palpable.
- Psoriasis may spread to involve any other sites although not usually the face.
- The guttate form, which is more common in children, consists of multiple small psoriasis lesions distributed mainly on the trunk
    - this acute form is often preceded by a streptococcal throat infection.
- There may be flexural (inverse psoriasis) in the body folds
    - groins, perineum, axillae, under breasts.
- There is nail involvement in 25% of cases
    - pitting, nail plate thickened, crumbling and opaque
    - discolouration resembling grease spots
    - nails become broken or loose and severely deformed.
- Psoriasis of palms and soles is thickened (hyper-keratotic) or pustular.
- Pustular psoriasis may be localised or generalised
    - *acute patients may be very ill and even die.*
- Erythroderma (generalised exfoliative dermatitis)
    - the most common causes of this are eczema and psoriasis.
- "Napkin psoriasis" typically involves the flexures and has a well-defined edge
- Psoriatic arthropathy (different patterns)
    - this is commonly found together with nail psoriasis.

> **MANAGEMENT**
> - Counsel regarding precipitating factors and chronicity.
> - For mild, non-progressive, asymptomatic lesions:
>   - no treatment is required.
> - Encourage sun exposure as tolerated
>
> **For flares (if delay experienced in obtaining a dermatological consultation)**
> - Coal tar 5%, topical ointment, applied at night
>   - may be used under plastic bag occlusion
>   - avoid use on the face, flexures and genitalia
>
> **For local plaques**
> - **REFER** for betamethazone 0.1% ointment applied 2 x daily.
> - Decrease according to severity to hydrocortisone 1%, then stop
>
> **Scalp psoriasis**
> - **REFER** for betamethasone 0.1% lotion (if available)
>   - apply once daily
>
> **Severe localised or generalised psoriasis**
> - **REFER**
>   - all patients to dermatologist
>   - patients with erythroderma for admission

CHRONIC PARONYCHIA

Chronic red swollen nailfold, lifted off the nail plate.

Due to hand contact with household detergents, washing powders and softeners.

> **MANAGEMENT**
> - Patients to wear rubber gloves when washing clothes, linen and kitchen utensils
> - Hydrocortisone 1% cream, massage into nailfolds at night until lesions have cleared.
> - If secondary infection is present, indicated by pain and tenderness in the nailfold, treat with an antibiotic i.e. flucloxacillin.

HORMONAL DISORDERS

ACNE VULGARIS

Chronic inflammatory disorder of an oil-producing gland in the skin (pilo-sebaceous follicle).

Causes
- Increased sebum secretion.
- There is obstruction of the canal of the gland, due to increased growth of the canal lining (keratinisation).
- This produces plugging of the hair follicle producing the comedone (primary lesion)
    - open = a blackhead
    - closed = a whitehead.
- Micro-organisms and their enzymes play a role in making the condition worse.
- Hormonal changes particularly during adolescence
- The leakage of sebum and keratin fragments into the dermis produces an inflammatory reaction and the formation of a papule or pustule.
- These papules and pustules may:
    - resolve without scarring
    - form deep pustules and nodules which may be followed by cysts and scars.
- Post-inflammatory hyperpigmentation may be disfiguring. This will gradually fade once the acne is controlled.

Clinical features
- Incidence
    - 80% of adolescents
    - males and females equally affected
    - worst cases in males
- The lesions of acne are the comedones and swellings in the skin which result from
    - a blocked duct
    - the swollen pilo-sebaceous gland
- These lesions may be papules, pustules, nodules, cysts or scars on the:
    - face
    - upper back and chest
    - upper arms (rare)
- Severe forms are common in HIV disease, and itching may be a feature

Mild acne
- Predominantly non-inflammatory comedones
- Few papules and pustules

Moderate acne
- Mixture of non-inflammatory comedones and inflammatory papules and pustules

Severe acne
- Presence of widespread nodules and cysts as well as many inflammatory papules and pustules

Influencing factors
- When premenstrual, the acne is made worse due to
    - fluid retention
    - blocking of pilo-sebaceous orifices
- Climate
    - sunlight is beneficial
    - there is improvement in summer, due to increased peeling of the skin
    - high humidity and temperature with cracking of the skin (maceration) and follicular obstruction may cause severe attacks
- Psychological factors make existing lesions worse
- Diet is controversial
    - it has not been proved but some people find that their acne is made worse by chocolates, fats, cheese and cola drinks
- Excessive scrubbing may rupture occluded follicles

MANAGEMENT
General measures
- Avoid greasy or oily topical products / cosmetics including moisturisers
- Increase peeling of the skin by sunlight, ultraviolet light
- Do not squeeze lesions.
- Regular normal cleansing with soap and water.

Medicine management
Reduce micro-organisms with antibiotics, given for a maximum of 3 months.
- Doxycycline is the first choice for inflammatory acne (not if risk of pregnancy) 100 mg daily
- Patients on oral contraceptives will need to use additional non-oestrogen contraceptive measures, i.e. condoms.

Inhibit abnormal keratinisation
- Topical retinoid eg. tretinoin gel / cream
    - doctor initiated

Mild acne
- Benzoyl peroxide 5% gel
    - apply in the morning to affected areas as tolerated.
    - wash off in the evening.
- If ineffective and tolerated increase application to 2 x daily.
- Avoid contact with eyes, mouth

OR

Tretinoin, topical
- apply at night to affected areas for at least 6 weeks.
- review patient after 6 weeks treatment.
- **minimize exposure to sunlight.**
- acne may worsen during the first few weeks.

Moderate acne
- Topical treatment as above

AND

For inflammatory acne:
- Doxycycline 100 mg daily for 3 months
    - review patient after 3 months treatment
    - it should be taken with meals
    - do not take together with iron preparations and antacids.
- Female patients who need oral contraception and have inflammatory acne can alternatively be initiated on cyproterone combined with oestrogen (combined oral contraceptive).

REFERRAL
- All severe cases
- Poor response to treatment

PIGMENTATION DISORDERS

HYPO-PIGMENTATION

ALBINISM

A recessive, genetic disease affecting skin pigmentation.

Clinical features
- Lack of melanin pigment in skin, hair and eyes
- This may result in
    - acute sunburn
    - chronic solar damage
    - multiple skin cancers
- Relatively common in the South African black population

MANAGEMENT
- Avoid sun by wearing hats and long-sleeved clothes, and by using umbrellas.
- Use sunscreens regularly e.g. zinc oxide ointment, titanium dioxide ointment/cream.
- Check skin regularly for signs of skin cancers such as new growths
- Wear sunglasses that preferably have UV filters
- Give guidance to patients, especially children, about the dangers of the sun.

VITILIGO

Acquired, localised loss of melanocytes, probably due to auto-immune destruction.

Clinical features
- Positive family history is common.
- It may appear at any age.
- They are well-circumscribed, usually symmetrical, white patches.
- The skin consistency is normal.
- It commonly affects extensor surfaces and areas around the mouth and genitalia.
- The hair may depigment as well.
- The course is unpredictable and it may
    - be static
    - have a generalised spread
    - have re-pigmentation.
- Diagnose clinically.
- Vitiligo on the labia has been associated with malignancy of the genital tract.

MANAGEMENT
- Screen for associated diseases
    - hypo-thyroidism in older persons
    - diabetes mellitus
    - anaemia
    - perform PAP smear if vitiligo of labia.
- Treatment is unsatisfactory.
- Avoid sun exposure when the sun is at its strongest (10 am – 3 pm)
- Do not use a sunscreen as moderate sun exposure is beneficial
- **REFER.**

POST-INFLAMMATORY DEPIGMENTATION

Causes
This may occur as a result of skin diseases such as:
- Leprosy
- Tinea versicolor
- Eczema

- Treat original disease.
- Use cosmetic covers.
- The skin colour gradually returns to normal.

HYPER-PIGMENTATION

POST-INFLAMMATORY HYPER-PIGMENTATION

Causes
This may occur as a result of skin diseases such as:
- Acne
- Eczema
- Impetigo
- Measles
- Herpes zoster

CHLOASMA

Causes
- Due to increased oestrogens in pregnancy
    - contraceptive pills
- It may be idiopathic

Clinical features
- More common in dark-skinned people
- Can occur in males
- Well-circumscribed, brown macules with a geographical, symmetrical outline
- The skin consistency is normal
- Occurs on forehead, cheeks, nose and upper lip

- Avoid the sun.
- Avoid the use of the contraceptive pill.
- Use sunscreens and cosmetic covers.

COSMETIC OCHRONOSIS

Causes
- Due to the use of bleaching creams
    - these are the so-called skin lightening or brightening creams containing hydroquinone

Clinical features
- Worse on sun-exposed parts of face
- The worst area is on the malar (cheek) region and around the eyes
- To begin with there is sooty pigmentation and small, black nodules develop later
- It is best seen when the skin is stretched

MANAGEMENT
Advise patient to:
- Use sunscreens and cosmetic covers
- Stop using skin lighteners
- Use safer cosmetics
- Avoid the sun eg. use hats, umbrellas

COMMON TUMOURS

BENIGN TUMOURS

VASCULAR NAEVI

Clinical features
Capillary naevi (haemangiomata)
- "Salmon patch"
    - common in neonates
    - shows as a pink stain over the occipital region and on the forehead and eyelids
    - usually fades
- "Port-wine stain"
    - large, persistent, bright purple macular lesion
    - tends to become nodular later in life

Angiomatous naevi (cavernous haemangiomata)
- Superficial
    - "strawberry mark"
    - appears when the baby is 2-3 weeks old
    - grows rapidly
    - collapses inwards (involutes) spontaneously within 4-7 years
    - tumour is raised, bright red in colour but goes white on pressure
- Deep, subcutaneous
    - appears as blueish, compressible swelling
    - does not resolve spontaneously

REFER if you are not sure of the diagnosis.

MELANOCYTIC NAEVI (MOLES)

Clinical features
- Some are present at birth (congenital) and are permanent.
- Most appear around puberty and subsequently disappear.
- More common in the white population
- Malignant change is rare, but more common in congenital types
- Moles are dark, flat or slightly raised, round or oval macules

MANAGEMENT
REFER for surgery
- Any mole which the patient complains about
- Any change from the normal appearance
    - increased size
    - irregular indented outline
    - extension into the surrounding skin
    - irregularly in the pattern of colour
    - nodule formation / or ulceration
    - itching or bleeding

SOLAR KERATOSIS

Clinical features
- Seen in the white population and albinos
- Superficial, non-infiltrated, hyper-keratotic (rough to the touch)
- Hyper-pigmented and ill-defined patches on sun-exposed parts
- A small percentage become malignant to form squamous cell carcinomas which are usually slow-growing and easy to treat

REFER.

MALIGNANT TUMOURS

SQUAMOUS CELL CARCINOMA

Malignant tumours derived from keratinocytes.

Clinical features
- The most common types occur on sun-damaged skin and arise from solar keratosis.
- Others may arise in chronic ulcers or scars.
- Lesions feel firm and hard.
- The surface may be hyper-keratotic or ulcerated.
- Metastases (to lymph nodes) may occur.

REFER any chronic sore or ulcer of the skin.

MALIGNANT MELANOMA

Malignancy of epidermal melanocytes.

Clinical features
- These may arise
    - in melanocytic naevi
    - spontaneously
- The increasing incidence is thought to be due to sun-exposure
- The back is the most common site in both sexes
- Large size, irregular, vague borders
- Irregular, mottled pigmentation

> **MANAGEMENT**
> **REFER** any pigmented spot or macule if:
> - There is any change in colour
> - Any ulceration
> - Any bleeding
> - Any itching
> - Any growth or extension
> - The patient is worried about the mole
> - The mole is on the sole of the foot
> - Pigmented band in nail plate (recent onset)

BULLOUS DISORDERS (BLISTERS OF THE SKIN)

Classification

Superficial blisters (epidermal)
- Impetigo
- Erysipelas
- Staphylococcal scalded skin syndrome
- Eczema, especially of palms and soles
- Pemphigus vulgaris (see opposite)

Less superficial blisters (sub-epidermal)
- Bullous pemphigoid
- Scabies in infants
- Porphyria
- Epidermolysis bullosa
- Drug eruptions
- Erythema multiforme and Stevens Johnson syndrome (see pages 257 and 258)
- Bullous insect bites

> **MANAGEMENT**
> - **REFER** any rash causing blisters
> - PHC sisters may treat
>   - bullous impetigo
>   - scabies
>   - insect bites

STAPHYLOCOCCAL SCALDED SKIN SYNDROME

This is a severe disease.

Causes
- An exotoxin produced by certain types of Staphylococci.

Clinical features
- Mainly occurs in infants.
- There is widespread reddening and blistering of the skin, which looks like burns.

> **REFER** for admission.

PEMPHIGUS VULGARIS

The cause is unknown.

Clinical features
- Occurs in middle and old age, mostly 40-60 years
- Relatively common in black South Africans
- Often presents with erosions in the mouth
- Flaccid skin bullae rupture early and progress to persistent erosions
- Often widespread or generalised
- All mucous membranes may be involved
- *Many patients die if untreated*

> **REFER.**

BULLOUS PEMPHIGOID

The cause is unknown.

Clinical features
- Occurs in the elderly, generally over 60 years
- Large bullae occur over wide areas, especially on upper arms and thighs
- The bullae are tense and dome-shaped and arise on reddened skin
- Mouth lesions are uncommon
- Remissions may occur

> **REFER.**

PORPHYRIA

There are two main types of genetic porphyrias in South Africa.
- **South African genetic porphyria**
- **Porphyria cutanea tarda**

Clinical features
Porphyria cutanea tarda
- This is a liver disease mostly due to alcohol in *genetically*

predisposed individuals, usually with haemochromatosis (iron overload)
- Common in black South Africans
- There are raised urinary porphyrins

In both types
- The formation of bullae followed by depigmented scars where bullae were situated
- Small, white cysts (milia) may be present in the areas of scarring
- Photosensitivity results in
    - hyper-pigmentation
    - a waxy, wrinkled, dark facial appearance
- There may be increased fragility of exposed skin, especially on the backs of the hands and face

---

MANAGEMENT
- **REFER** if severe.
- Advise patient
    - about stopping alcohol
    - to avoid the sun as much as possible
    - to avoid trauma of the involved skin.

SURGERY

SURGICAL PROBLEMS

HEAD INJURY

HOW TO ASSESS IF A HEAD INJURY IS SERIOUS

The cause of the head injury
- If the object which hit the head is softer than the head, then there is less likely to be serious injury
- If the object is hard more damage is likely
    - eg. a knobkierie

The effect on skull and scalp tissues
- The size, shape and severity of the wound may be a guide with direct trauma
    - with severe panga wounds to the head, the brain may be completely normal
    - in a motor vehicle accident which causes twisting of the head, there may be no external wounds at all, but severe brain damage (due to the brain stem twisting on itself)
- Exploring the wound may be of help
    - fractures may be obvious on inspection
    - the broken bits of bone may be felt with a sterile gloved hand
    - do not try to move the bone fragments

The most important criteria are the effect on the brain function
- Confusion or loss of consciousness is an important symptom
    - it implies definite brain damage needing careful assessment and observation
- Any other neurological sign is important
    - eg. any damage to the cranial nerves
- Examination of the ear drums is **vital** as base of the skull fractures can only be diagnosed by
    - bleeding behind the ear drum
    - epistaxis from the nose
- There may also be CSF flowing out of the ears or nose
    - this will test positive for glucose with a blood glucose test strip
- Changes in the size and unequal or loss of reaction to light of either pupil is a vital sign
- Rise in blood pressure, and slowing of the pulse and respiration suggest increased intracranial pressure and are important but late signs

Glasgow Coma Scale (GCS)
- This is used to assess the level of consciousness
- The score for each section is added up
- A score of 15 means the patient is fully conscious
- A score of 7 or less means the patient is in coma
- The score can also be used to test for any improvement or deterioration in the patient's condition
- The Glasgow Coma Scale should be recorded on all patients with a head injury and the results reported when the patient is **REFERRED**

Category of Response	Response	Score
Eyes open	Spontaneously	4
	When spoken to or on command	3
	To painful stimulus	2
	No reaction to any stimulus	1
	Untestable*	-
Verbal response	Talks normally and is fully orientated	5
	Confused and disorientated	4
	Inappropriate words eg. cursing or disorganised speech	3
	Incomprehensible words (makes sounds eg. moaning but no recognisable words)	2
	None (no sound even with painful stimuli)	1
	Untestable*	-
Motor response	Obeys commands	6
	Localises pain, does not obey, but attempts to push away a painful stimulus	5
	Flexion withdrawal (flexes arm in response to pain)	4
	Abnormal flexion (flexes arm at elbow and pronates making a fist)	3
	Abnormal extension of arm at the elbow (twists arm inwards at the shoulder)	2
	No response to pain at all	1
	Untestable*	-

*If untestable, this should also be noted, and the score altered eg x/10; x/11; x/6

MANAGEMENT

INDICATIONS FOR REFERRAL

REFER to hospital stat, with notes, in the following cases
- Definite history of loss of consciousness after the trauma
    - often patients are confused by the trauma, and may think that they lost consciousness, so it is important to get a report from a witness if possible (post-traumatic amnesia)
    - if the patient cannot remember, this suggests significant head trauma
- Any deterioration in the patient's condition, especially his / her mental state (eg as evidenced by a lower score on the GCS).

- Any change in the behaviour of the patient eg. increasing aggression, increasing restlessness, confusion and irritability may be due to
    - brain haemorrhage
    - other serious trauma
    - full bladder

  Note. it is important to check the whole patient
- Unconscious patient. **NB. Transport on his side**
- Any sign of raised intracranial pressure, especially
    - sluggishness of the pupil
    - changes in the size of a pupil
    - changes in the blood pressure, pulse, respiration
- Any other serious injury
    - **all** patients with a head injury **must** be suspected of having **a fractured neck** and given a neck collar immediately
- Special care should be taken with old people or alcoholics who may only show signs of intracranial bleeding late
    - it is safer to **REFER** them if there is any doubt
- Shock is very seldom due to head injury
    - other causes **must** be looked for eg. fractured pelvis
- Serious wound of the face or scalp
- Any suspected skull fracture, especially if it looks depressed
    - eg. due to a knobkierie
- A patient who may have a fractured base of skull as shown by
    - bilateral peri-orbital haematomas
    - bleeding from the ear(s) or blood behind the tympanic membrane
    - rhinorrhoea (tests positive for glucose indicating CSF leaking)
    - patients with bruising over the mastoid area
    - patients with subconjunctival haemorrhage especially if the bleed extends far posteriorly
- Children who had definately lost consciousness, even if they are conscious when you see them
- Patients with other associated injuries which will need hospital treatment
- Unexplained hypotension or hypertension
- Any localizing neurological signs
- Significant scalp bruising or swelling
- Suspected penetrating injury
- Any history of post traumatic memory loss (amnesia) at any time

If there is any doubt, it is essential to observe the patient for as long as possible

Check the following regularly at the clinic
- Level of consciousness
- Pulse
- BP
- Pupils
- Behaviour

REFER if during the observation the following occurs
- BP drops or rises by more than 20 mm Hg systolic
- Pulse slows by more than 20 beats per minute
- Pupils become unequal or unreactive to light
- Level of consciousness decreases
- Patient becomes more restless or fits
- If there are any other signs of deterioration

Note. A change in behaviour may be the only sign indicating a chronic subdural haemorrhage in elderly patients

Patients who can be observed at the clinic and allowed home later in the care of relatives
- No loss of consciousness at all and neurological examination normal
- The neurological system is completely normal and stable with no evidence of deterioration
- Ear drum and nose examination normal
- Children who have not lost consciousness
- Children who lost consciousness for a short period ie. less than a minute and
    - the condition is quite satisfactory and stable
    - it was more than 24 hours ago
- Children may go home provided that
    - the relatives have agreed to accept responsibility for the child and have **understood** how to assess the child's mental state
    - the relatives have a way of getting the child to hospital quickly if necessary
    - this is often better as relatives will have more time to observe the child than the nursing staff
- There is no need to refer a child or adult more than 24 hours after the injury, even if there has been loss of consciousness, provided they have none of the following
    - persistent severe headaches
    - drowsiness or sleepiness
    - behavioural changes reported
    - pupils unequal in size
    - any localizing neurological signs
- Ensure that the relatives know which are the symptoms and signs that mean the patient must be brought back urgently

SERIOUS HEAD INJURY

Ensure adequate airway and respiration and give oxygen.

Note. Suffocation and aspiration are the most common causes of death in unconscious patients with head injuries.

- If the unconscious patient is not intubated, he must be nursed in "the unconscious position", ie. on his side
- Apply a neck collar
    - if there is **any** possibility of a neck fracture
    - in all unconscious patients
- A neck collar can be made by folding up a towel or a piece of newspaper
    - without flexing the neck, put this around
    - fix it with a tie or bandage
- Look for other injuries

Other management
- Put up a drip and run slowly if the BP is normal or high
- Catheterize the bladder if the patient is unconscious
- Give tetanus toxoid 0,5 ml subcut. stat if there are any open wounds or burns

▼ **Note to doctor**
- If the Glasgow Coma Scale is 7 or less, intubate before transfer.
- If cerebral signs are deteriorating:
    - hyperventilate by bagging the patient
    - at a rate of 15-20 per minute
    - this lowers the PCO_2, and causes constriction of intracerebral vessels which lowers the intracerebral pressure
- If you have access to X-rays, obtain views of the cervical spine as well as the skull before transferring the patient ▲

Follow up of severe head injuries

It is an important responsibility of primary care personnel to help patients who have returned from hospital after a serious head injury.

These patients may

- Suffer from post concussion syndrome shown by
    - recurrent headaches
    - difficulty concentrating (this may seriously affect their ability at home or at work)
    - changes in behaviour and personality eg. easily angered
- These patients need help readjusting to normal life at home and work again
- **REFER** to physiotherapy, occupational therapy and social workers if available

LESS SEVERE HEAD INJURY

- Do a full neurological examination
- If there is any doubt, observe the patient until you are sure the condition is stable
- Discuss the diagnosis with the patient and relatives and advise them of the symptoms and signs of intracranial bleeding
- Give analgesics as necessary
- Check for lacerations and dress them
- Give tetanus toxoid if there is a wound
- Middle-aged and elderly patients can sustain venous bleeding some days after a minor head injury
    - this can result in mental confusion
    - this may be a sign of subdural haemorrhage
    - if it is suspected, **REFER** the patient to the nearest neurosurgical centre fairly urgently

SHOCK

Clinical features of shock

Shock may be difficult to diagnose.

Note. *The patient may be in significant shock with a normal blood pressure, maintained by a more rapid pulse and peripheral vasoconstriction*

The following may suggest that the patient is going into shock

- Patient complaining of dizziness, feeling lightheaded and wanting to sit or lie down
- Complaining of thirst or diminished urine output
- Signs of **severe shock** are changes in behaviour and becoming confused
- Cold extremities are a useful guide to the amount of blood available to the body
    - a useful tip is to check the temperature of the patient's nose
    - if it is colder than normal, it suggests shock
    - with successful resuscitation, the nose temperature will improve as the circulation improves
- Increased pulse rate
    - deciding whether the pulse is weak or not is difficult and not very accurate
- Increased respiratory rate suggests
    - acidosis
    - a sign of severe shock
- Drop in blood pressure is a sign of serious and advanced shock
    - ie. systolic blood pressure below 90 mm Hg in an adult

MANAGEMENT

- Stop any obvious haemorrhage
    - direct pressure is the safest and most effective
    - a narrow bandage may make the bleeding worse
- Check respiration and treat if necessary
- Do a rapid examination to find the main injuries
- Check for
    - decreased respiration sounds
    - dullness on percussion in the chest
    - increasing abdominal distention (this may indicate internal bleeding)
- Check the degree of shock. The following situations suggest severe shock
    - if the BP is below 90 mm Hg systolic in an adult, it is severe
    - if the extremities are cold

Intravenous fluids

Put up 2 drips

- In adults, use a size 14 or 16 cannula or a size 18 gauge (green) if nothing else is available
- In children and small babies, insert a canula into the back of the hand or put up a scalp vein drip

NB. Any drip is better than no drip!

IVI fluids can be divided into crystalloids and colloids.

Crystalloids

- normal saline is excellent to begin with, but large volumes eventually pass out of the blood stream and are lost into the tissue as oedema.
- Do not use more than 2 litres of crystalloid alone.

Colloids

- These also need to be given if the shock is severe
- They help to keep fluid in the blood vessels
- They should be used for infants, rather than crystalloids

Haemaccel

- This is better than plasma
- It is cheaper and has a longer shelf life
- It is free from the risk of transmitting diseases
- No time is lost in mixing it
- It has an equivalent colloid osmotic effect
- Give 4 units of 500 ml each
- This colloid may affect the blood bank being able to compat blood
    - always indicate on the request form that the patient has had it

Plasma

- This is no longer recommended for routine use in resuscitation
- Only use if nothing else is available
    - give 2 units

Other fluids

- 5% or 10% dextrose and maintenance solutions do not have a place in resuscitation
- Once 2 litres (4 units) of Haemaccel have been given, it is best to give further fluids in the form of blood, if available
- However, if the patient still needs to be transferred to hospital (or while waiting for blood)
    - further normal saline can be given rapidly until the blood pressure has risen to above 100 mm Hg systolic
    - give oxygen and elevate the legs

Amount of fluid needed

- The best way to estimate immediate fluid needs is to give 1 litre of fluid for each 20 mm Hg that the systolic BP is below 90 mm Hg
- However the fluid requirements must constantly be assessed as the patient may still be bleeding
    - as long as the BP is low, continue to give extra fluids **fast** IVI
- For children give approximately 20 ml / kg of colloid fast
    - reassess further fluid requirements
- Monitor urine output (catheterize)
- Beware of giving too much IV fluid to patients with head injuries who may have raised intracranial pressure
- Large volumes are also needed in major fractures eg. fractured pelvis
    - these patients should be given the same type of resuscitation as above

Guide to blood loss in shock

- Pelvic fracture   1,5 - 2,0 L
- Shaft of femur fracture   0,8 - 1,2 L
- Tibial fracture   0,5 - 0,8 L
- Humerus fracture   0,2 - 0,5 L
- Shoulder girdle fracture 1,2 - 1,5 L

NB. For compound fractures, **double** these estimates

Other management

- Give oxygen
- Elevate the legs
- Splint any suspected fractures to reduce bleeding
- Examine the whole patient
    - often patients will only complain of the most painful injury
    - they will not inform you of other injuries
- Antibiotics are not indicated in the acute stage
- **REFER** with notes of findings
- **NB.** It is important to record what IV solution has been used, and how much
- Tetanus toxoid 0,5 ml subcutaneously if there is an open wound

Monitor the response to treatment

It is important to assess the improvement in the shock

- Check the urine output
    - if necessary catheterize the patient on admission, so that the amount can be assessed all the time
- The patient's mental state is a valuable guide to decreasing shock
    - they should become less confused
- The temperature of the nose and hands should improve as the shock is corrected

STAB WOUNDS

Stab wounds are penetrating wounds inflicted with a sharp object.

- The most common object is a knife
- Other objects can be screwdrivers, wire spikes, pitch-forks, branches or glass
- The wounds penetrate to different depths and often it is impossible to tell
    - how deep the stab has gone
    - in which direction it has penetrated
    - which organs are affected

Possible effects of stabs

- Damage to structures
- Blood loss with all its complications, including shock and death
- Infection, including septicaemia and tetanus

MANAGEMENT

NB. If the knife is still in the wound, leave it alone and **REFER** for removal in theatre.

Suturing wounds

Wounds that a sister should NOT suture

- Crush injuries
- Human bites
- Bullet wounds
- Wounds that are not completely clean or are suspected of being contaminated with dirt
    - eg. motor vehicle accidents
- Stab wounds
    - more than 12 hours old on the body
    - more than 24 hours old on the face and head
- Animal bites - except if there is extensive gaping of tissues (see page 11)
- Chest stabs as this may cause a tension pneumothorax. It is better to
    - cover the wound with a clean bandage
    - **REFER**
- Wounds of the eyelids
- Wounds through the full thickness of the nose or ear

Wounds that a sister should suture

- Facial wounds
    - suture with 4/0 nylon using fine sutures catching the very edge of the skin
- Any cut into the fat or muscle below the skin
    - suture with chromic 2/0 as a deep suture
    - use nylon for the skin
- Animal bites where there is extensive gaping of tissues
    - insert a few stitches to pull widely separated tissues towards each other
    - leave a gap of 1 cm between sutures and wound edges

Recording length and position of wounds

- An accurate description of all wounds should be recorded in the notes
- Measure the length of wounds in centimetres
- For medico-legal purposes it is often easier to do this by drawing a diagram in the notes

For convenience use the following comparisons

- R2.00 coin   2,5 cm diameter
- match box   5 cm x 4 cm
- hand   7-8 cm wide at the base of the fingers
- wooden spatula   15 cm long

- It is important to note whether the wound is
    - clean cut, as from a knife or glass
    - jagged edged, as from blunt trauma
    - contaminated with dirt or not
- **Note.** Time elapsed (in hours) since the injury

Local anaesthetic

This may be prescribed by the PHC sister

The following local anaesthetic is available

- 1% lignocaine bottle of 20 ml
    - 10 mg / ml = 200 mg / bottle

- 2% lignocaine bottle of 20 ml
    - 20 mg / ml = 400 mg / bottle

The maximum dose of lignocaine is 3 mg / kg.
- Therefore, for a 60 kg adult the maximum dose is 60 kg x 3 mg / kg = 180 mg
    - 9 ml of 2% (20 mg / ml) gives 180 mg
    - 18 ml of 1% (10 mg / ml) gives 180 mg
- Only use 2% lignocaine for nerve blocks of the finger or toe
- For local administration to a large wound ½% is best
    - this is made from 1%, diluted with an equal amount of water for injection
    - it follows from above, that you can use up to 36 ml of this concentration in a 60 kg adult

Epinephrine
- Local anaesthetic works more effectively if epinephrine is added to it
- This causes local vasoconstriction which prevents blood flow from washing the anaesthetic away from the site of injection into the blood stream
- **Never** add epinephrine to local anaesthetic used for fingers, toes or the penis
    - the vasoconstriction action may result in gangrene

Maximum dose of lignocaine when epinephrine 1:200 000 is added is 5 mg / kg
- Therefore for a 60 kg adult the maximum dose of lignocaine plus epinephrine is 60 kg x 5 mg / kg = 300 mg
    - 15 ml of 2% (20 mg / ml) gives 300 mg
    - 30 ml of 1% (10 mg / ml) gives 300 mg
    - 60 ml of 0,5% (5 mg / ml) gives 300 mg

Suture materials
Steristrip
- In many instances and particularly in children, it is better to use Steristrip tape instead of sutures as this will
    - avoid the pain of suturing
    - result in a neater scar
- Clean the wound thoroughly and allow to dry
- Line up the edges carefully
- Place the strips perpendicular to the wound (across)
- Leave gaps between the strips to allow for drainage

There are many types of suture materials broadly classified into
- Absorbable
    - the material used is chromic
- Non-absorbable
    - the material used is silk and nylon
    - these will need to be removed after the wound has healed
- *Use the following materials and thicknesses*
    - chromic 2/0 to fat or muscle
    - nylon or silk 2/0 to skin
    - nylon or silk 4/0 to the face
    - chromic 4/0 inside the lip
    - chromic 2/0 to the tongue

Suture technique
The following points should be noted when suturing wounds
- Careful cleaning of the wound is essential (water is best)
    - all foreign matter should be washed away as it prevents healing
- Control of bleeding is important to prevent haematoma or infection later
    - direct pressure will stop the immediate bleeding
    - only remove clots prior to suturing
    - put in deep muscle stitches with chromic catgut to try and catch the bleeding points (these need to go to the bottom of the wound)
    - if you cannot control the bleeding, pack the wound and **REFER**
- Suture the full thickness of the wound, not just the top layer
- If the wound extends to the deep fat or muscle, this may need separate sutures
    - this prevents abscess and haematoma formation
- Do not tie the knots too tightly as this squeezes blood away from the area which
    - delays healing
    - promotes necrosis and gangrene
- Line up the edges carefully
    - the wound will not heal if there are "dog ears" or edges of skin folded into the wound
- Mattress sutures are safest as they turn the edges of the skin outwards

Removal of sutures
- Sutures should be removed after a week, except for
    - the face and neck where they can usually be removed after 4-5 days
    - the leg - 10 days
    - below knee - 2 weeks
    - wounds under tension eg. traumatic amputations of the finger - 2 weeks

Sutured wounds which ooze pus
- These wounds should
    - have some of the sutures removed to allow drainage
    - have the wound cleaned
    - be left open to heal
- Clean with Betadine or home-made saline solution
    - 1 litre water
    - 2 teaspoons salt

FACE AND NECK STABS

THE FACE

MANAGEMENT
Superficial facial lacerations may be sutured by the sister as long as they are not
- On the eyelid
- Right through the nose or ear
- Steristrips may be easier and leave less scar

THE NECK

- Stabs of the neck are potentially dangerous as major blood vessels and nerves are close to the skin and are easily damaged in this area
- Assessing the depth of wounds can be difficult and it is easy to make the mistake of thinking the wound is not deep
- Neck wounds should be properly explored in theatre

> **MANAGEMENT**
> - **REFER**, with notes of your findings, all stabs of the neck, unless you can be certain that it is a superficial one and no major structures have been damaged
> - If the patient is not in shock but the wound is in the neck region
>   - put up a drip on the opposite arm and let it run slowly
>   - give tetanus toxoid 0,5 ml subcutaneously
>   - pack wound with gauze
>   - do not sit the patient up until the wound is closed (risk of air embolus)

CHEST STABS

Clinical features

A patient with a haemo-pneumothorax may have some or all of the following

- Increased resonance (sound) to percussion on the affected side, with dullness at the base on the same side
- Abnormally soft breath sounds
- The trachea is usually not displaced
- Difficulty in breathing may occur
- Bubbling through the wound
   - this indicates that the lung has been punctured
- Coughing or vomiting blood
- Surgical emphysema (a feeling of crackling under the skin when you touch it)

> **MANAGEMENT**
> - Treat any life-threatening conditions, eg. shock or inadequate respiration, **before REFERRAL**
> - **REFER** all stabs of the chest for chest X-ray
>   - except for superficial skin snicks
>   - even if there are no abnormal chest signs
>
> ***If there is a haemo-pneumothorax***
> - Give oxygen
> - Drip the patient
> - Give tetanus toxoid
> - **REFER** stat with notes of your findings as this patient needs an urgent underwater chest drain
> - In a chest stab the knife may have been directed downwards and have penetrated the abdomen
>   - therefore the abdomen must be examined
>
> **NB.** Do **not** use a MAST suit in a patient with a chest injury

SUSPECTED TENSION PNEUMOTHORAX

Clinical features

The patient will have

- Acute distress and panic
- Cyanosis
- Low BP
- Trachea deviated to the opposite side
- Raised JVP (distended neck veins)
- Severe dyspnoea
- Decreased breath sounds on the affected side
- Resonance on percussion on the affected side

> **MANAGEMENT**
> **Safe method of relieving a tension pneumothorax**
> - Stick an IV catheter needle, eg. Jelco, into the front of the chest in the 2nd interspace, mid-clavicular line.
> - Remove the needle allowing the cannula to remain in position.
> - If there is a pneumothorax, the air will drain out.
> - Secure the cannula in position by strapping to the chest wall.
>
> **Other management**
> - Give oxygen
> - Drip the patient
> - Give tetanus toxoid
> - **REFER** stat with notes of your findings

STABBED HEART

Those patients who survive the immediate assault and do not die from massive haemorrhage, continue to bleed into the pericardial space (surrounding the heart).

This leads to a "cardiac tamponade".

The blood in the pericardial sac builds up pressure which squashes the heart and prevents it from working properly.

Clinical features

- The wound is usually seen in the precordial area or to the left or right of the sternum
- The patient is shocked with a low blood pressure
- There is a poor volume pulse
- Raised jugular venous pressure (JVP)
- Pulse disappears on inspiration (pulsus paradoxus)

> **MANAGEMENT**
> - **REFER** stat
> - If JVP is high, this suggests there is cardiac tamponade
>   - do not run fluids very fast as a cardiac arrest can be brought on
> - If JVP is low, treat as for shock (see page 271)

ABDOMINAL STABS

A stab to the abdomen could have been directed upwards and may have penetrated the chest through the diaphragm.

The chest should be carefully examined if there is any suspicion of this (eg. unexplained shock).

Clinical features

Features suggesting a penetrating wound of the abdomen

- Pain especially if
   - severe
   - getting worse
   - made worse by movement or breathing
- Nausea or vomiting
- Vomiting blood or passing blood per rectum
- Shock
- Increased respiratory rate, especially if shallow

- Increased pulse
- Pallor or a dry tongue
- Any impression of distension of the abdomen
    - regular measuring of the width of the abdomen with a tape measure will give a guide
    - do this at the same spot eg. the umbilicus
- A good test of peritoneal irritation
    - ask the patient to try and blow his / her stomach out
    - then suck it in as hard as possible
    - any tenderness on trying to do this suggests a penetrating wound
- Any tenderness, rebound or guarding
    - rebound can be tested by gentle percussion on the abdomen
- Decreased, absent or tinkling bowel sounds

NB.
- If there is any doubt, it is useful to observe the patient over some hours. If there is a penetrating injury, the patient's condition will get worse.
- Keep the patient fasted
    - a patient without serious injury usually becomes hungry.
- Avoid analgesia.

MANAGEMENT
Treat all life-threatening conditions, eg. shock or inadequate respiration, before REFERRAL.

- Drip the patient
- Give tetanus toxoid
- **REFER** with notes of your findings and treatment

If the patient is not shocked, the above investigations are negative and the patient has no difficulty in breathing, then

- Put up a drip and run it slowly
- Scrub up, put on sterile gloves, wash the wound
- Inject local anaesthetic around the wound (for guidelines, see stab wounds page 272)
- Feel inside the wound
- If the wound does penetrate through the muscle layer
    - **REFER**
- If the wound does **not** go deeper than the muscles and the base of the wound can be clearly seen or felt
    - suture
    - dress the wound
    - give tetanus toxoid

Follow up
- To check that the wound does not get infected

LIMB STABS

Clinical features

Check the following features

- If pulses are absent, it suggests that an artery has been cut
- Muscle power and movement. If the patient cannot use his muscles properly it can mean
    - cut muscles
    - cut tendons
    - cut nerves
    - cut artery causing ischaemia of the nerves and muscle
    - intense pain restricting movement
- Any abnormality of sensation eg. numbness, pins-and-needles, may be due to a cut artery or a damaged (but not necessarily cut) nerve
- If the stab is directly over the joint, there may be
    - swelling of the joint
    - pain and difficulty in bending the joint

MANAGEMENT
If any of the above features are found
- Give tetanus toxoid
- **REFER**

If none of the above features are found
It can be assumed that the wound did not damage any of these structures and can be managed as follows

- Scrub up
- Wash the wound
- Inject local anaesthetic into the wound (see the section on stab wounds page 272 for guidelines)
- Feel inside the wound
- If the stab is not deep:
    - suture
    - dress the wound
    - elevate the limb
    - give tetanus toxoid

Follow up
- To check that the wound does not become infected.
- For removal of sutures.

OPEN WOUNDS

Open wounds include:
- Traumatic wounds that are too septic to suture
- Leg ulcers
- Other ulcers

MANAGEMENT
General measures

Saline for dressings
- Saline is non-toxic and can be used
    - for cleaning wounds
    - for packing with gauze into cavities
    - for irrigating wounds to clean them when other medications are used
- Patients can also make up their own home-made saline solution for treating wounds
    - 1 litre of water
    - 2 teaspoons salt
- Betadine, Savlon, Dettol and other antiseptics may **delay** wound healing
- Many wounds even if they look septic, will respond well to home-care of frequent washing with saline

Chronic wounds
For chronic wounds that are not closing with povidone iodine (Betadine) try the following

Bactigras (chlorhexidine tullegras) dressing
- This may be applied and has the advantage over Tullegras as it is:
    - impregnated with chlorhexidine
    - available in single pieces in a sterile packet

Slightly septic wounds
- Clean well with normal saline
- Dress with Betadine or encourage frequent washing with home-made normal saline
- Do not spread Betadine all over a full square of gauze in order to treat a small wound as this
  - wastes Betadine, gauze and strapping
  - is likely to cause an allergic dermatitis in the surrounding normal skin if used over a long period of time

Dressings that are going green or blue
- This indicates a pseudomonas infection
- Treat the wound with a dilute vinegar solution (if available) at the clinic or at home

Very septic wounds
- Clean well with normal saline to remove pus
- Dress with Betadine while still septic
  - then dress with normal saline

If superficial slough is present
- Treat with Granuflex or Comfeel

If thick slough is present
- **REFER** for a surgical sloughectomy

If the ulceration has a foul smell
- Give metronidazole 400 mg 3 x daily for one week **or** apply directly to the wound
  - crush 2 g metronidazole (10 tabs)
  - pack the wound and cover with suitable dressing

Wounds for skin grafting
- Before **REFERRAL** for skin grafting, try to ensure that the wound is clean
- If a wound is likely to respond to a skin graft it should
  - be clean
  - have good granulation tissue
  - be a suitable size

Vitamin supplementation
- If the patient's nutritional status is poor
  - encourage the patient to eat a nutritious well-balanced diet with adequate protein, fruit and vegetables
  - give vitamins as well

HAND INJURIES

SUBUNGUAL HAEMATOMA

In an injury to a finger or toe from a direct blow, bleeding can take place beneath the nail. This can be extremely painful.

MANAGEMENT
- *Do not remove the nail*
  - it splints the damaged tissues underneath
  - it may fall off later by itself

Drill a hole through the nail
- Use a 20 or 21 injection needle and a gentle twisting motion
  - the point of the needle drills the hole
  - go right through until blood seeps back
- Blood can then be expressed from the hole
- If there is only a small bleed, one hole may be enough, but 3 or 4 often give better results
- A needle that is too small does not work as the blood blocks the hole
- It is not necessary to heat the needle first as modern needles are sharp enough to drill through fairly well, but if the needle is heated it is easier

If the finger is extremely painful
- It is kinder to first put in a digital block if you can
- If this is not possible, it is better to drill the hole anyway, rather than leave the patient with the pain

Drainage
- This can also be carried out if a fracture is present underneath
- The needle holes create a technical compound fracture so sterility is essential

CRUSH INJURIES OF FINGERS

MANAGEMENT
- These should not be sutured
  - suturing creates too much tension in the swollen tissues underneath
- Clean and dress with normal saline or Opsite / Granuflex if available or other suitable dressing (see open wounds page 275)
- Follow up
- Elevate

TRAUMATIC AMPUTATION OF FINGER TIP

MANAGEMENT
- Do not suture or interfere
- The best dressings are those that protect the wound, keep it moist and which do not stick to the newly growing tissue
  - a good dressing is a semi-occlusive plastic dressing eg. Opsite, Granuflex
- Apply TBCo to the adjoining skin to assist adhesion
  - the skin must be left to dry before applying the dressing

- Use overlapping strips of the dressing to help cover the curves.
- If an exudate forms:
    - this is usually not pus and is not important
    - if excessive, it can be aspirated with a needle and syringe
    - if there is an offensive smell, change the dressing
- The dressing can be left in place for a week
    - change more frequently if there is an offensive smell
- Advantages of using this dressing
    - it avoids damaging the new epithelium which happens with frequent daily dressings
    - wound healing is faster
    - fingertips regain normal sensitivity and fingerprints reform
    - swelling usually reduces very fast
    - the wound can be easily seen
    - the wound is well protected
    - even though expensive, it may save on dressings and infection

Reference:
Menner U, Wiese AMJ, Boomker D.
"Wound management using semi-occlusive dressings"
S.A. Family Practice 1995: 16: 328-335.

BRUISES AND ABRASIONS

BRUISES (CONTUSIONS)

A bruise is an injury to the skin or its underlying tissues, without any interruption in the skin surface.

Clinical features

- This is caused by bleeding into or below the skin
- No blood comes out and the skin is intact
- In lighter-skinned people it is usually seen as being a blue discolouration of the skin associated with swelling
- Later it turns greenish-yellow as the blood pigment is altered

MANAGEMENT
- No local medication needed
- Supportive bandage only if severe
- Paracetamol if required
- Ibuprofen 200 mg 3 x daily may be given instead of paracetamol in adults
- Use ice in the first 4 hours if available
- Elevate the affected area

ABRASIONS

An abrasion is a wound into the superficial layer of the skin, but not through the skin.

It is usually over an area of skin and not in a straight line eg.

- Skinned knees, when a child falls
- "Tram line abrasions" which occur as two parallel lines resulting from assault with a sjambok, stick or whip

- Give suitable analgesia orally
- Keep clean with home-made normal saline
- Cover with a suitable dressing

SEVERE BRUISES AND ABRASIONS

This type of injury may be due to a motor vehicle accident or a severe beating.

Even though there is no external blood loss, these patients may be bleeding severely into the tissues below.

MANAGEMENT
- Check the BP
- Put up a normal saline drip
- Give analgesia – they may need morphine if the pain is severe
- Give tetanus toxoid
- Ice or anything cold applied in the first 6 hours will decrease tissue damage
- **REFER**

NB.
- If the blood loss is severe, with extensive tissue damage, blood transfusions may be needed
- The patient may go into kidney failure from muscle breakdown products blocking up the kidneys
    - observe urine output
- Check for blood in the urine if a kidney injury is suspected
- Encourage as much oral fluid as possible to ensure good renal flow

CHEST INJURIES

FRACTURED RIBS

This is a common injury, but there can be serious or non-serious causes.

Serious causes

A crush injury such as from a motor vehicle accident with

- Multiple rib fractures
- Flail chest (see page 278)
- Haemo- or pneumothorax

> **MANAGEMENT**
> **REFER**
> - For a chest X-ray to
>   - confirm the diagnosis
>   - exclude pneumothorax
> - For appropriate analgesia
> - Maintain adequate ventilation with oxygen

Non-serious causes
Caused by a kick, punch, fall or a hit with a stick.

Clinical features
The following test will help to diagnose fractured ribs

Compression tenderness test
- The patient points to the area of pain
- Place a hand on the front and back, as far away as possible from the point indicated by the patient
- Squeeze the chest *gently* so as to press the ribs outwards
  - this can be done in more than one direction and at more than one level
- *If this causes pain at the place where the patient pointed, then there is a fracture, even if nothing can be seen on X-ray.*

Palpation of fracture
- You may be able to palpate the fracture
- Follow each rib down and sideways until the point of maximum tenderness is reached
- Record this as accurately as possible
- Fractures often occur in lower ribs below the diaphragm
  - these are almost impossible to see on X-ray, due to the liver shadow etc.
- If the tenderness is over the lower ribs, feel the abdomen
  - if there is damage to the liver or spleen, the abdomen will be tender, and guarding and rebound may be present
  - if this is present, **REFER** with a drip
- X-ray of ribs is not necessary to diagnose a rib fracture
- Fracture of 1 or 2 ribs can be diagnosed more easily clinically

> **MANAGEMENT**
> **REFER** if
> - There is respiratory distress
> - Breath sounds are decreased or unequal
> - There is tracheal deviation
> - Any suspicion of a haemo- or pneumothorax
> - Possible fracture of multiple ribs
>
> **Further management**
> Rib fractures can remain very painful for up to 3 weeks. The pain causes splinting of the ribs, which can also cause hypostatic pneumonia
> - Prescribe adequate analgesia for 2-3 weeks. Give paracetamol
>   - **plus** ibuprofen 400 mg 3 x daily after meals
>   - **or** naproxen 500 mg 2 x daily after meals

FLAIL CHEST

This results from an injury where 3 or more ribs are fractured in 2 places and there is a resulting loose segment. The underlying lung is also severely bruised, adding to the respiratory distress.

> - Give oxygen routinely
> - Give analgesia
> - **REFER** stat

MUSCLE INJURIES

PAINFUL MUSCLES AFTER INJURY

Exclude the possibility of a fracture.

Clinical features
- There is probably no fracture present if
  - the patient can use the limb
  - there is no tenderness on percussion in the long axis of the limb
- The problem is then bruising of the muscles and associated tissues
- See more details under the Musculoskeletal System (page 289)

> - Rest
> - Suitable analgesia

COMPARTMENT SYNDROME

Causes
- It is usually caused by swelling from trauma (fractures, haematomas, contusions) in a limb where expansion is limited due to the strong fascia
  - the increased pressure blocks adequate blood flow
- It also occurs with burns, tight dressings, casts and adder snake bites

Clinical features
- It usually occurs in the calf muscles
- It occurs less often in the thighs, buttocks, arms, forearms and hands

The 6 P's of Compartment Syndrome
- **pain** (severe)
- **pressure** (swollen tense compartment as compared with the same area in the opposite limb)
- **paraesthesia**
- **paralysis**
- **pulse** (usually palpable except in the advanced stages)
- **pink colour** (not pale, except in late stage)
- Late signs
    - pallor
    - cold

> **REFER** immediately for fasciotomy and decompression if you suspect it.

INFECTIONS

Note.
When there is a fracture, or a soft tissue injury, the pain will be present from the time of the injury and will improve over the next 4-5 days. If the pain starts or gets worse after 3-4 days, it suggests an infection at the injured site.

CELLULITIS

This is a spreading infection in the skin.

Clinical features
- It starts from a small wound, abrasion, sore or insect bite
- On history, the pain started in one small area, and gradually spread to involve a larger area
- When the cellulitis follows an injury, the pain usually starts some hours, or even a day or two, after the injury
- In a cellulitis, the pain is localised to a specific area of the body
    - if it is on a limb, the pain, heat and tenderness are often only on one side of the limb
    - if the opposite side of the limb is palpated, it is not tender

Differential diagnosis
- Osteomyelitis, especially in children (see under Musculoskeletal System, page 299)
- Septic arthritis
- Fractures
- Abscesses

MANAGEMENT
If there is **any** suspicion of osteomyelitis or septic arthritis, **REFER** immediately.

Medicine management
- If mild, give flucloxacillin or cephalexin 4 x daily for 5 days
    - adults 500 mg
    - children dosage according to age
- Moderately severe cases, give flucloxacillin or cephalexin 4 x daily for 10 days but review after 5 days
- Severe cases or rapid progression of erythema
    - **REFER** for intravenous antibiotics

- If penicillin-allergic, give azithromycin
    - adults and children >11 years 500 mg daily for 3 days
    - children <11 years (see pharmacopoeia for dosage)

REFER:
- if response is poor
- if the cellulitis is severe
- children who have significant pain, swelling or loss of function (to exclude osteomyelitis)

ABSCESSES / PUS FORMATION

Pus is formed by the body in response to infection. If pus cannot escape it collects in the tissues.
This is called an abscess.

Clinical features
Usually this is diagnosed too late.
Local signs of inflammation are
- Pain - commonly throbbing and severe enough to affect sleep
- Swelling
- Heat
- Redness
- Loss of function

Fluctuation
General signs of inflammation are
- Pyrexia (may be swinging)
- Malaise
- Tachycardia
- Tachypnoea

Areas where pus is very difficult to diagnose and only shows late
- Breast
- Bone
- Pulp space of fingers
- Ischio-rectal fossa

- Neck abscesses in children, especially of the glands underneath the sterno-cleido-mastoid muscle
    - these are commonly affected by infections of the mouth
- Thigh abscesses
- Anus

Diagnosis

Even if no obvious pus or fluctuation is seen, an abscess must be diagnosed on the following

- Pain severe enough to affect sleep
- Getting worse
- Throbbing in nature
- High body temperature
- More than 48 hours duration

MANAGEMENT

- In infection the object is to diagnose and treat before pus is formed
    - but if the patient presents when pus has already formed it should be drained
- Generally the mistake is to assume that there is no pus present
    - usually clinic patients come late and therefore pus is commonly present

The treatment of an abscess is not IMI antibiotics. It is drainage.

- In an abscess, antibiotics are only necessary if there is evidence of spread of the infection beyond the abscess
- For a small, localised superficial abscess, incision and drainage is the only treatment needed

*In assessing whether to drain an abscess in a clinic or **REFER** to hospital, take into account the following*

- The presence of a parent with a child (sending a child alone to hospital can be psychologically traumatic)
- Expected delay in transport and at the hospital before the I&D will actually be done
    - a few hours wait at the clinic may still be much shorter than at the hospital
- Check if a GA or formal block is essential
- If the patient is a child, the mother may have nobody to care for her other children at home

Incision and drainage (I&D)

Warn the patient that it is likely to be painful

- Ethyl Chloride Spray is suitable *only* for anaesthetising stretched-out, thin skin overlying a pointing abscess ie. skin less than 1 mm thick
- It can be used for any superficial abscess on the body, especially on the scalp
- Skin that is *dead white* over an abscess eg. in a paronychia, or a septic blister over a finger, is already "dead", and does not need any anaesthesia
- Abscess drainage is not always a simple procedure
- Abscesses in the following sites should be drained by a surgeon:
    - peri-anal
    - anterior and lateral neck abscess
    - central triangle of the face (formed by the corners of the mouth and nasal bridge)
    - pre-aurecular (adjacent to the facial nerve)
- Use a small incision over the area of fluctuation
- Insert a sinus forceps and open it within the cavity
- Release the pus
- Apply Betadine dressings
    - for first 3-4 days while the wound is very septic
    - then change to saline dressings
- Elevate the affected area

Drainage with a needle

- This is suitable only for
    - stye abscesses (see The Eye page 242)
    - pustules of less than 5 mm in size
    - buboes of chancroid and LGV in the groin

A very painful pointing abscess

- This may need **REFERRAL** for formal exploration under anaesthesia to drain it properly
- The patient's discomfort during transport and waiting can be greatly reduced by a simple stab puncture incision to
    - let out some pus
    - relieve the tension

Bigger abscesses

- These need to be drained more adequately
- Incisions that are just a slit in the skin, tend to close up in a few hours, before the infection has resolved
- The creation of a diamond shaped incision is preferable so that the pus can continue to drain out for a day or two

If a patient does not want an I&D of the abscess

- Advise them to apply frequent hot poultices
    - eg. a hot towel
    - this will encourage the abscess to drain on its own

▼ **Note to doctor**

Incision and drainage

Sedation for a child

Remember to allow enough time for the sedation to work

- Tilidine hydrochloride (Valoron) 50 mg / 0,5 ml
    - 1 drop per year of age plus 2 drops can be used
    - maximum 10 drops
- If morphine is being used to sedate a child for a procedure, use 0.1 - 0.2 mg / kg
- Once the procedure has been performed, the morphine can be reversed with naloxone (Narcan) 0,01 mg / kg or a proportion of adult dose 0,4 mg

Local anaesthetic

- If the skin overlying an abscess is thick enough to insert a needle into it
    - inject local anaesthetic directly into the skin over the abscess
- This anaesthetises it well enough to permit drainage of the pus, but it does not allow thorough cleaning out of the abscess cavity
    - a small local anaesthetic field block must be given for this, by injecting a diamond shape of local around the abscess

Abscess without cellulitis

- In many small abscesses, the pus is localised without surrounding cellulitis, and injecting around these localised abscesses is easy
- Local can also be infiltrated below the abscess (deep)
- *Lignocaine with epinephrine is best*, as the epinephrine vaso constricts the venous return and prevents spread of local and / or systemic infection
- A dental syringe with a cartridge of lignocaine 2% with 1:80 000 epinephrine is the easiest to use

Cellulitis around an abscess

- If there is marked cellulitis around an abscess, the above method is not suitable
- The abscess needs drainage
    - under IV sedation in the clinic

- **or REFERRAL** to theatre for drainage under general or formal regional anaesthesia ▲

FINGER AND TOE INFECTIONS

Finger and toe infections can be serious and need to be treated properly and followed up carefully.

> **REFER** if there is severe pain in extension of the finger as it indicates tendon sheath involvement.

ACUTE PARONYCHIUM

This is an infection in the nail fold.

> ### MANAGEMENT
> *For early cases*
> - Puncture with a No.18 needle to drain the pus
> - Give flucloxacillin or cephalexin 4 x daily for 5 days
>   - dosage according to age
>
> *REFER*
> - More severe infections
> - If on pressing the finger pad with a pencil, there is an area of localised tenderness
>   - this indicates an associated pulp space infection

FINGER AND TOE ABSCESSES

▼ **Note to doctor**
- These abscesses can often be drained under digital block anaesthesia. The block can be inserted in the doctor's consulting room and the patient then sent to the dressing room by which time the block should be working
- Use a dental cartridge **without epinephrine** or 4 ml of 2% lignocaine
- Raise a skin wheal on either side on the dorsum of the finger
  - then insert needle deeper, aiming down into the web spaces toward the volar side of finger
- The wheal of injected local should be in a triangle with its base on the top and its apex meeting below the finger
- It can be injected proximally to the MP joints or into the web spaces as far from the infection as possible
- In draining a paronychia, it is best to de-roof the abscess fully under a digital block
- Pulp space abscesses should be drained over the area of maximal fluctuation
- Give flucloxacillin 500 mg 4 x daily for 5 days ▲

INFECTED "BLISTERS"

These may represent a deep seated infection which has ruptured onto the surface.

> - Remove the blistered skin
> - If there is a sinus deep to the blister
>   - **REFER**

NECK ABSCESSES

These are often difficult to diagnose, especially in children. They often come as large, tender, deep swellings with no obvious evidence of pus.

> ### MANAGEMENT
> - Drainage of neck abscesses should **never** be done by dressing room nurses
> - If the child has symptoms that suggest pus, **REFER**
>   - if very superficial the doctor will drain them
>   - all others must be drained in theatre

LEG ULCERS

- Any damage to the deep veins of the legs may lead to damage to the superficial veins (underneath the skin)
- The superficial venous system becomes flooded with blood
  - as a result of this excessive load of blood, the superficial veins become dilated and over-distended (called varicose veins)
- The veins begin to leak plasma and red blood cells into the surrounding tissue because of the increased pressure
- This results in the superficial tissues of the lower leg becoming oedematous
- The red blood cells break down and leave iron deposits
- This sets up an inflammatory response with fibrosis and scarring
- Because of this damage, there is less blood supply to the skin
  - the skin therefore breaks down and ulcerates very easily
  - these ulcers heal with great difficulty

Clinical features
- The superficial tissues of the lower leg are
  - oedematous
  - chronically swollen
- The leg is
  - darker (hyper-pigmented) in colour, because of the iron pigment
  - firm, because of the protein and fibrosis.
- There may be associated cellulitis

Pressure bandages
- Compression bandages should be used in all below-knee leg ulcers, except where there is arterial insufficiency

- The pressure bandages work by compressing and squeezing the superficial veins of the leg flat
- This decreases the pressure in the skin and superficial veins
- All the blood has to travel in the deep venous system
- As a result the severe oedema decreases and the blood supply to the skin of the leg is improved
- Because of the improved blood supply, the ulcer heals well, **but the blood still has to be cleared from the deep venous system**
- The blood can only be cleared by the muscles of the calf pumping the blood up the leg
    - so patients must exercise as much as possible
- When sitting the leg should be elevated

When to use pressure bandages

Any ulcer due to deep vein incompetence
- They usually occur at or near the medial or lateral malleolus of the ankles
- There is usually a great deal of hard, non-pitting oedema of the area
- The area is very dark and shiny due to all the iron deposited
- Proximal or distal to the indurated area, the leg may be oedematous
- The actual varicose veins may not be visible because of all the oedema and induration

Ulcers due to hypertension and diabetes
- They may sometimes be helped by this treatment
- **NB.** Diabetics may have arterial disease, diagnosed by absent pedal pulses, and these patients must be **REFERRED**

Contraindications for use of pressure bandages

- *Any ulcer caused by arterial disease* must not be treated this way
- It is important to check for the presence of the dorsalis pedis and posterior tibial pulses in all patients with foot / leg ulcers
- See arteries, clinical features page 90
- If you suspect an arterial ulcer, or arterial insufficiency, **REFER.**

MANAGEMENT

If there is associated cellulitis:
- Treat with co-amoxyclav 875/125 mg 2 x daily for 5-10 days
- If penicillin-allergic, give azithromycin 500 mg daily for 3 days.
    - **plus** metronidazole 400 mg 3 x daily for 5-7 days

How to use pressure bandages

- Use Tubigrip from toes to knee and / or Elastocrepe (pink)
    - Elastoform cannot be used for compression
- Crepe bandage may be used if Elastocrepe is unavailable
- Give an extra Elastocrepe and measured Tubigrip stocking as TTO
    - the patient can wash those out at home and re-use them as long as they still have stretch
    - they only need replacing when the stretch is lost
- After the ulcer heals, the patient must continue to wear elastic stockings for the rest of his/her life, or else the ulcer will recur

---

Advice to patients

- The need for *steady continuous exercise* must be stressed
    - eg. a 5 km walk every day
- If this is not possible, the patient must
    - bend his / her feet up and down 5-10 x hourly while sitting
    - **or** stand up and lift the heels off the ground 9-10 x hourly
- If the leg is being treated with Granuflex or similar product, the bandage and the dressing can be left in place until it needs replacing
    - this may be at weekly intervals, or sooner if the Granuflex leaks
- For venous ulcers use paraffin gauze dressing
- At night the legs should be elevated
- Ideally patients should avoid sitting or standing in one place for any length of time. If they have to sit or stand, eg. at work
    - they must be encouraged to exercise continuously as suggested above
    - ie. moving their legs and their feet
- Legs with ulcers should be lifted up onto chairs
    - encourage patients to sit with their legs up on a chair or bench, while waiting to see you or the dressing room sister

Advice to dressing room staff

- Clean the wound well with normal saline and remove all pus and debris
- Chronic leg ulcers may be treated with Granuflex or similar product
    - 10 x 10 cm or 20 x 20 cm sizes
    - it can stay on for 4-7 days
    - it only needs to be changed after 1 week, or if it leaks

REFERRAL
- No improvement after 1 month
- All foot ulcers
- Ulcers with atypical appearance
- Venous ulcers that are persistently infected

SURGICAL LUMPS AND BUMPS

SEBACEOUS CYST / ABSCESS

Clinical features

- Sebaceous cysts occur commonly on the face as well as other parts of the body
- They are situated just under the skin
- A small opening (punctum) is often present in the overlying skin

REFER to surgeon for excision.

KELOIDS

Clinical features
- Keloids occur most frequently in scars
- Often seen on the back of earlobes (resulting from ear piercing)
- Also seen on the pre-sternal area

MANAGEMENT
- Small, or large flattish areas particularly in the pre-sternal area
    - use hydrocortisone ointment 1%
    - massage into the keloid 3 x daily
    - this relieves the itching
- **REFER** the following for intra-lesional injection of long-acting steroid
    - big, raised, flat areas eg. size of a large coin
    - nodular lumps the size of a pea
    - cosmetic reasons

HYPERTROPHIC SCAR FORMATION

This occurs frequently in healing burns or after skin grafts. The scar becomes thickened and raised.

MANAGEMENT
- They respond to sustained pressure applied over a long time
- Manage with Tubigrip sleeve if in an area where it can be applied giving good pressure eg. forearm and leg
    - to be worn for a few months
    - give extra Tubigrip as TTO so that sleeves can be changed, washed and replaced when worn out
- **REFER** difficult areas involved eg. face, axilla, trunk
    - to occupational therapist if available
    - **or** for surgery

LIPOMAS

Clinical features
- These are common benign tumours of adipose tissue
- They are subcutaneous and soft
- The edge slips away when pressed
- It is colder over the lipoma than the rest of the skin
- Multiple lipomas may be hereditary

MANAGEMENT
If non-painful:
- Advise patients that it is not serious and let them decide if they want it removed or not
- **NB.** The presence of the lump is not a reason for referring for surgery
    - many patients referred unnecessarily never arrive for surgery which results in irregular use of theatre time

REFER *for surgery if the lipoma is:*
- Painful
- Big
- Suddenly growing fast
- Causing a cosmetic deformity

INGUINO-SCROTAL REGION

IN CHILDREN

HYDROCELE

Clinical features
- Swollen scrotum
    - may sometimes shrink in size after sleeping lying down
- In a dark room, if a torch is pressed against the swelling, it often transilluminates (the light is seen to shine through the fluid in the scrotum)

MANAGEMENT
REFER
Over 1-year-old non-urgently, to specialist surgeon
- congenital hydroceles may close spontaneously before 18 months.
- Under 1 year old, only if very large

INGUINAL HERNIAS

Clinical features
- This is much more common in males
- A mass in the Inguinal region that "comes and goes"
- Often not visible in the clinic

- Examination
    - roll index finger across the abdominal wall in a line from the anterior superior iliac spine to the pubic tubercle
    - a slippery sensation may be felt as the finger crosses the cord structures - "silk glove sign"
    - the affected cord may be slightly thicker than on the other side
- It tends to occur more on the right side
- If you find a hernia in a female or on the left side in a male, check the other side for a possible hernia there

MANAGEMENT
REFER
- Urgently
    - under 1 year
    - if swelling cannot be reduced
- Non urgently
    - over 1 year
- In a neonate, if the mother reports that she saw a swelling, even if you cannot find it

EMPTY SCROTUM

This is very common.

Causes
- This can be due to retractile testes, where the testes are pulled up by a strong cremaster muscle, especially during cold weather
- May be due to a undescended testicle
- A good way to test if a testicle is present is to get the child to squat
    - this will often bring down a testicle

Clinical features
With retractile testes, both sides of the scrotum will be well developed.
In undescended testes, it may be obvious that one side is less developed than the other
- Try to milk the testis down into the scrotum by gently stroking a finger along the inguinal canal
    - stroke from the anterior superior iliac spine towards the pubic tubercle
- In this way the testis can often be drawn into the scrotum
- The hand must be warm
- If the testicle comes into the scrotum, it is retractile and no treatment is needed
- If it does not come down, it is undescended

REFER over 1 year olds with undescended testis to a paediatric surgeon.

TORSION OF TESTIS

Clinical features
- In infants there is a painless red / purple mass in the scrotum
- In older children severe pain, nausea and vomiting with sudden swelling of testicle
- There may be a history of trauma
- Unilateral pain
- Tender testis
- Testis appears elevated (high up in the scrotum)

MANAGEMENT
- Any male under the age of 18, with acute pain in the scrotum, must be treated as a suspected torsion, unless you can confirm the diagnosis of epididymo-orchitis
- **REFER** to hospital immediately
- Nil per mouth, to prepare for surgery

ORCHITIS

Causes
- Due to mumps especially prepubertal or pubertal
- Gonococcal if the child is sexually abused
- TB

Differential diagnosis
- Torsion of testis

- They are all difficult to diagnose
- **REFER** immediately

IN ADULTS

INGUINAL HERNIA

Clinical features
- There is a mass in the groin or in the scrotum
    - it is not possible to get above it
    - it comes and goes
- Cough impulse
    - the mass bulges or increases in size with the cough
- May have bowel sounds
- Sometimes only pain, without a mass

MANAGEMENT
- **REFER** for surgery when convenient
    - send details of any other conditions or medication that the patient is on
- **REFER** urgently if irreducible or strangulated (usually extremely painful)

HYDROCELE

Clinical features
- A scrotal swelling in elderly men
- It is possible to get above the swelling
- In a dark room, if a torch is pressed against the swelling, it often transilluminates (the torch light can be seen shining through the scrotum)

> **REFER** for surgery

ABDOMINAL WALL

IN CHILDREN

UMBILICAL HERNIA

This is a common problem.

> **MANAGEMENT**
> - If the hernia hole in the sheath and the skin are the same size, and the sheath hole is less than 4 cms (less than 3 fingers)
>   - it usually closes spontaneously
>   - no treatment is needed
> - If it is still present at 4 years
>   - **REFER** for surgery
> - A big skin sac with small sheath hole is dangerous as bowel can get stuck
>   - **REFER** for surgery
> - A massive hernia - ie. the sheath hole admits 3 or more fingers and the skin sac is the size of a tennis ball or bigger
>   - **REFER** for surgery

IN ADULTS

UMBILICAL HERNIA

> **REFER** as these are unlikely to close.

PARA-UMBILICAL HERNIA

Clinical features
- Situated above or below the umbilicus
- Palpable mass which may be reducible

> - **REFER** for surgery
> - When complicated, obstructed or irreducible
>   - **REFER** immediately

EPIGASTRIC HERNIA

Clinical features
- Occurs in children or adults
- There is pain between the umbilicus and xiphisternum
- Palpable mass which may be reducible

> **REFER** for surgery when convenient.

THE BREAST

BENIGN BREAST DISEASE

BREAST LUMP

"Breast mouse" or fibroadenoma is the most common cause of a breast lump.

Clinical features
- It is a small, well-defined, firm and mobile mass
- There may be multiple lumps
- It can occur from early puberty

> **REFER** for assessment.

FIBROADENOSIS

This is very common.

Clinical features
- There is an ill-defined lumpiness of the breasts which may be painful
- The pain is cyclical
- Sometimes a mass may be felt with the patient sitting, which disappears when she lies down

> **MANAGEMENT**
> - Reassure the patient
> - If the pain is generalised, give her ibuprofen
> - Re-examine 14 days after the period
> - If the pain is localised to a specific point or persists
>   - **REFER** for assessment

NIPPLE DISCHARGE

> - With any breast mass, ask if there is a nipple discharge
> - **REFER** if the nipple discharge is blood-stained or purulent.

MALIGNANT BREAST DISEASE

Clinical features
- The patient is usually over 35 years old
- Nipple discharge
- There may be an unexplained ulcer that does not heal
- Oedema of the breast
- Dimpling of the skin
- Nipple changes (deviation or inversion)
- A mass in the breast is found
  - it is ill-defined
  - it is attached to the skin
  - the presence of axillary or supra-clavicular nodes
  - fixation to the chest wall

> **REFER** for assessment.

BREAST DISEASE IN MALES

GYNAECOMASTIA

This is growth of breast tissue in males to any extent. It is caused by increased oestrogen levels and may occur in:
- Males with liver disease eg. due to alcoholism
- Males on hormonal treatment for prostate cancer
- Young men, between ages 15-25 (most common) and 80% resolve spontaneously in 2 years.
- Drugs particularly cimetidine, spironolactone and efavirenz.

> **MANAGEMENT**
>
> If alcoholism is the suspected cause, examine the testes
> - they are often small and tender
>
> **Bilateral gynaecomastia**
> - Pubertal breast enlargement
>   - reassure
> - If painful
>   - give paracetamol 2 tabs as required
> - All others
>   - exclude the above causes and breast cancer.
>   - if symptomatic and embarassing, refer for Danazol or other treatment.
>   - elderly males reassure.
>
> **Unilateral gynaecomastia**
> *Carcinoma of the breast is rare but very serious*
> - any breast lump in a male should be **REFERRED** immediately

Musculo-Skeletal System

GENERAL PRINCIPLES

DIAGNOSIS OF ORTHOPAEDIC PROBLEMS

- A useful way to look at an orthopaedic problem is to try to decide in which 1 of the 3 major groups the pathology is.
- These groups are:
    - bones
    - joints
    - tendons, muscles and any enthesis (tendon / ligament / joint capsule insertion into the bone).
- Sometimes the pathology may involve more than one of the above groups.

BONES

Bones usually need severe trauma before they get broken.

- However, sometimes a bone may break with only mild trauma, such as occurs with:
    - fractures of diseased bones eg. carcinoma often due to secondaries.
    - osteoporosis
    - stress fractures due to repetitive injury eg. fracture of a foot bone due to marching
    - disuse such as paraplegics.

Clinical features of a fracture

- Pain will be:
    - made worse by weight or pressure on the bone
    - relieved by rest or immobilisation.
- Palpation may show:
    - localised swellings of the bone
    - tenderness, particularly in the bone and not the surrounding tissues
    - irregularities or deformities of the bone.
- Percussion of the end of the bone (especially long bones) may localise the tenderness in a specific part of the bone
    - this will suggest that the pathology is in the bone itself, because the force of the percussion will have been sent mainly along the bone.
- Limitation of movement will be associated with the specific function and position of the bone involved, and so not all movements will be painful.

JOINTS

Clinical features

- The pain will be related to movement in **all directions.**
- There may be swelling because of increased synovial fluid in the joint
    - this may be easy to detect in some joints eg. fingers, knees.
- The fluid may be assessed by:
    - balloting the patella
    - fluctuation.
- Tenderness along the joint line, or over the specific joint, may be noted on palpation.
- Other joints of the body may be affected by the same disease process eg. rheumatoid arthritis.

TENDONS OR MUSCLES

Clinical features

- The patient will complain of pain only with **certain** movements or positions
    - a good example is the "painful arc syndrome" of the shoulder.
- This can be tested on examination by:
    - getting the patient to try to move the specific tendon or muscle and see if that produces the symptoms
    - the clinician can passively stretch the tendon or muscle and see if that produces the same symptoms.
- One way of testing is to keep the joint still and increase the tension in the muscles and tendons around the joint
    - either ask the patient to keep the joint still, or the examiner can hold the joint so that it cannot move, while the patient tenses the muscles around the joint (called isometric movements)
    - if there is **no pain**, then the problem is in the **joint**
    - if the patient feels the symptoms that they were complaining about
    - or if there is **tenderness around the joint**, then the problem is in the **tendons and muscles.**
- Direct palpation of the tendon or muscle shows specific local positive tenderness
    - eg. with ligament damage of the ankle.

PRINCIPLES OF MANAGEMENT OF TRAUMA

Any trauma or injury can initially be treated using the method of *R-I-C-E.*

R is for rest.
I for ice or anything cold.
- Cold lessens and prevents oedema, inflammation, and decreases pain.
- It can be wrapped in a cloth or a cold wet bandage and applied
    - within 12 hours of an injury
    - and should be left on for a $1/2$ hour.

- It can be used repeatedly for several days.
- Ice should not be applied directly to the skin as it may burn.

C is for compression
- The injured area should be compressed with a firm bandage to limit swelling.

E is for elevation
- The injured part should be elevated to decrease the oedema.

Rehabilitation
Physiotherapy and occupational therapy
Correct exercises, splinting, correct bandaging, special tools and aids for the muscles, and other techniques such as short wave diathermy may help to:
- relieve pain, decrease swelling and oedema
- strengthen tendons, muscles, joints and bones
- bring quicker healing and recovery
- prevent repeated damage
- help the person adjust to their work or home situation, despite the effects of the injury
- help the person adjust psychologically to the effects of the injury or disease:
- Physiotherapists and occupational therapists have special knowledge in these areas and can be of **great** assistance to the patient if their services are available.
- If they are not available, the PHC sister can give simple exercises and advice
    - some of the details of these will be given under specific problems in these guidelines.

Analgesia
- This can be given as well, and may assist if an anti-inflammatory drug is used eg. ibuprofen.

FRACTURES

- Definite diagnosis of fractures is often not easy.
- Some fractures can be obvious eg. if badly displaced.
- Quite commonly an injured limb that does not appear to be fractured clinically, has a fracture on X-ray.
- Other injuries may have all the symptoms and signs of fracture clinically, but have no fracture on X-ray.
- **Therefore have the patient X-rayed if there is any suspicion of a fracture, if at all possible.**

Clinical features
- Severe trauma
- Severe pain, especially if the pain persists more than a few days
- Severe swelling of the area
- Significant loss of function of the joint or limb involved
- Clinical evidence of deformity or angulation of the bones
- Symptoms or signs of neurological or arterial damage
- Localised tenderness over the fracture site can be a useful sign in bones which are easily palpated
    - eg. forearm bones in children.
- Percussion tenderness at the end of a bone
    - eg. if on percussion at the end of the finger, the patient localises the pain to an area of the metacarpal, it would strongly suggest a fracture.
- Crepitus in the broken bones may be noticed by the patient and given as a symptom on history
    - but you should never try to move or manipulate an area to try and detect crepitus
    - it is very painful and may make the fracture worse.
- Blisters may appear some days later on the skin.

Assessment of arterial damage
There are certain fractures that are likely to damage blood vessels. In any severe trauma, the blood supply to the limb **must** be assessed.

The most important injuries in this regard are:
- Displaced supra-condylar fractures of the elbow
- Knee dislocations
- Elbow dislocations
- Severe pelvic fractures

Method of assessing adequate blood flow
- Compare the normal side with the injured side.
- Check the colour and temperature of both limbs.
- Look for capillary refill on both sides
    - squeeze the finger or toe nail
    - then release the pressure
    - observe how quickly the flush of returning blood occurs (the colour returns).
- Check distal pulses
    - radial pulse in the arm
    - dorsal pedis in the foot.

NB. The circulation may be compromised (affected) if:
- the limb is cold
- there is loss of capillary refill flush.
- **REFER** the patient stat if you suspect poor circulation
    - even if the pulses are still present.

Assessment of nerve damage
Fractures and injuries may damage nerves passing through the area.

Method
- A quick and accurate method is to ask the patient if they have any symptoms of:
    - weakness
    - loss of function
    - loss or change in sensation in the area
- On examination check if any weakness, or loss or change of sensation is present.

If there is any suspicion of nerve damage the patient should be **REFERRED** *immediately.*

MANAGEMENT OF FRACTURES AND RELATED INJURIES
Injuries needing urgent REFERRAL

- Any suspicion of
    - a dislocation
    - arterial or nerve damage
    - fractured pelvis
    - fractured femur
    - cervical spine fracture
    - compound fracture
    - supra-condylar fracture of the elbow, if there is severe swelling
    - severely deformed fracture
- Be aware that it can be psychologically very traumatic for a small child to go to hospital alone for an X-ray.
- If there is no escort, only **REFER** the same day if:
    - the fracture is badly displaced
    - the limb has nerve or arterial damage (see above).
- Usually it is quite adequate to apply a backslab to the injured limb and to **REFER** the child when an escort is available.

Analgesia for fractures

- Analgesic requirements for fractures depends on:
    - the stability of the fracture
    - the amount of swelling present.
- Greenstick fractures, generally are not particularly painful once immobilized, and paracetamol is generally adequate.
- However, fractured ankles in adults and similar injuries, particularly where there has been a lot of tissue damage, may remain severely painful for a week or 2
    - the pain is also often experienced as being much worse at night, particularly on the first few nights
    - give paracetamol with or without tramadol tablets.

Advice to any patient after a POP is applied

- Elevate the fracture at home if possible for the night, especially if it is a fractured leg, hand or forearm.
- To come back the next day for a check of the circulation.
- Remember to provide crutches and to teach the patient how to use them properly so as to prevent brachial nerve damage due to pressure from the crutches on the nerve.
- Any stable fracture with a walking heel should not be walked on for the first 48 hours because the POP is not fully hardened yet.

Teach the patient the signs that the POP is too tight

- Pain when trying to move the fingers or toes
- Severe pain in the fracture area, not relieved by the pain tablets
- Swelling of the fingers or toes
- Excessive coldness of the fingers or toes
- Blueness of the fingers or toes
- If the patient is worried about the tightness
    - they should not just take more tablets
    - but should go immediately to the clinic or hospital, even if at night, as the POP may need to be split

Splitting a POP (bivalving)

- If there is any suspicion of the POP being too tight, it needs to be bivalved immediately.
- The POP must be split **down to the skin ie. all the POP wool must also be split.**
- Bivalving is done by:
    - removing a third of the circumference of the plaster (usually the anterior portion)
    - the removal of a third of the plaster should relieve the pressure and allow the skin to be checked
    - the two-thirds of plaster at the back should be strong enough to still stabilise the fracture.

How long to leave POP on

Healing of fractures depends on:

- The age of the patient
    - children's fractures usually heal very quickly, and the duration of immobilisation can be much less than in an adult.
- The position of the fracture.

Immobilisation

- Forearm fracture
    - adult, immobilize for 6 weeks
    - child of about 8, immobilise for 3 weeks
    - child of 4-5, immobilize for 2 weeks
- Ankle, immobilise for 6-8 weeks minimum
- Tibia, immobilise for 12 weeks minimum
- Fingers / hand, immobilise for 3 weeks **only**
- Feet, give crutches until pain free (usually about 4-5 weeks)

Leg fracture

- Once the period of immobilisation is over, children can usually be taken out of POP and left alone
    - they will spontaneously start to use the limb.
- Encourage the parents not to force the child to start walking
    - they will walk when they are ready
    - reassess in 2 weeks if not yet walking.
- In adults, remove POP and then assess the union of the fracture.

When to do a follow-up X-ray

Re-X-ray 1 week after reduction and again when the POP is removed in the following cases

- Displaced fractures, where reduction was needed
- All ankle fractures as they are potentially unstable

Assessment of union

- Assessment of fracture union is best done with an X-ray if possible.
- X-rays serve to confirm union particularly where
    - the fracture site cannot be palpated eg. femur neck fractures
    - there is doubt about the union.

Features suggesting a fracture is united

- No pain on using the limb for normal purposes.
- No tenderness of the fracture area on palpation
    - a united fracture should allow percussion over the area with a fist without being painful.
- The patient can walk in the case of a leg fracture, or can punch the examiner's hand without pain with an upper limb fracture.

If all these are satisfactory:

- The fracture can be considered to be united.
- The patient can be allowed home to continue with normal function.

If the fracture is still tender:

- Reapply the POP.
- If only mildly tender
    - apply an Elastocrepe bandage to the fracture site
    - keep the patient on crutches if it is a leg fracture.
- Reassess every 2 weeks until the fracture is no longer tender.
- If there is persistent failure to obtain union
    - **REFER** for assessment for possible surgical correction.

Note:
- Some fractures unite with scar tissue and not bone. This type of union may evidence the clinical features of union and be pain free.
- Only X-rays will show the lack of proper bony union.

Booking the patient off work

One of the most common reasons for misunderstandings between employers and employees, is that the employer:
- Does not know that the employee is sick and thinks that they have deserted when they do not arrive for work.
- Has unrealistic expectations of when the person may be able to return to work.

Certificate of sickness
- It is important to supply the patient, who is going to be off work for a long time, with a sick certificate early on, so that he / she can notify the employer.
- The patient may be able to return within a few days of the fracture depending on
    - the type of work the patient does
    - the type of fracture.
- It should state on the form that it is a provisional date, and that the fitness for returning for duty will be reassessed later on.
- If possible provide your telephone number so that the employer can contact you if there is any query.

JOINTS

JOINT PROBLEMS

SWELLING AND PAIN IN ONE OR MORE JOINTS

Important causes

Adults
- Minor causes eg.
    - local superficial infection eg. cellulitis
    - superficial trauma eg. bruising
    - bursitis
- Osteo-arthritis
- Rheumatoid arthritis
- Gout
- Connective tissue disease
- Osteoporosis
- Septic arthritis
- Gonorrhoea
- Tuberculosis
- Tumours

Children
- Trauma
- Rheumatic fever arthritis
- Juvenile rheumatoid arthritis
- Septic arthritis
- Tuberculosis
- Osteomyelitis
- Diseases of the epiphyses eg. Perthes' disease
- In very young children
    - septic arthritis (rare)
    - trauma eg. after a fall
    - congenital or birth trauma
    - congenital syphilis should always be considered

MANAGEMENT

REFER patients, not previously investigated, with any of the following

- Signs of inflammation in one joint (mono-arthritis) or more than one joint (polyarthritis)
    - ie. swelling, effusion, heat, redness
    - unless clinically obvious gouty arthritis eg. involvement of the metatarsophalangeal joint of the big toe
- Arthritis or arthralgia associated with features outside the joint eg.
    - anaemia
    - fever
    - erythema nodosum
    - tenosynovitis
    - significant weight loss
- Severe inflammation of one joint (suspect septic arthritis)
- Significant swelling of a joint for which you cannot find a cause
- Significant loss of movement of a joint for which you cannot find a cause
- Complete loss of movement of a joint, particularly if combined with severe pain, means **severe** disease, and needs **REFERRAL** stat
- General signs of infection, temperature greater than 38°C
- If there is evidence of fluid in the joint (effusion), particularly if this
    - is acute
    - has not been investigated before
    - seems to be getting worse
    - is not responding to previous management
- Any loss of sensation or neurological damage
    - eg. after a prolapsed (slipped) intervertebral disc
- Any lumps or bumps
    - unless the cause is known eg. ganglion
    - especially if they are painful
- Any suspected damage to an artery
- Any suspected damage to a tendon
- Any injury of the hands, fingers or knees unless
    - it is very minor
    - you are sure of your diagnosis and management
- Any patient
    - with an injury at work who may claim from Workman's Compensation
    - who is a police case
    - whose ability to work is significantly affected
- Any joint or limb pain in a young child or new born as
    - the causes are likely to be serious
    - examination of young children is difficult
- Any suspected wound into a joint

OSTEO-ARTHRITIS

This is a condition where the cartilage of a joint degenerates resulting in changes in the joint and local bone.

Causes
- It is commonly associated with obesity, excessive use, previous trauma and old age.
- There is also a primary form of the disease, which results in a more generalised osteo-arthritis.

Clinical features
- It is a disease of the joints **only** and does not affect the rest of the body.
- The symptoms are gradual in onset.
- The joints most frequently involved are
    - those that bear weight (knees, hips and lumbar spine)
    - the cervical spine
    - distal inter-phalangeal joints of the fingers.

- In the majority of patients the disease is confined to one joint or only a few joints, and one joint may be more involved than others.
- There is pain on movement of the affected joint
  - made worse by prolonged activity
  - relieved by rest.
- Inflammation in the joint is common and may be spontaneous or follow minor twists or injuries
  - if this is a feature, pain will be present at rest or even at night.
- Stiffness may be present in the morning, lasting less than 30 minutes.
- There is often bony enlargement but little or no deformity of the joint.
- Limitation of movement of the affected joint or joints.
- There may be repeated effusions into the joints, especially the knees
  - this causes swelling, which is usually mild.
- Increased crepitus may be felt.
- There is often associated muscle wasting
  - muscle wasting leads to joint injury because of the loss of normal muscular control - see osteo-arthritis of the knee joint (page 321).
- In generalised osteo-arthritis, there is involvement of the small joints of the fingers (excluding the metacarpo-phalangeal joints)
  - this occurs in old age
  - it is associated with the development of bony thickening on the back (dorsal) aspects of the end finger joints (called Heberden's nodes)
  - it may be associated with deformity, but seldom produces disability.
- Cervical spine involvement may
  - be a cause of headache
  - produce neurological symptoms and signs due to nerve entrapment. eg. pain radiating to the arm or loss of sensation in a part of the arm.

MANAGEMENT

The primary objectives of treatment are:
- Reduction of pain and inflammation
- Preservation of function
- Preventing or decreasing further damage

At each visit try and assess how well the pain is controlled
- How severe the pain is, especially if it is affecting sleep
- How much the osteo-arthritis is affecting the patient's home and work situation
- Diet adherence, if overweight
- Any side effects of the drugs
- If the drugs are controlling the pain

On examination check for the following
- Signs of inflammation
- Degree of mobility

REFER patients with:
- Chronic severe pain which is seriously affecting their life and which is not responding to analgesics for
  - assessment for possible joint replacement surgery which may greatly relieve the pain
- Cervical spine involvement for:
  - physiotherapy
  - soft neck collar (with acute episodes)
- Neurogenic compression

General measures
- Weight reduction, if overweight
- Exercise, non-weight bearing and postural
- Quadriceps strengthening should be considered for OA knee

- Rest during acute painful episodes
- Patients with osteo-arthritis of the knees to use
  - soft-soled shoes for walking
  - or foam rubber inner soles
- They should be encouraged to use a walking stick for long distances
- Physiotherapy and /or occupational therapy

Medicine management
Analgesics and anti-inflammatory drugs are indicated.

Pain without inflammation
- Paracetamol will usually provide sufficient analgesia
  - 1 g 3-4 x daily, as required
  - if the patient responds, reduce the dose to 500 mg 3-4 x daily, as required
  - give methyl salicylate ointment

Pain with inflammation or no response to the above
- Inflammation is shown by:
  - joint tenderness and increased warmth on palpation
  - joint effusion

- **ADD** Ibuprofen 400 mg 3 x daily or diclofenac 25 mg 3 x daily after meals as needed for 7 days
  - max dose of diclofenac 50 mg 3 x daily
- Once the acute inflammation has lessened, try to reduce the treatment
  - give the lower dose of ibuprofen i.e. 200 mg 3 x daily, or paracetamol alone
- If NSAID is not tolerated
  - **or** in high-risk patients >65 years
  - **or** with a history of peptic ulcer disease
  - **or** on concomitant aspirin, warfarin or corticosteroids:

Then add lansoprazole 30 mg daily while the patient is on the NSAID.

REFERRAL
- Uncertain diagnosis
- Intractable pain
- Frequent recurrent episodes of pain with inflammation
- For consideration of joint replacement

GOUT

Clinical features
- It mostly affects males, usually over 40 years of age and often obese.
- In women the onset is usually post-menopausal.
- It is characterised by:
  - recurring acute arthritis early on, usually of one joint only (mono-articular)
  - chronic deforming arthritis later on.
- It occurs mostly in the first (metatarso-phalangeal) joint of the big toe
  - in most patients this is the site of the first attack.

- Other joints commonly involved
    - ankle
    - instep
    - heel
    - knee
    - metacarpo-phalangeal joints of the hands
- Bursae such as the olecranon may be involved
- The acute attack
    - may be precipitated by a sudden rise in serum urate from alcohol, diuretics or low-dose aspirin
    - may follow initiation of treatment with allopurinol (Zyloprim)
    - may follow surgery or severe systemic illness or dehydration.
- In acute gout
    - the affected joint is hot, red and swollen with shiny, overlying skin
    - inflammation may extend beyond the joint
    - it is very painful and tender
    - only one joint at a time is affected.
- In chronic gout
    - many joints may be damaged
    - they may not be acutely painful.
- Attacks tend to recur with increasing frequency
    - later the arthritis may become chronic with progressive loss of function
    - gross joint deformities may occur especially of the fingers and toes.
- Tophi (nodular deposits of urate crystals) are occasionally seen
    - they are found in the cartilage of the ear, joints, bursae and tendon sheaths, e.g. olecranon bursae, dorsum of the toes
- Gout and hyper-uricaemia are frequently associated with
    - obesity
    - increased blood lipids
    - hypertension
    - diabetes
    - ischaemic heart disease.

MANAGEMENT

- Take blood for serum uric acid.
- The diagnosis is reliably suggested by finding a raised serum uric acid level greater than 0.42 mmol/L in the presence of the typical symptoms and signs.

Note:
The serum uric acid level may be normal during an acute attack, and may range between 0.3 and 0.42 mmol / L.

Acute attacks
General measures
- Cold compresses help to ease the pain.
- Encourage high fluid intake.
- Bed rest until the acute pain has lessened.
- Immobilise the affected joint.
- Avoid alcohol.
- Avoid aspirin.
- Avoid high purine-containing foods (kidney, liver, sardines, anchovy).
- Encourage weight loss, if overweight.

Medicine management
- Give ibuprofen 400 mg stat
    - then 400 mg 3 x daily for 5 days after meals.
- **Or** give diclofenac 50 mg immediately
    - then 25 mg 3 x daily for 5 days after meals

If NSAIDs are contra-indicated, eg warfarin therapy, kidney dysfunction

- Give prednisone 40 mg daily for 5 days (doctor initiated)

- Check in 5 days if not improved

Prevention of acute attacks / chronic gout
Allopurinol

Indications
- Recurrent acute attacks of gouty arthritis ie. more than 2 per year
- History of urate kidney stones
- Presence of tophi
- Structural damage e.g. presence of deformities

Contraindications
- Acute gout: do not use allopurinal during, or for 2-4 weeks after, an attack.
- Kidney impairment
    - kidney function should be checked routinely in the older patients.

Interaction
- There is increased risk of a skin rash when used together with amoxicillin.

Precaution
- Treatment should be withdrawn if a skin rash or fever appears which may precede a serious hypersensitivity reaction.

Starting treatment (**REFER** to doctor)
- To prevent the acute attack of gouty arthritis which may follow starting treatment with allopurinol:
    - treatment is commenced together with moderate doses of ibuprofen, (400 mg 12 hourly after meals) until the maintenance dose of allopurinol is reached.

Doses
- Allopurinol
    - initially 150 mg daily
    - increased to 300 mg daily depending on response as reflected by serum urate levels
    - average dose 300 mg daily
    - maximum dose 400 mg daily.
    - in the elderly and patients with kidney impairment (eGFR 30-60 ml / min start at 50 mg daily)
- Encourage high fluid intake.
- Aim to reduce serum urate to less than 0.35 mmol/L and optimally to <0.3 mmol / L.
- Do not stop allopurinol if an acute attack occurs
    - give treatment for the acute attack

Note:
Thiazide diuretics must be avoided in acute attacks. In patients with chronic gout, diuretics must be used in the lowest dose possible.

REFERRAL
- No response to treatment despite adequate adherence
- Suspected secondary gout
- Non-resolving tophaceous gout

RHEUMATOID ARTHRITIS

Clinical features
- This is a disease of the whole body
    - it shows itself mainly as a chronic inflammation of the synovium of multiple joints.
- The onset is usually gradual with joint pain, stiffness and symmetrical swelling of a number of peripheral joints.

- The course is typically chronic with periods of worsening and improving.
- Pain and stiffness are:
    - worse in the morning (for longer than 1 hour)
    - better during the day
    - stiffness may recur after daytime inactivity.
- Most often the proximal small joints of the fingers and toes are the first to be affected ie.
    - metacarpo-phalangeal (knuckles)
    - proximal inter-phalangeal
    - but not the distal inter-phalangeal joints.
- Later the disease may progress to involve the:
    - wrists, elbows, shoulders, knees
    - but almost any synovial joint may be involved.
- It is usual for at least 3 joint areas to be affected simultaneously.
- Disease of one joint only is **not** common.
- In its acute form there may be systemic symptoms including fever, weight loss, fatigue and malaise.
- As the disease advances, progressive joint destruction results in:
    - limitation of movement
    - subluxation
    - deformities.
- A dangerous complication is subluxation of the atlanto-axial cervical spine joint
    - this may result in damage to the spinal cord with the development of quadriplegia
- Characteristic deformities include:
    - symmetrical swelling of the proximal interphalangeal joints (spindling)
    - subluxation of the metacarpophalangeal joints with ulnar deviation of the fingers
    - radial deviation of the wrist
    - "swan neck" and "button-hole" finger deformities
    - "z" deformity of the thumb
    - hammer toe deformity

Features outside the joint include
- Anorexia, weight loss, fatigue and malaise
- Muscle weakness and wasting, occurring next to inflamed joints and more diffusely (widespread) as part of the systemic disturbance.
- Tenosynovitis and bursitis as tendon sheaths and bursae are also lined with synovium and are therefore affected by the disease.
- "Triggering" of the fingers may be associated with nodules in the flexor tendon sheaths which can progress to
    - permanent flexion contractures
    - tendon rupture.
- Subcutaneous nodules most commonly situated over bony prominences such as the elbow, scalp, scapula, as well as on the fingers and toes.
- Median nerve compression in the carpal tunnel giving rise to the carpal tunnel syndrome.
- Anaemia which is commonly a feature of chronic disease
    - this may be secondary to gastrointestinal blood loss from treatment with analgesic anti-inflammatory drugs.
- Increased susceptibility to bacterial infections, including pulmonary tuberculosis.
- Raynaud's phenomenon
    - this is spasm of the digital arteries brought on by cold and emotion
    - the fingers are numb and tingling
    - they are extremely sensitive to cold.
- Pericardial and pleural effusions
- Peripheral neuropathy and nerve entrapment due to the deformities
- Lymphadenopathy
- Dry eyes that feel sandy
- Dry mouth - a feeling of sand in the mouth and no saliva under the tongue

Confirmation of the diagnosis
- To be done by a specialist/rheumatologist. (ACR/Eular criteria (2010))
- No test is specific.
- Rheumatoid factor (quantitative test)
    - may be negative in up to one-third of patients.
    - patients with high titres tend to have more severe and progressive disease with extra-articular manifestations.

Monitoring of disease activity
- Disease activity is reflected by elevated ESR or elevated CRP (C-reactive protein)

MANAGEMENT
General measures
Articular rest
- During the active phase the affected joints should be rested as far as possible.
- It may be helpful to immobilize a very painful or inflamed joint (eg. the wrist or elbow) by applying
    - a POP backslab
    - an Elastocrepe bandage (pink).
- Rest-splints may also be used to prevent deformities
    - eg. wrist splint to prevent radial deviation

Occupational therapy
- For education on joint-care and to assist those who have difficulty in carrying out routine tasks (cooking and eating).

Medicine treatment
- **All newly diagnosed patients must be referred for specialist management with disease modifying antirheumatic drugs (DMARDs)**
- For control of acute symptoms whilst awaiting referral for specialist management (Doctor initiated)
    - Diclofenac 25 mg 3 x daily after meals.
    - **or** ibuprofen 400 mg 3 x daily after meals.
    - continue for no longer than 3-6 months.
- For control of acute symptoms during disease flares and in severe extra-articular manifestations e.g. scleritis (Doctor prescribed):
    - Diclofenac 25 mg 3 x daily after meals for 2 weeks
    - **or** ibuprofen 400 mg 3 x daily after meals for 2 weeks
- If NSAIDs are contraindicated e.g. warfarin therapy, renal dysfunction (Doctor prescribed):
    - Prednisone 7.5 mg daily for a maximum of 2 weeks.
- In high-risk patients, i.e. patients > 65 years of age and those with a history of peptic ulcer disease or on concomitant aspirin, warfarin or corticosteroids:
    - give lansoprazole 30 mg daily whilst the patient is on an NSAID.

> **REFERRAL**
> - All patients early for confirmation of diagnosis and management.
> - For confirmed rheumatoid arthritis, NSAIDs will be continued by a specialist as bridging therapy until DMARDs have taken effect.
> - Known rheumatoid arthritis patients with acute disease flares.

SEPTIC ARTHRITIS

Causes
- The infection is usually blood borne from a distant focus and then settles in a joint
    - there is no history of trauma.
- It can also follow penetrating injuries.

Clinical features
- Any severely inflamed joint where the patient will not allow the joint to move **at all** must be considered to be a septic arthritis.
- Large joints are most frequently affected eg. knee, hip
- Systemic symptoms of infection
    - high fever
    - rigors
    - headache
    - malaise
    - ill patient
- Local features of infection
    - severe pain in the joint, throbbing and affecting sleep
    - severe tenderness on palpation
    - severe limitation of movement in any direction
    - the joint is hot, red and swollen

Differential diagnosis

Abscess over the joint
- Commonly the knee
- Patients may have a pre-patellar bursa abscess in front of the knee, which does not involve the knee joint itself.
- The diagnostic feature will be that the joint movement will be nearly normal.

Cellulitis around a joint
- When this occurs, the pain, redness and tenderness are usually localised to only **one** side of the joint.
- Joint movements are fairly normal.

> **MANAGEMENT**
> - Put up a normal saline drip.
> - **REFER** immediately.
> - If referral in children is delayed for longer than 2 hours
>   - give ceftriaxone IVI/IMI
>   80 mg / kg

GONOCOCCAL ARTHRITIS

Clinical features
- More common in young females
- Often starts at the time of menstruation
- One or two joints usually affected
    - most often the wrists, fingers, knees and ankles
- Purulent discharge from the cervical os is often present and is the diagnostic feature
- Tenosynovitis is also common in gonorrhoea

> - **REFER** for hospitalisation.
> - For tenosinovitis or arthritis:
>   - ceftriaxone 1 g IV daily for 1 week

VIRAL INFECTIONS

This is commonly associated with mild joint pain for a short time (polyarthralgia).

It is common in patients with influenza.

> **MANAGEMENT**
> - Analgesics.
> - Reassurance.
> - The patient must come back if it gets worse, for further investigation.

TUBERCULOSIS

This is a common disease, and will become more common with increasing incidence of AIDS in the community.

It should be considered in any chronic swelling of any joint, particularly of the spine.

Clinical features
- Gradual swelling and pain in any joint of the body, particularly spine, long bones.
- There will usually be the other features of tuberculosis eg.
    - history of previous tuberculosis or a close contact
    - weight loss, night sweats, chronic cough.
- Usually a single large joint is affected.
- Joint pain, swelling and restriction of movement.
- Suspect it in any child with chronic pain or deformity (gibbus) of the spine or any joint.

> **REFER** if you suspect it.

COMPARISON OF THE CLINICAL FEATURES OF DIFFERENT TYPES OF ARTHRITIS

	OSTEO-ARTHRITIS	RHEUMATOID ARTHRITIS	ACUTE GOUT
Age	40 years +	20-40 years	Men = 40 years + Women = 50 years +
Pain	Increased with use of the joint	Decreased with movement and warmth	Constant
Stiffness	Morning stiffness less than 30 minutes	Morning stiffness more than 1 hour	-
Small joints of hands • Metacarpophalangeal • Proximal interphalangeal • Distal interphalangeal	- + +	+ + -	+ - -
Large joints • Weight bearing • Non-weight bearing	+ -	+ (knee) +	+ (mainly ankle & knee)
Spine • Cervical • Lumbar	+ +	+ -	- -
Extra-articular features • Tenosinovitis • Bursitis	- -	+ +	- +

BONE DISORDERS

OSTEOPOROSIS

This is a common bone disease.

Causes
- Old age (bone density declines in all people after middle-age)
- Lack of exercise
- Post-menopausal due to decreased oestrogen
- Inadequate dietary calcium
- Small slim build
- Smoking and excess alcohol
- Steroid treatment

Clinical features
- It affects mainly the spine and long bones.
- It causes compression fracture and collapse of the vertebrae, and leads to fracture of the femoral neck, upper end of the humerus and lower end of the radius.
- It is more common in post-menopausal women.
- There are fractures after only minimal trauma.
- Intermittent backache (pain comes and goes)
    - later persistent pain in a patient who is generally well.
- Loss of height and thoracic kyphosis (hump of the aged).

MANAGEMENT
- Adequate calcium intake is needed, particularly in women nearing middle-age
    - encourage all patients to drink a glass of milk a day if at all possible.
- Elderly people should try to keep as active as possible so as to prevent disuse osteoporosis.
- Weight loss if obese
- Analgesics for pain - aspirin / paracetamol
- Ibuprofen and diclofenac are **not** indicated unless osteo-arthritis is also present
- Physiotherapy
- Regular exercise slows the development of osteoporosis
- Avoid smoking and excessive alcohol
- Children, especially teenagers, should have enough calcium eg. 1-2 glasses of milk per day
- Women at risk of developing osteoporosis should be encouraged to use replacement hormones after menopause
    - eg. conjugated oestrogen and medroxy progesterone
    - provided there are no contraindications

REFER if:
- Symptoms are severe
- Present in early post-menopausal period

Medicine management
- The PHC sister may continue the treatment of patients (confirmed cases only) on calcium carbonate (Titralac) started by the doctor.

OSTEOMYELITIS

Clinical features
- This is more common in children.
- Usually there is no history of trauma.
- The infection commonly is blood-borne and comes to settle deep in the middle of the bone below the epiphysis (metaphysis).
- The surrounding soft tissue becomes tense, hot and swollen and may look like a cellulitis.
- Common sites are the upper tibia, lower femur and lower tibia.
- Sudden onset of severe pain in or around the joint.
- Pyrexial
    - cannot use the limb (pseudo-paralysis)
    - the joint is swollen
    - maximum tenderness is **next** to, but not **in**, the joint.
- Joint movements are painful and restricted
    - tenderness and swelling all around the joint ie. not only on one side.

Positive long axis percussion
- Hit the sole of the heel sharply with the tips of your fingers.
- If this causes pain in a localised part of the leg (usually the upper or lower end of the tibia)
    - the problem is in the bone
    - either a fracture or an osteomyelitis is likely.

Differential diagnosis
- Cellulitis of the limb is very similar
    - but in osteomyelitis, the inflammation will be seen to be deeper and the patient will be more ill
    - but if there is **any** doubt, the patient must be **REFERRED**.

MANAGEMENT
REFER stat if you suspect osteomyelitis.
- Arrange for consent for emergency surgery from a parent.
- Put up a normal saline drip.
- Keep nil per mouth, apart from stat treatment.
- Start antibiotic therapy
    - cloxacillin 500 mg IVI or IMI
    - **or** ceftriaxone 80 mg / kg IV or IM as a single dose
    - maximum IM dose at one injection site = 1 g
- Give analgesia.
    - morphine 0.1 mg/kg IM

THE SPINE

SPINE PROBLEMS

FEATURES WHICH SUGGEST A SEVERE SPINE PROBLEM

■ HISTORY OF WHAT CAUSED THE PAIN

- A severe injury eg. a motor vehicle accident
- Head injuries are often associated with neck injuries
- In older people, especially women with osteoporosis of the spine, even minor trauma may result in fractures of the vertebral body

NB. In patients with multiple injuries, spinal and neck fractures are easily missed in the rush to treat the other injuries.

■ SEVERITY OF THE PAIN

- Generally if patients complain of severe pain, especially children, there is likely to be significant disease present.
- Severe disease will usually cause difficulty with normal work or home responsibilities.

■ DURATION OF THE PAIN

- Any pain for more than 3 weeks should be reassessed to look for worsening neurological symptoms or signs.
- Back pain is a very common complaint with many causes **outside** the spinal column
    - it is vital to check the abdomen, pelvis and hips before assuming that the problem is in the spinal column or the back.

■ RANGE OF MOVEMENT

- Very valuable information can be obtained by watching the patient get undressed
    - it tests a large range of back movements
    - the patient is usually unaware that he / she is being observed, so movements are more natural and honest than when in a more formal examination situation.
- Serious limitation of movement suggests serious disease.

■ LOCALISED PAIN OR TENDERNESS

- Direct pain or tenderness in the midline over the spinous processes of the vertebrae may be a sign of serious disease
    - this is the bony part of the spine which is most easily seen and felt in the back

■ EVIDENCE OF DAMAGE TO THE SPINAL CORD OR SPINAL NERVES

Changes in sensation
- There may be change in sensation or loss of sensation, in either or both arms or legs, or in any part of any limb.
- This may be:
    - a shooting pain
    - "pins and needles" felt in parts of the arm or hand in cervical spine disease.
- The patient may be able to say which movements or position of the neck cause these sensations.

Change in the power of the arms or legs
- Ask the patient if they have noticed any weakness in either of the arms or legs eg.
    - difficulty with walking is a particularly valuable guide to leg and lower spinal problems
    - dropping objects out of one hand
    - unable to dress properly.
- The weakness may be in one limb, both limbs, or parts of the limb.

Straight-leg raising test
- This is done by lying the patient on his / her back, and then trying to raise each leg, with the knee straight, as high as possible.
- If the one leg cannot lift as high as the other, it suggests nerve root entrapment
    - normally a leg should lift to 90°.
- However, sometimes a reason for the patient not being able to raise the leg is that he/she gets pain in the back of the thigh
    - this is due to tightness of the ham-string muscles
    - the difference between this and spinal cord disease is that the patient with tight ham-string muscles will complain of the pain in the back of the thigh only.
- Decreased straight-leg raising on the opposite side to the pain is a sign of serious disc prolapse.

■ EVIDENCE OF AN ABNORMAL SHAPE TO THE NECK OR SPINE

- The presence of kyphosis.
- The presence of a gibbus (very prominent spine of a vertebra).
- The presence of a bend or twist to the spine (scoliosis).

■ DIRECT TENDERNESS OF THE SPINOUS PROCESSES

- Tenderness in the midline may be a sign of serious bone disease of the spine.

How to test for this
- Palpate for tenderness
    - press in the midline of the back, over the bony prominence of the spine (spinous process)
    - start at the top of the spine
    - press on each vertebra in turn

> **REFER** if any of the above are found, unless:
> - Previously investigated.
> - There has been no deterioration.

BACKACHE AND X-RAYS

Low backache
- Routine lumbosacral X-rays to investigate low back ache, without any suspicious features, are not indicated in Primary Care / General Practice. This is because only 1:2500 patients present with unexpected disease.
- There is generally no indication for surgery in patients with mechanical backache without any neurological fallout
    - routine X-rays and orthopaedic referral are not indicated.

REFER for X-ray
- Patients with symptoms and signs suspicious of malignant disease
    - pain getting worse in spite of treatment
    - increasing neurological fallout signs
      ie. loss of sensation, motor weakness, limited straight leg raising, pain radiating down into one or both legs, loss of bowel or bladder control
    - ESR raised above 50
    - recent onset of pain in an elderly person
- Patients with suspected lumbar disc prolapse have neurological fallout that is severe enough to consider surgery
    - mild weakness or mild sensation loss is not an indication for surgery
    - 95% of lumbar disc prolapse injuries respond to conservative treatment in 8 weeks and surgery is not indicated
- Middle-aged women with chronic backache should have an X-ray to exclude spondylolisthesis.

Thoracic spine backache
REFER for X-ray
- Thoracic backache in low socio-economic group patients who are at risk for developing tuberculosis is an indication for early **REFERRAL.**
- Any persistant backache in children.

Back pain following injuries
- Any patient who has had severe trauma eg. following an MVA needs routine urgent X-rays of
    - cervical spine
    - pelvis
    - chest
- The lumbar and thoracic spine need an incredible amount of trauma to cause a displacement of the vertebrae. Urgent X-ray of the thoracic or lumbar spine is only needed in the presence of
    - paralysis of the lower limbs
    - loss of bowel or bladder control
- In all other cases a decision as to whether or not to X-ray the thoracic and lumbar spine can be deferred until after
    - all other injuries have been attended to
    - the cervical spine has been X-rayed
- If the cervical spine is normal, the patient can then sit up, or stand if there are no leg fractures, and can then be re-examined
    - a better clinical decision can then be made as to whether these X-rays are needed or not.

NECK INJURY

Suspect a neck injury in:
- Any unconscious patient after trauma, especially if there is evidence of a head injury
- Any conscious patient with a painful neck following trauma eg.
    - MVA (whiplash mechanism)
    - assault to head
    - a fall on the head
    - a dive into a pool and hit his/her head on the bottom

Clinical features
- See as above for features of serious problems
- If the injury does not appear to be serious and the patient presents some days after the injury, check carefully for
    - the range of movement
    - any weakness or lack of control of the movements

> **MANAGEMENT**
>
> **REFER for urgent cervical spine X-rays if:**
> - There is any evidence of serious damage.
> - There is any weakness or lack of control of the movements.
> - The injury is acute.
>
> **If the injury is acute**
> - Do **not flex** the patient's neck.
> - Apply a neck collar while the neck is kept extended.
> - During any attempt to apply a neck collar or to move the patient, use the following technique
>   - stand at the head of the patient looking towards the patient's feet
>   - place your hands over the patient's ears, with the thumbs up
>   - pull the head **straight** in the long axis of the body ie. by pulling away from the feet, as if dragging the patient by the head
>   - **NB.** The neck must not be bent or flexed in **any** way.
> - If no collar is available
>   - fold a newspaper or a towel so that it is about 10 cms wide
>   - wrap it around the neck and fasten it with a belt or a tie (not too tight).
> - Any acute injury to the neck with or without severe pain or limitation of movements, should be immobilised in a hard collar and **REFERRED** for X-ray and assessment.

▼ **Note to doctor**
- X-ray views that should be requested are:
    - AP
    - lateral or swimmer's view
    - C1-C2 (open mouth).
- **NB.** Do not take stress views following a suspected whiplash injury. ▲

NECK PAIN IN A CHILD

The following are causes for neck pain in children.

■ MENINGITIS

- Meningitis must always be considered first in a child complaining of an acute pain in the neck.
- See page 221 for clinical features.

■ LYMPH NODE ENLARGEMENT

- Acute tonsillitis
- Infections in the mouth
- Infections of the scalp (impetigo)

Clinical features

- Pain on moving the neck
- The infection is usually obvious and the enlarged glands easily palpated in the neck

> - Manage the infection.
> - See ENT (page 40) and The Skin management of impetigo (pages 249-250).

■ STRESS

- Emotional eg. at school
- Physical due to over-exertion
- The clinical features will be similar to those of fibrositis (see page 306)

> Manage as for stress.

■ INJURIES

- Especially contact sports, such as rugby
- Clinical features and management as for adults above

■ TUBERCULOSIS

Tuberculosis of the spine must always be thought of when a child complains of a chronic neck pain.

Clinical features

- Chronic progressive pain and limitation of movement of the neck.
- Other features of tuberculosis may be present eg. failure to thrive, as seen on the Road to Health Card.
- An important sign is deformity or prominence of the cervical spine (gibbus).
- Direct tenderness on palpating the spinous processes in the midline.
- Signs of damage to the spinal cord and nerves
    - eg. loss or change in sensation or power in the arms or legs.

> **REFER** to specialist.

■ ACUTE INFECTION IN THE SPINE
(PYOGENIC SPONDYLITIS)

Causes

- May be due to typhoid.

> **MANAGEMENT**
> **REFER**
> - Stat if there is:
>   - any evidence of spinal cord damage
>   - definite tenderness on palpation of the spinous processes
> - If you suspect tuberculosis or an acute infection

■ ACUTE WRY NECK (ACUTE TORTICOLLIS)

Causes

- The most common cause in children is an infection of the mouth or throat
- Acute slipping out of place (subluxation) of an intervertebral facet joint
- Cervical or submandibular lymph node enlargement
- Fibrositis

Clinical features

- The patient complains of:
    - acute onset of severe pain in the neck
    - inability to turn the neck
- No pre-existing neck problem
- Sudden onset which usually starts after sleep
- One side of the neck is painful
    - pain may start at a particular point on one side of the neck vertebrae and then radiates
- The neck is usually tilted to the side of the pain
- Movements of the neck are severely limited
- It is important to check for infectious causes such as:
    - tonsillitis
    - enlarged neck glands

> **MANAGEMENT**
> - Neck collar
> - Give an anti-inflammatory
>   - eg. ibuprofen 200-400 mg 3 x daily for 5-7 days
> - **REFER** if not improved.

NECK PAIN IN AN ADULT

Causes

- Fibrositis (see page 306)
- Stress with spasm of the neck muscles
- Facet joint subluxation (acute wry neck)
    - see above
- Severe osteo-arthritis of the cervical spine
- After trauma
- Infections in and around the neck eg. tonsillitis with enlarged cervical glands

- Myocardial infarction or angina pectoris with referred pain to the neck
- Bone diseases of the cervical spine such as tuberculosis or tumours
- Rheumatoid arthritis especially of the atlanto-axial joint.
- Cervical rib

MANAGEMENT
- REFER stat if:
  - there is any suspicion of acute nerve damage
  - previous nerve damage has become worse
  - you suspect a serious cause
- If the nerve damage has been investigated before, and it is not getting worse, referral is not necessary
  - continue with previous treatment.
- Treat for any causes that you can manage.

OSTEO-ARTHRITIS

Clinical features
- Crackling noises may be noted by the patient when moving the neck
  - this strongly suggests osteo-arthritis
  - this is similar to the crepitations found in the osteo-arthritic knees
- A humped back may be noticed if osteoporosis is present
  - there will be increased prominence of the bend of the spine, forcing the head to bend forward
- There will be decreased movements
- Pressure on the cervical nerves may cause weakness or abnormal sensation in any part of the arms or hands
- X-rays may show osteophytes
  - but the bone changes on X-ray usually do not accurately reflect the amount of pain a patient is likely to have
  - they are essential only to exclude bone tumours or tuberculosis as a rare cause of neck pain

---

MANAGEMENT
- Analgesics, anti-inflammatories
  - see under osteo-arthritis page 293
- Apply a cervical collar
  - fill a length of stockinette with cotton wool (or orthopaedic wool)
  - tie firmly (not tightly) around the neck
- Home neck manipulation can be taught to the patient (see below)
- REFER for physiotherapy if available

Home neck manipulation
There are a few simple movements that patients can be taught to do themselves at home to relieve their neck pain.

Rotating the head
- Touch the chin onto the left shoulder.
- Straighten the head and point the chin upwards lifting it as high as possible.
- Swing the chin around to the opposite shoulder.
- Bring the chin down to touch the opposite shoulder.
- Bring the chin back to the first shoulder keeping it as low as possible.

THORACIC PAIN IN A CHILD

Causes
- Tuberculosis
- Other infectious diseases eg. typhoid causing an abscess in the spinal bones
- Trauma
- Scoliosis
- Scheuermann's disease
- Pain from chest or heart disease

REFER all children with thoracic spine pain, unless you can be sure it is due to a minor cause.

SCHEUERMANN'S DISEASE

Causes
- This is due to damage to the epiphyses in the vertebrae in children who are still growing.

Clinical features
- Age 13-16
- It may be brought on by excessive pressure and exercise
  - eg. playing as a rugby forward
- Pain in the thoracic spine which is
  - mild to moderate
  - chronic
- Rounded back
- Exclude a scoliosis (see page 309)
- The active disease lasts about 2 years
  - slight rounding of the back may persist

REFER if you suspect this disease to confirm the diagnosis.

THORACIC PAIN IN AN ADULT

This is not a common area for backache.

Causes
- Fibrositis
- Herpes zoster, either a first episode or a recurrence
- Chest disease
- Heart disease
- Reflux oesophagitis
- Serious causes include:
  - tuberculosis
  - carcinoma, especially secondary deposits
  - severe osteoporosis with collapse of a vertebra
  - acute infection causing an abscess

REFER unless you can be sure the cause is not serious.

ACUTE BACKACHE

CAUSES OUTSIDE THE SPINAL COLUMN

- Referred pain from
    - the bowel
    - gynaecological diseases
    - male urogenital disease, especially acute or chronic prostatitis
    - hip disease
    - kidney disease

> See the various sections for details of the diseases and management.

CAUSES IN THE JOINTS OF THE PELVIS

Clinical features

- Pain in the joints of the pelvis is a common cause of lower back pain, especially in:
    - older people
    - pregnant women
    - after delivery
- The patient may describe it as lumbago or sciatica.
- It will be worse on standing and weight-bearing.
- The patient may be aware of a possible cause eg. a motor vehicle accident, a recent delivery of a child.
- The patient may then be able to localise the part of the pelvis experiencing the pain.
- Palpation all along the area of the sacro-iliac joint or pelvis may reveal specific tenderness
    - in an obese person this may be difficult and will require quite firm pressure.
- If on direct pressure on this area the patient says that it is similar to the pain they are complaining about, then this suggests pelvic joint disease.

Common sites of pain

- The sacro-iliac joint
    - this is a few centimetres lateral to the base of the spine
- The symphysis pubis
    - local tenderness on palpation in the anterior midline of the pelvis over the symphysis

Features suggesting a more serious cause

The patient may have carcinoma or tuberculosis

- Sudden onset in middle-aged or older patient
- Other features such as
    - weight loss
    - progressive worsening of the pain
    - raised ESR
- Chronic pain which has remained unchanged, or is intermittent, is unlikely to be due to a serious cause.

MANAGEMENT

Sacro-iliac joint disease

Serious causes

REFER if a serious cause is suspected for X-ray.

Non-serious causes

- Weight loss may be helpful in an overweight patient
- **REFER** to physiotherapy if available
- Give analgesics, starting with paracetamol first (see osteo-arthritis page 293)

Symphysis pubis pain

- If this is during pregnancy or follows delivery
    - bed rest until the pain has settled and the symphysis has reunited
    - give analgesics, eg. paracetamol, NSAID

FRACTURE OF THE THORACIC OR LUMBAR SPINE

Clinical features

- History of severe trauma or a fall from a height
- A fracture of the spine must be suspected if there is marked localised tenderness over one or more of the spinous processes of the vertebra
- More obvious prominence of a part of the spine

> **REFER** if you suspect a fracture.

LIGAMENT DAMAGE IN THE LOWER BACK

Clinical features

- Localised pain may occur as a result of poor posture and inadequate back muscle exercises
- The common area where this occurs is where the back muscles attach to the posterior iliac crest
- Backache, localised to one side of the midline
- Point tenderness on deep palpation
    - either in the triangle between the iliac crest and the lumbar vertebrae (ie. to the lateral side of the sacrum)
    - **or** along the upper posterior edge of the iliac crest
- No neurological symptoms or signs
- No radiation of the pain

MANAGEMENT

- Physiotherapy if available
- Rest and avoidance of the exercise which caused the problem if possible
- Analgesics eg. ibuprofen
- If there is no adequate response to the above, and it is causing severe disability, **REFER** for Depo-Medrol and local anaesthetic injection
    - directly into the point of maximum tenderness
    - this may give dramatic relief

FIBROSITIS

Fibrositis of the lower lumbar muscles is very common. This is a chronic muscle spasm.

Causes

- It commonly occurs after any sudden, severe exercise eg. sport, lifting things or working in a garden
- It often follows stress eg. when somebody is studying, anxious or depressed
- Cervical spine or shoulder "fibrositis" may also be due to nerve compression in the cervical spine
    - especially in older people with cervical spine osteo-arthritis

Clinical features

- It can occur almost anywhere in the muscles of the body
- It commonly presents as painful, tender nodules in the upper edge of the trapezius muscles of the shoulders or between the scapulae, where the scapula muscles attach to the spine
- It is sometimes associated with severe headaches, which spread from the shoulders and neck into the occipital region
- The patient complains of severe pain
    - made worse by any movement of the muscles
    - relieved by rest and heat
- The pain often only starts 1-2 days after the exercise
- Pain on movement of the joint
    - eg. with scapula fibrositis there is pain on movement of the shoulders
- Severe local tenderness of the affected muscles on palpation
    - palpation over the vertebral processes of the spine will be painless
- There will be a gradual onset of pain and stiffness some days after strenuous exercise
- There may be a history of
    - having done a lot of back exercise a day or two before the onset of the pain
    - stress or anxiety
- The tenderness is away from the midline
- There will be no evidence of nerve damage
- The pain will improve after 2-3 days

Differential diagnosis

- Carcinoma or tuberculosis of the spine may also give symptoms similar to fibrositis

Trigger points in fibrositis

- Where a person has pain over a wide area, careful palpation may show that there is one specific point that is more tender than the rest of the area
- This is called a trigger point

The pain radiates from this point to the surrounding areas
- Trapezius (most common)
    - often tender in the suboccipital region
- Supra-spinatus origin
    - over the medial upper edge of the scapula
- Rhomboid
    - medial to the scapula
- Buttock
    - anterior fold of gluteus medius
- Neck
    - low cervical C 4 - 6
- Back
    - low lumbar L 4 - S 1

MANAGEMENT
- **REFER** if:
    - a patient has any associated neurological signs such as sensory loss
    - the symptoms are related to neck movement
    - there is tenderness on direct palpation of the vertebral processes
- Reassure the patient
- Give paracetamol
- Give ung meth sal to use with gentle massage
- Heat can be of benefit
- **REFER** for physiotherapy if available
- Trigger points may respond dramatically to an injection of local anaesthetic (with long-acting steroid) into the point of maximum tenderness

---

SLIPPED FACET JOINT

This occurs with a sudden movement of the spine, causing a part of the lining of the joint (synovium) to be trapped in the joint between 2 vertebrae.

Clinical features

- This looks very similar to a prolapsed intervertebral disc, but there will be **no** neurological symptoms or signs as no nerves are damaged
- There is acute onset of backache after
    - lifting an object
    - sudden movement

MANAGEMENT
- Bed rest
- Analgesics
- Manipulation of the spine by a physiotherapist or chiropracter can give instant relief

---

PROLAPSED INTERVERTEBRAL DISC (SLIPPED DISC)

Discs degenerate with age and a weakened disc may be unable to resist body weight and is liable to bulge or rupture. Prolapsed disc material may press on the dura (causing backache) or on nerve roots (causing backache or sciatica or both).

Clinical features

- Usually young or middle-aged male patients
- Sudden onset of severe back pain usually when trying to get up after bending down
    - the patient will be able to describe in detail exactly when and how it started
    - he may not have been able to get up off the floor
    - he may have pulled himself up by means of the furniture
    - he may have used his hands on his knees to push himself up
- Pain is so bad that he cannot walk properly
- The pain may
    - radiate down one or both legs
    - be associated with weakness or loss of sensation

- be associated with incontinence of urine or faeces if severe
- follow hard work involving use of the back eg. picking up heavy weights at work
- be brought on by minor movement eg. coughing or bending down
- He will walk bent forwards a little and with his buttocks pushed out backwards, or his knees bent so as to make his spine vertical
- There will be spasm of the muscles of the back
- The back is held very stiff and straight
- Bending forwards or backwards is limited
- The patient will have particular difficulty in straightening up after bending down
- There may be
  - loss of sensation or weakness of the foot
  - weakness of ankle movements
- There will be limited straight-leg raising (see page 301)

Differential diagnosis

In the younger patient
- Slipped interfacet joint
- Severe fibrositis of the back
- Infections of the spine eg. tuberculosis, typhoid
- Causes outside the spine eg. genito urinary disease, bowel disease

In middle-aged or older patients
- A tumour of the spine, primary or secondary
- Osteo-arthritis causing nerve entrapment
- Osteoporosis, especially in elderly women causing fracture or the lower lumbar vertebrae

MANAGEMENT

Reasons for REFERRAL

REFER if:
- The pain radiates down one or both legs which suggests that there is significant nerve compression
- There are any neurological symptoms or signs of nerve compression eg. weakness, sensory loss
- The pain is very severe
- There are repeated episodes
- You suspect severe underlying disease eg. a tumour
- There is failure to respond to conservative treatment for at least 10 days
- There is decreased straight leg raising on the opposite side to where the main pain or radiation is being felt

If the patient can be managed at the clinic

General measures
- Discuss with the patient likely causes of the prolapse and how to prevent it recurring.
- Advise the patient to sleep on a hard surface eg.
  - to put a wooden board under the bed
  - to put the mattress on the floor.
- The patient may be more comfortable lying with a pillow behind his or her knees.
- If the patient has to travel by car or minibus, a small pillow put in the small of the back encourages the normal lordosis and helps to relieve the pain.
- Teach the patient how to pick up objects from the floor
  - bending at the knees and the hips
  - keep the back straight and vertical.
- If obese, weight loss will help to take strain off the lumbar spine.
- If stress is an aggravating factor, try and help the patient deal with it.
- Book off work for 2 weeks.
- Strict bed-rest at home for 2 weeks.
- Reassess after 2 weeks.

If improved:
- Discuss with the patient about when to return to work
  - this will depend on his occupation.

*If **no** improvement:*
- **REFER.**
- Physiotherapy can be of great assistance to
  - relieve the pain and muscle spasm with heat and infra-red and other techniques
  - limit further prolapse of the disc into the spinal canal
  - develop the muscles of the back and stomach.
- An occupational therapist will be able to give assistance in dealing with the home and work situation as a result of the back problem.

Medicine management
- Give ibuprofen 400 mg 3 x daily for 7-10 days after meals
  - **or** diclofenac 50 mg 3 x daily for 2 days after meals
  - then 25 mg 3 x daily for 6-8 days after meals
- **Plus** paracetamol 2 tabs 3 x daily as needed

When should X-rays be done?
- In middle-aged and older patients, X-rays should be done in the following cases to make sure that the cause of the symptoms is not another serious disease
  - if onset of pain is less than a year before
  - if the pain is getting progressively worse
  - if there are other symptoms or signs of severe disease eg. weight loss, prostatic symptoms in a male.
- Generally X-rays will not help to prove the diagnosis as no significant changes will be seen.

Exercises
- Simple exercises can easily be taught to the patients.
- The exercises themselves often help to relieve pain and lessen the need to give strong analgesics.
- Remember to warn the patient that he / she will have to carry on with these exercises regularly for the rest of his / her life
  - this is to keep the stomach and back muscles strong
  - this is to prevent further prolapsed intervertebral discs.

For the back muscles
Stand with your back against a wall or a flat surface.
- Place your hand in the hollow of your lower back.
- Tighten the muscles of your bottom and push the hollow of your lower back into the wall
  - this will hold your hand tightly between your back and the wall.
- Hold this position for a few moments
  - then relax.
- Repeat this 5 times, 3 x a day.
- Slowly increase to 10 times a day.

Again stand with your back against a wall or a flat surface.
- Place your hand in the hollow of your lower back.
- Push your shoulders as hard and as high up the wall as possible.
- Your hand should now have much more space available.
- Hold this position for a minute
  - then relax.
- Repeat this as often as possible during the day.

Lie face down on the floor.
- Place your arms at your side with your finger-tips just under your hips.
- Lift both your legs off the floor while keeping your knees straight
    - this should be high enough so that both knees are lifted off the floor.
- Hold this position for the count of 5.
- Lower your legs
    - then relax
- Repeat this 5 times, 3 x a day.

For the stomach muscles
The abdominal muscles need to be strong as they are an important front support for the spine.

Lie flat on your back with your knees bent and feet on the floor.
- Keep your feet firmly fixed on the floor
    - **do not** hook them under any heavy object or get anyone to hold them down
- Flatten the hollow of your lower back hard into the floor
- Hold this position and stretch your arms out in front of you
- Slowly raise your head and shoulders off the floor until your shoulders are just off the floor
    - it is not necessary to sit up completely as this may hurt your back
- Hold this position to the count of 5
- Slowly lower your head and shoulders
- Relax your lower back
- Repeat this 5 times, 3 x a day

Lie flat on your back with your knees bent and your feet on the floor.
- Flatten the hollow of your lower back into the floor
- Hold the lower back in this position while you place your chin on your chest
- Stretch your right arm across your body so that you touch the outer side of your left thigh with your right hand
    - your right shoulder should be lifted up off the floor
    - now lower your arm and shoulder
    - relax
- Again flatten the hollow of your lower back into the floor
- Hold the lower back in this position while you place your chin on your chest
- Now stretch your left arm across your body so that you touch the outer side of your right thigh with your left hand
    - your left shoulder should be lifted up off the floor
    - now lower your arm and shoulder
    - relax
- Repeat these movements to each side 5 times, 3 x a day
- Slowly increase to 10 times, 3 x a day

How to lift anything heavy
The most common reason for backache, is that heavy objects are lifted up using the back to do all the work. This places tremendous strain on the lumbar vertebral discs and ligaments.

- Get as close as possible to whatever has to be lifted
- Bend your knees as much as possible
- **Keep your back straight and upright**
- Pick up the object while you keep your lower back straight as you straighten your knees
- Stand up using your **legs** and **knees** to do the lifting
- *Get help in lifting anything heavy*
- *Try and avoid repeated lifting of heavy objects.*

LUMBAR OSTEOARTHRITIS (SPONDYLOSIS)

Long-standing prolapse disturbs the mechanics of the facet joints which leads to degenerative changes in the joints, producing osteoarthritis.

Clinical features
- Backache is usually gradual in onset and relieved by rest
    - sometimes acute attacks of backache or sciatica occur if more disc material prolapses
- Lumbar movements (flexion and extension) are limited
    - there may also be leg signs of nerve root pressure (see straight-leg raising test page 301)
- Often tender areas are felt in the back.

MANAGEMENT
- Give paracetamol 1g (2 tabs) 3 x daily when necessary.
- During acute episodes add:
    - ibuprofen 200-400 mg 3 x daily after meals
- Advise patient on:
    - exercises to strengthen back muscles
    - correct method of picking up weights
    - a hard board under the mattress
    - weight loss if the patient is overweight
- **REFER** if the condition does not respond to the above treatment to make sure there is not a more serious cause, especially in the older patients
    - e.g. carcinoma of the prostate

CHRONIC LOW BACKACHE

This is a common problem.

Causes
- It is usually the end result of the poor posture and inadequate back muscle exercises
    - this causes chronic lower lumbar ligamentous strain (postural back pain)
    - it is probably due to weak muscles not protecting the ligaments from strain
- It is more common in urban dwelling people who
    - do not get enough exercise to maintain the muscles of the back
    - have not developed a good walking posture by having to carry and balance things on their heads as the rural community do
- Travel in motor cars is a common precipitating cause
    - this is because the back loses its normal forward bend (lordosis) when seated in a car or taxi seat
    - any bumps or trauma while travelling will then damage the unprotected back
- Depression
    - this may be the only cause of the backache
    - more commonly it makes genuine backache worse
- Anxiety eg. fear of sexually transmitted infections
- Women are particularly prone to this condition after menopause because of loss of vertebral bone due to osteoporosis

- Osteo-arthritis of lumbar intervertebral joints
- Other serious causes are multiple myeloma, metastases eg. from prostate carcinoma.

In men, important causes to look for are:
- Prostatitis, usually chronic
- Impotence from any cause

In women, important causes to look for are:
- Chronic gynaecological disease eg.
    - carcinoma of the cervix must be considered in middle-aged women
    - chronic pelvic infection
- Uterine fibroids
- Endometriosis
- Retroverted uterus
- Uterine prolapse
- Spondylolisthesis

Clinical features
- Middle-aged or elderly
- Usually female
- Often overweight
- Pain in the lower back which is
    - vague and not localised
    - chronic and recurrent
    - related to posture and movement
    - worse during the day and relieved with rest
    - responds quite well to paracetamol and "rubbing medicine"
- Men may complain of "loin pain" and hold their hands over the lumbar and kidney area
- No neurological symptoms or signs
- The pain can be localised to the lumbo-sacral area
- No specific point tenderness on palpation
    - the tenderness is over the whole of the lower lumbar area including the lumbar muscles

MANAGEMENT
General measures
- Physiotherapy
    - this can be of great benefit and must be encouraged if available
    - if not available, teach the patient exercises for the back and stomach muscles (see pages 307 and 308)
- Depression, stress and loneliness may make the pain worse
    - if these are helped with advice, counselling and support, there may be very little need for the use of drugs to relieve pain
- Where backache is provoked by the daily activities which the patient cannot avoid, **REFER** for an orthopaedic (Freeman's) corset
    - the use of a corset must be combined with back and abdominal muscle exercises, (otherwise the muscles will become increasingly weak)
    - it is best not to wear a corset continuously, but only during those days when strenuous activity is expected
- Treat any other possible causes outside the spine eg. gynaecological disease.

Prevention
This disease can be prevented by:
- Regular back exercises
- Developing a good posture
- Walking instead of travelling by car!

Medicine management
- Often these patients have other chronic diseases eg. hypertension and diabetes.
- They often have chronic joint pain in other joints, particularly knees. Therefore be careful of:
    - interactions of different drugs
    - side effects of the drugs.
- Use the mildest and safest analgesics first
    - the safest is "rubbing medicine" eg. ung meth sal
- Analgesics. As there is no active inflammation present, start treatment with
    - paracetamol or aspirin 2 tabs 3 x daily as needed
- Only if no response, treat with ibuprofen 200-400 mg 3 x daily after meals

When to REFER for X-ray
- Generally X-rays are not of much benefit in older people
- However X-rays should be done if:
    - there is any suspicion of a serious cause (see page 302)
    - the pain is not responding to treatment, especially in older people
    - there are other systemic signs of illness eg. weight loss.

CROOKED BACK

This is more a disease of children, but the deformity will persist into adulthood.

Causes
- Tuberculosis of the spine
- Disease or deformities in the pelvis or legs may result in the spine appearing to be crooked.
- In elderly people, especially women, osteoporosis can result in severe forward bending and collapse of the spine.
- Ankylosing spondylitis
- Excessive obesity may give this appearance

SCOLIOSIS

Causes
- Congenital or acquired disease of the spine. If possible, all children should be screened for this problem because
    - with early treatment, the results are excellent
    - with late treatment, deformity may be permanent

Clinical features
- This condition can only be seen if the child is undressed and the back carefully inspected.
- Check if the line of the spinous processes (the visible bones of the back) are in a straight line up and down.
  Note. The child may make the spine look straight by tilting the pelvis, so that the spine is straight but the pelvis and legs are crooked.
- In scoliosis the spine is bent to the side in an S-shape
- Often starts age 10-12
- Usually no pain
- Presents with a twisted or crooked back or peculiar gait
- The position of the scapula may be seen to be at different heights on the two sides.

- There may be a skin crease in the lower back on one side and not on the other.
- When the patient **bends over forwards**, the deformity persists

Differential diagnosis
Compensatory scoliosis
- This is due to a disease outside the spine such as a short leg.
- As a result, the spine is held bent to compensate for the difference in the length of the legs.
- This can be tested by making the child bend forwards
  - if the crookedness in the back disappears, then it was a compensatory scoliosis

> **REFER** a scoliosis, in a child or adolescent, as it may need investigation and specialised treatment.

HUNCH BACK

Causes
- A common cause is tuberculosis of the spine
- Old age

Clinical features
- The spine is deformed and the back is bent forward
- The patient is undressed and the hump of the back is usually obvious.

Complications
- Recurrent chest infections
- Chronic obstructive airways disease and possibly cor pulmonale.
- Obstetric problems and obstructed labour
- Difficulty doing manual labour
- Psychological and emotional problems

> **MANAGEMENT**
>
> **REFER** If the condition is acute.
>
> *If it is a chronic problem that has been investigated*
> - Check for chest infections or other complications
> - Treat as necessary
> - **REFER** for
>   - physiotherapy to decrease the chance of recurrent chest infections by improving breathing and aeration of the lungs
>   - occupational therapy, if available, to assist with work and home-related problems

THE ARM

SHOULDER PROBLEMS

PAIN IN THE SHOULDER

Causes
Sudden pain
- Acute trauma
- Referred pain from the neck
- Referred pain from another organ
    - the heart to the left shoulder
    - abdominal organs to the right shoulder (eg. gall bladder, ectopic pregnancy)

Gradual or chronic pain
- Damage to the tendons of the shoulder (see painful arc syndrome and bicipital tendonitis below).
- Fibrositis around the scapula
- Chronic cervical spine disease
- Referred pain from a carpal tunnel syndrome
- Chronic bone disease eg. tuberculosis, carcinoma
- Osteo-arthritis of the shoulder joint (rare)

Pain when moving the arm sideways and upwards (abduction and elevation)
- This is strongly suggestive of damage to the supraspinatus tendon
    - usually called a rotator cuff syndrome (see opposite)

Pain on movement of the shoulder in all directions
- This suggests a disease of the shoulder joint eg. due to an arthritis
- Severe trauma to the shoulder or surrounding structures eg. the clavicle
- Frozen shoulder

Pain not related to movement of the shoulder
- This suggests referred pain from
    - the heart
    - diaphragm
    - gall bladder
    - lungs eg. pneumonia
    - cervical spine disease
    - liver disease
    - ectopic pregnancy

MANAGEMENT
- **REFER** if you suspect a serious cause
- Treat for each cause according to guidelines given under each section

In an older person
People over the age of 40, get stiff joints very quickly after an injury.

- Early mobilisation is needed after any injury to the shoulder or humerus
    - this should start within 2 weeks after the injury
- The arm can be supported in a collar and cuff, and the patient must begin to move the shoulder.
- This is done by swinging the arm in a circular manner ie. abduction and circumduction of the arm.
- This can often be performed most easily if the patient bends his body over, towards the injured side, so that the elbow swings freely away from the body.

ROTATOR CUFF SYNDROME

Causes
- The main tendon of the muscles which abducts the shoulder, (supraspinatus tendon) passes through a narrow passage between the acromion and the head of the humerus, on its way to attaching to the humerus lower down.
- This tendon can become inflamed and swollen by the constant friction of moving through this passage (tendonitis).
- Inflammation may also resut from an injury causing a partial (usually small) tear.

Clinical features
- It is more common in people over the age of 45
- There may be a history of:
    - recent, unusual, repeated use of the shoulder
    - recent or previous trauma to the shoulder.
- There may be localised tenderness below the acromion process or further forward
- If the tendon was partly torn, there may be weakness in trying to lift the arm sideways and upwards (abduct).

The classic feature is "the painful arc"
- This usually shows itself as pain when abducting
- The patient moves the arm easily and painlessly at the beginning of the movement.
- As the arm moves further up, the patient suddenly feels pain and cannot move the arm further.
- If the arm is then taken up closer to the head, the pain disappears.
- The arm can move freely in other directions
    - forwards and backwards

BICIPITAL TENDONITIS
- May follow unaccustomed use, e.g. rigorous tennis in patients over the age of 30
- If the biceps tendon is involved, there may be tenderness in front of the upper arm where the tendon travels in the bicipital groove
- The patient feels pain when moving the arm forward and when the elbow is flexed against resistance.

MANAGEMENT
REFER
- If you suspect that the supraspinatus tendon has been torn completely recently (gross weakness of abduction)
- If there has been severe trauma
- If the patient does not respond to conservative treatment
- If it is severely affecting work
- For physiotherapy or occupational therapy if available for:
    - heat (infra-red and short-wave diathermy)
    - exercises

Other management
- Rest in an armsling
- Analgesics and NSAIDs, e.g. ibuprofen 3 x daily for 5 days
- Reassure and explain the cause
- Encourage the patient to gently use the arm, avoiding painful movements as much as possible.
- Apply local heat

If the pain persists despite the above treatment
- **REFER** for injection of local anaesthetic and steroid (Depo-Medrol)
    - it may give dramatic relief, especially if the problem is chronic

DISLOCATED SHOULDER

Clinical features
This is a clinical diagnosis.

X-rays are usually not necessary unless there has been severe trauma

- The patient will be unable to:
    - abduct the arm at all
    - put the hand of the affected side on the top of the opposite shoulder (adduction).
- A swelling may be seen or palpated in front of the shoulder, anterior and medial to the normal position of the head of the humerus.
- Looking at the side of the dislocated shoulder (deltoid area), it will be seen to have lost the normal, round, outward bulge.
- On palpation, the head of the humerus will not be felt under the deltoid.
- Occasionally posterior dislocation may occur

MANAGEMENT
A dislocated shoulder must usually be reduced by a doctor.

However a nurse may try the following, which does not require sedation
- Let the patient lie face down on an examination couch with the injured arm hanging down for 10 minutes
- The shoulder may reduce spontaneously
- If it does not
    - **REFER** to doctor for reduction

Recurrent dislocations
- These cause progressive damage to the shoulder joint
- **REFER** for surgery

FRACTURED CLAVICLE

Causes
- This usually occurs a result of a fall on the outstretched hand
- The diagnosis is usually easily made on clinical examination

Clinical features
- The patient complains of pain over the clavicle when the arm is moved in any direction
- A tender lump may be seen or palpated in the clavicle
- It is important to check for nerve and arterial damage by checking the pulses and sensation in the arm
- An X-ray is not necessary as it does not give extra information

MANAGEMENT
- Apply a broad arm (triangular) sling to support the upper arm
    - do not use a collar and cuff which drops the shoulder
- Immobilise for 3-4 weeks
- If the patient is a manual labourer, put him off work for 2 months

FRACTURED HUMERUS

Clinical features
- Severe deformity, swelling and bruising of the humerus may be obvious
- Localised tenderness of the humerus on percussion over the elbow.
- Clinical deformity
- Finger extension should be checked in order to exclude a nerve lesion

- Apply a forearm sling - not a collar and cuff
- Give analgesics
- **REFER** for X-ray

ELBOW PROBLEMS

ELBOW PAIN IN A CHILD

Causes
- The most common cause is trauma which may be:
    - mild eg. pulled elbow
    - severe eg. supra-condylar fracture.

- Infections of the skin or deeper tissue
    - osteomyelitis may occur occasionally
- Arthritis such as rheumatic fever

See the relevant sections for management.

"PULLED ELBOW"

Causes
- This is caused by the child being lifted up by one arm, especially if a lot of force is used
    - this causes the head of the radius to slip out of its normal position (subluxation) and become impacted in the round ligament.

Clinical features
- No swelling and only mild tenderness of the elbow
- Able to flex and extend the elbow quite well, with only mild limitation of movement.
- Pain when the child tries to turn the palm upward (supinate)

If you suspect a pulled elbow
- Give paracetamol
- **REFER** to reduce the transient radial head subluxation

SUPRACONDYLAR FRACTURE

Clinical features
- This is a common injury in children
- Usually there will be a history of a fall onto the hand with the elbow bent.
- Depending on the amount of damage to the elbow, there will be varying amounts of pain, swelling and limitation of movement.
- A backward shift just above the elbow is apparent.
- A very important complication in elbow injuries is damage to the brachial artery as it passes close to the elbow.
- It is therefore essential to check the circulation

How to check arm circulation
See details on page 290 - assessment of arterial damage.
- The swelling around the arm may be so severe that feeling for the pulse at the wrist is difficult.
- The circulation can then be checked by the perfusion in the fingers

MANAGEMENT
- **REFER** stat if there is any suggestion of damage to the arterial supply of the arm.
- **REFER** all displaced fractures.

When an X-ray is needed
- X-ray of the injured elbow in a child is only indicated if there is swelling of the elbow or loss of movement.
- Apply a collar and cuff **under** the clothes for 3 weeks.
- Give paracetamol for pain.

- If the elbow cannot be sufficiently flexed, apply a broad arm (triangular) bandage or a posterior plaster slab.
- After 3 weeks, the child is encouraged to regain elbow movements gradually and without force
    - never allow movements to become painful

ELBOW PAIN IN AN ADULT

Causes
- Tennis elbow (tenosynovitis)
- Referred pain from a carpal tunnel syndrome
- Rheumatoid arthritis
- Gout

TENNIS ELBOW AND GOLFER'S ELBOW (TENOSYNOVITIS)

Causes
- Repetitive rotary movements of the elbow
    - eg. repetitive twisting of the wrist
- Excessive use
- Carrying heavy objects
- Tennis

Clinical features
- Pain localised to the lateral side of the elbow (tennis elbow) or to the medial side (golfer's elbow)
    - this sometimes radiates down the forearm
- Pain with certain movements eg. pouring out tea, turning a stiff door handle.
- The pain is worse on gripping anything with the hand
- There is localised tenderness just below the lateral or medial epicondyle of the elbow.
- The elbow looks normal

MANAGEMENT
- Rest
- Anti-inflammatory eg. ibuprofen 200-400 mg 3 x daily for 5-10 days
- **REFER**
    - to physiotherapist if available
    - for Depo-Medrol injections if improvement is slow
    - for surgery if above fails

FOREARM PROBLEMS

FOREARM PAIN IN A CHILD

Causes
- Commonly caused by minor injury which is not usually significant
- Fractures are also common

- If it is only painful during supination of the forearm, it may be due to "a pulled elbow" (see page 313).
- If the child is having recurrent injuries, consider possible child abuse.

> **MANAGEMENT**
> - If marked tenderness and / or **any** swelling is found in any part of the forearm
>   - give an analgesic
>   - apply a crepe bandage
>   - **REFER** for X-ray
> - If there is mild tenderness, with **no** swelling
>   - apply a broad arm bandage
>   - give an analgesic
>   - advise the escort to bring the child back if the condition does not improve within 2 days
> - If nil is found on examination
>   - give paracetamol syrup only for the pain
>   - advise the escort to bring the child back in 2 days, if the condition does not improve

FRACTURES OF THE FOREARM (RADIUS OR ULNA)

Clinical features
- The area where the fracture is will be:
  - swollen
  - very tender.
- The bend in the bone or bones may be obvious
- There will be limited movement, especially pronation or supination (turning the hand down or up).
  - but should not be attempted especially if deformity is obvious
- It is not always easy to be sure if a fracture is present or not.

> - **REFER** if there is any suspicion of a fracture
> - Splint the arm – broad arm bandage
> - Give analgesics for pain

WRIST PROBLEMS

WRIST INJURY IN A CHILD

Causes
- Minor injuries and bruises
- Undisplaced greenstick fracture of the lower end of the radius is a common injury.

Clinical features of greenstick fractures
- There will usually be a history of a fall
- There will usually be the features suggesting a fracture as above.
- The forearm can often be clearly palpated as the swelling is usually slight
  - so displacement can be excluded clinically

> **MANAGEMENT**
> - **REFER** for X-ray if there is any swelling or deformity.
>
> *Painful wrist movements but no swelling or deformity*
> - Apply a POP backslab for 3 weeks
>   - a full POP is necessary if a bone is broken or angulation is present

WRIST INJURY IN AN ADULT

Causes
- The most common injury is a Colles' fracture, especially in older people.
- However it is important to **always** check for a possible **fracture of the scaphoid**
  - this is easily missed unless specifically looked for clinically, because X-ray changes may only appear 2 weeks after the fracture
- The classic sign of a scaphoid fracture is
  - definite tenderness between the 2 large tendons at the back of the base of the thumb
  - this is called the "anatomical snuff box"

> **REFER** for application of a scaphoid POP if there is any suspicion of a fractured scaphoid (see page 316)

COLLES' AND COLLES'-LIKE FRACTURES

This is a fracture of the lower end of the radius.

Clinical features
- This is a fracture which occurs in adults, especially older adults, after a fall
- There will be pain and swelling of the wrist
- The deformity of the wrist is similar to the shape of a dinner fork
  - the lower radius is displaced backwards and radially

> **MANAGEMENT**
> - **REFER** for X-ray and management if you suspect a fracture
> - Give analgesics and a sling to relieve pain

If the patient is in severe pain
- This will be because of the pressure of the displaced segments on the neurovascular structures.
- The fracture must be reduced **stat** under adequate anaesthesia.

*If the patient is **not** in severe pain*
- This is usually the case
- Urgent **REFERRAL** is not necessary
- Apply a dorsal slab **without** reduction for 48 hours
- Elevate the arm at home
- **REFER** for reduction of the fracture after 48 hours when the swelling has gone down

WRIST PAIN

Causes
- Carpal tunnel syndrome
- Trauma
- Ganglion
- Tenosynovitis eg. De Quervain's disease (see below)
- Fractured scaphoid
- Rheumatoid arthritis or gout

CARPAL TUNNEL SYNDROME

This is due to median nerve entrapment at the wrist in the carpal tunnel.

Causes
- The median nerve passes through the tunnel formed by carpal bones and the transverse carpal ligament in company with the flexor tendons of the fingers.
- Compression of the median nerve is produced by any process that causes swelling in the carpal tunnel.
- This occurs when a woman has a high level of oestrogen and progesterone, eg.
    - pregnancy
    - use of oral contraceptives
- This also occurs in premenstrual and menopausal women.
- Physical activities involving the wrists, eg. sewing, knitting.
- Also sometimes seen in:
    - rheumatoid arthritis
    - diabetes mellitus
    - hypothyroidism
    - acromegaly

Note. A similar syndrome of nerve entrapment may occur at the ankle producing burning, tingling and numbness of the plantar surface of the foot and toes (tarsal tunnel syndrome).

Clinical features
- Severe pain in the wrist
    - radiating up the arm
    - worse at night
- Patients may present initially with pain in the elbow or shoulder.
- Symptoms are:
    - relieved by letting the arm hang down
    - made worse by flexing the wrist.
- There is often loss of sensation or "pins and needles" in the 1st, 2nd, 3rd fingers and half the 4th finger.
- They may also find that they keep dropping things from their hands.
- There is tenderness over the median nerve at the wrist.
- Putting the back of the hands together and pushing them closer may produce the same pain.

MANAGEMENT
- Explain the cause and reassure the patient.
- Patients with only sensory symptoms:
    - splint wrist in dorsiflexion with a volar POP slab for 1 week
    - give ibuprofen 200-400 mg 3 x daily for 5-10 days.
- **REFER** for a corticosteroid injection or possible surgery if:
    - symptoms persist
    - motor abnormalities are evident eg. hand weakness.

GANGLION

Clinical features
- This is a swelling arising from a joint capsule or tendon sheath
- It usually occurs at the back of the wrist or ankle
- There is a small, painless or slightly painful, cystic swelling usually found on the back of the hand or wrist.
- If it is attached to a tendon, it will move with movements of the tendon.
- It can also occasionally occur at the front of the wrist, palm or fingers.

MANAGEMENT
- If the swelling is mild, and causing no symptoms
    - reassure, as often the ganglion disappears after some months
- If the swelling is causing mild symptoms, apply a crêpe bandage for 1-2 weeks
- If the swelling is large or causing severe symptoms:
    - **REFER** for possible surgery
    - warn the patient that ganglions come back in 25% of cases, even after surgery

DE QUERVAIN'S TENOSYNOVITIS

Causes
- It is usually due to overuse of the thumb eg. excessive use of scissors, wringing clothes

Clinical features
- Severe pain on the radial side of the lower forearm, especially when moving the thumb away from the palm (extension).
- Pain is relieved by:
    - rest
    - keeping the thumb still.
- Pain becomes progressively worse if the patient continues with the action causing the problem.
- Marked localised tenderness of the tendons of the thumb just above the wrist.
- Pain when the examiner tries to stop the patient from moving the thumb away from the palm (resisted extension)
- Pain when the examiner pushes the thumb across the palm (passive adduction).

MANAGEMENT
- Stop the action causing the problem
- Give ibuprofen 200-400 mg 3 x daily for 5-10 days
- Splint wrist with crépe bandage, or POP slab if the pain is severe.
- If necessary **REFER**
  - for a doctor's letter to be put off work, or to get other duties at work
  - for physiotherapy if available
- If no response **REFER**
  - for an injection of long-acting steroid
  - **or** operation

SCAPHOID FRACTURE

- Results from a fall on the outstretched hand
- Pain above the thumb at the wrist between the thumb tendons.
- Pain when the examiner bends the hand backwards (passive extension).
- Localised tenderness between the thumb tendons at the wrist (anatomical snuffbox).
- Pain when gripping

REFER.

▼ **Note to doctor**
It is often difficult to see a fracture of the scaphoid on X-ray. If there is doubt, a scaphoid POP is applied. The patient should be re-X-rayed after 2 weeks (out of plaster) when a fracture can be seen more easily. ▲

HAND AND FINGER PROBLEMS

THUMB PAIN

Causes
- Osteo-arthritis is common in people who use their hands a great deal.
- Trauma with dislocations or fractures
- Infections
- Inflammation in the tendons (De Quervain's tenosynovitis)

MANAGEMENT
- **REFER** all problems of the thumb, unless you are sure it is minor
- Permanent damage to the thumb is a very serious handicap
  - **all diseases of the thumb should be treated as serious**
- Physiotherapy is important to regain full function

SWOLLEN, PAINFUL HAND

It is important to realise that the skin of the palm is so tightly attached that it does not swell as easily as the back of the hand.

Causes
- Infections
- Foreign body
- Trauma
- Gout

MANAGEMENT
These should be treated with great care.

REFER if:
- There is suspicion of an abscess
  - throbbing pain
  - pain present for more than 2 days
  - pain so severe that it affects sleep
- There is decreased function of the fingers
- There is a history of a foreign body
  - it is sometimes tempting to try and dig out foreign bodies
  - this can result in more damage as often they are very difficult to find
- You suspect a fracture or tendon injury.
- There is no obvious minor cause.

SWOLLEN, PAINFUL FINGER

Causes
- Infections eg.
  - paronychia
  - infections of the tendon sheath
- Bites, especially human
- Dislocations or fractures

MANAGEMENT
*Any infection of the fingers should be viewed as being extremely serious. It should be **REFERRED** unless it is very minor.*

Human bites are particularly dangerous (see page 11).

Mobilisation of hand and finger fractures
- Finger joints tend to get stiff after 2 weeks immobilisation, due to contracture of the joint capsules and ligaments.
- The hand should be bandaged in the position of function, as if holding a ball, with the knuckles straight and the fingers partially flexed.
- The maximum immobilisation should be 2 weeks
- After that the person must start to move the fingers
- A good exercise is to squeeze a sponge throughout the day
- Remember that the fracture is not fully united after 2 weeks
  - a manual labourer may need to be off work for 8 weeks, before the hand is fully functional again

THE LEG

UPPER LEG PROBLEMS

HIP PAIN IN A MIDDLE-AGED OR ELDERLY ADULT

Causes where there is no history of injury

*If the cause of the hip pain is not obvious from examining the hip, then it may be **referred pain**.*

- Osteo-arthritis of the hip joints is the most common cause
- Gynaecological causes should always be considered in women
- Inflamed glands in the groin
- Tenosynovitis, bursitis or nerve entrapment around the thigh
- Lumbar spine disease eg. prolapsed intervertebral disc
- Disease of the sacro-iliac joint
- Peripheral vascular disease with ischaemia of the leg
- Inflammation in the tendons of the back muscles attaching to the iliac crests.
- Avascular necrosis of the hip

OSTEO-ARTHRITIS OF THE HIP JOINT

Clinical features

- It is particularly common in overweight women
- It may follow a previous injury
- The pain is usually
  - made worse by exercise
  - relieved by rest
- Night pain occurs as a later symptom
- Stiffness of the joint occurs later in the disease
- Early cases have pain without limitation of movement
- Late cases have limited movement of the joint

MANAGEMENT

General measures

- Weight reducing diet if overweight
- A walking stick may help to take some weight off the joint and relieve pain.

Exercises

- This is to strengthen the surrounding muscles
- Strengthen the hip abductor muscles
  - lie next to a wall
  - open the legs so that the leg is pushed sideways against the wall
  - keep the pressure for ½ minute
  - then relax
  - repeat this 5 times
  - do the exercise 3 x daily at first
  - increase the number of times by 5 every four days until this exercise can be done 50 times
- Strengthen the hip adductor muscles
  - squeeze the 2 legs together for ½ minute
  - repeat as above
- Strengthen the quadriceps muscle at the front of the thigh
  - see page 322

If physiotherapy and occupational therapy are available, **REFER** *for further rehabilitation and assistance with coping at work and home.*

Medicine management

- Analgesics
  - start with paracetamol 2 tabs 3 x daily as needed
  - see Joints page 294 for further details

Indications for REFERRAL for possible surgery

- Severe limitation in the range of movement
- Severe pain
  - not responding to drugs
  - seriously affecting the person's life and work and sleep

AVASCULAR NECROSIS OF THE HIP

Clinical features

- This commonly occurs in men between the age of 30-50 years who drink heavily.
- It may also result from prolonged or high-dose oral steroid therapy.
- There is pain in the thigh, which becomes progressively worse.

- Stop drinking to prevent progression of the necrosis in both hips
- **REFER** for X-ray to confirm the diagnosis

HIP PAIN FOLLOWING AN INJURY

FRACTURED PELVIS

Clinical features

- History of major trauma
- Usually other injuries are also present
- Any movement of the thigh is tender
- Palpation of the lower abdomen may be tender
- Marked tenderness if direct pressure is exerted
  - on the symphysis pubis
  - over the iliac crests

- The patient may be severely shocked, depending on how bad the fracture is.
- The patient may have:
    - retention of urine
    - haematuria
    - rupture of the urethra.

> **MANAGEMENT**
> - Treat for shock (see page 271)
> - **REFER**
> - Send for a MAST suit if available and inflate it
> - If a MAST is not available, then fasten a draw sheet or dressing towel tightly around the pelvis to support it.
> - Do not remove tight jeans or corset as the patient may suddenly go into shock.
> - Observe and record the urine output

FRACTURED NECK OF FEMUR

Clinical features
- Usually an elderly woman
- Often fairly minor trauma eg.
    - the patient tripped
    - the patient fell for no obvious reason
- The patient is unable to get up after the fall
- Upper part of the thigh is swollen
- The leg is shortened
- A useful sign is that the foot of the fractured leg lies flat pointing outwards

NB. Be careful, because in rare cases, the broken pieces may be impacted and the patient may
   - still be able to walk
   - appear not to have a fracture

> **REFER** for reduction and internal fixation of the fracture.

FRACTURED FEMUR

Clinical features
- History of a severe injury eg. MVA
- The patient cannot walk on the leg
- The thigh is very tender and swollen
- The leg is shortened
    - lying in external rotation (the foot pointing outwards)
    - at an angle
- Tenderness felt in the femur on percussion under the foot

> **MANAGEMENT**
> **REFER** for probable surgery (internal fixation)
> - Put up a drip as more than 2 litres of blood can be lost into tissues (see page 271)
> - Apply a Thomas splint to the leg if available
> - If a Thomas splint is not available
>   - fasten the 2 legs to each other from the top of the leg to the bottom
>   - **or** apply any kind of wooden splint to the side of the thigh and upper leg
>   - fasten at the top to the pelvis and below to the leg

BRUISING OF THE THIGH MUSCLES

Clinical features
- History of moderate injury eg. pedestrian hit by a car that was not travelling very fast.
- The patient will be able to walk into the clinic
- Only one side of the thigh is swollen and tender
    - usually the lateral side

> **MANAGEMENT**
> - Reassure
> - R.I.C.E. therapy if seen within 12 hours (see pages 289-290)
> - Give analgesics
> - If the swelling is severe, apply a supportive bandage
> - X-ray is not necessary
> - Encourage fluids to help the kidneys clear breakdown products of the muscle and blood

HIP PAIN IN A CHILD OR TEENAGER

Causes
- Slipped upper femoral epiphysis
- Degeneration of the femoral head epiphysis (Perthes' disease)

SLIPPED FEMORAL EPIPHYSIS

Clinical features
- It occurs between ages 9 and 18 years
- More common in boys
- The patient is often obese but may be unusually tall and thin
- Mild pain in hip or knee

Later features
- The patient's trunk leans towards the affected side when the weight is taken on walking.
- There is external rotation of the leg
- There is decreased internal rotation and abduction of the hip joint.

PERTHES' DISEASE

Clinical features
- It occurs between ages 3-11 years
- It is four times more common in boys than in girls
- The patient may have pain in the hip or referred pain to the knee.
- Sometimes there is a limp without pain
- Some movements are decreased
    - abduction in flexion (opening the legs with the hips flexed)
    - internal rotation
- Other movements are full and painless

MANAGEMENT
REFER
- Any child or teenager with a limp or pain in hip or knee for more than a week.
- For an X-ray of hip joints and possible surgery

SUDDEN ONSET OF SEVERE HIP PAIN IN A CHILD

Causes
- Septic arthritis of the hip joint is the most important cause (see page 297 for clinical features).

REFER
- If there is **any** suspicion that this may be the diagnosis
- For an aspiration of the joint and IVI antibiotics

KNEE PROBLEMS

SWOLLEN OR PAINFUL KNEE AFTER AN INJURY

Causes
It is useful to establish if the injury is due to
- A direct hit which is more likely to cause a fracture
    - eg. a motor vehicle accident
- A twisting injury which is more likely to cause tearing of ligaments and cartilages (menisci)
    - eg. a sporting injury

DIRECT TRAUMA

This may result in:
- A fracture of the patella
- Supracondylar fractures of the femur or condylar fractures of the femur or tibia.
- A dislocation of the patella

Clinical features
- Usually a history of moderate to severe trauma
- Swollen knee
- Mild or moderately limited movements, depending on the degree of trauma.
- There will be only mild heat

Test for fluid
One hand compresses the suprapatellar pouch while the index finger of the other pushes the patella sharply backwards. If fluid is present, the patella is felt striking the femur and bouncing off
- this is called a "patellar tap"
- this indicates fluid in the knee joint, either blood or an effusion

MANAGEMENT
REFER if
- There is any suspicion of fluid in the knee
- The knee is very swollen
- The patient complains of instability in the knee
- You suspect a fracture
- There is severe pain or tenderness in any part of the knee, especially over the patella, femur or tibia
- There is significant loss of movement of the knee
- A wound could be penetrating into the joint

NB. Apply a temporary supportive bandage **before referral.**

If there are none of the above, and the injuries appear not to be serious:
- Give a supportive bandage
- Give analgesics
- Tetanus toxoid if there is a wound
- Advise the patient to come back if the knee does not improve within a week.

TWISTING KNEE INJURY

Causes
- Patient hit from the side by another player eg. during soccer
    - while running with weight on that knee at the time of the collision
- Patient tripped while turning at speed with the foot fixed and caught, and the knee twisting.

Clinical features
If the injury was mild
- The knee may move normally and have no signs of injury

If the injury was more severe, there may be some or all of the following

Possible effusion into the knee
- Swelling of the knee
    - immediately, due to bleeding after the injury
    - later after some hours, due to an effusion
- Positive patellar tap

Instability of the knee
- The patient may notice this especially when walking down steps
    - this suggests damage to the internal ligaments (cruciate ligaments)
- Positive tests for instability of the collateral ligaments around the knee

Tenderness
- Along the joint line
- Along the medial or lateral anterior aspect of the joint line
    - this suggests damage to the medial or lateral meniscus
- Above or below the knee where the collateral ligaments insert medially and laterally on the lower femur and the upper tibia
    - this suggests a sprain or tear of the collateral ligament

MANAGEMENT
Knee injuries are not easy to diagnose.

If there is any doubt it is better to put on a Robert Jones bandage and **REFER** when convenient.

REFER
- For any of the criteria given above
- If there is any suggestion of instability in the knee
- If you suspect a torn meniscus or torn ligaments

If the knee is stable and the above are not obvious.
- Apply cold to the area
- Give ibuprofen 200 mg 3 x daily
- Encourage exercises to strengthen the quadriceps muscles.
- Reassess in 2 weeks time
- All knee injuries and fractures of the tibia and femur will develop quadriceps atrophy and need quadriceps exercises (see page 322).

Robert Jones bandage
- This is the best method of bandaging for injuries around the knee.
- It consists of the application of 3 layers of wool and 3 layers of bandage.
- The thickness of the bandage should be 5 cm
- It should extend from 15 cm above the knee to 15 cm below the knee
  - that is a total of 30 cm
- If only very thin ortho wool is available, 4 layers may be needed to give the 5 cm thickness.
- Elastoform can be used for the inner layers
- Elastocrepe (pink) should be used for the outer layer
- In areas where crepe bandage is available, it can be used instead of Elastocrepe.
- Put the layers on in the following order from the skin outwards:
  - wool
  - Elastoform
  - wool
  - Elastoform
  - wool
  - Elastocrepe

The obese thigh
- Application of the bandage is difficult in a patient with an obese thigh (a funnel shaped leg) without any normal slight narrowing above the knee.
- The top of the bandage needs to be attached to the skin of the thigh.
- Use vertical strips of elastoplast to prevent the bandage from falling.
- **NB.** Never apply elastoplast around the whole diameter of any limb
  - it may cause severe obstruction to the blood flow and the lymphatics

Note. The patient will have difficulty putting the trousers back on again
  - the trousers may need to be slit

LUMPS AROUND THE KNEE

PRE-PATELLAR AND INFRA-PATELLAR BURSAE

Clinical features
- These occur in people who have to do a lot of kneeling eg.
  - domestics
  - parsons
  - housewives
- There is increased fluid in the bursae (sacks of fluid) around the knees
  - those affected are at the front of the knee over the patella
  - they are not at the back of the knee
- There is swelling over the patella
- Unless it is infected it is not painful
- There is no limitation of knee movement
- The mass is fluctuant and is just underneath the skin

Complications
- The patient can develop:
  - a cellulitis
  - an abscess of the bursa (see page 321).

MANAGEMENT
- Advise patient of the cause
- If small
  - apply a firm bandage
  - kneeling is to be avoided
  - **REFER** for aspiration and Depo-Medrol injection if not improved
- If big and the patient wants it removed
  - **REFER** for surgery

SWOLLEN KNEE DUE TO INFECTION

Causes
Serious
- Septic arthritis (see page 297 for clinical details and management)
- Osteomyelitis (see page 299 for clinical details and management)

Less serious
- Cellulitis
- Bursitis of the pre-patellar bursa

Clinical features
The following will suggest a serious cause
- Severe signs of general infection such as an ill patient, high fever and pulse rate, rigors.
- Loss of movement of the knee
  - in a serious cause, there will be very limited or no movement of the knee at all
  - a valuable sign of a less serious cause is that, although the knee may look very inflamed, there is still moderately good, or almost completely normal movement
- Bone and percussion tenderness will be usually present in a serious cause, but will be absent in a less serious cause.

INFECTED PRE-PATELLAR BURSA

Clinical features
- Often a history of a precipitating cause eg. having to kneel a lot cleaning floors.
- Pain, warmth and tenderness in front of the knee, directly over the patella.
- No tenderness or pain at the back of the knee
- The knee can still be flexed and extended with only mild limitation of movement.

MANAGEMENT
- Treat with antibiotics
  - flucloxacillin 250-500 mg 4 x daily for 5 days
- Give paracetamol 2 tabs 3 x daily
- Reassess in 2 days to make sure that a pre-patellar abscess is not developing.

PRE-PATELLAR ABSCESS

Clinical features
- As above, but more severe
- Systemic symptoms of:
  - increased pain which is throbbing and affects sleep
  - more severe fever, tachycardia and malaise.
- Local signs
  - increase in tenderness
  - fluctuation may be present
  - the abscess may be pointing

REFER for incision and drainage.

PAINFUL LUMP JUST BELOW THE KNEE

OSGOOD SCHLATTER'S DISEASE

Causes
- This is due to repeated pulling of the patella tendon onto its attachment, on the front of the tibia.

Clinical features
- It is found between ages 10-16 where the bones have not yet fully formed (called a traction apophysitis).
- It occurs at the insertion of the patellar tendon into the tibial tubercle.
- It is quite common
- They present with a painful lump below the knee on the front of the upper tibia.
- There is often a history of excessive exercise for some weeks before the pain begins eg.
  - running
  - jumping
  - athletics
- The pain is worse with:
  - moving the knee
  - the specific exercise that they have been doing recently.
- A useful guide is that there is localised tenderness on palpation of the tibial tuberosity
  - the tuberosity is also seen and felt to be more obvious
- The pain is worse if the quadriceps are tensed as in extension of the knee against resistance.
- X-rays should be done to confirm the diagnosis.

MANAGEMENT
- Encourage rest and stop sport
- Reassure that the condition settles down on its own at the end of the growth spurt.
- Paracetamol 1-2 tabs 3 x daily as required
- In very severe cases, the leg can be immobilized in a POP cylinder for 2 months.

MILDER AND MORE CHRONIC PAIN AND SWELLING OF THE KNEE

Causes
- Rheumatoid arthritis
- Gonococcal arthritis
- Osteo-arthritis
- Tumour of the bone or joint
  - these are rare but must not be missed, especially in children

Differential diagnosis
- Tuberculosis can look very similar to any of the above causes
  - often gross muscle wasting and sinuses may be seen
  - always look for any signs which may suggest it

- See Joints for the management (pages 293-294)
- **REFER** any patient with an effusion for which there is no obvious cause, especially in a child

OSTEO-ARTHRITIS OF THE KNEE JOINT

Clinical features
- This is the most common place for osteo-arthritis
- It is particularly common in overweight women
- It may follow:
  - a previous injury
  - operation to the knee.
- Pain in the knee is the main symptom
- The pain is usually:
  - made worse by exercise
  - relieved by rest.
- Night pain occurs as a later symptom
- Stiffness of the joint may be prominent in the morning or after immobility but usually lasts less than 1 hour
- The patient may feel that the knee is unstable, especially when going down stairs.
- Swelling and an effusion may occur, especially after the knee is stressed eg. after exercise.
- Crepitus (crackling) is felt when a hand is placed over the knee during flexion or extension.
- There is wasting of the quadriceps muscle of the thigh
  - ie. the muscles are thinner
- In some cases there may be limited flexion and extension of the knee.
- Advanced osteoarthritis may result in a deformity of the knee, especially bow-legs (varus) deformity.

MANAGEMENT

General measures
- Weight reduction
- A walking stick may help to take weight off the knee
- Quadriceps exercises to strengthen the muscles that support the knee.
- If physiotherapy and occupational therapy are available, **REFER** for further rehabilitation and assistance with coping at work and home.

Quadriceps exercises
- The quadriceps becomes weak and thin very quickly if there is any knee pain
    - early and regular exercise is needed if there is any injury
- If the muscle is very weak, the patient can start by holding the knee straight on the bed and then trying to lift the leg as often as possible during the day until it is strong enough to go on to the next step (below).
- Place a brick in any kind of bag that can be hung from the ankle
- Lift the leg up and down without bending the knee
- As the weight of the brick is lifted up, so the quadriceps muscle will be felt to contract.
- If the leg is weak, the patient may only manage 2 times at first
    - then do the exercise 3 x daily for the first week
    - then increase each week
- Do this every day as many times as possible
    - up to 50 elevations

Bandaging
- Bandage the knee
- A knee guard which can be brought privately is useful
- Crepe or Elastocrepe (pink) bandage can also be used

NB. A supportive bandage must only be used intermittently (now and again) when there is stress to the leg eg.
- a lot of walking
- stressful work
- If it is used continuously, the quadriceps muscles rely on the bandage to do their work
    - they atrophy further
    - this makes the whole situation worse

Indications for REFERRAL for surgery
- If the person is having severe pain which is not relieved by the strongest analgesics available.
- If the pain is seriously interfering with work or coping at home.
- If the pain is affecting sleep

Medicine management
- See Joints page 294
- **NB.** Any joint that needs NSAIDs or analgesics needs physiotherapy for the surrounding muscles.

CROOKED KNEES

KNOCK-KNEES

■ IN CHILDREN (GENU VALGUM)

One way to remember genu valgum is as "gum stuck together"

Clinical features
- This condition is so common that it may be considered to be normal
    - it appears at age 2-3 years
- In some patients however, underlying disease is evident such as
    - bone softening (rickets)
    - bone injury, especially to the growth plate
    - stretched ligaments
- The deformity has usually recovered by the age of 7 years
- There may be associated flat feet but the child is otherwise normal
- The joint is normal

MANAGEMENT
- Reassure the parents that the legs usually straighten with time.
- Surgical correction is usually not necessary, unless the deformity persists after 10 years of age.
- **REFER** for X-ray if
    - it is severe
    - you suspect a serious cause
- Suspect rickets due to calcium deficiency in any child if:
    - the knock-knees do not show signs of correction after age 4 years
    - knock-knees appear for the first time between 4-18 years.
- **REFER** for:
    - assesment of the cause
    - corrective surgery if severe

■ IN ADULTS

Causes
- Osteo-arthritis is an important cause
- Previous disease such as rheumatoid arthritis or trauma

MANAGEMENT
- If mild, reassure the patient that it is usually not a serious problem
- **REFER** for surgical correction if
    - the deformity is severe
    - it is causing severe pain

BOW-LEGS (GENU VARUM)

The knees are widely separated and the legs are round as if going round a barrel (varum sounds like round).

Causes
- Rickets
- Blounts disease (congenital genu varum)
- In adults an important cause is osteo-arthritis

Clinical features
- This is usually a benign condition
- The amount of separation between the knees should be measured and watched to check progress.
- This can be done in the following way:
    - the patient must be standing
    - put the ankles together so that the medial malleoli of the ankles are touching
    - measure the distance between the insides of both knees.

MANAGEMENT

In children
- Reassure the paretns that most children recover with time
- **REFER** if the distance between the knees is more than 5 cm

In adults
- Severe genu varum may be a sign of advanced osteo-arthritis of the knees which may benefit from surgery
    - **REFER**

LOWER LEG PROBLEMS

SEVERE PAIN IN THE CALF

Causes

There are 2 important non-traumatic causes
- Deep vein thrombosis (see page 89)
- Peripheral vascular disease (see page 90)

Other causes
- Compartment syndrome due to trauma (see page 278)
- Shin splints
- Cramps

SHIN SPLINTS

Causes
- This is usually due to excessive exercise, especially running long distances.
- This causes stress and tearing of the tendon attachments of the muscles of the leg
    - especially on the lateral side (peroneus muscles)

Clinical features
- History of severe pain on the lateral side of the leg
- The pain starts after running a long distance
- The pain may be so bad that the person has to stop running

MANAGEMENT
- Advice about good running shoes which relieve the tension on the muscles.
- Rest the muscles until the pain no longer occurs on exercise
    - this may take 3 weeks or more
- Protect the muscles by
    - correct training methods
    - not trying to run too far when not fit
- **REFER** for physiotherapy if available

CRAMPS

Causes
Often the cause is not easy to find

Some common causes
- Lack of potassium or magnesium as a result of diuretics
- Peripheral vascular disease (see page 90)
- Over-use of the muscles during the day
- Calcium deficiency is often blamed and patients can sometimes benefit from calcium tablets
    - but no genuine calcium imbalance can be shown
- Peripheral neuropathy which may be due to:
    - diabetes
    - alcohol abuse
    - antiretroviral medicines for AIDS
    - TB medication
- Neurological disease
    - especially of the spinal cord

MANAGEMENT
- Treat the cause if there is an obvious one
- Discourage smoking and alcohol
- Potassium replacement in a patient using diuretics
    - this is easiest done by eating more fruit which also supplies magnesium
    - Slow K tablets can also be used
- If severe in patients with peripheral neuropathy, **REFER** for amitriptyline 25 mg nocte.

INJURIES TO THE LOWER LEG

Clinical features
- The bones of the lower leg are strong and it usually needs severe trauma to cause a fracture.
- Features suggesting a fracture (see page 290)
- Check circulation and possible nerve damage
- In children the clinical features may be much less obvious

MANAGEMENT
- **REFER**
    - if there is any doubt
    - for X-ray to make sure that a fracture is not present
- Treat any less severe cause

ANKLE PROBLEMS

PAIN IN THE ANKLE

Causes
Non-traumatic
- Osteo-arthritis following previous injury
- Gout
- Infective causes eg. osteomyelitis
- Rheumatoid arthritis

> For clinical features and management see Joints pages 293-294.

Traumatic
- Ankle joint sprain (ligament damage)
- Fractured ankle

> For clinical features and management see below.

ANKLE INJURIES

- The ankle has 3 ligaments on each side (anterior, posterior, and central) to attach it to the underlying bones of the foot.
- Any twisting or trauma to the ankle is likely to injure these structures.
- Because these ligaments are strongly attached to the underlying bones, severe force on these ligaments may also break the underlying bones.

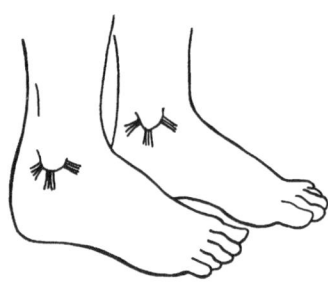

Clinical features
The clinical features make it usually fairly easy to decide on what treatment is likely to be needed.

When to X-ray
- Tenderness over either of the bony prominences of the ankle (malleoli) strongly suggests the need for an X-ray to exclude a fracture.

When to apply a POP
- Tenderness over the insertion of the ligaments suggests torn ligaments.
- If more than 2 ligaments are tender, the patient will need to be put in a POP walking plaster, even if there is no evidence of a fracture.
- Any stress on the damaged ligaments during the initial phase of healing will interfere with the quality of healing.
- Ankle injuries should be immobilised properly in POP casts or special braces for not less than 4 weeks.
- Following this the ankle should be protected against stressing for a further 6-8 months with ankle guards.

ANKLE FRACTURES

Clinical features
- Ankle moderately or severely swollen
- Patient can often still walk, but with discomfort
- If the bony prominences of the malleoli are carefully palpated with one finger, ie. pressure exerted directly over the bony points
    - there will be tenderness over one or both of the malleoli
- The swelling and tenderness may be so great that it is impossible on palpation to clearly tell what is damaged.
- Clinical diagnosis can be confirmed on X-ray

> **MANAGEMENT**
> **REFER** for
> - X-ray and management if there is **tenderness** over one or both malleoli
>
> **Fitness for work**
> *An ankle that has been in POP for 6-8 weeks will still be stiff when the POP is removed.*
> - The type of work and how to get there will decide when a patient can return to work
>   - a person who travels by car from his home to a clerical job may be able to work, while still in POP
>   - a person who has a long walk to the taxi or train may not be ready to start work until 3 weeks after coming out of POP
> - After the POP is removed, the patient may need to walk with crutches for the first 2 weeks while the joint slowly loosens up.
> - **REFER** for physiotherapy, if available, as this can:
>   - help strengthen the muscles
>   - loosen up the joint
>   - improve the patient's ability to walk and cope at work.

PAIN BEHIND THE ANKLE

PARA-TENDONITIS OF THE ACHILLES TENDON

Clinical features
- Pain around the Achilles tendon at the back of the ankle, especially when walking and climbing stairs.
- Tenderness over the Achilles tendon
- Tenderness when the gutter between the tendon and the back of the ankle is squeezed.

> - Rest and strapping
> - Give ibuprofen 200-400 mg 3 x daily for 5-10 days
> - **REFER** for physiotherapy if available

FOOT PROBLEMS

INJURY TO THE HEEL

Causes
- A fall from a height onto the heel can cause a fractured heelbone (calcaneus).

Clinical features
- If it is just bruising, the symptoms and signs will be mild
- Features suggesting a fracture of the calcaneus
    - a bruise appears in the sole
    - swelling at the sides of the heel
    - very tender
    - the patient cannot walk

> - **REFER** for X-ray if there is any suggestion of a fracture
> - If it is a bruise, treat with analgesics and a bandage

PAIN BEHIND THE HEEL
(ACHILLES BURSITIS)

Causes
- This is usually due to bad shoes rubbing on the skin

Clinical features
- Occurs commonly in women
- Tenderness at the back of the heel, where the back of the shoe is in contact with the heel.
- If bursitis has developed, a swelling will be seen or palpated low down in the heel.

> **MANAGEMENT**
>
> Mild cases
> - Protect the back of the heel with strapping
> - Advise about shoes
> - Give analgesics
>
> More severe cases
> - **REFER** for surgery if the bursa is causing significant symptoms.

HEEL PAIN IN A CHILD AGED 8-13 (SEVER'S DISEASE)

Causes
- Pain at the back of the bony part of the heel is caused by excessive pulling on the point of attachment of the Achilles tendon into the calcaneus bone (traction apophysitis)
    - this is usually due to sport

Clinical features
- Pain after exercise, which is relieved by rest
- It is tender over lower part of the calcaneus, (the big bone at the back of foot) where Achilles tendon inserts.

> **MANAGEMENT**
> - Reassure the patient that the problem settles down at the end of the growth spurt.
> - Stop the sport if this is the likely cause
> - **REFER** for physiotherapy if available
> - Paracetamol 1 tab 3 x daily as required
> - Raising the heel of the shoe a little may relieve some tension on the point of attachment

PAIN UNDERNEATH THE HEEL

Causes
- Plantar fasciitis
    - the plantar fascia is a thick fibrous band that ties the calcaneus to the metatarsal bones, holding the foot in an arch
- Painful heel fat pad due to mild trauma, incorrect foot wear or walking too much.
- Calcaneal spur due to calcification of part of the plantar fascia
    - this occurs in middle-aged people
    - it causes very severe knife-like pain on weight-bearing and walking.
- Gout

Clinical features
- Pain is felt on walking or standing
- There is tenderness below the heel
    - when pressed from below
    - when the heel is squeezed from side to side, the pain is felt below the bone
- An X-ray of the foot is necessary, if you suspect a calcaneal spur.

> **MANAGEMENT**
>
> Mild cases
> - Symptomatic treatment with analgesics
> - Better shoes
>   - an inner sole may help
> - **REFER** for physiotherapy if available
>
> More severe cases
> - **REFER** for further assessment.

SWELLING OR PAIN IN THE FOOT

Causes
- Trauma, bruising or fracture of a metatarsal bone
- Infections
- Gout
- Rarer causes
    - nerve tumours
    - bone tumours

> Treat as for the cause.

FRACTURED METATARSAL BONES

Causes
- The bones of the foot are usually injured by a weight falling on them eg. a brick.

Clinical features
- The foot is severely swollen and tender
- It is often not easy to diagnose whether it is just a bruise or a fracture
    - but this is not important, as the treatment for both is the same

MANAGEMENT
- **Crutches for 2 months if a fracture is present**
    - **this is the most important part of the treatment**
- Bandage the foot with Elastocrepe / Tubigrip so that comfort is maintained as the swelling goes down
- Elevate the foot
    - in clinic or at hospital overnight, if there is severe swelling
    - at home, if mild or moderate
- **REFER** for physiotherapy if available
- Book off work
    - for 2 weeks, if a clerical worker
    - for 2 months, if a manual labourer

Note.
- POP application is of only slight benefit because it does not immobilise the foot bones.
- Soft tissues of the foot compress and arches deflect under body weight, even if in POP.

FRACTURED FIFTH METATARSAL BASE

Causes
- This injury results from a "twisted ankle", but the injury is actually in the foot, not the ankle.
- The tip of the base of the 5th metatarsal bone is pulled off (avulsed) when there is a sharp jerk on the tendon attaching there (peroneus brevis tendon)
    - because of this muscle pull, the fracture may not heal well.

Clinical features
- History of a twisted ankle
- No tenderness over the ankle
- Tenderness only over the lateral side of the foot, where the 5th metatarsal base can be clearly palpated in a thin foot.
- Confirm diagnosis with an X-ray of the **foot, not** the ankle

MANAGEMENT
- Crutches for 6 weeks
- Elastocrepe bandage to the foot
- A POP with a walking rubber is not necessary, as the bones of the foot displace inside a POP if weight is placed on the foot.
- Give ibuprofen 400 mg 3 x daily for 5-10 days
- If the fracture has not united well after 6 weeks, it should be **REFERRED** for surgical internal fixation.

FLAT FOOT

This is where the inside (medial) border of the foot lies close to the ground.

Clinical features
Note. All children have flat feet for the first 2 years.
- A useful way to diagnose whether a flat foot is present is to get the patient to walk barefoot with wet feet
    - this will leave the imprint of the foot
    - a flat foot will show as a foot print of the whole of the sole
    - a normal foot will show just the lateral border of the sole

Flexible flat feet
- The foot is flat when the patient stands
- It is normal when not weight-bearing
- The arch is present when standing on tip toe

Rigid flat feet
- The arch is never present

MANAGEMENT
Mild flexible flat feet in children
- This requires no treatment
- Give reassurance

Moderate or severe flat feet
- **REFER** for
    - physiotherapy
    - arch supports and heel wedges
- Encourage low heeled shoes

More complex rarer causes
- **REFER** if you suspect these

PAIN UNDER THE SOLE OF THE FOOT

Causes
- Metatarsalgia
- Plantar warts
- Corns and callosities

CORNS

- These are hard thickenings of the skin over the toes
- They are caused by shoes that are too tight

MANAGEMENT
- Correct shoes with enough space at the front
- Wear open shoes or sandals, or go barefoot as much as possible.
- Apply ung acid salicylate to the hardened skin
- **REFER** to podiatrist if available

CALLOSITIES

Causes

- Usually this is due to wearing poorly fitting shoes or shoes with worn out inner soles
    - this causes irritation and thickening of the skin of the sole of the foot
- Abnormalities of the foot can cause the metatarsal heads to be more prominent under the feet and cause pressure which results in callosities eg. rheumatoid arthritis.

MANAGEMENT

- The thickened skin must be removed with a scalpel in the clinic.
- Apply acid salicylate daily, only to the hardened skin
    - take care not to apply it to normal skin
- Encourage correct foot wear such as open shoes or sandals with lower heels.
- Encourage walking barefoot as much as possible
- **REFER** to a podiatrist (chiropodist) if available for metatarsal bar for shoes.

Abnormal foot alignment
- **REFER** to
    - a physiotherapist
    - **or** a podiatrist
    - **or** an orthopaedic surgeon if it is severe

METATARSALGIA

This is pain in the metatarsal region (the widest part of the foot before the toes).

Causes

- Pain in the muscles of the forefoot due to the foot being cramped up inside a shoe which is too small.

Clinical features

- A dull, aching pain under the front of the foot, made worse by standing or walking for a long time.
- Palpation of the forefoot under the metatarsal heads shows tenderness.

MANAGEMENT

- Advise the patient about the cause of the problem
- Encourage the patient to use shoes which allow the forefoot to spread out, and give the muscles more room.
- Encourage walking barefoot to develop the muscles of the forefoot.

PLANTAR WARTS

For clinical features see The Skin page 253.

MANAGEMENT

- Treat with application of ung acid salicylate, which can be applied many times to the wart
    - apply a plaster over it
- As the person walks, the acid salicylate will penetrate more deeply.

- This is a very slow treatment, but is better than either excision or cautery
    - these treatments can result in a painful scar
- For other methods of treatment see The Skin page 253.

SWOLLEN OR PAINFUL TOES

Causes

- Trauma
- Infection

FRACTURE OF A TOE

Clinical features

- Trauma to the toes is quite common
    - it is often a crush injury
- Features suggesting a fracture or dislocation are:
    - history of quite severe trauma
    - severe swelling or pain in the toe
    - difficulty walking due to the pain
    - tenderness on percussion of the end of the toe.

MANAGEMENT

- With most trauma to the toes, the treatment is conservative
    - R.I.C.E therapy as immediate treatment (see pages 289-290)
- For fracture of a single toe, "buddy strap" the toe (not too tightly) to an adjacent toe for 3 weeks

If the pain is severe and the person cannot walk
- Crutches
- A walking below-knee POP may be needed if:
    - there are multiple fractures
    - the person cannot cope with the crutches alone
- The POP should extend beyond the end of the toes

INFECTIONS

- These are usually due to trauma, especially if the person is walking barefoot, or has cut himself while cutting toe nails.
- Fungal infections occur between the toes, particularly at the little toes. This is more common in:
    - people who wear closed canvas shoes where the toes are kept moist and warm
    - people who keep their socks on day and night
- The fungal infection can cause fissuring, pain and bleeding between the toes.
- Foreign bodies are more common in the foot and toes
    - especially in those who walk around barefoot

MANAGEMENT

Beware of infections of the toes or feet in
- Diabetic patients
- Patients with peripheral vascular disease
- The infection is often much worse than it looks on the surface.

*These patients should be **REFERRED**, unless the infection is very minor and is responding well to clinic treatment.*

Fungal infections
- See The Skin page 253

Other infections
- These are usually minor
- Give dressing and reassurance
- Advise the patient to bathe the foot 3-4 x daily in a solution of 1 cup of water and ½ teaspoon salt.
- If the infection is severe, amoxicillin and / or flucloxacillin may be needed.

Foreign body in the foot or toe
- If the foreign body is still definitely in the foot and can be clearly seen or felt, it may be possible to remove it at the clinic.
- Patients are often afraid that the foreign body will move to other parts of the body
    - reassure them that this will not happen
- However if it is deep or difficult to remove, the patient should be **REFERRED**
    - needles and pieces of metal may penetrate deeply, and can be very difficult to find
    - these need X-ray and proper theatre facilities, and removal should **not** be attempted at a clinic.

PAINFUL FIRST METATARSO-PHALANGEAL JOINT (FIRST JOINT OF THE BIG TOE)

Causes
- Hallux valgus with or without a bunion
- Gout

BUNION

Clinical features
- If shoes with very narrow-pointed fronts are worn for a long time, the big toe gets pushed more and more across towards the little toe (hallux valgus).
- The metacarpo-phalangeal joint becomes more and more dislocated.
- Thickening of the skin and a bursa develop over this joint
- This is called a bunion and may become inflamed

MANAGEMENT
- Encourage patients to buy correct shoes
    - rounded toes are more comfortable
    - open shoes or sandals are good
    - avoid pointed shoes which help to cause this condition
- Where necessary lose weight
- Walking barefoot may help a little
- In mild cases, podiatrists can help
- **REFER** for possible surgery if the toe is markedly deformed and is causing severe symptoms.

GOUT OF THE BIG TOE

For clinical features and management see gout pages 294-295.

MATERNITY

ROUTINE ANTENATAL CARE

NORMAL PREGNANCY

- Women commonly come to the clinic to find out if they are pregnant or not.
- They may not immediately say this is the reason
- They may present with vague complaints, and you may need to ask them if they are concerned about pregnancy.

Clinical features
- Missed menstrual period (amenorrhoea)
- The woman's own opinion about whether she is pregnant is of value, especially if she has had previous pregnancies.
- Nausea and vomiting
    - the so called "morning" sickness
- Tender engorged breasts with painful nipples, more marked than during the normal menstrual cycle.
- Frequency of micturition
- Constipation

Urine pregnancy tests
- Modern pregnancy tests are very accurate and can indicate pregnancy as early as the time of the first missed period.
- A pregnancy test is useful for a woman:
    - who has symptoms of pregnancy without a palpable uterus
    - if ectopic pregnancy is suspected.

MANAGEMENT
- If the woman is pregnant
    - **REFER** immediately to book at antenatal clinic.
- If in doubt, ask her to return to you in 2 weeks time for another pregnancy test.
- **REFER** if there are any complications with the pregnancy eg. pain or bleeding

---

THE FIRST ANTENATAL VISIT

CONFIRMATION OF PREGNANCY

Many women visit general primary care outpatients' departments, and ask to be examined or tested to confirm pregnancy.

- If found to be pregnant, they should immediately book in for antenatal care.
- Where no antenatal care facilities are available, these women should be **REFERRED** to the nearest and most convenient antenatal clinic as soon as possible.

THE MATERNITY RECORD

- The antenatal chart is contained in the maternity record.
- The record is given to the mother at the first antenatal visit, and kept with her until delivery.
- The antenatal chart is the only document that is needed to record pregnancy details in uncomplicated pregnancies
    - duplication of information from the chart is a waste of time and money.
- There should however be a record in the clinic of all antenatal attendances, as prescribed by the provincial government or local health authority.

NB.
The card is being phased out, so antenatal care is entered on the national maternity record. The antenatal chart is included in the maternity record.

IMPORTANT ASPECTS TO ASSESS

Estimate the gestational age
This is a vital step as almost all decisions on obstetric care are based on gestational age. This is best estimated early in the pregnancy.
- Try to establish the first day of the last menstrual period
- Assess the gestation by careful examination of the abdomen.
- Measure the symphysis fundal height

It may be necessary to **REFER** for ultrasound scan if:
- it is impossible to chart gestational age
- palpation or measurement differ by 4 or more weeks from the dates based on LMP.

Check for problems
- Assess if there are any diseases or factors likely to interfere with the pregnancy.
- First check for these factors on history
    - most antenatal charts provide check-lists or blocks to help with history taking.
- Do a complete physical examination.
- Record a baseline weight at the first visit.

Ultrasound scanning

- This is not routinely preformed in South African antenatal clinics.
- However, ultrasound scanning at ≤24 weeks is a very useful indicator of gestational age.
- Always ask the woman if she has the results of an ultrasound as done by a private practitioner.

The five warning signs

Advise the woman of the five warning signs of pregnancy complications:

- Severe headache
- Vaginal bleeding
- Reduced foetal movements
- Drainage of liquor
- Abdominal pain

Screen for tuberculosis

Perform GeneXpert sputum testing for any woman with:
- Cough
- Weight loss
- Drenching night sweats
- Fever

Urine testing

- Test the urine for protein and glucose

Blood tests

- Bloods must be taken for
    - haemoglobin
    - rhesus blood grouping.
- RPR syphilis test should be done at the clinic using a rapid test, so that the results are available before the pregnant woman leaves.
- HIV testing should be offered to all women
    - counselling and informed consent is essential.
- CD4 and viral load tests as prescribed in guidelines.

Other tests

- Tell the woman about tests that are not done routinely in the clinic.
- If she wants these tests she will have to have them done at her own expense at a private health facility.
- These will include:
    - baseline ultrasound scans without medical indication
    - urine culture
    - rubella serology
- Women over 35 should be **REFERRED** for ultrasound scan if less than 24 weeks pregnent.

Routine treatment and supplements

- Folate
    - given from conception
    - give 5 mg - one tablet daily
    - this helps prevent foetal neural tube defects
- Iron
    - given from conception
    - give tablets in a dose equivalent to 60 mg elemental iron daily, eg. ferrous sulphate 200 mg daily
    - this helps prevent anaemia
- Calcium
    - given from conception
    - give elemental calcium 1 000 mg daily (eg. Titralac 3 tablets twice daily)
    - this helps prevent complications of pre-eclampsia

Tetanus toxoid

- Assess the need for giving prophylactic tetanus toxoid
- If the woman is likely to return to her rural home for delivery, tetanus immunisation should be given.
- If she has never been immunised against tetanus, give tetanus toxoid 0,5 ml IMI, three doses, at least one month apart.
- If the mother has received immunisation in a previous pregnancy, or as a child, give one dose as a booster.

Pregnancy risk

- To qualify for 'Basic Antenatal Care', there should be no risk factors.
- The presence of risk factors will need **REFERRAL** to hospital for further antenatal care.
- See risk factors below.

PREGNANCY RISK FACTORS

Check list of risk factors requiring referral or hospital delivery

Obstetric history

- Previous stillbirth
- Previous neonatal death
- Previous low birth weight baby (<2.5 kg)
- Previous large baby (>4.5 kg)
- Previous pregnancy admission for hypertension or pre-eclampsia/eclampsia
- Previous Caesarean section
- Previous myomectomy
- Previous cone biopsy
- Previous cervical cerclage

Current pregnancy

- Diagnosed or suspected multiple pregnancy
- Age <16 years
- Rhesus isoimmunisation in previous or current pregnancy
- Vaginal bleeding
- Pelvic mass
- Diastolic blood pressure ≥90 mmHg or systolic blood pressure ≥140 mmHg

General medical conditions

- Diabetes mellitus
- Heart disease
- Kidney disease
- Epilepsy
- Asthma on medication
- Active tuberculosis
- Known 'substance' abuse including alcohol
- Undernutrition or wasting - mid-upper arm circumference less than 23 cm
- Any severe medical condition

Risk factors requiring hospital delivery

- Previous postpartum haemorrhage
- Parity ≥5

Further risk factors that arise during antenatal care

- Anaemia not responding to iron tablets
- Uterus large for dates (>90th centile symphysis-fundal height)
- Uterus small for dates (<10th centile symphysis-fundal height)
- Symphysis-fundal height decreasing
- Breech or transverse lie at term
- Extensive vulval warts that may obstruct vaginal delivery
- Pregnancy beyond 41 weeks
- Abnormal glucose screening (GTT or random blood sugar)
- Reduced foetal movements from 28 weeks

ANTENATAL VISITS

There should be five antenatal visits in a low-risk pregnancy: early booking (<12 weeks); 20 weeks; 26 weeks; 32 weeks; 38 weeks; and 41 weeks (if still pregnant).

CHECK LIST FOR BASIC ANTENATAL CARE ACTIVITIES

Check list for basic antenatal care activities at each antenatal visit. If the first visit is later than 12 weeks, all activities for the '<12th' week visit should be undertaken at that time, regardless of gestation.

Weeks of gestation	<12	20	26	32	38
History taken	X				
Clinical examination	X				
Estimated date of delivery calculated	X				
Blood pressure taken	X	X	X	X	X
Maternal height and weight	X				
Haemoglobin test	X				X
RPR performed	X				
Rapid Rh performed	X				
Counselled and voluntary testing for HIV*	X			X	
Tetanus toxoid given	X				
Iron and folate supplementation given	X	X	X	X	X
Calcium supplementation given	X	X	X	X	X

* *HIV is repeated at 32 weeks if first test is negative*

Weeks of gestation	<12	20	26	32	38
Information on emergencies given	X	X	X	X	X
Antenatal card completed, given to women	X	X	X	X	X
Clinical examination of anaemia		X	X	X	X
Urine test for protein		X	X	X	X
Uterus measured for growth		X	X	X	X
Instructions given for delivery and transport				X	X
Advice on lactation and contraception				X	X
Detection if breech and referral					X
Reminder to bring card when in labour					X
Give follow-up visit for 41 weeks at hospital					X

▼ **Note**

Staff should follow any national guideline updates. ▲

PROCEDURE AT SUBSEQUENT VISITS

- Ask about any problems
- Ask about foetal movements
- Measure the blood pressure carefully and accurately
- Measure the symphysis-fundal height (SFH)
- Record the weight
- Check the foetal lie and presentation
    - start palpation at the fundus
    - feel for the back
    - and lastly feel for the presenting part using a pelvic grip
- Check the foetal heart
- Check for protein and glucose using a urine dipstix test
- Repeat haemoglobin at 30-32 and 38 weeks
- Repeat HIV every 12 weeks if HIV test is negative.

Measurement of SFH

- The measurement of SFH is most useful between 20 and 36 weeks of pregnancy
    - it may be used as part of the gestational age assessment at the first visit
    - it may later be used to screen for abnormalities of uterine growth
- Using a tape-measure, measure the distance from the upper border of the symphysis pubis in the midline, to the highest point of the uterus
    - measure in centimetres
    - the highest point of the uterus need not necessarily be in the midline

- The SFH is best drawn onto a graph in the column corresponding to the known or presumed gestational age. This should have been assessed at the first antenatal visit
    - upper and lower limits of normal (90th and 10 centile lines respectively) are usually provided on the antenatal card graphs
- Measurements above the 90th centile (large for dates) and below the tenth centile (small for dates) indicate possible abnormalities and require referral for ultrasound assessment

Causes of large for dates uterus
- Wrong dates
- Multiple pregnancy
- Polyhydramnios
- Very large fetus
- Uterine fibroids
- Hydatidiform mole

Causes of small for dates uterus
- Wrong dates
- Intra-uterine growth restriction (IUGR)
- Intra-uterine death
- Oligohydramnios

INDICATIONS FOR SPECIAL TESTS

Pregnancy ultrasound assessment
- Doubt about gestational age after clinical assessment
    - possible twins, hydramnios, IUGR, incorrect dates
- Foetal movements not felt after 20 weeks, and foetal heart not heard
    - suspected intra-uterine death
- Significant risk for IUGR, eg. chronic hypertensive
- Significant risk of a large baby (macrosomia), eg. diabetic
- Previous or family history of congenital abnormalities
- Risk of foetal chromosomal defect, eg. mother with a previously affected baby
- Poor obstetric history (two or more previous pregnancy losses)
- History of antepartum haemorrhage
- Breech presentation after 34 weeks

ANTENATAL PROBLEMS

MANAGEMENT OF COMMON ANTENATAL PROBLEMS

PROTEINURIA

Clinical features
- Proteinuria of one plus or more should make you suspicious of:
    - pre-eclampsia
    - urinary tract infection

MANAGEMENT
- Repeat blood pressure measurement
- Test a mid-stream urine specimen (MSU) for protein

Proteinuria and hypertension
- If proteinuria and hypertension are found, the mother most likely has pre-eclampsia.
- If proteinuria persists in the absence of hypertension, check for a urinary tract infection
    - use a dipstix to test for leucocytes and / or nitrites.
- If there is no evidence of a urinary tract infection, check the woman again in a week.

VOMITING

Causes
- Try and find the cause such as
    - food
    - stress
    - medication, eg. iron tablets, use of emetics or laxatives.
- It may just be normal morning sickness
    - this is especially common in a first pregnancy.

MANAGEMENT
- It is important to check for any urinary tract infection
    - test the urine for nitrites or leucocytes with a dipstix.
- Examine the abdomen for tenderness or distension
- Mothers with mild vomiting may be reassured
    - suggest frequent small meals with little fat.
- Metoclopramide 1 tab (10 mg) 3 x daily if vomiting more severe (not in first trimester)
- Pyridoxine 25 mg 3 x daily

Indications for REFERRAL to hospital
- Not responding to clinic treatment
- Cannot eat or drink anything
- Pyrexia greater than 37,5°C or tachycardia greater than 100 bpm
- Appears ill or dehydrated
- Abdominal pain or tenderness
- Haematemesis

HEARTBURN (ISILUNGULELO)

Clinical features
- The woman herself may recognise this
- She may complain of chest pain which is burning or colicky and related to food.

Other causes for chest pain
- Chest infection
- Muscular pain
- Pulmonary embolism if pain is severe

MANAGEMENT
- Advise the woman to
    - elevate the head of the bed
    - avoid bending down if possible.
- If severe symptoms prescribe available PPI, e.g. lansoprazole 30 mg daily when needed

CONSTIPATION

MANAGEMENT
- Reassure that mild constipation is normal in pregnancy
- Discourage the use of laxatives generally
    - however if necessary lactulose can be given 15 ml 2 x daily at first; then 15 ml daily as a maintenance dose.
- Recommend a high fluid intake, with plenty of fibre eg.
    - fruit, vegetables and bran.

NON-SPECIFIC ACHES AND PAINS OF JOINTS OR MUSCLES

This may be due to the effects of increased hormones in pregnancy. Swelling and laxity in joints and ligaments occurs.

MANAGEMENT
- Hot compresses or water-bottles may help
- Give rubbing medicine eg. ung methyl salicylate
- Only oral paracetamol can be recommended
    - 2 tabs (1g) 3 x daily if necessary

VARICOSE VEINS

- Prescribe elastic stockings
- Recommend elevation of the legs

OEDEMA

Causes
Important causes to look for are:
- Pre-eclampsia
    - check for hypertension and proteinuria.
- Heart failure
    - the woman will usually have noticed increased breathlessness, especially with exertion or when lying down.
- Unilateral oedema may indicate
    - a deep venous thrombosis
    - local trauma
    - infection
- Oedema of the hands or face may be a warning of pre-eclampsia

MANAGEMENT
- **REFER** if you suspect any of the above causes.
- If the woman has oedema of the hands and face, consider referral or follow-up after 2-3 days.
- If none of the above causes are present, then reassure the mother that this is normal in pregnancy.

RASHES

Causes
- Always consider chickenpox, herpes zoster and syphilis as causes
- Also consider rashes caused by antiretroviral drugs.
- Often rashes are due to applications to the skin, eg.
    - Vaseline, glycerine, disinfectants such as Savlon.

MANAGEMENT
- **REFER**
    - infectious diseases
    - rashes that don't respond to simple measures
    - rashes associated with antiretroviral drugs
- Applications to the skin
    - treat with aqueous cream or ung emulsificans

HEART DISEASE

The most common form of heart disease in South Africa is rheumatic mitral valve stenosis and/or regurgitation. Research has shown that good history-taking will detect almost all cases of heart disease in pregnancy. Physical examination for a murmur is less accurate.

History suggesting heart disease
- Shortness of breath on mild to moderate exertion
- Shortness of breath when lying flat
- Palpitations
- Chest pain
- Haemoptysis
- History of recurrent joint pain as a child or of diagnosed rheumatic fever.

Clinical features
- Rapid heart rate (more than 96/minute)
- Irregular heart rate
- Shortness of breath at rest or on mild movement, eg. getting onto the examination couch
- Excessive oedema

MANAGEMENT
- Women with any of the above features should be **REFERRED** to a nurse or doctor skilled in clinical examination of the heart.
- If the findings are further suggestive of heart disease, the mother should be **REFERRED** to a specialist.

DIABETES MELLITUS

GESTATIONAL DIABETES

This is diabetes detected for the first time during the pregnancy, or that has only occurred during a previous pregnancy.

Diagnosis
- Diabetes is confirmed by a glucose tolerance test (GTT)

- a 75 g oral GTT is performed, preferably at 26-28 weeks.

Indications for GTT
- Glycosuria on two or more visits
- A previously abnormal GTT
- Other women at risk for gestational diabetes, where a GTT may be considered, include
  - mothers with a history of previously giving birth to a large baby
  - maternal obesity
  - age over 35
  - a first-degree relative with diabetes mellitus.

Glucose Tolerance Test
- The GTT is performed using 75 g glucose given orally after an overnight fast
- Give glucose in 250-300 ml water
- Blood is taken just before taking the glucose
- Bloods are taken again one and two hours afterwards

REFER to hospital if at least one of the following is found:
- Fasting ≥5.1 mmol/l
- One hour ≥10.0 mmol/l
- Two hour ≥8.5 mmol/l

MANAGEMENT
- On diagnosis, all gestational diabetic mothers must be **REFERRED** for admission to hospital
  - preferably a specialist diabetic pregnancy unit.
- Control of the blood sugar level is essential by diet
  - if necessary using insulin injections or oral hypoglycaemic tablets.

PRE-GESTATIONAL DIABETES

These are women who are known to have been diabetic outside of pregnancy.

MANAGEMENT
- These women should be evaluated by a doctor.
- Admission is usually needed
  - if the blood glucose control is good, this may not be necessary.
- Very early antenatal booking is essential, for prevention and treatment of complications as a result of the diabetes.

EFFECTS OF DIABETES ON PREGNANCY

- Increased risk of intra-uterine death
- Increased risk of a very large baby and complications at delivery
- Increased risk of neonatal complications, eg. jaundice, respiratory distress, hypoglycaemia
- Increased risk of pre-eclampsia
- Increased risk of foetal congenital abnormalities

EFFECTS OF PREGNANCY ON DIABETES

- Increased risk of uncontrolled diabetes with ketoacidosis
- Increased risk of kidney damage
- Increased risk of eye damage

EPILEPSY

PROBLEMS WITH PREGNANCY AND EPILEPSY

- Pregnant epileptic women have an increased risk of giving birth to children with congenital abnormalities.
- This risk is further increased with certain drugs, eg. valproic acid, phenytoin and carbamazepine.
- The altered metabolism of anti-epileptic drugs in pregnancy results in a higher risk of convulsions occurring in pregnant women.

MANAGEMENT
- Antenatal care is best given in a specialist unit, where the best drug dosing can be carried out
  - routine procedures and labour can be conducted by midwives.
- Carbamazepine is the drug of choice.
- Drugs should only be changed by specialists
- Breast feeding should be encouraged
  - the mother should be taught simple precautions, such as sitting down when feeding in case she has a fit.

ASTHMA

Asthmatic attacks only occur very rarely during labour. Pregnancy has no predictable effect on the severity of asthma.

MANAGEMENT
- The drugs used for control of asthma are believed to be safe in pregnancy, eg.
  - oral and inhaled corticosteroids, beta 2-stimulants and ipratropium.
- Treatment should not be stopped during pregnancy
- Asthmatic attacks must be prevented as they may cause foetal hypoxia and intra-uterine death.
- Pregnant women with uncontrolled (wheezing) asthma should be **REFERRED**.

ANAEMIA

Anaemia is defined by the World Health Organisation as a haemoglobin (Hb) level of less than 11 g/dl. For practical reasons, many obstetricians use a cut-off of 10 g/dl as the level where action should be taken.

Screening for anaemia
Measure level at the first antenatal visit.

MANAGEMENT

Levels of haemoglobin

Hb 10 g/dl or more
- Give elemental iron 60 mg tab daily, eg. ferrous sulphate 200 mg daily
- Repeat Hb at 32 and 38 weeks

Hb less than 8 g/dl
- **REFER** to hospital or to a specialist clinic for investigation

Hb between 8 and 10 g/dl:
- **REFER** if:
  - ≥ 36 weeks pregnant
  - short of breath or with gross oedema
  - known to have a history of anaemia eg. sickle-cell disease
  - malaria is suspected
  - woman on AZT
- Start treatment with ferrous sulfate 200 mg 3 x daily with Vitamin C 100 mg 3 x daily and folic acid 5 mg daily.
- Repeat Hb after 3 weeks and expect Hb increase if adherence is good.
  - Hb should increase by 1.5 to 2.0 g/dl in 3 weeks.
- **REFER** if no adequate increase in Hb and 32 or more weeks pregnant.

Note: Anaemic mothers who cannot tolerate iron should be **REFERRED** to hospital or specialist clinic.

Advice to anaemic mothers
- Encourage honesty about adherence with medication.
- Encourage mothers to eat meat (iron) and tomatoes or fruit (Vitamin C).
- Discourage eating ash or soil and too much tea or coffee as these may interfere with iron absorption.
- Advise taking iron tablets during meals to decrease gastritis, nausea and vomiting.
- Do not take iron at the same time as calcium.

SEXUALLY TRANSMITTED INFECTIONS (STIs)

VAGINAL DISCHARGE

Clinical features
- Often the patient herself will note that the discharge is abnormal
  - she may sometimes confuse the normal increased discharge (leucorrhoea) with an abnormal discharge
  - leukorrhoea is a profuse, non-offensive and off-white discharge that is normal in pregnancy.
- Symptoms suggesting an infection are burning, offensive discharge, yellow colour, a fishy smell after sexual intercourse.

Diagnosis
- If possible perform a speculum examination on all patients complaining of discharge.
- Discharge coming through the os of the cervix is suggestive of gonorrhoea or chlamydial infection.

■ CANDIDIASIS
- This usually shows as a non-offensive, irritating, white discharge with plaques.

Treat with a single-dose imidazole (eg. clotrimazole 500 mg) PV pessary stat.

■ TRICHOMONIASIS
- This may be seen as a non-specific, yellow/green, bubbly and/or offensive discharge.

Treat with metronidazole 2 g orally stat, except before 10 weeks gestation.

■ BACTERIAL VAGINOSIS
- This appears as a greyish, sticky, homogeneous discharge
- Sometimes the discharge has a fishy smell, which the patient may notice particularly after sexual intercourse.

Treat with metronidazole 2 g orally stat.

■ GONORRHOEA / CHLAMYDIAL CERVICITIS
- This can be diagnosed if there is a mucopurulent cervical discharge seen on speculum examination.

SYNDROMIC MANAGEMENT
- Treat patients with:
  - ceftriaxone 250 mg IM as a single dose
  - **plus** metronidazole 2 g as a single oral dose
  - **plus** azithromycin 1g as a single oral dose
  - **plus** if candida present (curd-like discharge, erythema): give clotrimazole vaginal pessary 500 mg single dose at night

---

VULVAL WARTS

Causes
- These are caused by human papillomavirus and are sexually transmitted.
- They generally enlarge and multiply during pregnancy and all treatments are unsatisfactory, or unsafe in pregnancy.

MANAGEMENT

- Uncomplicated warts need no special treatment in pregnancy
  - they usually resolve in the puerperium.
- Offensive vaginal discharge should be treated with metronidazole 2 g orally stat, or 400 mg 2 x daily for 7 days.
- Very extensive warts need hospital delivery, and occasionally Caesarean section.

POSITIVE TPAB AND RPR TESTS

Untreated syphilis in pregnancy will kill 20% of babies infected.

MANAGEMENT

- Treatment is benzathine penicillin 2,4 million units IMI weekly for 3 doses at weekly intervals
  - if allergic to penicillin, **REFER** to hospital or to an experienced doctor to undertake penicillin de-sensitisation.
- Treatment for the partner should be strongly encouraged
- Repeat TPAB and RPR 6-8 weeks after the last dose of penicillin to exclude re-infection
  - if the RPR titre is greater than it was before treatment, then re-treat as a possible repeat infection with one further injection (including the sexual partner).
- Treponemal tests (eg. TPAB, TPHA)
  - they are used as a screening test and to rule out a false positive RPR
  - they remain positive for life despite treatment

HIV AND AIDS

HIV testing should be offered to all pregnant women. Informed consent and full pre- and post-test counselling is essential. HIV-positive pregnant women can be managed at primary care clinics.

Testing for HIV
- Rapid testing must be carried out

Counselling
Issues in counselling HIV-positive pregnant women.

- Establish what the woman knows about HIV.
- Give information on how the virus is transmitted.

Note:
Be aware of updated HIV care guidelines as these may change.

- Discuss the progression of disease and the possibility of a long, symptom-free period.
- Describe the symptoms and signs of the progression to AIDS.
- Discuss the effect of pregnancy on HIV infection.
- Explain the risk of transmission of HIV from the mother to the baby, and how this may be reduced.
- Discuss benefits, risks and importance of adherence to antiretroviral treatment.
- Discuss the importance of CD4 count and viral load monitoring.
- Discuss how to to inform her male partner if the test is positive.
- Discuss condom use to prevent transmission to sexual partners.
- Discuss future fertility plans
  - offer postpartum sterilisation as a choice

MANAGEMENT

Antenatal care
- *This is in addition to the routine antenatal care.*
- *All women should be counselled and tested for HIV.*

First antenatal visit
HIV positive and not on ART (known and newly diagnosed)
- Clinical assessment for TB and WHO staging.
- If no active psychiatric illness or history of kidney disease:
  - start TEE (TDF, FTC, EFV) same day
  - send blood for serum creatinine and CD4 count

1 week later
- If creatinine <85 micromol / L
  - continue FDC as a lifelong treatment
- If creatinine >85 micromol / L
  - **stop** FDC
  - **REFER** urgently to doctor for initiation of alternative lifelong triple regimen (usually AZT, 3TC, EFV) and investigation and management of kidney disease

Viral load monitoring
- First viral load to be done 3 months after ART initiation.
- Review results within 2 weeks
  - if virally suppressed (CD4 <1000), continue on current regimen
  - if not virally suppressed (CD4 >1000), adherence problems or viral resistance, then get expert advice for the management of the woman
- Repeat viral load after 3 months and then 6 monthly throughout pregnancy and breastfeeding
  - return to annual viral load monitoring only once she has stopped breastfeeding.

HIV infected on ART
- Continue ART regimen
- Send blood for viral load at booking
- Review results within 2 weeks

Labour and delivery
Known HIV-positive women are managed in the same way as those who are HIV negative or HIV unknown, except for the following:
- Avoid artificial rupture of membranes early in labour.
- Prevent prolonged labour.
- Avoid vacuum extraction if possible.

Newly diagnosed in labour (unbooked women and previously diagnosed HIV negative)
- Provide nevirapine 200 mg as a single oral dose
  - **plus** zidovudine (AZT) 300 mg 3 hourly during labour
- After delivery, mother to be given TDF/FTC as a single oral dose (can be given same time as NVP).

Postnatal care
- Make sure that contraception advice is given.
- Counsel about safe feeding practices
  - advise exclusive breastfeeding
- Arrange follow-up for wellness assessment and cervical smear 6 weeks after delivery.
- Initiate ART if newly diagnosed HIV positive in labour
- Continue ART regimen for patients already on lifelong ART and viral load monitoring (6 monthly during breastfeeding)

HIV-exposed infant (see Neonatal Care, page 353)

URINARY TRACT INFECTION

CYSTITIS

Clinical features
- This is suspected with symptoms such as frequency of micturition or dysuria.
- It should be suspected if there are abnormal findings on urine dipstix testing
  - nitrites, protein and leucocyctes are suggestive of infection
  - leucocytes may be due to other causes such as a vaginal discharge
  - protein may be found in pre-eclampsia.

If there is good evidence of a cystitis
- Nitrofurantoin 100 mg 4 x daily for 7 days

PYELONEPHRITIS

- The woman looks ill and usually has abdominal pain
- The temperature is high
- The urine may show leucocytes and nitrites
- If the urine is positive and there is definite renal angle tenderness, pyelonephritis should be diagnosed
  - **REFER** to hospital for admission and intravenous antibiotics.

PULMONARY TUBERCULOSIS (PTB)

Clinical features
- PTB should be suspected in any woman who has a cough for more than 3 weeks.
- It is more suggestive if there is also failure to gain weight, or actual weight loss, haemoptysis, chronic fever, chronic tiredness or chronic chest pain.
- These women should be **REFERRED** for investigation

MANAGEMENT
- Of the modern drugs used for treatment of PTB, only streptomycin is contra-indicated in pregnancy.
- Rifampicin, isoniazid, pyrazinamide and ethambutol may all be used in the normal doses irrespective of the gestational age.
- Antenatal care and delivery need not necessarily take place in hospital
  - mothers who are clinically well may visit and deliver at a midwifery clinic
  - the PTB must be managed and the treatment supervised by their local clinic.
- If the mother is on treatment, breast feeding is safe and should be encouraged.

HYPERTENSION

Clinical features
- This is a diastolic blood pressure of
  - 90 mm Hg or more on two occasions at least 4 hours apart
  - or diastolic BP of 110 mm Hg or more measured on one occasion
  - or a systolic blood pressure ≥140 mm Hg on two occasions at least 4 hours apart

- Proteinuria is significant
  - if one plus or more is found
  - on two dipstix specimens
  - taken at least four hours apart

The importance of protein in the urine

The presence of proteinuria with hypertension as defined above is suggestive of pre-eclampsia.

Definitions

Pre-eclampsia (gestational proteinuric hypertension, pre-eclamptic toxaemia)

Hypertension with proteinuria, which arises after the 20th week of pregnancy.

Severe pre-eclampsia
- Pre-eclampsia, where the diastolic blood pressure is 110 mm Hg or more, on two occasions, at least 4 hours apart **or** systolic blood pressure is 160 mm Hg or more on 2 occasions at least 4 hours apart.
- **Or** 120 mm Hg at least once.
- **Or** there is proteinuria persistently +++ or more.

Imminent eclampsia

Typical clinical findings in pre-eclamptic women, which may precede eclampsia are:

- Severe headache
- Visual disturbance
- Severe epigastric pain
- Hyperreflexia (ankle clonus >3)

Eclampsia
- Generalised tonic-clonic seizures occurring after the 20th week of pregnancy associated with hypertension and proteinuria.

Maternal risk factors for the development of pre-eclampsia
- Chronic hypertension
- Kidney disease
- Diabetes mellitus
- Previous pregnancy complicated by hypertension
- Non-proteinuric hypertension during the current pregnancy
- Family history of hypertension or pre-eclampsia
- Age >35 years
- Primigravida
- Obesity
- Multiple pregnancy
- Hydatidiform mole

Complications of pre-eclampsia
Maternal
- Eclampsia
- Cerebro vascular accident
- Abruptio placentae
- Kidney failure
- Pulmonary oedema
- HELLP syndrome
- Subcapsular liver haemorrhage

Foetal
- Pre-term birth resulting from early induction or delivery
- Intra-uterine growth restriction
- Foetal distress during labour
- Intra-uterine death

MANAGEMENT
General principles
- Pre-eclamptic mothers must be admitted to hospital
- The only known treatment for pre-eclampsia is delivery
- Antihypertensive drugs (nifedipine, methyldopa) are useful for blood pressure control, but do not stop the progression of the disease.
- Depending on the severity of the condition, an attempt may be made to delay delivery to allow the fetus to mature.
- Women with severe pre-eclampsia, eclampsia or imminent eclampsia usually require immediate delivery
- Pregnancies with non-proteinuric hypertension may be managed conservatively
    - they are allowed to go to term, unless they develop superimposed pre-eclampsia.
- All women with hypertension during pregnancy should be **REFERRED** to hospital or to a doctor experienced in the management of these disorders.

Hypertensive emergencies at primary care level
Eclampsia
- Ensure adequate airway, turn patient on side and give oxygen
- Give magnesium sulphate 4 g in 200 ml normal saline
    - this must run fast
    - it must be followed by 200 ml normal saline to run at 100 ml/hour
- Add magnesium sulphate 5 g IMI in each buttock (total dose 14 g)

- Insert an indwelling urinary catheter
- If convulsions cannot be controlled, give diazepam 5-10 mg IVI or rectally
- **REFER** to hospital by ambulance

Imminent eclampsia or severe pre-eclampsia
- Give magnesium sulphate 4 g in 200 ml normal saline
    - to run fast
    - it must be followed by a normal saline drip to run at normal rate
- Add magnesium sulphate 5 g IMI in each buttock (total dose 14 g)
- Insert an indwelling urinary catheter
- **REFER** to hospital by ambulance

MULTIPLE PREGNANCY

Look for a multiple pregnancy at all antenatal visits, in all women, unless they have had an ultrasound examination. Women with suggestive clinical findings should be referred for an ultrasound scan. A diagnosis will then be made.

Suggestive clinical findings
- Large for dates uterus
- More than two foetal heads or buttocks palpated
- If able to feel the back on both sides
- Two or more foetal hearts audible
- Foetal head small for the size of the uterus

Complications
Maternal
- Pre-eclampsia
- Exaggerated symptoms of pregnancy
- Anaemia
- Antepartum haemorrhage
- Postpartum haemorrhage

Foetal
- Prematurity
- Intra-uterine growth restriction
- Congenital abnormalities
- Intra-uterine death
- Malpresentation

All multiple pregnancies should have antenatal care and delivery at a hospital.

BREECH PRESENTATION

Breech presentation is not considered to be abnormal before 34 weeks.

Causes of breech presentation after 34 weeks
- Foetal abnormality, eg. hydrocephalus
- Polyhydramnios
- Multiple pregnancy
- Uterine abnormality, eg. fibroids

Complications of breech presentation
- Cord prolapse
- Foetal head entrapment with asphyxia or death
- Foetal birth injuries

> **MANAGEMENT**
> - All mothers with breech presentation after 34 weeks should be **REFERRED** for ultrasound assessment.
> - External cephalic version (ECV) will be considered for those women with breech presentation at 37 weeks
>   - ECV should only be performed in a hospital with facilities for emergency Caesarean section.
> - Elective Caesarean section at term is the safest method of delivery for babies with breech presentations.

> **MANAGEMENT**
> - These above categories should be referred for
>   - a screening sonar for gestational age
>   - consultation at a genetic counselling clinic.
> - Further management will be decided there
> - The usual procedure for antenatal diagnosis is an amniocentesis
>   - this is best performed at 16 weeks, and not later than 24 weeks

POST-TERM PREGNANCY

- This is defined as pregnancy of gestational age above 42 weeks
    - however it is often a problem to decide if the women's dates for the last menstrual period are correct.
- Encourage women to come to antenatal clinic early in the pregnancy
    - this makes it easier to get the correct date and gestation
    - it helps to prevent miscalculations about post-term pregnancy.
- If you suspect post-term pregnancy, review the gestational age and antenatal care to exclude errors in assessment.
    - ask again about any ultrasound scans done by private practitioners.

> **REFER** to hospital pregnancies suspected to be 41 weeks or more. Such pregnancies will be assessed for possible induction of labour.

CONGENITAL DISORDERS

Indications for antenatal diagnosis
- Early antenatal attendance makes intra-uterine diagnosis and management of congenital disorders easier and more effective
    - it is best if done before 24 weeks gestation.
- The following categories of pregnant women are at increased risk for foetal chromosomal or genetic abnormalities
    - maternal age greater than 35 years
    - a previous baby with a congenital disorder
    - a family history of genetic disorder.

ANTEPARTUM HAEMORRHAGE (APH)

This is bleeding from the genital tract from 20 weeks of pregnancy up to delivery of the baby. Bleeding before 20 weeks is considered to be a miscarriage, or may be due to non-obstetrical causes.

Presence of fresh blood or clots suggests a more serious obstetrical cause.

Causes
Painless bleeding
- Think of placenta praevia, especially if there is heavier bleeding.
- Infections of the cervix, vulva and vagina may be painless or painful.
- There may also be a history of bleeding after intercourse
- Carcinoma of the cervix must be considered

Pain with the bleeding
- Think of an abruptio placenta

SEVERE APH

Clinical features
- The patient is pale, has tachycardia or hypotension.
- Fresh blood or clots may be passed.

Causes
- This is almost always caused either by
    - placenta praevia (no pain, live baby, soft uterus)
    - abruptio placentae (abdominal pain, no foetal movements, hard uterus).

> **MANAGEMENT**
> - All women with suspected antepartum haemorrhage, should be referred to hospital by ambulance
>   - the only exception is mild APH caused by cervical manipulation.
> - Vaginal examination may cause severe bleeding so should be avoided.
> - Insert a large bore intravenous cannula, number 16 or 18.
> - Start a fast drip of normal saline or Ringer-lactate
> - Take a blood specimen in a plain tube and attach it to the drip line, for cross-match.
> - Insert an indwelling urinary catheter
> - **REFER** urgently to hospital by ambulance

RHESUS INCOMPATIBILITY

Antenatal screening
- Use tests which can be done at the clinic such as Rapidtest Rh
- If the mother's blood is Rh positive, nothing more needs to be done because the baby is at no risk.
- If the mother's blood is Rh negative, blood must be sent for antibody testing
    - if antibodies are found with titre 1:16 or more, at over 26 weeks, the mother is referred
    - if antibodies are not found or are of titre less than 1:16, repeat specimens should be sent at 26, 32 and 36 weeks gestation.

Previous history
- It there is a history of a previous severely affected infant, do not wait for Rh testing
    - **REFER** the mother immediately as the baby may need urgent intra-uterine blood transfusion.

MANAGEMENT
Antenatal
- If antibodies are found (see under screening), **REFER** to hospital where ultrasound tests will be done to look for evidence of foetal anaemia.

Postnatal
- After cutting the cord at delivery, allow the placental end to bleed freely.
- Any woman who is Rh negative should be given anti-D 100 mcg intramuscularly within 72 hours of any delivery
    - this includes abortion.
- If this is missed, anti-D might still be effective if given up to 1 week after delivery.

LABOUR AND DELIVERY

DIAGNOSIS OF LABOUR

The earlier in labour the woman comes to the labour ward, the more difficult it is to be sure whether she is in definite labour or not.

The diagnosis of labour can be easily made when there are:
- Painful uterine contractions **plus**
  - progressive dilatation and effacement of the cervix, **or**
  - a definite show, **or**
  - rupture of the membranes.

Definition of the phases of labour
The following rules are for practical guidance. Exceptions do occur and are identified with experience.
- The latent phase is defined as labour with the cervix dilated 3 cm or less.
- The active phase is defined as labour with the cervix dilated 4 cm or more.

EARLY AND FALSE LABOUR

Clinical features of early true labour
- The cervix shows shortening (effacement) on repeat assessment.
- Contractions become more frequent, more painful and more regular.
- There is usually a show that precedes the first vaginal examination.

Signs suggesting another illness or a problem in labour
- Raised temperature
- Raised respiratory rate
- Raised pulse
- Increased foetal heart rate

Other possible causes of lower abdominal pain which should be considered
- Urinary tract infection
- Colic
- Gastroenteritis
- Use of enemas

MANAGEMENT
- On admission, check the length and dilatation of the cervix
  - this is to assess whether the woman is really in labour
  - if so, is she in the latent phase or the active phase?
- Allow the woman to walk around.
- She can eat or drink if she wants to

Reassess after 4 hours:
- If the pains have stopped, she can be discharged
- If the pains persist and the cervix has shortened or dilated, then labour can be diagnosed.
- If the pains persist and the cervix remains unchanged, consider other causes of abdominal pain
  - if these have been excluded, give pethidine 100 mg IMI with hydroxyzine 100 mg IMI.

Reassess after another 4 hours:
- If pains have stopped, she can be discharged
- If pains persist and pregnancy is at 37 weeks or more, a diagnosis of prolonged latent phase is made
  - rupture the membranes and expect labour to progress.
- If pains persist and membranes cannot be ruptured, (HIV positive) or pregnancy is less than 37 weeks
  - **REFER** to hospital or for expert advice.

ESTABLISHED LABOUR FOR LOW-RISK WOMEN

MANAGEMENT
- Women may eat during the latent phase and take fluids during the active phase.
- An intravenous drip does not need to be put up routinely.
- Women should be allowed to walk around, sit or stand, whichever suits them best.
- One person (partner, friend or relative) should be allowed to stay during the labour and delivery
  - this makes the delivery less painful
  - it improves the mother's bonding with the child
  - it improves breastfeeding.
- All important observations, whether by doctors or midwives, must be made on the partogram (see page 346)
- All HIV-negative women must be retested for HIV in labour.

The latent phase
- Observe hourly heart rate, contractions and foetal heart rate (FHR)
- Observe 4-hourly temperature, BP and pad-checks
- Perform 4-hourly abdominal and vaginal assessment

- If the latent phase exceeds 8 hours, try to find the reason
  and take appropriate action
    - rupture of the membranes
    - consultation
    - or **REFERRAL** to hospital.

Common reasons for a prolonged latent phase
- Full bladder
- Uterine inertia
- Malpresentation
- Cephalopelvic disproportion

The active phase
- Observe half-hourly heart rate, FHR, contractions and pad-checks
- Observe 4-hourly BP and temperature
- Perform 2-hourly abdominal and vaginal assessment
- Chart the progress on the partogram

The partogram
- The alert and action lines are pre-drawn on the partogram
- The most important observations are
    - foetal head descent in fifths
    - cervical dilatation
    - moulding.
- If the alert line is crossed, perform amniotomy (if HIV negative) and look for a cause of poor progress.
- If the action line is crossed, **REFERRAL** to hospital is essential.

Note:
- The alert line is drawn at a slope of 1 cm/hr, starting from the first cervical dilatation of 4 cm or more.
- The action line is drawn 2 hours parallel and to the right of the alert line.

Analgesia in labour

Opiate analgesia
- The standard regimen is pethidine 100 mg IMI with promethazine (Phenergan) 25 mg IM, given 4 hourly when necessary.

Other forms of analgesia
- Nitrous oxide and oxygen (Entonox), and epidural analgesia, are very effective.
- They are generally not available at primary care level in South Africa.

COMMON LABOUR PROBLEMS

PRE-LABOUR RUPTURE OF THE MEMBRANES (PROM)

This is rupture of the membranes before the onset of labour pains.

Diagnosis
The woman may describe anything from a watery discharge to the bursting of a large volume of liquor onto the floor.
Rupture must be confirmed by the following examinations:
- Ask the woman to cough
    - check if there is any amniotic fluid coming out of the vagina.
- Using a sterile speculum for examination, fluid may be seen coming through the cervical opening
- The fluid is likely to be amniotic fluid if there is
    - a blue colour on testing with litmus paper
    - a pH of 7 or more using a urine dipstix.
- If you are unsure, despite the above tests, observe for at least 4 hours.
- If there is doubt, **REFER** for ultrasound assessment of liquor volume and/or admission to hospital.

MANAGEMENT
Management depends on gestational age or foetal weight estimation (by clinical methods or ultrasound).

- Pregnancy 24-33 weeks, estimated foetal weight 500 g to 2 000 g
    - **REFER** to hospital.
- Pregnancy 34 weeks or more, estimated foetal weight greater than 2 000 g, with labour pains:
    - assess for cervical dilation and manage as for labour.
- If not in labour, insert an intravenous line
    - give amoxicillin 1g IV
    - give metronidazole 400 mg orally
    - **REFER** to hospital

PRE-TERM LABOUR

This is labour that occurs before 37 weeks' gestation.

MANAGEMENT

Pregnancy 24-33 weeks, estimated foetal weight 900-2 000 g
- Give betamethasone 12 mg IMI stat.
- Give salbutamol 0.2 mg IVI stat slowly.
- **REFER** to hospital.

Pregnancy 34-36 weeks, estimated foetal weight greater than 2 000 g
- **REFERRAL** to hospital is not necessary.
- Give amoxicillin 500 mg orally 8 hourly and metronidazole 400 mg 8 hourly until delivery.
- Manage labour and delivery as for term pregnancy.

FOETAL DISTRESS IN LABOUR AND MECONIUM STAINING OF THE LIQUOR

Foetal distress should be suspected in the following circumstances:

- Persistent foetal tachycardia (greater than 160 bpm)
- Foetal heart decelerations persisting after the end of contractions (late decelerations).
- Persistent foetal bradycardia (less than 110 bpm)
- Thick meconium staining of the liquor

MANAGEMENT
- Do a vaginal examination to make sure there is no cord prolapse or second stage labour.
- Turn the woman on the side, usually the left lateral.
- Give oxygen 40% mask at 10 l/min.
- Start an intravenous drip with normal saline 1 000 ml at 125 ml/hr.
- Give salbutamol 0.2 mg IVI stat slowly.
- **REFER** urgently to hospital by ambulance.

CORD PROLAPSE

Risk factors for cord prolapse
- Malpresentation
- Preterm labour
- Polyhydramnios
- Multiple pregnancy
- High head at the time of rupture of membranes

MANAGEMENT
If the foetus is alive, the pregnancy more than 26 weeks, and delivery is not imminent:

- Give oxygen with a 40% mask at 10 l/min.
- Insert an indwelling urinary catheter
    - fill the bladder with 500 ml normal saline.
- Start an intravenous drip with normal saline 1 000 ml at 125 ml/hr.
- If there are uterine contractions, give salbutamol 0.2 mg IVI stat slowly.
- Turn the woman on her side with pillows under her hips.
- If the presenting part is deeply engaged, use the knee-elbow position.
- Reassure the woman
    - explain that a Caesarean section is going to be necessary.
- **REFER** urgently to hospital by ambulance.

SECOND STAGE OF LABOUR

This is defined as the stage of labour from full dilatation of the cervix to delivery of the baby.

MANAGEMENT
- Midwives should be prepared to conduct the second stage in almost any position that the woman requests
    - eg. sitting, kneeling, standing, squatting, on her back (supine), lateral.
- Bearing down should be encouraged only if
    - the woman has an urge to push
    - the foetal head is fully engaged and on the pelvic floor.
- The foetal heart rate should be checked between contractions to exclude foetal distress.

Indications for REFERRAL
- No maternal urge to bear down after one hour of full dilatation of the cervix
- Failure to deliver the baby after 45 minutes of bearing down in a nullipara
- Failure to deliver the baby after 30 minutes of bearing down in a multipara.

SHOULDER DYSTOCIA

- This emergency is almost always associated with delivery of a big baby (weighing 3.5 kg or more; with symphysis-fundal measurement greater than 40 cm).
- When vaginal delivery of a large baby is expected, shoulder dystocia should be anticipated
    - appropriate action can then be planned.

Risk factors
- Obese woman
- Previous large baby
- Previous shoulder dystocia
- Prolonged late first or second stage
- Diabetic mother

Complications
- Foetal humeral fracture
- Foetal brachial plexus injury
- Foetal birth asphyxia and brain damage
- Foetal death
- Maternal perineal injuries

MANAGEMENT

1. Immediately move the woman to the end or edge of the bed, to provide posterior room for delivery of the baby.
2. With the woman on her back, fully flex both hips so that the knees almost touch the shoulders (MacRoberts' position)
    - the woman can help by holding up her thighs.
3. With an assistant pushing on the abdomen from the top, push the baby's head downwards as far as possible toward the anus
    - this helps to deliver the upper shoulder (anterior) from behind the symphysis pubis
    - repeat once if necessary.
    - do not stretch the baby's neck as it may cause brachial plexus injury.
4. If you cannot get the shoulder out, the next step is to try and deliver an arm
    - the easiest arm to deliver is the one at the back (posterior vagina)
    - grip the arm as near the hand as possible
    - bring it round in front of the chest and out of the vagina
    - delivery will usually be achieved.
5. If this fails, the next manouvre is to try and twist the baby out
    - this is done by pulling on the back (posterior) shoulder, and rotating the shoulder through 180°
    - this brings the impacted anterior shoulder out from under the symphysis
    - it is brought into the posterior hollow of the pelvis at a lower level than the symphysis where there is more room
    - this should make it easier to pull out the shoulder or arm.
6. If this fails, get the woman to turn into the "all-fours" position (knee-elbow position), and try again to deliver the posterior arm.

- If all these steps fail, the prognosis for the baby is poor
- Any further procedures to deliver a dead baby (eg. cutting the collar bone) should be undertaken in hospital under sedation or general anaesthesia.

THIRD STAGE OF LABOUR

MANAGEMENT

- Active management is the routine.
- Put the baby in dry towels on the mother's abdomen
- Give syntocinon 10 units IMI as soon as the baby is delivered
    - the possibility of a twin must be excluded by palpating the abdomen
- As soon as the uterus contracts, start Brandt-Andrews controlled cord traction
    - upward counter pressure on the uterus is carried out.
    - rub the uterus well after the placenta has been expelled
- Wait for one minute after delivery of the baby before clamping and cutting the cord.

RETAINED PLACENTA

If the placenta has not been expelled within 30 minutes of delivery:

- Do a vaginal examination to try and find out if
    - the placenta is still in the uterus (truly retained)
    - it has come into the vagina, and can be eased out
- Start an IV infusion of 1 litre normal saline with 20 units syntocinon at 240 ml/hr.
- Insert an indwelling urinary catheter.
- If there is heavy vaginal bleeding and the placenta is still in the uterus
    - **REFER** to hospital urgently by ambulance.
- If the placenta remains in the uterus after 1 hour of syntocinon infusion, irrespective of bleeding
    - **REFER** to hospital urgently by ambulance.

RETAINED PRODUCTS OF CONCEPTION

MANAGEMENT

- The expelled placenta must be examined thoroughly.
- No special treatment is necessary for retained membranes alone.
- A missing cotyledon or lobe requires urgent referral to hospital for evacuation in theatre.

POSTPARTUM HAEMORRHAGE (PPH)

PPH means a blood loss of more than 500 ml, or excessive blood loss with evidence of shock (heart rate high, blood pressure low).

MANAGEMENT
- Immediately rub up a uterine contraction and get help
- Start an IV infusion of 1 litre normal saline with 20 units oxytocin, running fast, using a 16 or 18 G cannula.
- Take blood in a plain tube and attach it to the intravenous line, for cross-match at hospital.
- For persistent severe bleeding, insert a second IV infusion, using an 18 G or 16 G cannula.
- Insert an indwelling urinary catheter and keep the bladder empty
- Find the cause
    - atonic uterus, retained products, lacerations, coagulopathy.
- **REFER** urgently to hospital by ambulance
    - continue to try to stop the bleeding
    - replace the blood loss.
- The following measures may help to stop the bleeding while waiting for transport
    - syntometrine 0.5 mg IMI stat
    - manual evacuation of the uterus
    - local pressure on vaginal or perineal lacerations
    - continuous massage of the uterus
    - compression of the aorta against the mother's spine.

EPISIOTOMY AND PERINEAL TEARS

Indications for episiotomy
These are in approximate descending order of importance:
- Breech presentation
- Tight perineum
- Foetal distress in the second stage
- Ineffective bearing down in the second stage

Note. It is not necessary or helpful to do a routine episiotomy on all primiparous mothers.

MANAGEMENT
Episiotomy and suturing procedure
- Mediolateral episiotomies are acceptable
- Local anaesthetic must always be given before episiotomy and perineal repair
- Lignocaine 1% (maximum dose 20 ml) is the standard local anaesthetic agent.
- Chromic catgut or polyglactin (Vicryl) are acceptable suture materials.
- After repair, always feel inside the rectum for any sutures and remove the vaginal tampon
    - if a suture is felt in the rectum, the suture must be cut and removed
    - if the suture is left it might cause a rectovaginal fistula.
- Check carefully to make sure the anal sphincter is not torn (third-degree tear)
- Third-degree tears require emergency referral to hospital by ambulance, for repair in theatre.

THE PUERPERIUM

ROUTINE POSTNATAL CARE

MANAGEMENT
- Normal meals are given
- Well babies room-in with their mothers
- Breastfeeding assistance and advice is given
- Advice is given on perineal hygiene
- The mother may want contraceptive advice
    - she should be helped with this as much as possible.
- The HIV, RPR and Rhesus group results must be checked or the tests repeated if necessary

DISCHARGE FROM THE CLINIC

A mother may be discharged six hours after vaginal delivery if:

- There is no excessive vaginal bleeding (clots)
- There is no offensive lochia
- Her temperature is not above 37.5°C
- Her pulse rate does not exceed 100 bpm
- Blood pressure is normal
- She feels well enough to go home
- The baby is healthy

Note: If there are any problems with the mother or child, they should be referred to a doctor or to hospital.

FOLLOW-UP VISITS

- Ideally, mothers should be visited at home daily in the first week of the puerperium.
- Where this is not possible, they may be discharged with a note to attend their clinic 3 days after delivery.
- At that visit their general condition, breasts, uterine involution, perineum and lochia are examined
    - problems are also discussed and advice given
    - the babies are also checked.

COMMON POSTNATAL PROBLEMS

PUERPERAL SEPSIS (ENDOMYOMETRITIS)

Clinical features
- Pyrexia
- Uterine tenderness and/or offensive lochia

MANAGEMENT
- **REFER** urgently to hospital for intravenous broad-spectrum antibiotics.
- For more information see under Female Reproductive System, page 202.

PERSISTENT VAGINAL BLEEDING (SECONDARY PPH)

Causes
- Puerperal sepsis
- Retained products of conception
- Breakdown of lacerations or suture lines

This requires **REFERRAL** to hospital for investigation and specific treatment.

The Maternity chapter (pages 331-351) has been written by Professor Emeritus E Buchmann, Consultant, Department of Obstetrics, Chris Hani Baragwanath Hospital, Johannesburg

NEONATAL CARE

NEONATAL CONDITIONS

Indications for REFERRAL
- If you are worried about the baby's condition
- A respiratory rate above 60 per minute or any evidence of respiratory distress
- Twitching or tremor
- An Apgar Score of less than 6 / 10 at 5 minutes
- Blood glucose 40 mg% (2,2 mmol / L) or less *after* initial management with glucose
- Small for gestational age (see page 356)
- A big baby over 4,5 kg
- Any significant congenital abnormality
- Cyanosis or anaemia
- Any abnormal bleeding
- Hypothermia
- Failure to suck in a neonate
- Failure to cry, or an abnormal cry
- Membranes ruptured for more than 24 hours
- Offensive smelling liquor
- Significant birth injuries eg. Erb's palsy

HIV-EXPOSED INFANT

This refers to an infant whose mother is HIV infected, and in whom HIV infection has not been confirmed or excluded.

MANAGEMENT

Children <18 months of age (HIV PCR test)
- Perform PCR testing on all HIV-exposed infants at birth, and if negative:
    - repeat at 10 weeks if the infant is given ARV prophylaxis (NVP) until 6 weeks of age
    - and at 10 and 18 weeks if the child is given 12 weeks of prophylaxis
- If any test is positive, confirm with a second HIV PCR test
    - initiate treatment while awaiting the second PCR test result.
- If the child is breastfed and the 10- or 18-week test is negative, testing should be repeated 6 weeks after complete cessation of breastfeeding
    - if the child is >18 months, a rapid test or ELISA can be done
- If an exposed child reaches 18 months of age and has not had a positive HIV PCR test or positive HIV infection diagnosis, a rapid test should be done.
- If at any time the child has evidence suggesting HIV infection, even if this is <10 weeks of age, the child should be tested for HIV infection (PCR).

Children >18 months of age (HIV rapid / ELISA tests)
- If the first rapid test is positive, confirm the result with a second rapid test using a kit from a different manufacturer (preferably on different blood specimens).

NB.
- HIV rapid tests may be less reliable in children with advanced disease.
- If the rapid test is negative and the clinical findings suggest HIV infection, send blood for HIV ELISA.

Infant regimens

Mother is started on ART early in pregnancy, i.e >4 weeks before delivery
- Give NVP at birth
- Then daily for 6 weeks

Mother is started on ART late during pregnancy, i.e. <4 weeks before delivery, or at delivery
- Give NVP at birth
- Then daily for 12 weeks

Mother has viral load at booking
- Mother has VL <1000:
    - give NVP at birth
    - then daily for 6 weeks
- Mother has VL >1000 and failing 1st line and is initiated on 2nd line:
    - >4 weeks before delivery: give AZT + NVP to the infant for 6 weeks
    - <4 weeks before delivery: give AZT for 6 weeks and NVP to the infant for 12 weeks

Mother is newly diagnosed <72 hours after delivery
- Mother to be initiated on ART
    - give infant NVP immediately
    - then daily for 12 weeks

Mother is newly diagnosed >72 hours after delivery
- Infant is breastfed or breastfeeding stopped <1 week previously:
    - infant AZT + NVP started and mother initiated on ART
- HIV PCR sent and obtain result within 7 days
- If negative HIV PCR, stop AZT
    - give NVP for 12 weeks
    - check PCR at 10 weeks and 18 weeks
- If positive HIV PCR, Initiate infant on ART
    - confirm with a second HIV PCR

Infant not breastfed and has not breastfed in the previous week
- Initiate mother on ART.
- Do HIV PCR and get results within 7 days
    - if negative HIV PCR, check PCR at 10 weeks of age
    - if positive HIV PCR, initiate infant on ART and confirm with a 2nd HIV PCR

JAUNDICE

*Jaundice may be either **physiological** or **pathological**.*

*Most cases of neonatal jaundice are **physiological** and have the following features*

- It appears at 3 days *not* sooner
- It does not exceed 14 mg% (240 umol / L) bilirubin
- It is usually only noticed clinically on the 3rd day or later

Causes

Pathological jaundice

- Rh incompatibility
- ABO incompatibility
- Infections eg.
  - syphilis
  - septicaemia
  - urinary tract infection
  - toxoplasmosis
  - rubella
- Cephalhaematoma
  - the re-absorption of bilirubin from the red blood cells in the haematoma often raises the blood levels enough to present as jaundice
- Hypo-thyroidism (cretinism) may present with jaundice as the only feature

There are many other less common types of jaundice including certain congenital abnormalities of the liver and bile ducts.

Assessment

- Jaundice is best seen by pressing on the tip of nose or upper lip, then checking the colour as the blood flows back.
- Checking of the eyes is *not* accurate because the jaundice only
  - appears there some time after the blood level has increased
  - goes away after the blood level has dropped
- Jaundice of the soles of the feet often means the child needs referral

■ KERNICTERUS

- Pathological and physiological jaundice may result in kernicterus if the bilirubin is allowed to rise to high levels
- This occurs when bilirubin crosses the blood-brain barrier and affects certain parts of the brain resulting in brain damage
- This manifests as a form of cerebral palsy, sometimes associated with mental retardation

Clinical features of kernicterus

- Floppy baby
- Poor feeder
- Convulsions
- Opisthotonus (stiffening posteriorly)
- Later spasticity, chorea, athetosis
- Mental retardation

MANAGEMENT

It is impossible to accurately assess the degree of jaundice clinically.

Clinical jaundice appears later than the rise of blood and brain levels of bilirubin.

Do not take chances.

Indications for REFERRAL

- Any baby with jaundice in the first 2 days of life
- All babies with prolonged jaundice (>14 days)
- All sick babies with jaundice
- **REFER** all babies (of any age) where
  - there is any doubt about the severity
  - the jaundice gets worse or persists

If no facilities are available

If no facilities are available for testing for serum bilirubin, treat conservatively and observe the baby if

- The child is above 2 kg
- The jaundice only appeared on or after the 3rd day
- The baby is clinically completely well and is sucking satisfactorily
- The jaundice appears to be mild
- There is no jaundice of the soles of the feet

Phototherapy

Ultraviolet light (UV) in sunshine or UV lamps make bilirubin water soluble so that it can be excreted.

- In a full term baby aged 3 days or older, phototherapy should be started if the bilirubin is above 14 mg% (240 umol / L)
- In premature babies, or if jaundice starts before the 3rd day, phototherapy (and admission) should be considered at lower levels 5 -10 mg% (85 - 171 umol /L)
- If phototherapy fails, an exchange transfusion may be needed so the baby should be **REFERRED** to hospital
- In situations where phototherapy facilities are not available, **REFER** as above
- In a full term normal weight baby, 3 days or older, exchange transfusion should be considered if bilirubin is 25 mg% (428 umol / L)
- In premature babies, or jaundice before the 3rd day, exchange transfusion should be done if the bilirubin reaches 15 mg% (257 umol / L)

Phototherapy unit protocol

All first visits

Day 3-7
- If serum bilirubin (SB) is *less* than 14 mg% (240 umol / L)
  - check SB the following day
- If SB is *more* than 14 mg% (240 umol / L)
  - start or continue phototherapy

Day 8 and older
- If SB is *below* 14 mg% (240 umol / L)
  - discharge with advice to keep the baby in direct sunlight

Repeat visits

- Use phototherapy for all babies with SB >14 mg% (240 umol / L)
- If SB is 18 mg% (308 umol / L) or more
  - **REFER** for exchange transfusion
- **REFER** all babies with prolonged jaundice

OEDEMA

Causes

- This may be a normal effect of a breech delivery
- It is also common in premature babies
- The above 2 causes resolve spontaneously (disappear on their own)
- There may be a more serious cause

REFER within 1-2 days if
- You suspect a serious cause
- You have any doubt about the cause

HYPOTHERMIA

This is a sign of a seriously ill child.

MANAGEMENT
- Do an immediate blood glucose test and treat according to the results
- **REFER** stat
- Cover with a blanket and apply heat from an electric pad or hot water bottle, taking care not to burn the child
- An easy and effective way of warming is to put the child against the mother's bare skin
    - wrap them both in blankets
    - keep them in a warm room

FLOPPY CHILD

This is a serious problem.

Clinical features
- The child is unable to move properly, or cannot support his / her head
- When picked up the baby will be floppy like a doll, and the limbs will droop

MANAGEMENT
- Check the blood glucose
- Give emergency treatment of oxygen if it is an acute problem just after birth
- **REFER** stat if this has not been investigated before

ABNORMAL BLEEDING FROM ANY SITE

Causes
- The most common cause is haemorrhagic disease of the new born, due to Vitamin K deficiency

MANAGEMENT
- Give 1 amp (1 mg) Vitamin K IMI stat
- **REFER** stat any abnormal bleeding or bruising in the
    - baby's skin
    - umbilicus
    - mouth

BABY OF A DIABETIC MOTHER

Babies of diabetic mothers are usually large (greater than 4 kg) and can be hypoglycaemic.

They have many problems as a result of the mother's diabetes.

Many of these problems can be life-threatening

MANAGEMENT
- Check the blood glucose, and treat accordingly
- Routinely give a feed
    - breast milk is better than dextrose water
- **REFER** within 1-2 days

Indications for routine blood glucose checks
- Child of a diabetic mother
- Preterm infants
- Asphyxia neonatorum
- Small for gestational age (SGA)
- Big baby over 4 kg
- Respiratory distress
- Twitching, tremor or suspected fits
- Hypothermia
- High pitched cry or suspected brain damage
- Floppy child

Management of blood glucose checks

If the blood glucose test is 1,2-2,5 mmol / L
- Give an oral feed of dextrose 10%
    - dilute 4 ml dextrose 50% in 16 ml water for injection
    - give 5 ml/kg eg. a baby weighing 3 kg will get 15 ml of solution

If the blood glucose test is below 1,2 mmol / L)
- Give dextrose 10% 5 ml/kg directly into the vein slowly
- *Repeat blood glucose test every half an hour*
- **REFER**
- Repeat as above if blood glucose remains below 2.5 mg % while waiting for the baby to be transported to the hospital.

BABY OF AN EPILEPTIC MOTHER

These babies should have no special problems.

MANAGEMENT
- Breast feeding should be encouraged as this will help to give the woman confidence that she can be a normal mother
- It will also protect the baby from diseases, and encourage the bonding between the two of them
- If she has frequent fits, or she is worried about her fits affecting the child, advise her to feed sitting or lying down if possible and in the presence of another person
- **REFER** if there are any problems antenatally or postnatally

SMALL FOR GESTATIONAL AGE BABIES (SGA) (OR UNDERWEIGHT FOR GESTATIONAL AGE – UWGA)

This is defined as a birth weight of less than 2,5 kg in a full term baby.

Causes
Maternal causes
- Severe PIH
- Severe hypertension
- Kidney disease
- Tuberculosis
- Severe systemic illness
- Smoking
- Drugs
- Alcohol

Foetal causes
- Twins
- Congenital abnormality
- Congenital infections
    - syphilis
    - toxoplasmosis
    - rubella
    - cytomegalovirus
    - herpes simplex

Associated problems
- *Labour*
    - foetal distress
- *Delivery*
    - birth asphyxia
    - meconium aspiration
- *Post delivery*
    - hypoglycaemia
    - hypothermia
    - infections
    - polycythaemia (from chronic hypoxia)
    - poor intellect, such as foetal alcohol syndrome

MANAGEMENT

Babies weighing less than 2 kg
- **REFER**

Babies weighing 2-2,5 kg

Check the general condition carefully
- If any problem is suspected, **REFER**
- If the child is well, sucks strongly and is active
    - **REFER** to doctor if available to check
    - if doctor not available, keep the child at the clinic for at least 4 hours, and observe
    - perform a blood glucose test with blood from a heel prick
    - give oral glucose if the blood glucose is below 2,5 mmol / L
    - babies that are well can go home, but ensure follow up at home if possible

---

CONGENITAL SYPHILIS

Clinical features
Suspect congenital syphilis if any of the following are present
- "Snuffles" - blocked nose with considerable discharge which may be bloody
    - the nostrils may be rubbed raw (excoriated)
- "Pseudo paresis" - the infant fails to move a limb (usually an arm) due to pain
    - an X-ray will show bone involvement due to syphilis
- Skin rashes
    - peeling or blisters especially of the palms and soles (this is different from the more generalized body peeling seen in dysmature neonates)
    - condylomata lata (moist perianal warts)
    - copper-coloured rash
- Large liver and spleen, with or without jaundice
- Anaemia
- Purpura
- Rhagades in the neonate (cracks around the mouth, especially at the corner of the lips)
- Fits
- Hydrocephalus

- **REFER** within 1-2 days, all suspected cases of congenital syphilis
- See guidelines for RPR-positive mothers page 339

HEAD PROBLEMS

CLEFT PALATE

MANAGEMENT
REFER when convenient to speech and hearing clinic for oral plate
- Assessment of possible surgery
- Assistance with breast feeding if needed
    - consider spoon-feeding expressed breast milk

TONGUE TIE

This condition relieves itself and no treatment is needed.

SUBCONJUNCTIVAL BLEEDING

This is a benign condition.

Clinical features
There is fresh, red bleeding between
- The sclera (white part of the eyeball)
- The conjunctiva

MANAGEMENT
- It can be treated by reassuring the mother that it will clear up in 6-8 weeks
- Any blue bruising or discolouration of the eyelids suggests a more extensive bleed
    - these should be **REFERRED** stat
    - it may be due to a sub-aponeurotic haemorrhage

UNABLE TO SEE

This is a serious problem

It may be noticed at birth, as newborns often show evidence of reacting to visual stimuli. The mother may tell you that something is wrong.

REFER when convenient
- If you or the mother **suspect it**
- Even if you cannot be sure on clinical examination

UNABLE TO HEAR

This is a serious problem

It may be noticed at birth, by the midwife or by the mother. A normal baby often shows evidence of reacting to sound and auditory stimuli.

MANAGEMENT
- **REFER** when convenient
    - if either you or the mother suspect the problem
    - as it needs special tests to be sure
- Any delay in the treatment can seriously affect speech development

DISCHARGE FROM THE EYES

This is potentially a serious problem.
- The pus beneath the eyelid may erode the cornea and cause a perforation
    - blindness may result
- Ideally no child should develop this condition as it is preventable by the routine prophylactic treatment at birth with chloromycetin eye ointment.

Causes
- The most common cause is an infection acquired from the mother's vagina during delivery, often
    - gonococcal
    - chlamydial

See The Eye page 238 for management

DISCHARGE FROM THE EARS

Causes
- It may be due to a suppurative otitis media
- Often it is difficult to be sure of the cause

REFER stat
- If you cannot be sure of the cause
- If you suspect otitis media

DISCHARGE FROM THE NOSE

Causes
- There may be several causes of this
- A viral upper respiratory tract infection is a common cause

MANAGEMENT
Newborn babies are always nose breathers. They cannot breathe through their mouths.
- If the baby is not able to breathe properly at all, a number 0 oral airway must be inserted and strapped in place
    - the baby should then be **REFERRED**

- *If the infection is severe or chronic*, then suspect neonatal syphilis
    - **REFER** within 1-2 days
- If the discharge has been checked and is not due to a serious cause, the mother can be advised to manage the problem in the following way
    - wet the discharge with some normal saline
    - remove the mucus with cotton wool swabs or cotton wool ear buds
    - the safest and most effective method is for the mother to try and suck the mucus out with her own mouth or with a syringe

SWELLING OF THE HEAD

CEPHALHAEMATOMA

Clinical features
- This is confined by suture lines so that the swelling occurs on one side of the head and does not cross the sutures
- Scalp haemorrhages develop from the trauma at birth
- It may take up to six weeks to disappear

MANAGEMENT
- Management is conservative
- Do not aspirate the cephalhaematoma
- Give reassurance to the mother
- However there is an increased chance of jaundice, so the child should be
    - carefully observed for this
    - **REFERRED** if it occurs

CAPUT SUCCEDANEUM

Clinical features
- This is swelling of the head due to oedema which crosses the sutures
- It usually subsides within 48 hours without treatment

SUB-APONEUROTIC HAEMORRHAGE

Causes
- It is usually due to haemorrhagic disease of the newborn
- It may also result from a difficult delivery by forceps or vacuum

Clinical features
- There is a boggy (spongy) swelling of the scalp extending **across** the sutures
- There may also be a blue discolouration of the upper eyelids, behind the ears or neck

These babies should be **REFERRED** stat.

CHEST PROBLEMS

COUGH

Any cough in a neonate implies that the child has pneumonia, even if there are no other symptoms or signs.

NB. Babies that are given water feeds or supplementary feeds, especially from a bottle, are more susceptible to chest infections.

MANAGEMENT
- Warn the mother of the danger of using bottle feeds or giving water
- For management see the Respiratory System (see pages 63-64)

BIRTH ASPHYXIA

Asphyxia is a state where there is a lack of oxygen circulating to the brain.

Causes
- Prenatal maternal hypoxic conditions
    - pneumonia
    - severe heart failure
    - eclamptic fit
- Placental insufficiency
    - severe PIH in the mother
    - placenta partially separated
    - long and severe labour which causes reduced placental blood flow with each contraction
- Severe Rh incompatibility

Foetal causes
- Severe foetal anaemia (eg. as in severe Rh incompatibility)
- Cord accidents
    - knotting of the cord
    - pressure on the cord
    - prolapsed cord
    - cord around the neck

Clinical features

The following are the clinical warning signs of birth asphyxia

In labour
- An irregular foetal heart
- Foetal bradycardia below 110 / min or tachycardia above 165 / min
- Delay in recovery of the foetal heart rate after each contraction
- Thick green meconium-stained liquor

At delivery
- An Apgar score less than 6 at 5 minutes
- Failure of the baby to start breathing on its own after
    - clearing the airways
    - moderate stimulation

THE APGAR SCORE

	SCORE 0	SCORE 1	SCORE 2
HEART RATE	Absent	Below 100/min	Above 100/min
RESPIRATORY RATE	Absent	Weak	Good crying
MUSCLE TONE	Flaccid	Some flexion of extremities	Well flexed
REFLEX IRRITABILITY	No response	Grimace	Cough or sneeze
COLOUR	Pale blue	Body pink extremities blue	Completely pink

MANAGEMENT

What to do if the newborn baby does not start breathing immediately.

Evaluation of the infant

- Ask yourself these questions:
  - is the baby breathing adequately (not just gasping)?
  - is the baby's heart rate above 100 beats per minute?
  - is the baby centrally pink?
- If the answer to all these questions is "yes", the baby does not need resuscitation.
- The baby is reassessed in this way every 30 seconds during the resuscitation.
- If the baby is improving, then the intervention, eg. bagging, can be stopped.
- If the baby is not responding or getting worse, then further intervention is needed (eg. start chest compression).

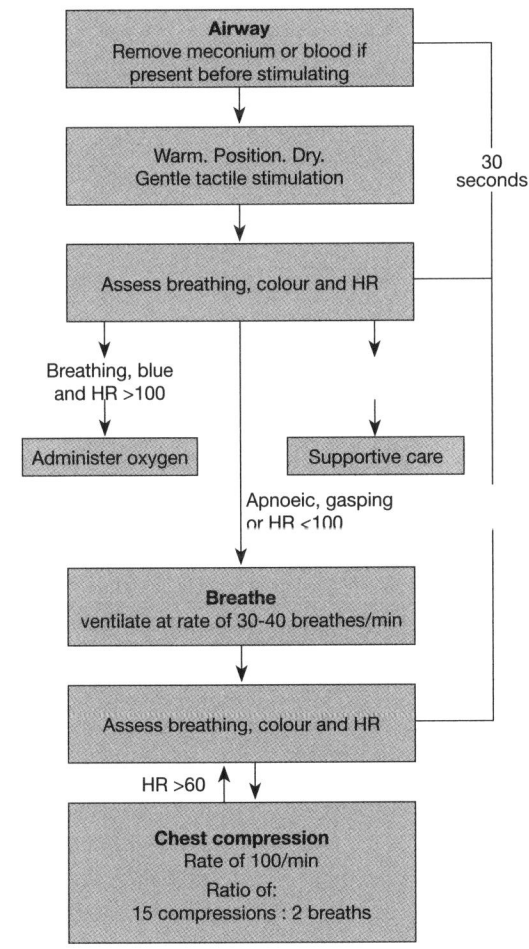

How to do external cardiac massage on a baby

- Put the baby on a firm surface
- Compress the sternum gently to a depth of about 2 cm using the index and middle finger, placed 1 finger breadth below the inter-nipple line
- The rate should be 100-120 per minute
- Excessive force may cause damage to the liver or break the ribs or sternum
- Be careful not to use unnecessary force because you are anxious
- This must be combined with effective ventilation of the baby's lungs
- Give 15 cardiac compressions to every 2 respirations

How to do artificial respiration on a baby

Mouth to mouth resuscitation
- This is quite effective
- Care must be taken about infections from the health worker to the baby (or from the baby to the health worker)
- Use a mask or mouth piece, or plastic protective airway if available
- Close either the nose or mouth and blow into the other at 40 breaths per minute
  - use only the air in your mouth and cheeks to avoid over-distending the neonate's lungs

A bag and mask
- This is effective if used properly
- It is vital to hold the mask firmly over the baby's face so that air does not escape
- Place the hand over the mask with the index and middle finger hooked under the jaw (a good method)
- Check if the chest is moving well while pumping
- Sometimes you must try various positions before good ventilation is achieved
- The rate of pumping should be 30-40 per minute
  - pumping too quickly is harmful and limits air entry
- If oxygen is available, attach it to the mask
  - eg. Laerdal and Ambu masks

Nasal catheter
- This is a useful and effective method
- Place a small nasal catheter (about 5 cm) into one nostril
- Connect it to an oxygen supply which has a safety valve
  - eg. a water manometer to prevent excessive pressure
- If no valve is available, be careful not to use high pressures which may burst the lungs
- Close the baby's mouth and then pinch the nose 30-40 times per minute
- Check that there is effective respiration by observing the chest movement

Endotracheal intubation
- This is the most effective method if you have the necessary knowledge
- The easiest tube to use is the one with a shoulder (Cole type)
  - for a baby of less than 1500 g, use a 2,5 mm tube
  - for a baby 1500-2500 g, use a 3 mm tube
- One way to assess the size is to use a tube which is the same diameter as the baby's small finger
- When intubating, it is easier if the head is not extended too much
- Put the baby on a firm surface with the head tilted down slightly
- Use a neonatal straight-bladed laryngoscope
- Place the tip at the back of the tongue
  - if the blade is correctly placed, the epiglottis and opening into the larynx can be seen

- Slight pressure over the front of the neck makes the larynx easier to see
- Once the tube has been inserted it is *vital* that the lungs are checked to hear if there is air entry into both the left and right lungs
- It is easy to push the tube too far so that it ends up in the right main bronchus
    - this can be checked by listening with a stethoscope over both sides of the chest
    - listening over the stomach will also reveal if the tube is in the oesophagus as bubbles of air will be heard
- Do not let the baby deteriorate if intubation is difficult
    - give oxygen by mask in between attempts at intubation
- If the stomach begins to blow up as a result of the artificial respiration, it may obstruct movement of the diaphragm
    - this can be relieved by passing a narrow catheter into the stomach and aspirating the air
    - leave it open while continuing artificial respiration

IV infusion

- *Two people begin and continue with cardiac massage and respiration*
- *A third person puts up the drip on the baby's limb*
    - the hand is easiest
    - the umbilicus often results in infection
    - only use the scalp or umbilicus if you cannot manage anywhere else
- Use a Jelco / Abbocath number 24 (yellow) as this is the easiest
- If this is unavailable, use a number 22 (blue) or a scalp vein needle
- Use a drip set Buretrol with a 60 drops / ml micro dropper
- Drip rate
    - 3 kg baby at 7 ml per hour ie. 7 micro drops per minute
    - 2 kg baby at 5 micro drops per minute
    - 1 kg baby at 3 micro drops per minute

Note. Newborns need only 60 ml of fluid / kg / 24 hours.

Medicine management

- Epinephrine 1:1,000. This can be given IV only if the heart rate remains below 60 beats per minute despite the above treatment
    - dilute 1 ml of epinephrine 1:1000 in 9 ml of sterile water
    - give 0,1 ml per kg slowly IVI or via ET tube
    - eg. a 3 kg child will need 0,3 ml

NB. Epinephrine should **not** be given by the intra-cardiac route

- *Use 10% dextrose water*
    - dilute 2 ml dextrose 50% in 8 ml sterile water
    - give 2 ml / kg body weight IVI slowly
    - eg. a 3 kg baby will need 6 ml of the dextrose solution.
- Give sodium bicarbonate (8,5%) at 1 cc / kg body weight diluted in an equal amount of water, very slowly IVI
- If mother has had pethidine, give neonatal Narcan 0,02 mg / ml
    - ie. 2ml IVI
    - 1 ml for a premature baby

NB. *Do not over-hydrate the baby by leaving the drip running too fast!*

- When the baby is stable, make a drip of Non-Potassium Cocktail or give Neonatolyte

- 5 % dextrose water	200 ml
- 50 % dextrose water	20 ml
- 10 % calcium gluconate	2,6 ml
- 20 % sodium chloride	2 ml
- 50 % magnesium sulphate	0,3 ml

NB. Any solution containing potassium, (eg. ½ strength Darrows) should be avoided in the newborn less than one week old. The immature kidney fails to excrete loads of potassium and water adequately.

Outcome of resuscitation

- Usually the baby begins to breathe regularly and can then be nursed in a warm incubator or a crib in a warm room
- Keep the child in a head box with oxygen until the baby stabilises and remains pink
- **REFER** the baby if you suspect any other problems (see following pages)
- Failure of spontaneous respiration, even after resuscitation for more than one hour, may mean that
    - the baby was badly asphyxiated
    - very little is likely to be gained by continuing resuscitation longer
- Fortunately there are more successes than failures. Babies appear to be more resistant to asphyxia, and may be normal mentally even after severe neonatal asphyxia
- If the baby dies, it helps the grieving process to allow the parents to see and hold the dead child
- Often a priest or a professional counsellor are the best people to assist the parents with the loss of the child

RESPIRATORY DISTRESS SYNDROME (RDS)

Clinical features

- Respiratory rate of above 60 per minute
- Recession
- Grunting
- If severe, the child may be cyanosed
- There may be difficulty with feeding

REFER any baby with any of the RDS symptoms, with oxygen if available.

HYALINE MEMBRANE DISEASE

This is a disease of preterm babies usually below 33 weeks.

Causes

- The preterm infant lacks mature surfactant (a substance which reduces surface tension in the lungs and helps breathing)
- This means that with each breath the baby takes inspiratory effort is increased
- The second problem is that the preterm baby has leaky tissue surfaces
- As a result, there is leakage of protein substances from the capillaries into the alveoli
- This causes a thick lining, called the hyaline membrane, which prevents exchange of oxygen and carbon dioxide in the lungs

MANAGEMENT
- **REFER** to hospital
- Keep the baby warm while transporting
- Give 3 cc of 50% dextrose water by naso-gastric tube
- Give oxygen by a head box if the baby is breathing regularly
- If not breathing regularly, pump regularly, with the Laerdal neonatal resuscitator, while waiting for transfer

MECONIUM ASPIRATION

When a foetus is distressed during labour, the anal sphincters can relax and meconium passes into the amniotic fluid. The foetus may swallow this meconium-stained liquor or hold it in the mouth.

If there is inadequate suctioning when the head is delivered, the meconium may be inhaled which results in the following.

Chemical pneumonitis
- This is due to chemical burning of the alveoli by bile acids and salts
- This causes the alveoli to become inflamed which harms the gas exchange

Persistent foetal circulation
- This is due to increased lung pressure forcing blood from the right to left sides of the heart
- The blood bypasses the lungs and this results in cyanosis

Obstruction of small bronchioles
- Particles of meconium obstruct the bronchioles
- This can reduce the number of alveoli for gas exchange (if extensive)
- It can also trap air in the alveoli
    - over-inflated alveoli may burst and cause a fatal spontaneous pneumothorax

MANAGEMENT
NB. 20% of babies with meconium aspiration die
- Suction the mouth, then the nose, **before** you deliver the shoulders
    - keep the head down while doing this
    - this encourages the meconium to drain out
- Delay resuscitation until as much meconium as possible is cleared from the airway
- After delivery, suction the mouth and the back of the throat gently
    - do not do repeated suctioning as this may delay respiration
- If some one present has any experience in tracheal intubation, then the trachea should be cleared of any meconium before air is blown into the lungs
    - this is done by suctioning under vision from the laryngoscope
- If the baby is not breathing spontaneously, bagging with oxygen should begin after clearing the airways,
- If the baby is tachypnoeic (a respiratory rate greater than 60 per minute), fluids should not be given orally unless dextrose is needed for hypoglycaemia
- Give oxygen via a funnel / mask
- **REFER** stat
- If the meconium is thin and the baby is well, there is no need for **REFERRAL**

PNEUMONIA

A baby can be born with infection of the lungs in addition to other organs.

Conditions where infection should be suspected in the foetus include the following

Prolonged rupture of membranes (PROM)
- This means a rupture of amniotic membranes of over 24 hours before the baby is born

Offensiveness
- Babies with an unpleasant smell of the skin, or liquor

Maternal amnionitis
- A mother with tachycardia, pyrexia and a tender uterus is almost certainly infected
- She may or may not have an offensive vaginal discharge
- Both mother and baby need treatment

REFER stat.

TRANSIENT TACHYPNOEA IN THE NEWBORN

- Some babies become slightly breathless shortly after birth
- This results from residual amniotic fluid in the lungs which was not squeezed out during delivery
- The lymphatic system slowly absorbs this fluid in about 8 hours and then the baby breathes more easily

REFERRAL for frequent observation of the baby is all that is required.

SWOLLEN BREASTS

- Some babies have enlarged, lactating breasts
- This is normal and is due to the effect of the maternal hormones

> - Reassure the mother
> - Discourage her from squeezing the baby's breasts

ABDOMEN PROBLEMS

VOMITING

The most common cause is irritation due to liquor still in the stomach.

> **MANAGEMENT**
> - Feed the baby with breast milk or dextrose water
> - If there is vomiting a second time
>   - do a gastric washout via a naso-gastric tube with warm normal saline until the fluid drawn back is clear
> - If the vomiting persists
>   - repeat the gastric washout
>   - **REFER** stat
> - *Any baby with bile-stained vomitus **must** be **REFERRED** stat as there is an intestinal obstruction*

SEPSIS OF THE UMBILICAL CORD

Clinical features
- Any baby with redness or inflammation extending from the umbilicus on to the surrounding abdominal wall implies a spreading cellulitis
- **This can be rapidly fatal**

> **REFER** stat.

UMBILICAL GRANULOMA

Clinical features
- This is when the umbilicus does not heal well
- It leaves a chronic, red, granulomatous ulcer

> - Cauterize with a silver nitrate stick.
> - Protect normal skin (eg. wih Vaseline)

OMPHALOCELE IN NEONATES

This is a large hernia through the abdominal wall.

> - Pass a NG tube and allow free drainage
> - Cover omphalocele with gauze, wet with saline
> - **REFER**

VAGINAL BLEEDING

New born girls may have a blood-stained vaginal discharge due to the effect of the maternal hormones.

> Explain to the mother that
> - This is normal
> - The bleeding will stop in a day or two

INGUINAL AND SCROTAL SWELLINGS

This is a serious problem.
Important causes include an inguinal hernia.

> **REFER** within 1-2 days.

DIFFICULTY PASSING URINE

Common causes include a minor phimosis due to the trauma of nappies.

MANAGEMENT

If the baby is managing to pass urine with some ballooning of the foreskin, but with a reasonable flow, it can be treated as follows

- Advise to keep nappies off as much as possible
- Avoid strong soaps and fabric softeners as these tend to irritate the foreskin
- Using the metal nozzle of the tube, apply chloramphenicol eye ointment 3 x daily into the foreskin
- Do *not* try to retract the foreskin as this causes bleeding and possible permanent scarring of the foreskin with attachments to the glans
    - this may need surgical excision

*If the obstruction is more serious, or if the baby is having difficulty passing urine, **REFER** within 1-2 days.*

BOWEL ATRESIA

Clinical features

- This usually presents as bile-stained vomiting
- There may be signs of intestinal obstruction

REFER stat.

IMPERFORATE ANUS

REFER stat.

LIMB PROBLEMS

CLUB FEET

REFER when convenient.

EXTRA DIGITS

MANAGEMENT

- If the extra digit is only attached to the main finger by a narrow stalk, it can be tied with nylon or silk at the base
    - it will then drop off on its own

- If the stalk is thick, or has definite structures in it such as muscle or bone
    - **REFER** when convenient for surgical removal

LIMB PARALYSIS

Clinical features

- The baby will not be able to move that arm
- Erb's and Klumpke's palsy are common in difficult deliveries such as impacted shoulder
- Usually the whole arm will be paralysed in a brachial plexus injury
- Check that it is not a pseudo paralysis due to syphilis

REFER when convenient for
- Appropriate management
- Physiotherapy

FRACTURES

- These can be sustained during a difficult delivery such as impacted shoulders or a difficult extended breech
- Common fractures are those of the *clavicle, humerus and femur* (in that order)
- Suspect a fracture when there is a painful limb

REFER within 1-2 days.

CONGENITAL HIP DISLOCATION

- This is an important condition to look for in *all* new borns and at the 6 week postnatal check because with early treatment, good results are obtained.
- Late diagnosis and treatment may result in permanent disability

Clinical features

- A fairly reliable test is to place the fingers of each hand over the greater trochanter of each femur
- Now flex the hips and rotate them outwards
- If a click is felt over either of the hips, it suggests that the hip is dislocating

If you suspect a dislocation **REFER** when convenient.

TROPICAL DISEASES

MALARIA

Cause
Parasites of the genus Plasmodium that are transmitted from an infected person to a healthy person by the bite of an Anopheles mosquito.
- There are 4 species of *Plasmodium*
    - *P. falciparum*
    - *P. vivax*
    - *P. ovale*
    - *P. malariae* (rare)
- In southern Africa *P. falciparum* is the common variety. It is the most dangerous form because of the high frequency of severe and fatal complications
- *P. vivax* occurs in low prevalence and is confined to a few areas only

Clinical features
- History of exposure in a malaria endemic area
- Incubation period for *P. falciparum* is an average of 10-21 days
- Incubation periods of up to 12 months can occur with any of the other forms
- Headache
- Tiredness
- Muscle and joint pains
- Fever
    - suspect malaria in any patient with pyrexia of unknown origin in a malaria endemic area, or in a traveller who has just returned from a malaria area
    - the temperature may be present on alternate days in some cases. It is, however, often constant in early *falciparum* malaria
    - fever may be absent in some patients living in endemic areas
- Sweating
- Shivering attacks
- Gastrointestinal symptoms (nausea, loss of appetite, abdominal pain, vomiting, diarrhoea)
- Dry cough
- Splenic enlargement
    - common in endemic areas where people are subjected to repeated episodes of malaria
    - less common in South Africans who travel to a malaria area and get a first episode of malaria
- Liver pain with liver enlargement

Complications of *falciparum* malaria
- Cerebral malaria (headache, drowsiness, convulsions, delirium, coma)
- Hyperpyrexia
- Severe haemolytic anaemia
- Pulmonary oedema (not of cardiac origin)
- Acute kidney failure with production of dark urine (blackwater fever)
- Acute hepatitis with jaundice
- Hypoglycaemia
- Circulatory collapse and shock
- Diarrhoea and dysentery

Diagnosis
- By microscopy of a thick blood smear that has been stained with Giemsa stain
- By rapid test, if available eg. a plasma reagent dipstix
    - test any person resident in or returning from a malaria area **and** who presents with fever usually within 3 months of exposure
- In areas where there is predominantly one type of malaria present, eg. *P. falciparum* in southern Africa, a clinical diagnosis of *P. falciparum* may be made, when blood microscopy is not available
- In areas where both *falciparum* and another type (usually *vivax*) are present, a microscopic diagnosis is essential as the management differs for the different types
- A slide may be taken and treatment for *P. falciparum* started immediately if there is likely to be a delay in obtaining results
    - eg. if a blood slide has to be sent in from a rural area with delayed transport to the nearest microscopist
    - once the microscopic results are obtained the patient can be retreated if indicated

MANAGEMENT
MALARIA PREVENTION (self-provided care)
Malaria can be prevented by
- Preventing mosquitoes from biting people
- Taking medication to prevent the disease developing if a person is bitten by a malaria-carrying mosquito

General measures
- Advice for people living in malaria endemic areas, or who intend travelling to a malaria area eg.
    - Mpumalanga
    - northern KwaZulu-Natal
    - Limpopo
    - Mozambique
    - Zimbabwe
- Only visit malaria areas during the dry season if possible
- People for whom malaria attacks may be very dangerous, should preferably **not** visit malaria areas
    - pregnant woman
    - children under 5 years
    - elderly people
    - immuno-compromised people eg. HIV disease
    - people taking steroids for any disease eg. severe asthma, collagen diseases or rheumatoid arthritis
- Wear long-sleeved shirts and long trousers between dusk and dawn in malaria areas
- Apply mosquito repellent sparingly on exposed skin
    - use Peaceful Sleep, Tabard, Mylol
    - apply to the hands, ankles and face
    - if you are wearing a short-sleeved shirt, apply to the back of elbows and forearms

- do not get repellent into eyes or mouth
- do not apply repellent to hands of small children as they may then touch their mouths
- do not use for long periods in small children
- avoid the use of repellent in children under 6 months of age - the DEET can get absorbed and give dose-related cerebral problems
- Sleep under a mosquito net preferably impregnated with repellant
  - make sure that the net is tucked underneath the mattress so that there aare no gaps through which mosquitoes can enter
  - remember that a mosquito can bite through a mosquito net if any part of your body is in contact with the net
  - apply permethrin, deltamethrin or Peripel 55R insect repellent to the net if not already impregnated in the net
- Soak the mosquito nets in one of the above solutions using 1 sachet to 0,5 litres for nylon nets and 1 sachet to 2 litres for cotton nets
  - soak for 2 minutes, then wring out
  - wear gloves if possible while wringing out
  - leave in shade to dry then hang up
  - repeat every 6 weeks
  - these substances are poisinous if ingested
- Use mosquito coils at night
- Stay indoors at night wherever possible
- Seal windows with screens
  - if not available, windows should be kept closed at night
- Spray rooms, especially bedrooms, with an aerosol insecticide at dusk after closing the windows

Medicine preventative measures

- There is no 100% effective chemo-prophylaxis and therefore the non-drug measures above should be used as well.
- Drug preventative measures are n ot necessary if they will be visiting highly developed towns of cities eg. in Asia, and the traveller is unlikely to leave buildings at night.
- For visits to cities in Central Africa, however, chemo-prophylaxis should be used.
- During the drier months (June to September) the risk of contracting malaria is low and measures to prevent mosquito bites should provide sufficient protection in all the malaria areas in South Africa.
- There are certain parts of the world where malaria parasites are no longer sensitive to chloroquine
  - in these areas, chloroquine no longer can be used alone to prevent malaria.
- The medication to be used to prevent malaria depends on whether a person is visiting a chloroquine-sensitive or chloroquine-resistant area.
- All areas in Southern Africa are now regarded as chloroquine-resistant areas.

The following is the currently recommended chemoprophylaxis

Dosage schedule

Adult dose	Start before entering area	Maintenance	Stop after leaving area
mefloquine 250 mg	1 week	weekly	4 weeks
doxycycline 250 mg	1 day	daily	4 weeks
In children			
mefloquine • Not recommended for children less than 5 kg 5-19 kg 62,5 mg 20-30 kg 125 mg 31-45 kg 187,5 mg Over 45 kg 250 mg			
doxycycline • Not recommended for children under 8 years. • Children over 8 years – 2 mg / kg daily.			

Note.
- Doxycycline can cause gastrointestinal intolerance. It should therefore be taken with a meal or swallowed with a full glass of water.
- It is not recommended to use doxycycline for more than 4 months.
- State facilities do not provide prophylactic treatment.
- It is recommended that people intending to travel to high-risk areas take the relevant prophylactic therapy.

Special cases
- The standard prophylactic medications have interactions with various other medications that patients may be taking chronically
- Contraindicationss exist for the prophylactic medications in certain diseases or special conditions

The combinations below should be avoided:

Condition	Do not use
Acne patients on minocycline	minocycline - use doxycycline
Breastfeeding	doxycycline
Heart disease	mefloquine
Epilepsy	mefloquine
Severe hepatic or renal impairment	mefloquine
Immuno-compromised patients	do not visit malaria areas because of increased risk of severe malaria
Porphyria	doxycycline
Pregnancy	doxycycline, mefloquine (in first trimester)
Neuropsychiatric disease eg. depression of psychosis	mefloquine
Where fine motor coordination needed eg. divers, pilots	mefloquine
Children under 5 kg	mefloquine
Children under 8 years	doxycycline

Medication	Do not use
Antacids	doxycline
Chloroquine for other diseases eg. rheumatoid athritis	mefloquine

Iron	doxycycline
Oral contraceptives	doxycycline
Warfarin	mefloquine
Quinolones eg ciprofloxacin	mefloquine
Cardioactive drugs eg beta-blockers calcium anagonists digoxin	mefloquine

MALARIA MANAGEMENT

Most patients who live in endemic areas, and have malaria that has been diagnosed early in the course of the disease, can be satisfactorily treated as outpatients.
In other areas patients should be referred for treatment

Features indicating severe or complicated malaria
- Severe generalised weakness
- Impaired consciousness, convulsions
- Hypoglycaemia (blood glucose less than 4 mmol / L)
- Repeated vomiting
- Reduced urine output and raised serum creatinine
- Respiratory distress and/or cyanosis
- Severe anaemia
- Jaundice
- Shock
- Acidosis
- Haemoglobinuria/black urine

Medicine management
Falciparum malaria
Ideally treatment in a non-endemic area should be started in hospital.

Uncomplicated *falciparum* malaria
- If unsure of the species, treat as for *P. falciparum* malaria
- Give artemether-lumefantrine (Coartem) 20/120 mg.
- Administer with fat-containing food / full cream milk to improve absorption.

Adults and children over 12 years
4 tabs orally stat and repeat after 8 hours; then 2 x daily for 2 days.

Children
- 8-12 years: 3 tabs orally stat and repeat after 8 hours; then 2 x daily for 2 days.
- 3-8 years: 2 tabs orally stat and repeat after 8 hours; then 2 x daily for 2 days.
- 1-3 years: 1 tab orally stat and repeat after 8 hours; then 2 x daily for 2 days.

REFER URGENTLY:
- Patients not responding to oral treatment within 48 hours

After first dose of artemether/lumefantrine:
- All patients with any signs of severe malaria
- All children less than 2 years of age
- Pregnant women
- Patients with co-morbidities such as HIV, diabetes, etc.
- Patients >65 years of age

Suspected or confirmed severe malaria
- Do an HGT or similar blood test.
- Put up a 5% dextrose drip.
- If blood glucose is low (< 2.5 mmol / L), give IV bolus of 10% dextrose water 5 ml / kg rapidly.

Adults
Quinine 20 mg / kg mixed in 500 ml 5% dextrose water **over 4 hours**, starting immediately, and **REFER** urgently.
- Rapid administration can cause cardiotoxicity and is **dangerous** and should be avoided
- Monitor blood glucose levels frequently
- A repeat IVI infusion of 10 mg quinine salt / kg diluted in dextrose may be run in 8 hours after the start of the loading dose if transport to hospital is delayed.

Children
- Quinine 15-20 mg / kg diluted in 5-10 ml / kg of 5% dextrose water **over 4 hours**, starting immediately
- Quinine can be given IM 15-20 mg/kg
    - dilute dose in normal saline to between 60-100 mg/ml
    - inject half the volume immediately as a single dose in each antero-lateral thigh

REFERAL
Urgent: All patients

Vivax malaria

Adults
- Chloroquine 1,5 g over 3 days
    - 4 tabs stat on day 1 (600 mg)
    - then 2 tabs 6 hours later (300 mg)
    - day 2, give 2 tabs (300 mg)
    - day 3, give 2 tabs (300 mg)
- Followed by primaquine 15 mg base / day (2 tabs) x 14 days

Children
- Chloroquine 10 mg / kg initially
    - then 5 mg / kg taken 6, 24 and 48 hours after the first dose
- Followed by primaquine 0,25 mg / kg daily x 14 days
- In children under 2 years, only use chloroquine, no primaquine

Note.
- Do not use primaquine in patients with a history of or proven G6PD deficiency
- Once treatment has started, repeat blood slides should be performed every 2 days until they are negative

Malaria in pregnancy
- Pregnant patients should preferably be managed as inpatients in hospital
- Pregnant women in endemic areas who have had malaria previously, may not manifest all the classical signs of malaria (eg. fever) and may therefore have a delayed diagnosis
    - they may develop anaemia
    - this may be very dangerous during delivery
    - any pregnant anaemic woman in an endemic area should be regularly screened for malaria
- The following medications are contra-indicated during pregnancy
    - doxycycline
    - Fansidar
    - primaquine
- Pregnant women are particularly susceptable to quinine-induced hyper-insulinaemia and hypoglycaemia
    - a 5% dextrose drip should therefore be put up if the first dose of treatment is given at the clinic
- **REFER** urgently for admission to hospital

MENTAL HEALTH

MENTAL HEALTH

When a patient presents with abnormal behaviour or when mental illness is suspected, it helps with diagnostic decisions to try to classify the type of mental illness. This will help to make as clear a diagnosis as possible.

Note: In children mental illnesses are quite common, especially with the effects of HIV, violence, migration and poverty. The history and examination in children is similar to that for adults as set out below. However, both the examination and the diagnosis may be more difficult.

If mental illness is suspected in a child, it is safer to refer the child for more specialist assessment. This may be to a psychiatric sister or a psychiatrist.

There are four major groups of mental illness. Assessing which one the patient falls under makes decisions about management much easier.

The four major groups

- **Mental disorder due to a physical illness**
    - it may present acutely, is then called delirium and is due to illnesses such as malaria, meningitis and brain tumours
    - it may develop more slowly and progressively, and is then called a dementia, such as Alzheimer's dementia.

- **Psychoses** either:
  Acute such as
    - acute toxic psychosis
    - an acute psychotic episode in someone with schizophrenia
    - a manic episode in someone with bipolar mood disorder
  Chronic (Schizophrenia)

- **Mood and anxiety disorders** such as depression, bipolar mood disorder, acute stress disorder, post- traumatic stress syndrome, panic attacks, adjustment disorder with depressed mood, conversion phenomenon (hysteria).

- **Substance misuse such as:**
    - substance use disorder, substance-induced mood disorder, substance-induced psychosis, alcohol withdrawal.

Checklist for diagnosis:
- **D** – Drugs (Intoxication and withdrawal) e.g. Wernicke's encephalopathy
- **I** – Infections e.g. pneumonia, sepsis, peritonitis, meningitis
- **M** – Metabolic e.g. hypoglycaemia, liver failure, kidney failure
- **T** – Trauma e.g. chronic subdural haematoma
- **O** – Oxygen deficit (including hypoxia, carbon monoxide poisoning)
- **P** – Pre-existing neurological disease e.g. epilepsy, dementia

Clinical features

Clinical features suggesting delirium/dementia are found in the normal general and neurological examinations.

On general history and examination
- There may be symptoms of the illness.
- Fever, headache, vomiting are important symptoms
- Vital signs may show abnormalities, such as raised temperature, pulse and respiratory rate.
- Restlessness and agitation
- Hallucinations
- Autonomic symptoms such as sweating, tachycardia and flushing
- patients may be hypo-active with reduced responsiveness to the environment

On neurological examination there may be:
- **Changes in the level of consciousness**
- Changes in the orientation to time and place.
- Changes in the ability to do calculations
- Changes in recent memory e.g. not being able to remember five objects forward
- Cranial nerve abnormalities e.g. double vision, ophthalmoplegia (eye muscle paralysis)
- Changes in cerebellar function e.g. tremor, ataxia.
- Loss of sensation or power in a limb

> **MANAGEMENT**
> - **REFER** for medical assessment
> - For agitated and acutely disturbed patients - see below (Aggressive Disruptive Behaviour in Adults)

MENTAL DISORDER DUE TO A PHYSICAL ILLNESS

This should be the first cause to look for in a patient who presents with abnormal behaviour.

Causes
Delirium is a sudden onset state of confusion in which there is impaired awareness and memory and disorientation.
There are many possible causes including extracranial causes

AGGRESSIVE DISRUPTIVE BEHAVIOUR IN ADULTS

Aggressive behaviour includes verbally abusive language specific verbal threats, intimidating physical behaviour and/or actual physical violence to self, others or property.

Causes

Physical

- Acute medical illness, delirium and its causes, epilepsy,

intracerebral lesions, traumatic brain injury.
Psychiatric
- Psychosis, mania, agitated depression, developmental disorders (e.g. intellectual disability and autism), severe anxiety.

Substance misuse
- Alcohol, cannabis, drug intoxication or withdrawal

Psychological factors
- High levels of impulsivity and antagonism, hypersensitivity to rejection or insult, poor frustration tolerance and maladaptive coping skills all contribute to aggression and rage.

MANAGEMENT

General measures
- Be prepared
  - Be aware of high risk patients e.g. those known with previous violence, substance misuse, state patients.
- De-escalate and contain
  - Be calm, confident, kind and reassuring
  - Maintain a submissive posture with open hands; do NOT turn your back
  - Do NOT argue, confront delusions or attempt to touch the patient
- Be vigilant for delirium, medical and other causes while calming the patient.

Medicine treatment
Oral treatment:
- Diazepam, oral, 5 mg immediately
- **or** midazolam, buccal, 7.5-15 mg immediately, using the parental formulation.

If alcohol use is suspected

ADD
- Thiamine, oral, 300 mg immediately and daily for 14 days

If oral treatment fails after 30-60 minutes,

OR

If the patient refuses oral sedation:

IM treatment
- Midazolam, IM, 7.5-15 mg immediately.
  - repeat after 30-60 minutes if needed

OR
- Haloperidol, IM, 5 mg, immediately
  - repeat after 30-60 minutes if needed

AND
- Promethazine, IM, 25-50 mg (25 mg in the elderly)

NB Always monitor vital signs of a sedated patient

Monitor particularly for respiratory depression

REFERRAL
- Urgent: All cases

PSYCHOSES

ACUTE PSYCHOSIS

Characterised by recent onset of psychotic symptoms such as hallucinations, delusions, disorganised or illogical speech, agitation or bizarre behaviour and extreme and labile emotional states.

These symptoms may be preceded by a period of deteriorating social, occupational and academic functioning.

Clinical features
The history from the relative is very important as the patient may deny any abnormalities.

Features suggesting a psychosis are:
- Abnormal speech is often a valuable first sign. A psychosis affects the normal cerebral function:
  - the person cannot think logically so speech is characteristically illogical or disorganised
  - the speech may jump from topic to topic with no sensible connection, called "word salad"
- Delusions - fixed, unshakable false beliefs, which are often bizarre:
  - believing that someone is interfering with their thoughts
  - people want to poison them
  - someone is beaming electrical waves into their brain from "overhead cables" or "outer space"
  - feelings of being controlled by some outside force may occur
  - there may be paranoia; believing someone is trying to deliberately hurt them
- Hallucinations - perceptions without adequate corresponding external stimuli e.g:
  - hearing voices (may be threatening or controlling)
  - visual perceptions - e.g. seeing pink elephants
  - tactile - feeling insects crawling on the skin; this is often due to alcohol or drug abuse
- Taste and smell abnormalities may be due to epilepsy, especially temporal lobe causes.
- The person's behaviour or dress may be grossly inappropriate.

MANAGEMENT

General measures
- Ensure the safety of the patient and health care workers
- Minimise stress and stimulation (do not argue with psychotic thinking).
- Avoid confrontation or criticism, unless it is necessary to prevent harmful of disruptive behaviour.

Medicine treatment
- See above: Aggressive disruptive behaviour in adults (general measures and medicine treatment)

OR

- If known to have schizophrenia, and has used antipsychotics previously and is non-aggressive:
  - give zuclopenthixol acetate, IM, 50 mg immediately

REFERRAL
All patients

CHRONIC PSYCHOSIS

SCHIZOPHRENIA

This is a mental disorder, characterised by a disintegration of thought processes and emotional responsiveness.

Clinical features

Two or more of the following positive or negative symptoms, each present for much of the time during a 1-month period:

Positive symptoms
- Hallucinations, mainly auditory
- Delusions
- Disorganised or illogical speech, which is a manifestation of a thought process disorder
- Grossly disorganised behaviour or catatonic behaviour (person stays stuck in one position).

Negative symptoms
- Being quiet, withdrawn, non-emotional (blunted affect)
- Lack of wanting to do anything (avolition)
- Lack of wanting to speak (alogia)
- Social and/or occupational dysfunction

Making a diagnosis
- The diagnosis of schizophrenia should be confirmed by a psychiatrist

Note:
Very rare for schizophrenia to present for the first time in patients over 40 years of age.

MANAGEMENT

General measures

NB. Consultation with a community psychiatrist is essential to confirm the diagnosis and to initiate treatment.

Effective psychotherapy includes:
- Family therapy
- Rehabilitation may be improved by:
  - assertive community programmes
  - supported employment

Medicine treatment
- Specialist initiated.
- Review patients every six months by a psychiatrist.

First episode
- Haloperidol, oral, 1 mg daily, increasing to 5 mg daily
- Once stabilised, administer as a single dose at bedtime.

The elderly
- Initial dose 0.5 mg 2 x daily
- Increase the dose more gradually until symptoms are controlled or until a maximum dose of 5 mg is reached.
- Once stabilised, administer as a single dose at bedtime.

If extrapyramidal side-effects occur
- Switch to resperidone (rather than add orphenadrine)
  - initial dose 2 mg daily
  - increase to 4 mg daily, if poor response after 4 weeks

Patients already stabilised on chlorpromazine
- Maintenance dose 75-300 mg at night

Long-term depot therapy where adherence is a problem or patient preference
- Flupenthixol decanoate (Fluanxol depot), IM, 20-80 mg every 4 weeks
  - initial dose 20 mg

Or
- Zuclopenthixol decanoate (Clopixol depot), IM, 200-600 mg every 4 weeks
  - initial dose 100 mg

Extrapyramidal side-effects (EPSEs)

EPSEs can occur with even the lowest effective dose of antipsychotic medication.

Common EPSEs include:

Acute dystonia: Severe, sustained muscle spasms, usually of the head and neck which can cause:
  - twisting movements
  - abnormal posture
  - abnormal eye position
  - laryngospasm

Note: these can occur within a few minutes to days after administering medicines such as haloperidol.
- **Drug-induced Parkinsonism**: Tremor, rigidity, shuffling gait, delayed responses, mask-like faces and a pill rolling tremor.
- **Akathisia:** Severe motor restlessness, e.g. pacing, rocking, marching, crossing and uncrossing legs.

NB: Haloperidol and other high-potency agents are more likely to cause EPSEs. The low-potency agent, chlorpromazine is less likely to cause them.

Medicine treatment
- **Acute dystonic reaction**

Adults
- Biperiden, IM slow IV, 2 mg immediately
  - may be repeated every 30 minutes
  - maximum of 4 doses within 24 hours

Or
- Promethazine, IM, 50 mg immediately

Children
- Biperiden, 0.1 mg/kg, as a single dose and refer.

Or
- Promethazine, IM, 0.5 mg / kg as a single dose and refer.

Parkinsonism
- Orphenadrine, oral, 50 mg 3 x daily whilst awaiting specialist review.

Akathisia
- Propranolol, oral, 10 mg 8 hourly whilst awaiting specialist review.

Referral
- All children urgently
- All patients for review of psychotropic medication

MOOD DISORDERS

This is when a person experiences unusual moods and emotions. The mood may be depressed, sad, angry, elated, manic or any of these in combination.

Classification of mood disorders

Depressive disorders
- Depression is characterised by low mood and a reduced capacity to enjoy life.

Bipolar mood disorder
- A lifelong illness in which the patient has recurrent episodes of depression and a history of one or more manic episodes (severely elevated mood with excessive activity and risk-taking behaviour).

Mood disorder due to a general medical condition
- The mood disturbance is secondary to an underlying medical condition e.g. HIV, TB, malignancy, chronic pain conditions.

Adjustment disorder with disturbances of mood
- Depressive symptoms as a response to a major crises or event.

Substance induced mood disorder
- The mood disorder is secondary to a substance use or withdrawal such as abuse of alcohol, drugs or cannabis.

DEPRESSIVE DISORDERS

Clinical features

The person may present with a depressed mood or diminished interest and pleasure in activities.

In addition there are the following symptoms:
- Somatic
    - change in appetite and sleep
    - reduced motivation
    - loss of energy
- Psychic
    - sadness
    - feelings of worthlessness
    - guilt
    - social withdrawal
    - diminished concentration
    - indecisiveness
    - thoughts of death and suicide

MANAGEMENT

Management objectives
- Monitor symptoms
- Conduct a risk assessment to establish risk in patients with possible suicidal ideation.
- Provide medicine treatment and/or psychotherapy.
- Address relevant psychosocial stressors.

General measures
- Supportive measures should be provided.
- Exclude underlying medical conditions and optimise treatment for comorbid medical conditions e.g. HIV, TB, hypothyroidism, diabetes.
- Broader stressors may need to be addressed
- Stress management/coping skills -refer to counselling services
- Marital and family issues -refer to counselling services/social worker if abuse.
- Accommodation and vocational issues – refer to labour/ social development.
- Assess social support and refer to a social worker if financial difficulty.

Medicine treatment
- **NB** Ask about suicidal ideation in all patients, particularly adolescents and young adults before initiating an antidepressant.
- Adolescents with depression should only be treated by a psychiatrist due to the increased risk of suicide.

SSRI e.g. Fluoxetine
- Initiate at 20 mg alternate days for 2 weeks
- Increase to 20 mg daily after 2-4 weeks
- Delay dosage increase if increased agitation/panicky feelings occur.
- If only a partial or no response after 8 weeks, **REFER**.

OR

If fluoxetine is poorly tolerated

Alternative SSRI e.g. Citalopram, oral
- Initiate at 10 mg daily for the first week
- Then increase to 20 mg daily.

Caution with SSRIs
- SSRIs may cause agitation initially.
- This typically resolves within 2-4 weeks.

- **If a sedating antidepressant is required:**

Tricyclic antidepressant e.g. Amitriptyline
- Initial dose: 25 mg, oral, at bedtime
- Increase by 25 mg per day at 4-5 day intervals
- Maximum dose: 150 mg per day

Caution with tricyclic antidepressants
- Tricyclic antidepressants can be fatal in overdose.
- The elderly are more sensitive to side effects and need lower doses.
- Avoid tricyclic antidepressants in patients with heart disease, urinary retention, glaucoma and epilepsy.

Note:
- Continue treatment for a minimum of 9 months
- Consider stopping only if patient has had no/minimal symptoms and has been able to carry out routine daily activities.
- Concomitant generalised anxiety disorder (extend treatment to at least 1 year).
- Previous episode/s of depression (extend treatment to at least 3 years).
-

REFER if:
- Suicidal thoughts
- Major depression with psychotic features
- You suspect bipolar disorder
- Failure to respond to available anti-depressants
- Pregnancy and lactation
- Children and adolescents

BIPOLAR MOOD DISORDER

This is a lifelong illness characterised by recurring periods of depression and either a current or previous episode of mania.

Clinical features

An episode of mania is typically characterised by an elevated mood evidenced by:
- Increased energy / activity
- Talkativeness
- Reduction in the need for sleep
- Feeling of extreme happiness lasting days to weeks, which might also be associated with an underlying irritability
- Grandiose and/or religiose delusions

Depressed mood has the following features:
- Low or irritable mood
- Negative thinking (hopelessness, guilt, unmotivated)
- Lack of enjoyment
- Reduced energy, slowness
- Increased or decreased appetite
- Suicidal thoughts and/or attempts
- Cognitive impairment

MANAGEMENT
General measures
- Hospitalisation may be required during acute mania.
- Psychotherapy, usually after the manic episode, has been controlled with medication.

Management of manic episodes
General measures
- Reduce stimulation and maintain a structured routine.
- Delay individual from making important decisions.

Acute medicine management
- See medicine management of Aggressive disruptive bahaviour in adults (page 373)
- **REFER** to psychiatrist for initiation of an antipsychotic therapy, eg. risperidone
    - once patient can adhere to therapy, follow by a mood stabiliser, eg. oral lithium or oral valproate.

Management of depressive episodes
- **REFER** to psychiatrist for initiation of fluoxetine in the morning and olanzapine at night.
- If the patient is on a mood stabiliser, the dose must be optimised.

ADJUSTMENT DISORDER WITH DEPRESSED MOOD

- Depressive symptoms as a response to a major crisis or event and is the reaction of normal people to the "ups and downs" of life
- Usually lasts < 6 months unless the stressor persists

MANAGEMENT
General measures
- Counsellling
- **REFER** for psychotherapy

Medicine management
This is indicated for severe somatic symptoms, e.g. severe headache, insomnia and depressed mood.
- Diazepam 2.5-5 mg as a single nighttime dose for 5-10 days.
  Or
- Amitryptyline 25-50 mg as a single nighttime dose for up to 1 month.

SUBSTANCE-RELATED DISORDERS

SUBSTANCE-USE DISORDERS

Substance use disorder is medical and physical symptoms caused by the use of one or more substance despite significant substance-related problems (including abuse and dependence)

GENERAL MEASURES
- Reassurance and support of the patient and family.

MEDICINE TREATMENT
- For severe anxiety, irritability and insomnia:
    - Diazepam, oral, 5-10 mg as a single dose daily for 5-10 days

REFERRAL
- Severe alcohol dependence.
- Past history of withdrawal seizures or Delirium Tremens.
- Pregnancy.
- Opioid substance use disorder.
- Significant polydrug use.
- Lack of support at home or homelessness.
- Previous failed community detoxification attempts.

SUBSTANCE-INDUCED MOOD DISORDER

This is a mood disorder secondary to a substance use or withdrawal such as abuse of alcohol, drugs e.g. cannabis.

GENERAL MEASURES
- Remove the causative substance.
- May require acute detoxification
- If symptoms persist after 2 weeks, treat the mood disorder.
- See Mood disorders Page 375.

SUBSTANCE-INDUCED PSYCHOSIS

Psychosis secondary to a substance use or withdrawal such as abuse of alcohol, drugs e.g. cannabis.

GENERAL MEASURES
- Most patients with substance-induced psychosis can be managed without medication.
- Ensure the safety of the patient and health care workers
- Minimise stress and stimulation (do not argue with psychotic thinking).
- Avoid confrontation or criticism, unless it is necessary to prevent harmful of disruptive behaviour.

Medicine treatment
- See Page 374: Aggressive disruptive behaviour in adults (general measures and medicine treatment)

REFERRAL
- All patients

ALCOHOL WITHDRAWAL (UNCOMPLICATED)

- This is a syndrome that occurs when an alcohol dependent individual abruptly stops or significantly reduces alcohol consumption.

The symptoms include:
- Autonomic (sweating, tachycardia, tremors)
- Gastrointestinal (anorexia, nausea, vomiting)
- Cognitive (poor concentration, anxiety restlessness)

MANAGEMENT

Medicine treatment
- Thiamine, oral, 300 mg daily for 14 days

Plus
- Diazepam, oral, 10 mg immediately
- Then 5 mg 6 hourly for 3 days
- Then 5 mg 12 hourly for 2 days
- Then 5 mg daily for 2 days
- Then stop

REFERRAL
- See referral criteria of substance use disorder (page 377)

ANXIETY AND STRESS-RELATED DISORDERS

Anxiety is an emotional response to a perceived or anticipated stress. It is diagnosed as a disorder when it is excessive or persistent and impacts daily functioning.

ACUTE STRESS DISORDER / AND POST-TRAUMATIC STRESS DISORDER

Clinical features

- Psychological manifestations include excessive worry, mood changes, irritability, tearfulness and difficulty concentrating.
- Physical symptoms include headache, neck and back muscle tension, abdominal cramps, nausea, palpitations, sweating, a choking feeling, shortness of breath, chest pain, dizziness, numbness and tingling of the hands and feet.
- Anxiety in people with intellectual disability may present with aggression, agitation and demanding behaviour.

MANAGEMENT

General measures
- Assess severity of the condition
- Maintain an empathetic and concerned attitude
- Educate the patient and family regarding the nature of the condition.
- Refer to local support groups.

Medicine treatment
Patients with severe conditions should be assessed by a doctor.

SSRI e.g. Fluoxetine
- Initiate at 20 mg alternate days for 2 weeks
- Increase to 20 mg daily after 2-4 weeks
- Delay dosage increase if increased agitation/panicky feelings occur.

OR

If fluoxetine is poorly tolerated
- Alternative SSRI e.g. Citalopram, oral Initiate at 10 mg daily for the first week
- Then increase to 20 mg daily

Caution with SSRIs
- SSRIs may cause agitation initially.
- This typically resolves within 2-4 weeks.

NB Ask about suicidal ideation in all patients, particularly adolescents and young adults before initiating an SSRI. If suicidal ideation present, refer before initiating SSRI.

Note: Continue treatment for a minimum of 9 months Consider stopping only if patient has had no/minimal symptoms and has been able to carry out routine daily activities.

REFFERAL
- High suicide risk
- Poor response to treatment

PANIC ATTACK / AND PANIC DISORDER

Clinical features
- Acute onset of intense anxiety accompanied by a sense of dread, usually for no apparent reason.
- Usually accompanied by physical symptoms, e.g. rapid pulse, palpitations, shortness of breath, dizziness, sweating.
- Recurrent episodes of panic attacks (panic disorder)

MANAGEMENT

General measures
- Psychology e.g. cognitive-behaviour therapy
- Always consider the possibility of an underlying medical condition e.g. thyrotoxicosis or substance-related disorder

Medicine treatment

For panic attack:
- Diazepam, IV, 5-10 mg as a single dose. Followed by diazepam, oral, 5 mg daily for 7-10 days

REFFERAL
- All patients

Pharmacopoeia

PHARMACOPOEIA

ACYCLOVIR

Therapeutic action: Antiviral medicine

Indications: Herpes virus infections, particularly in immuno-compromised patients.

Precautions: Doses should be reduced in renal impairment.

Adverse effects:
Headache, dizziness, nausea and diarrhoea may occur.

Dose

Adults

- *Herpes simplex ulceration:* 400 mg 3 x daily for 7 days
- *Herpes zoster:* if fresh vesicles are present, and preferably within 72 hours of onset: 800 mg 5 x daily for 7 days
- *Chickenpox: immuno-compromised patients and all cases with severe chickenpox:* 20 mg/kg (maximum 800 mg/dose) 4 x daily for 7 days

Children:

- *Herpes simplex infections of the mouth and perioral:*
  - 1-3 months   50 mg
  - 3-6 months   80 mg
  - 6-18 months   100 mg
  - 18 months-3 years   120 mg
  - 3-7 years   160 mg
  - 7-11 years   200 mg
  - 11-15 years   300 mg

ALBENDAZOLE (Zentel)

Therapeutic action: Anthelmintic

Indications:
- Roundworm (Ascaris), pinworm (threadworm), whipworm
- Hookworm
- Tapeworm (Taenia) and cutaneous larva migrans (sandworm)
- Microsporidiosis in patients with AIDS

Contraindications: Pregnancy and lactation

Adverse effects:
Side effects are uncommon with doses recommended for intestinal worms.

Dose:
- *Adults and children over 2 years:* 400 mg as a single oral dose
- *Children 1-2 years:* 200 mg (10 ml suspension) as a single oral dose
- *Sandworm and tapeworm:* 400 mg daily for 3 consecutive days
- *Microsporidiosis:* 400 mg 2 x daily for 4 weeks

ALLOPURINOL (Zyloprim)

Therapeutic action: Uric acid production inhibitor

Indications: Long-term treatment of hyperuricaemia

Contraindications:
Should be avoided in acute gout and severe renal impairment.

Adverse effects:
- Acute gout and kidney stones may be precipitated.
- Hypersensitivity reactions, including urticaria and various skin rashes and sometimes severe toxic syndrome with fever, hepatitis or other organ involvement and eosinophilia (DRESS).

Drug interactions:
Increased incidence of skin rashes when amoxicillin / ampicillin is combined with allopurinol.

Dose:
- Initially 100-150 mg daily
- Average dose: 300 mg daily.
- *Renal impairment:* Lower doses should be used.

AMITRIPTYLINE (Tryptanol)

Therapeutic action: Tricyclic antidepressant

Indications:
- Management of depressive illness
- Additional therapy for pain relief in chronic pain syndromes
- Nocturnal enuresis in children over 6 years of age, after exclusion of organic pathology

Precautions:
- Prostatic enlargement
- Closed angle glaucoma
- Arrhythmias
- Epilepsy
- Impaired liver function

Adverse effects:
- Commonly anticholinergic effects including dry mouth, blurred vision, constipation and difficulty with micturition
- Appetite stimulation and weight gain
- Produces varying degrees of sedation and is best given as a single night-time dose
- Precipitation of seizures in epileptics and mania in patients with bipolar mood disorders
- Tolerance to many of the side-effects may develop during prolonged therapy

Drug interactions:
Antihistamines, antipsychotics and anticholinergic-type antiparkinson agents increase anticholinergic effects

Dose:
- *Adults:*
  - initially 25-50 mg at night
  - if necessary the dose may be increased by 25 mg per day at weekly intervals to 150 mg daily
- *In the elderly:* not recommended
- A single bedtime dose is best for most patients.
- A period of 2-4 weeks therapy is required before antidepressant action becomes evident.
- *Nocturnal enuresis:*
  - *6-12 years* 10-25 mg at bedtime
  - *over 12 years* 25-50 mg at bedtime
- *Chronic pain syndromes:*
  - initially 25 mg at night
  - increase if necessary by 25 mg at weekly or monthly intervals to 75 mg at night

AMLODIPINE (Norvasc)

Therapeutic action:
- Long-acting calcium channel blocker
- Dominant effect is arterial vasodilatation

Indications: Hypertension; angina pectoris

Precautions and contraindications:
- Acute myocardial infarction

Adverse effects:
- Dizziness, palpitations
- Pedal oedema is a frequent side effect

Pregnancy: Safety not established

Lactation: Safety not established

Dose:
- *Initial dose*: 5 mg daily
- *Maximum dose*: 10 mg daily

AMOXICILLIN (Amoxil)

Therapeutic action: Broad-spectrum penicillin

Indications:
- ENT infections
- Respiratory tract infections
- Soft tissue and skin infections

Contraindications: Penicillin-allergic patients

Adverse effects:
- Maculo-papular and urticarial rashes. Maculopapular rashes are common in patients:
   - with renal impairment
   - receiving allopurinol
- Urticarial rashes are more likely to be associated with true penicillin allergy

Drug interactions:
Increased risk of skin rash if allopurinol and amoxicillin are used together.

Dose:
For otits media, sinusitis and pneumonia:
- Amoxicillin 45 mg/kg/dose 2 x daily
- 1-3 months   200 mg
- 3-6 months   250 mg
- 6-18 months   400 mg
- 18 months-3 years   500 mg
- 3-5 years   750 mg
- 5-7 years   1000 mg
- 7-10 years   1250 mg

For children 10 years and older and adults:
- 1000 mg 3 x daily

- *Prevention of infective endocarditis for dental procedures*:
   - *adults:* 2 g orally 1 hour before the procedure
   - *children 5-10 years:* half adult dose
   - *children <5 years:* quarter adult dose

ASPIRIN (Disprin)

Therapeutic action:
- Analgesic, antipyretic, anti-inflammatory
- Inhibits platelet aggregation and blood clotting

Indications:
- *Adults:*
   - relief of mild to moderate pain and for pyrexia
   - prevention of clot extension in acute myocardial infarction
   - prevention of strokes and of thrombo-embolism after myocardial infarction
- *Children:* Chronic inflammatory diseases eg. juvenile rheumatoid arthritis

Contraindications:
- Patients with peptic ulceration, GIT bleeding, bronchial asthma, gouty arthritis and the more severe degrees of hypertension
- Patients on anticoagulants (warfarin)
- Acute, febrile illnesses in children or adolescents (danger of Reye's syndrome)

Adverse effects:
- Gastric irritation and may cause abdominal pain, nausea and vomiting
- GIT bleeding, either occult bleeding or acute haemorrhage
- Bronchospasm especially in asthmatics
- Urticaria and angio-oedema
- Tinnitus and decreased hearing

Drug interactions:
- Increases the pharmacological effects of the sulphonylureas, insulin, sulphonamides (including co-trimoxazole) and warfarin

Dose:
- *Prophylaxis of thrombo-embolism:* 75-100 mg daily
- *Acute stroke:* 300 mg as an oral stat dose

ATENOLOL (Tenormin)

Therapeutic action: Cardio-selective beta-blocker

Indications:
- Prevention of angina pectoris and repeat infarction
- Hypertension

Contraindications:
Avoid in asthma or COAD, untreated heart failure, pregnancy or lactation, pulse rate less than 60 / minute.

Precautions:
- Use with care in cardiomegaly (without clinical failure), diabetes mellitus, peripheral vascular disease and in renal impairment.

Adverse effects:
Bradycardia, bronchospasm, impotence, cold extremities, worsening of heart failure and masking of the symptoms of hypoglycaemia

Dose:
- *Hypertension:* 50 mg daily
- *Angina:* 50 mg daily

AZITHROMYCIN (Zithromax)

Therapeutic action: Macrolide antibiotic

Indications:
- Alternative to penicillin in penicillin-allergic patients
- Sexually transmitted infections

Contraindications:
- Avoid in patients with liver disease

Adverse effects:
- Gastrointestinal upsets including nausea, vomiting and diarrhoea

Drug interactions:
- May reduce the efficacy of oral contraceptives

Dose:
- *Adults and adolescents over 11 years of age:* 500 mg daily for 3 days.

- *Children:* 10 mg / kg daily for 3 days
  - 1-3 years   120 mg
  - 3-5 years   160 mg
  - 5-7 years   200 mg
  - 7-11 years   250mg
- *Genital chlamydia and gonorrhoea infections:* 1-2 g as a single oral dose (2 g when not used in combination with a cephalosporin).

BECLOMETHAZONE / BUDESONIDE

Therapeutic action: Inhaled corticosteroid

Indications:
- Chronic persistent asthma and acute asthma
- Prophylaxis and treatment of allergic rhinitis

Adverse effects:
- In asthma oropharyngeal candidiasis is a frequent occurrence. Rinsing the mouth with water after inhalation may be preventive.
- In allergic rhinitis transient burning or stinging may occur. Only aqueous preparations should be used.

Dose:
- *Adults:*
  - *Chronic asthma:* 100-200 mcg 2 x daily
  - *Severe symptoms:* initially 400 mcg 2 x daily
  - *Allergic rhinitis:* 50 mcg (1 spray) into each nostril 2 x daily.
- *Children:*
  - *Chronic asthma:* 50-100 mcg 2 x daily
  - *Severe symptoms:* initially 200 mcg 2 x daily
  - *In allergic rhinitis:* 50 mcg (1 spray) into each nostril 2 x daily.

BENZOYL PEROXIDE GEL

Indication: Acne vulgaris

Adverse effects:

Redness and scaling is common during the first few weeks. This usually becomes less severe with continuous use.

Skin application:
- Initially apply on alternate days.
- Increase frequency to daily once tolerance to irritant effect develops.
- Proper skin cleansing before application enhances efficacy.

BENZYL BENZOATE (Ascabiol)

Indications: Scabies and pediculosis (lice)

Contraindications:
- Infants and small children unless diluted
- Septic scabies
- Open wounds, abraded skin or eczema
- Avoid contact with eyes, face, neck

Adverse effects: Skin irritation and burning

Application:

Scabies:
- Apply after bathing at night.
- Apply to the whole body omitting the head and neck.
- Leave on for 24 hours.
- *Small children:* dilute 1:1 with water.
- *Infants:* dilute 1:3 with water (3 parts water).
- Repeat application once within 5 days

Pediculosis (not head lice):
- Apply to the affected areas.
- Leave on for 24 hours.
- Repeat once a week for up to 3 weeks.

BIPERIDEN (Akineton)

Therapeutic action: Anticholinergic agent

Indications:
Acute dystonia associated with drug-induced parkinsonism

Precautions:
- Dosage should be reduced:
  - in the elderly
  - in patients with ischaemic heart disease, heart failure, prostatic hypertrophy

Adverse effects:
Parenteral administration may produce transient postural hypotension or disturbance of coordination.

Dose:
- 2 mg IMI or slow IVI which can be repeated every 30 minutes
- Maximum of 4 doses within 24 hours

CALAMINE LOTION

Indications:
Itchy skin conditions eg. chickenpox, insect bites, herpes zoster

Adverse effects:
- Prolonged use may cause excessive dryness of the skin
- Very poisonous if swallowed

Application: Apply to affected areas 4-6 hourly

CARBAMAZEPINE (Tegretol)

Indications:
- Epilepsy in non-HIV infected patients of all ages
- Used for the management of:
  - generalised tonic-clonic epilepsy (primary or secondary to a focal discharge)
  - partial seizures (simple or complex including temporal lobe seizures)
- Trigeminal neuralgia
- Diabetic or post-herpetic neuralgia
- Mood stabiliser in bipolar disorders

Precautions:
Pregnancy
Initial dose must be kept small to avoid acute side effects eg. dizziness, nausea.

Adverse effects:
- Skin reactions including erythema, photosensitivity reactions, urticaria and Stevens Johnson syndrome.
- Drowsiness, dry mouth, nausea and anorexia but these often subside spontaneously after 1-2 weeks of treatment.

Drug interactions:
- Avoid concurrent use with antiretroviral drugs and monitor levels carefully when using together with other anticonvulsants.
- Azithromycin and INH may inhibit carbamazepine metabolism and lead to carbamazepine toxicity.

Dose:
Epilepsy
Adults:
- Start with 100 mg 2 x daily (for 1 week)
- Then 200 mg 2 x daily
- If seizures remain uncontrolled, increase by 200 mg/day at weekly/monthly intervals
- Maximum dose 600 mg 2 x daily

Children:
- Start with 2 mg/kg 3 x daily for 2 weeks
- Then increase to 5 mg/kg 3 x daily according to response
- Maximum dose 10 mg/kg 2 x daily

Pain syndromes
Adults:
- Initially 100 mg 2 x daily for 1 week
- Then 200 mg 2 x daily
- Increase by 100 mg twice daily at weekly intervals until pain is relieved
- Maximum dose 400 mg 2 x daily

CEFTRIAXONE

Therapeutic action: Cephalosporin antibiotic

Indications:
- Gonorrhoea both complicated and uncomplicated
- Pneumonia
- Meningitis
- Acute pyelonephritis

Precautions and contraindications:
- Previous, severe hypersensitivity to any penicillin
- Any severe reaction to a cephalosporin
- Do not administer if calcium-containing IV fluids administered within the previous 48 hours.

Adverse effects:
Cross-sensitivity may occur in 5-16% of patients allergic to penicillin

Dose:
- *Adults:*
  - gonorrhoea: 250 mg IMI as a single dose
  - meningitis: 2 g by IV infusion prior to referral
  - other severe disease: 1 g IV / IM as a single dose prior to referral
- *Children:*
  - 80 mg/kg as a single dose for meningitis or other severe disease prior to referral

- 0-1 month	225 mg
- 1-3 months	300 mg
- 3-6 months	440 mg
- 6-12 months	625 mg
- 12-18 months	750 mg
- 18 months-3 years	800 mg
- 3-5 years	1 000 mg
- 5-15 years	1 500 mg
- 15 years and above	2 000 mg

CEPHALEXIN

Therapeutic action: Cephalosporin antibiotic

Indications:
- Staphylococcal and streptococcal skin and soft tissue infections
- Urinary tract infections but resistance now widespread

Precautions, contraindications and adverse effects:
As for ceftriaxone.
- *Adults and children over 7 years:*
  - 500 mg 4 x daily
- *Children:*

- 0-3 months:	62.5 mg 4 x daily
- 3-18 months:	125 mg 4 x daily
- 18 months-7 years:	250 mg 4 x daily
- 7 years and above:	500 mg 4 x daily

CHLORPHENAMINE
(Chlortrimeton, Allergex)

Therapeutic action: Antihistamine

Indications:
- Allergic disorders such as allergic rhinitis, urticaria or angioedema
- Pruritic conditions such as eczema, chickenpox

Precautions and contraindications:
- Use with caution in patients with asthma, glaucoma, prostatic hypertrophy, pregnancy and lactation.
- Should not be used together with alcohol.
- Use with caution in children under 2 years of age

Adverse effects:
- Drowsiness, especially if used with alcohol or sedatives

Dose:
- *Adults and children >11 years:* 4 mg (1 tablet) 3 x daily
- *Children:*

- 2-3 years	3 ml 3 x daily
- 3-5 years:	4 ml 3 x daily
- 5-7 years:	5 ml 3 x daily
- 7-11 years	7.5 ml 3 x daily

CIPROFLOXACIN

Therapeutic action: Quinolone antibiotic

Indications:
- Gastrointestinal infections
- Urinary tract infections

Contraindications:
- Should be avoided in pregnancy and lactation
- Patients under 18 years of age unless benefits outweigh risks.

Drug interactions:
- Increased plasma theophylline concentration
- Antacids containing aluminium, magnesium or calcium may reduce absorption of the quinolone

Adverse effects:
- Generally well tolerated.
- Most common are GIT disturbances, such as nausea, vomiting and diarrhoea

Dose:
- Uncomplicated cystitis: 500 mg 2 x daily for 3 days
- *Complicated cystitis:* 500 mg 2 x daily for 7 days
- *Acute inflammatory diarrhoea (dysentery):* 500 mg 2 x daily for 3 days
- *Paediatric dose:*
  - where benefits outweigh the risks (e.g. acute inflammatory diarrhoea) 15 mg/kg/dose 2 x daily for 3 days

CLOTRIMAZOLE (Canestin)

Therapeutic action:
- Broad-spectrum antifungal agent
- Limited effectiveness against vaginal trichomoniasis and bacterial vaginosis

Indications:
- Vulvo-vaginal and cutaneous candidiasis
- Dermatophytosis (including tinea affecting intertriginous areas eg. crural region)
- Tinea versiculor and erythrasma
- Symptomatic relief of vaginal trichomoniasis and bacterial vaginosis in the first trimester of pregnancy

Dose:
- *Vulvo-vaginal candidiasis:*
  - insert one 500 mg pessary high into the vagina at night as a single dose

Skin application:
- Apply to affected areas 2-3 x daily. Use sparingly in intertriginous areas
- In tinea treatment is continued for 2 weeks after the condition has cleared

CO-AMOXICLAV (Augmentin)

Therapeutic action: Broad-spectrum penicillin

Indications:
- Urinary tract infection
- Chronic leg ulcers
- Animal and human bites
- Pneumonia with underlying medical conditions

Contraindications: Penicillin-allergic patients

Adverse effects:
- Maculo-papular and urticarial rashes. Maculopapular rashes are particularly common in patients:
  - with glandular fever or renal impairment
  - receiving allopurinol
- Anaphylaxis (rare)
- Urticarial rashes are likely to be associated with true penicillin allergy

Drug interactions: Increased risk of skin rash if allopurinol and amoxicillin are used together.

Dose:
- *Adults and children over 11 years*: 875 / 125 mg 2 x daily before meals
- *Children under 11 years with UTI:* 15-25 mg/kg/dose 8 hourly

COMBINED ORAL CONTRACEPTIVE

Therapeutic action:
- Inhibits ovulation
- Increases viscosity of the cervical mucus
- Decreases endometrial receptivity to implantation

Indications:
- Contraception
- Dysfunctional uterine bleeding
- Menorrhagia
- Dysmenorrhoea
- Endometriosis
- Secondary amenorrhoea

Contraindications:
- Myocardial infarction, angina pectoris, pulmonary embolus, DVT, hypertension or previous CVA, active or recent liver disease
- Abnormal uterine bleeding, carcinoma of the breast, cervix or uterus, malignant melanoma, leukaemia
- Psychosis or depression (or a history of severe depression)
- Uncontrolled diabetes, hyper-lipidaemia
- Avoid in women over 35 years who have risk factors for cardiovascular disease, or who are smokers

Precautions:
Heavy smokers, diabetes, hyper-lipidaemia, hypertension, obesity, gall bladder disease, epilepsy, mental retardation or disorder, varicose veins, migraine

Adverse effects:
- Headache and migraine may occur.
- Gynaecological effects include spotting, breakthrough bleeding, amenorrhoea, post-use anovulation (for about 3 months).
- Chloasma and hair loss may occur.
- Acne improves in some patients but may be worse in others.

Drug interactions:
- Hepatic enzyme induction by the anti-epileptics, griseofulvin and rifampicin may lead to enhanced metabolism of the oral contraceptives and reduce their efficacy.
- Antibiotics may alter intestinal flora and result in loss of efficacy.
- The efficacy of antihypertensive and oral hypoglycaemic agents is decreased and their combination with combined oral contraceptives should be avoided.
- Theophylline clearance may be reduced increasing the risk of theophylline toxicity.

Administration:
Pills should be taken at the same time every day, according to the package.

CO-TRIMOXAZOLE (Purbac, Bactrim)

Therapeutic action:
- Broad-spectrum antibiotic
- Combination of trimethoprim and a sulphonamide

Indications:
- Primary prophylaxis of opportunistic infections in the WHO clinical stages III and IV in HIV disease
- Treatment and prophylaxis of *P carinii pneumonia*

Precautions and contraindications:
- Contra-indicated in sulphur-sensitive patients and patients with liver disease or severe renal impairment.
- Should be avoided in infants under 6 weeks of age.

Adverse effects:
- Skin rashes, often minor, in sensitive patients
- Less commonly severe reactions such as the Stevens Johnson syndrome or toxic epidermal necrolysis
- Occasionally GIT disturbances eg. nausea, vomiting

Drug interactions:
- Increases the action of sulphonylureas and thus may produce hypoglycaemia.
- May increase phenytoin blood levels and the anticoagulant effect of warfarin.

Dose:

Prophylaxis in HIV disease and P. carinii pneumonia

- *Adults and children over 10 years:*
  - 2 tabs (800/160 mg) daily
- *Children:*
  - 6 weeks -3 months 2.5 ml
  - 3 months-3 years   5 ml
  - 3-10 years   10 ml

DIAZEPAM (Valium)

Therapeutic action:
Anticonvulsant, muscle relaxant and mild tranquillizer

Indications:
- A supplement in the treatment of acute, painful musculo-skeletal conditions
- The management of acute alcohol withdrawal
- Intravenously or rectally to stop status epilepticus
- Anxiety states

Precautions and contraindications:
- Avoid in patients with severe hepatic disease (danger of hepatic encephalopathy), bronchial asthma and chronic obstructive pulmonary disease.
- Use with caution in the elderly because of the risk of over-sedation, respiratory depression, disorientation and ataxia, and in those patients with anxiety, secondary to an

underlying depressive disorder.
- Intravenous diazepam may cause respiratory arrest.
- Prolonged treatment requires gradual withdrawal to avoid withdrawal effects.

Adverse effects:
- Drowsiness and over-sedation, particularly in the elderly
- Less frequently depression, disorientation, confusion and ataxia

Drug interactions:
Additive CNS depressant effects with alcohol, antipsychotics, antihistamines and other CNS depressants

Dose:
- *Oral:* 5 mg 1-4 x daily (average dose 5 mg daily)
    - duration of therapy should preferably not exceed 7-10 days
- *Intravenously:* 0,1 mg / kg = 0,2 ml / 10 kg.
    - give 2 mg (0,4 ml) per minute to a maximum of 10 mg (adults)
- *Intra-rectal administration in status epilepticus:*
    - 6 months-1 year: 2,5 mg (0,5 ml)
    - 1-5 years: 5 mg (1 ml)
    - 5-8 years: 7,5 mg (1,5 ml)
    - 8-14 years: 10 mg (2 ml)

DOXYCYCLINE (Cyclidox, Doxyclin)

Therapeutic action: Broad-spectrum antibiotic

Indications:
- Syphilis
- Chlamydial genital and gynaecological infections
- Rickettsial diseases including tick bite fever
- Chronic bronchitis exacerbations
- Malaria prophylaxis
- Acne

Precautions and contraindications:
Children under 8 years of age

Adverse effects:
- GIT effects such as nausea, vomiting and epigastric pain
- Erythematous or maculopapular skin rash

Drug interactions:
- Chelation with calcium, magnesium and iron decreases absorption
- May reduce efficacy of oral contraceptives

Dose:
- *Adults and adolescents over 14 years of age*: 100 mg 2 x daily
- *Children 8-14 years of age*: 100 mg daily
- *Malaria prophylaxis*: 100 mg daily
- *Acne*: 100 mg daily

EFAVIRENZ (EFV)

Therapeutic action:
Non-nucleoside reverse transcriptase inhibitor.

Indications:
Used in HIV infection in combination with at least two other antiretroviral drugs.

Contraindications:
- Pregnancy – potential teratogenic effect
- Severe liver disease

Precautions: Patients with a history of mental illness.

Dose:
- *Adults:*
    - 600 mg at bedtime
    - for body weight less than 40 kg, give 400 mg
- *Children:*
    - 200-400 mg dose according to body weight
    - not recommended for children under 3 years or under 10 kg

Adverse effects:
- Dizziness, insomnia, abnormal dreams, impaired concentration, depression
- Mild to severe skin rash
- Hepatoxicity

ENALAPRIL (Renitec)

Therapeutic action:
- ACE-inhibitor
- Vasodilator, antihypertensive
- Produces vasodilation by inhibiting the conversion of angiotensin I to angiotensin II (the latter is a powerful vasoconstrictor)
- Inhibits production of aldosterone and therefore has a natruretic and diuretic effect

Indications:
- CCF with poor left ventricular function
- Hypertension
- Nephropathy, especially diabetic

Contraindications: Avoid in pregnancy

Precautions:
- To avoid hypotension, start with a small dose.
- This applies particularly to patients:
    - in heart failure
    - receiving high-dose diuretic therapy
    - who are elderly
- Use with caution in kidney impairment

Adverse effects:
- Persistent dry hacking cough - the most common side effect - requires the drug to be stopped
- Angioedema - this also requires drug to be stopped
- Hypotension (orthostatic)
- Taste disturbance

Drug interactions:
- Enalapril is a potassium-sparing agent
- Potassium supplements and potassium-sparing diuretics, eg spironolactone, should be used with caution in patients receiving enalapril
    - this is because hyper-kalaemia may occur.

Dose:
This should be individualised

Initial dose	Average dose	Maximum dose
Hypertension		
10 mg daily	10 mg daily	10 mg 2 x daily or 20 mg daily
Heart failure		
5 mg 2 x daily	10 mg 2 x daily	10 mg 2 x daily

FERROUS SULPHATE

Therapeutic action: Iron supplement

Indications:
Treatment and prophylaxis of iron deficiency

Precautions:
- Poisoning due to iron salts is common
- It is important to keep iron tablets out of reach of young children
- Should not be administered for longer than 6 months.

Adverse effects:
GIT intolerance including nausea, epigastric pain, diarrhoea or constipation and black stools

Drug interactions:
Absorption is decreased by doxycycline, antacids and mineral supplements eg. calcium.

Dose:
- *Therapeutic:* 1 tab 3 x daily
- *Prophylaxis in pregnancy and lactation:* 1 tab daily

FLUCLOXACILLIN (Floxapen)

Indications:
Staphylococcal infection commonly of the skin, soft tissue and bone

Contraindications: Penicillin sensitivity

Adverse effects:
- Hyper-sensitivity reaction
- GIT disturbances eg. nausea, anorexia

Dose:
- *Adults and children over 7 years of age:* 500 mg 4 x daily

FLUCONAZOLE

Therapeutic action: : Imidazole antifungal with widespectrum fungistatic activity

Indications (at primary care level):
- Secondary prevention of cryptococcal meningitis in patients with AIDS
- Oesophageal, bronchial and pulmonary candidiasis
- Tinea capitis and severe tinea in other areas
- Fungal nail fold infection

Contraindication: Pregnancy - avoid in first trimester

Dose:
- *For prevention of relapse of cryptococcal meningitis:* 200 mg daily
- *For oesophageal candidiasis:* 200 mg daily for 21 days
- *For extensive tinea corporis and pedis:*
  Adults: 200 mg daily for 14 days
- *For tinea capitis:* 200 mg weekly for 6 weeks
  Children:
    - *6 months-3 years:* 50 mg/day
    - *3-7 years:* 100 mg/day
    - *7-11 years:* 150 mg/day
    - *>11 years:* 200 mg/day
    - given as a single dose for 28 days
    - mix contents of the capsule/s with unheated food or fluid

FUROSEMIDE (Lasix)

Therapeutic action: Loop diuretic

Indications: Heart failure, kidney failure, cirrhosis with ascites

Precautions:
- Use with caution in patients with diabetes and gout.
- The elderly are particularly susceptible to excessive dehydration and hypotension.

Adverse effects:
- Can cause hypo-kalaemia, especially in the elderly, in patients on a potassium depleted diet and in cirrhosis.
- Can cause hyper-uricaemia, hypo-magnesaemia, hypo-calcaemia.
- Can cause hypo-natraemia, especially if the oedema is reduced quickly.

Drug interactions:
NSAIDs, especially indomethacin, may reduce the diuretic efficacy of furosemide by causing sodium and fluid retention.

Dose:
- Usually 40-80 mg / day in a single dose or in two divided doses
    - to avoid nocturia, the second dose is best taken in early evening (5-6 pm)
    - higher doses may be needed in kidney failure
- Potassium chloride (Slow-K) supplementation is usually not indicated. It may need to be avoided or reduced in patients:
    - on treatment with spironolactone (Aldactone) or ACE-inhibitors at the same time
    - with kidney failure

GLIBENCLAMIDE (Euglucon, Daonil)

Therapeutic action: Sulphonylurea oral hypoglycaemia drug

Indications: Type 2 diabetes mellitus

Precautions and contraindications:
Avoid in patients with severe renal impairment or liver disease.

Adverse effects:
GIT disturbance with nausea, epigastric discomfort and heartburn

Drug interactions:
- Hypoglycaemic effect is increased if used together with aspirin, sulphonamides, cimetidine and warfarin.
- Increased risk of hypoglycaemia if used together with alcohol.
- Beta-blockers may cover up the warning symptoms of hypoglycaemia and non-cardio-selective beta-blockers
    - eg. propranolol may produce hypoglycaemia.
- Hypoglycaemic effect is diminished with drugs that
    - induce hepatic metabolising enzymes eg. phenobarbitone and phenytoin
    - are associated with impaired glucose tolerance eg. thiazides, furosemide and oral contraceptives.

Dose:

Initial dose	Intermediate dose	Maximum dose
2,5-5 mg mane	5 mg mane 5 mg nocte	10 mg mane 5 mg nocte

GLIMEPERIDE (Diaglim, Euglim)

Therapeutic action: Sulphonylurea oral hypoglycaemic medicine

Indications: Diabetes mellitus Type 2

Precautions and contraindications: Avoid in patients with renal impairment (eGFR <60 ml / min) or liver disease.

Medicine interactions:
- Hypoglycaemic effect is increased if used together with aspirin, sulphonamides, cimetidine and warfarin.
- Beta-blockers may cover up the warning symptoms of hypoglycaemia
    - e.g. during exercise, may produce hypoglycaemia
- Hypoglycaemic effect is diminished with medicines that:
    - induce hepatic enzymes, e.g. phenytoin, rifampicin
    - are associated with impaired glucose tolerance, e.g. thiazides, furosemide and oral contraceptives

Dose:

Initial dose	Intermediate doses	Maximum dose
1 mg daily	2-3 mg daily	4 mg daily

HALOPERIDOL

Indications:
- Psychotic disorders, particularly schizophrenia and mania
- Agitated or aggressive behavioural disturbance, especially when associated with a medical disorder.

Precautions and contraindications:
- Parkinson's disease and those patients who have previously developed drug induced extrapyramidal effects.
- Use with caution in depression, epilepsy and hyperthyroidism.

Adverse effects:
Extrapyramidal effects are common particularly dystonic reactions and motor restlessness.

Drug interactions:
- Lowers convulsion threshold in epileptic patients
    - lower dose may be required
- Antagonises effects of anti-parkinsonian agents eg. levodopa.

Dose:
- *Psychotic disorders:*
    - initial dose 1 mg daily (0.5 mg 2 x daily in the elderly)
    - increasing to 5 mg daily
    - once stabilised administer as a single dose at bedtime

- *Acute psychotic disorders:*
    - IMI 5 mg
    - may be repeated after 1 hour if needed
    - maximum dose 10 mg in 24 hours

HYDROCHLOROTHIAZIDE

Therapeutic action: Diuretic and antihypertensive

Indications: Hypertension, heart failure

Contraindications:
- More severe degrees of renal or hepatic impairment
- Pregnancy and lactation
- Uncontrolled gout

Adverse effects:
- Hyperuricaemia - may precipitate gout
- Hyperglycaemia (avoid high doses)
- Hyperlipidaemia (avoid high doses)
- Hypokalaemia (avoid high doses)
- Occasionally photosensitivity and hypersensitivity rashes

Dose:
- *Hypertension:* 12.5 mg in the morning
- *Heart failure:* 25-50 mg in the morning

HYOSCINE (Buscopan)

Therapeutic action: Antispasmodic, anticholinergic

Indications: Abdominal colic

Contraindications:
- Should be avoided in patients with urinary retention, glaucoma or ileus.
- Use with caution in patients with prostatic hypertrophy.

Adverse effects:
Dry mouth, blurred vision, tachycardia, urinary retention and constipation

Dose: *Adults*: 10 mg 3 x daily

IBUPROFEN (Brufen)

Therapeutic action:
Non-steroidal anti-inflammatory drug (NSAID)

Indications:
Used to relieve a wide spectrum of inflammatory and painful conditions eg. arthritic disorders, post-traumatic inflammation.

Precautions and contraindications:
- Should be avoided in patients with peptic ulceration and GIT bleeding.
- Use with caution in bronchial asthma, heart failure, hypertension, renal or hepatic impairment.

Adverse effects and drug interactions: As for aspirin

Dose:
- 200-400 mg 3 x daily after meals
- *In the elderly and in patients with cardiac, renal or hepatic impairment:* 200 mg 3 x daily
- *Acute gout:* 400 mg 3 x daily until pain and inflammation have subsided.

NB. Not recommended for children except in selected cases eg. rheumatic illnesses

IPRATROPIUM

Therapeutic action: Anticholinergic bronchodilator

Indications: Chronic bronchitis, asthma

Cautions: Prostatic hypertrophy, closed angle glaucoma

Adverse effects: Dry mouth and a bitter taste

Dose:
- *Adults:*
    - aerosal inhalation 2 puffs 3 x daily
    - nebuliser solution 0,5 mg (diluted to 5 ml with normal saline) 4 hourly
- *Children:*
    - nebuliser solution 0,25 mg (diluted to 5 ml with normal saline) 4 hourly

ISONIAZID (INH)

Indications:
- Treatment of tuberculosis (in combination with other agents).
- Prophylaxis of tuberculosis

Contraindications:

- Pre-existing liver disease
- Alcohol abuse
- Previous hypersensitivity reactions to INH
- Pregnancy (unless CD4 count <100)

Adverse effects:
- Hepatotoxicity.
- Neurotoxicity that presents mainly as peripheral neuropathy and ataxia; reversed by pyridoxine administration.
- Skin rashes occur in a small percentage of patients, including acne.

Drug interactions:
- Anti-epileptic drugs e.g. phenytoin, carbamazepine and theophylline: plasma levels are increased and dosage may need to be reduced
- Aluminium containing antacids: diminished absorption of INH; patients should be advised to take the agents 2 hours apart.

Dose:
Tuberculosis
- *Adults*: 5 mg/kg/day in a single dose: maximum 300 mg/day
- *Children*: 5-10 mg/kg/day: maximum 300 mg/day

Prophylaxis (monotherapy)
- 5 mg/kg/day: maximum 300 mg/day (adults)
- 10 mg/kg/day: maximum 300 mg/day (children)

ISOSORBIDE

Indications: Relief and prophylaxis of angina

Contraindications:
Aortic stenosis, mitral stenosis

Adverse effects:
Headache, transient flushing, tachycardia

Dose:
- *Pain:* Sublingual 5 mg every 5-10 minutes as needed to a maximum of 4 tablets.
- *Acute pulmonary oedema:* sublingual 5 mg immediately and repeat every 5-10 minutes if needed.

LAMIVUDINE (3TC)

Therapeutic action: Nucleoside reverse transcriptase inhibitor

Indications:
Used in HIV infection in combination with at least two other antiretroviral drugs.

Adverse effects:
- Generally well tolerated
- Nausea, vomiting, abdominal pain
- Pancreatitis

Dose:
- *Adults:* 150 mg 12 hourly or 300 mg daily
- *Children:* 4 mg/kg 12 hourly

LAMOTRIGINE (Lamictin)

Indications:
- Partial epilepsy with or without secondary generalised tonic-clonic seizures
- Primary generalised tonic-clonic seizures
- Preferred antiepileptic drug in adult HIV-infected patients on ARV therapy because of fewer significant interactions

Contraindications: Impaired kidney or liver function

Adverse effects:
- Skin rashes, usually maculopapular and manifesting within 4 weeks of initiating therapy
    - occasionally progressing to severe hypersensitivity reactions e.g. Stevens-Johnson syndrome
- Blurred vision, nystagmus, dizziness, drowsiness
- Headache, ataxia, irritability, aggression, tremor

Drug interaction:
- Drugs which induce hepatic enzymes e.g. carbamazepine, phenytoin, lopinavir/ ritonavir
    - metabolism of lamotrigine significantly increased with decreased plasma levels and half-life
- No interaction with oral contraceptives reported

Adult dose:
- Initially 25 mg daily for 2 weeks
    - then 50 mg daily for 2 weeks
- Thereafter increased by up to 50 mg every 2 weeks according to response
- Usual maintenance dose: 100-200 mg daily as a single dose.
- When switching to lamotrigine from other anti-epileptic drugs:
    - the dose of lamotrigine is titrated up at 2-weekly intervals as above
    - once a maintenance dose is reached, the other anti-convulsant can be stopped
- Patients on lopinarir / ritonavir - initial dose and subsequent dose increases will need to be doubled

LANSOPRAZOLE (Lanzor)

Therapeutic action: Proton pump inhibitor that suppresses gastric acid secretion

Indications:
- Management of peptic ulcer disease and gastro-oesophageal reflux
- Long-term prevention of relapse of gastro-oesophageal reflux disease (GORD)

Contraindications:
- Severe liver disease

Adverse effects:
- Diarrhoea, headache and skin rashes

Dose:
- 30 mg once daily for 2 weeks
- Long-term management of reflux oesophagitis: 15 mg daily

LEVONORGESTREL (Norlevo)

Indications: Prevention of pregnancy following unprotected intercourse

Adverse effects:
- Headache and migraine may occur

Dose:
- 1.5 mg (2 levonorgestrel 0.75 mg tablets) as a single dose taken as soon as possible
    - preferably within 72 hours of unprotected intercourse
    - not more than 5 days later

LOPERAMIDE (Imodium, Gastron)

Therapeutic action: antipropulsive

Indications: Acute and chronic diarrhoea e.g. HIV/AIDS patients.

Contraindications:
- Dysentery
- Dehydration

- Children and the elderly

Adverse effects:
Fluid retention in the bowel (due to reduced peristalsis) may mask and aggravate dehydration.

Adult dose:
- Acute diarrhoea, oral, initially 4 mg followed by 2 mg after each loose stool until diarrhoea is controlled.
    - maximum 12 mg / 24 hours
- Chronic diarrhoea, usually 4-8 mg daily in divided doses.
- If no response occurs within 10 days, treatment is unlikely to be effective.

LOPINAVIR / RITONAVIR (Kaletra, Aluvia)

Therapeutic action: Protease inhibitor

Indications: Treatment of HIV infection in combination with at least 2 other anti-retroviral medicines.

Medicine interactions:
As a result of enzyme induction by rifampicin:
- In children with combined TB and HIV initiated on, or already taking, LPV/r, add extra ritonavir to boost the dose (1:1).
- Adults co-infected with HIV and TB, the dose of LPV/r should be doubled slowly over 2 weeks (to 800 / 200 mg twice a day).

Adverse effects:
- Diarrhoea occurs frequently.
- Lipodystrophy and metabolic disorders - high potential.
- Elevated serum transaminases.

Dose:
Adults: Lopinavir 400 mg + ritonavir 100 mg 12 hourly with food.

MEBENDAZOLE (Vermox)

Therapeutic action: Anthehmintic

Indications:
Roundworm (Ascaris), pinworm (threadworm), whipworm, hookworm

Contraindications:
- Pregnancy and lactation
- Side effects are uncommon with doses recommended for intestinal worms

Dose:
- *Adults and children over 2 years*: 500 mg as a single oral dose
- *Children 1-2 years*: 100 mg (5 ml) 2 x daily for 3 days

MEDROXYPROGESTERONE (Provera, Depo-provera)

Indications:
- Depo-progesterone for hormonal contraception
- Menopausal symptoms
- Endometriosis
- Secondary amenorrhoea

Precautions and contraindications:
- Undiagnosed vaginal bleeding
- Neoplasm of the breast or genital tract
- Acute or chronic liver disease
- Arterial thrombosis (myocardial infarction or stroke)
- Use with care in patients with depression

Adverse effects:
- Heavy or prolonged menstrual bleeding, irregular menses, spotting or amenorrhoea occur frequently
- Breast tenderness
- Bloated abdomen
- Mood changes

Drug interactions:
- Not affected by antibiotics
- Enzyme-inducing drugs, eg. anti-epileptics, increase the rate of metabolism and reduce the efficacy of medroxyprogesterone.

METFORMIN (Glucophage)

Therapeutic action: Biguanide oral hypoglycaemic drug

Indications: Type 2 diabetes mellitus

Contraindications:
Avoid in patients with severe kidney (eGFR < 30 ml/min) impairment, severe liver disease, uncontrolled heart failure, alcoholism and pancreatitis.

Adverse effects:
- GIT disturbances eg. anorexia, diarrhoea are common but usually short term
- Lactic acidosis usually only occurs if there are predisposing factors (see contraindications)
    - symptoms include nausea, vomiting, hyperventilation, malaise, abdominal pain

Drug interaction:
Increased risk of lactic acidosis with the simultaneous use of alcohol

Dose:
- Initially 500-850 mg once daily
- Increase by 500-850 mg at monthly intervals if required
- Maximum dose: 850 mg 3 x daily
    - 850 mg 2 x daily in patients predisposed to lactic acidosis e.g. alcoholism, pancreatitis

METHYLDOPA (Aldomet)

Therapeutic action:
- Centrally-acting antihypertensive drug - as a sympathetic blocking agent
- Usage has declined as it impairs the quality of life

Indications: Hypertension in pregnancy and during lactation

Contraindications:
- Avoid in patients with hepatic disease, a history of mental depression or Parkinson's disease.
- Use with caution in moderate or severe alcoholism.

Adverse effects:
- Can cause fatigue, drowsiness, dry mouth, nasal congestion, postural hypotension and dizziness.
- Drowsiness may disappear with continued administration.
- Other effects include depression, decreased libido and impotence and decreased ability for mental concentration and decision making.

Drug interactions:
NSAIDs and tricyclic anti-depressants may reduce the efficacy of methyldopa.

Dose:
- Initially 250 mg 3 x daily
- Increase to 500 mg 3 x daily after 1-2 weeks if necessary
- Maximum dose 750 mg 3 x daily

METOCLOPRAMIDE (Maxolon)

Therapeutic action:
- Enhances gut motility (movement)

- Anti-emetic

Indications:
- Reflux oesophagitis
- Nausea and vomiting associated with conditions such as gastrointestinal infection, drug-induced conditions including cancer chemotherapy and uraemia
- Hiccoughs (Hiccups)

Contraindications:
Avoid in patients with epilepsy, Parkinson's disease or mechanical bowel obstruction.

Adverse effects:
- Drowsiness and fatigue
- May cause extra-pyramidal side effects particularly in children, young adults and the elderly. Dystonic reactions eg. trismus, opisthotonus and torticollis are more common in children and young adults.

Drug interactions:
- The sedative effects are increased by alcohol.
- The risk of extra-pyramidal side effects is increased if antipsychotic agents eg. phenothiazines are used at the same time.

Dose: *Adults:* 10 mg 3 x daily

METRONIDAZOLE (Flagyl)

Therapeutic action: Anti-protozoal and anti-bacterial agent

Indications:
Anaerobic infection including: salpingitis, chronic leg ulcers, necrotising ulcerative gingivitis, peritonsillar abscess, giardiasis and trichomoniasis

Precautions and contraindications:
- Use with caution during lactation, and only if esential. Breast feeding should be withheld for 48 hours after single dose therapy.
- Not to be used with alcohol.
- Avoid in patients with active CNS disorders or blood dyscrasias.
- Giardiasis
- Trichomoniasis

Adverse effects:
- Nausea, anorexia, headache and a metallic taste in the mouth
- May have an "antabuse-like" action when alcohol is used at the same time.

Dose:
- *Adults and adolescents over 15 years*:
  - *anaerobic infection*: 400 mg 3 x daily usually for 7 days
  - *urogenital trichomoniasis and bacterial vaginosis*: 2 g as a single oral dose (avoid in the first trimester of pregnancy)
  - *giardiasis*: 2 g daily for 3 days
- *Children with dental abscess, animal and human bites*:
  - 7.5 mg / kg / dose 3 x daily
- *Children under 12 years with giardiasis and urogenital trichomoniasis*:
  - 1-3 years 500 mg/day
  - 3-7 years 600-800 mg/day
  - 7-10 years 1 g/day
  - **for 3 days** for giardiasis
  - **as a single dose** for trichomoniasis

MIDAZOLAM (Dormicum)

Therapeutic action: Anticonvulsant, sedative and anxiolytic

Indications:
- Anxiety states
- Buccally or intramuscularly to stop status epilepticus
- Orally or intramuscularly in adults with:
  - acute confusion and aggressive, disruptive behaviour in adults
  - acute psychosis
  - manic episodes in bipolar mood disorder

Precautions:
Use with caution in the elderly or debilitated patients.

Adverse effects:
- Drowsiness and over-sedation, particularly in the elderly

Dose:
- *Oral*: 7.5-15 mg, preferably at bedtime
  - 7.5 mg in the elderly or debilitated
- *Buccally in status epilepticus in children*:
  - 0.5 mg/kg/dose as a single dose
  - use midazolam for injection 5 mg in 1 ml
  - administer into the buccal cavity (between gum and cheeks on the dependent side)

  Note: Buccal midazolam should not be used in infants <6 months of age
- *IM in status epilepticus, acute confusional states, aggression*:
  - adults: 10 mg as a single dose

NEVIRAPINE (NVP)

Therapeutic action:
Non-nucleoside reverse transcriptase inhibitor

Indications:
Used to treat HIV infection in combination with at least two other antiretroviral drugs, and for prevention of mother-to-child transmission in HIV infected patients.

Precautions:
Hepatic and renal impairment

Adverse effects:
- *Hepatotoxicity* (potentially life-threatening) usually occurring in first 8 weeks: monitor liver function every 2 weeks for 2 months, then every 6 months
  - discontinue if significant liver function abnormalities occur.
- *Rash* (including Stevens Johnson syndrome) usually in the first 8 weeks: discontinue if severe rash or if accompanied by mucosal involvement or fever
- Fever, nausea, headache

Dose:
- *Adults:* 200 mg once daily for first 14 days, then (if no rash present) 200 mg twice daily.
- *Prevention of mother-to-child transmission:*
  - expectant mother 200 mg as a single dose at onset of labour, only if not on ART (whether for treatment or prophylaxis)
  - baby: 4 mg/kg daily for 6 or 12 weeks, depending on relevant risk to the infant for contracting HIV from the mother.

NICOTINAMIDE (VITAMIN B3)

Indications: Pellagra

Dose: *Adults and children:* 100 mg daily

NORDETTE

Therapeutic action: Combined oral contraceptive

Indications:
- Contraception
- Dysfunctional uterine bleeding
- Dysmenorrhoea
- Premenstrual tension
- Secondary amenorrhoea

Contraindications, adverse effects and drug interactions:
As for combined oral contraceptive

Dose:
- *Contraception:* One pill taken at the same time every day
- *Dysfunctional uterine bleeding:*
  - one active pill taken 3 x daily for 1 week
  - then daily (including placebos in the pack) for 3-6 months
  - only the once daily dose is necessary if the bleeding is mild

NYSTATIN (Mycostatin)

Therapeutic action: Antifungal active against Candida albicans and other candida species

Indications:
Monilial infections of the mouth, GIT, vagina and skin

Dose:
Liquid: 1 ml 4 x daily as a mouth rinse and to swallow

OESTROGEN CONJUGATED

Indications:
- Hormone replacement therapy in peri- and postmenopausal women to relieve symptoms
- To prevent and possibly treat the long-term effects of the menopause

Contraindications:
- Oestrogen-sensitive malignancies such as breast and endometrial carcinoma
- Deep vein thrombosis and pulmonary embolus
- Active liver disease
- Abnormal uterine bleeding

Dose:
- *Oral:* 0.3-0.625 mg daily

Treatment should be reviewed annually. If it has been stopped and symptoms recur, resume treatment. The average duration of menopausal symptoms is about 5 years. In women with intact uteri the addition of a progestogen is needed (cyclically for 10 days every 3 weeks).

ORPHENADRINE (Disipal)

Therapeutic action: Anticholinergic agent

Indications:
- Parkinson's disease
- Drug-induced parkinsonism

Precautions and contraindications:
- Should be avoided in patients with urinary retention or closed angle glaucoma.
- Should be used with caution in patients with heart failure, prostatic hypertrophy, ischaemic heart disease or hiatus hernia.

Adverse effects:
- Dry mouth
- Blurred vision
- Tachycardia
- Constipation
- Urinary retention

Dose: 50 mg 2 x daily

PARACETAMOL (Panado)

Therapeutic action: Analgesic and antipyretic

Indications: Fever or mild to moderate pain

Contraindications: Avoid in liver disease

Dose:
- *Adults and adolescents over 14 years:* 1 000 mg (2 tabs) 3-4 x daily
- *Children:*
  - under 1 year: 2.5 ml 3-4 x daily
  - 1-5 years: 5 ml 3-4 x daily
  - 5-8 years: 10 ml 3-4 x daily
  - 8-14 years: 1 tab 3-4 x daily

PENICILLIN

Therapeutic action: Narrow-spectrum bacteriocidal antibiotic

Indications:
- Streptococcal tonsillitis/pharyngitis
- Syphilis and meningococcal meningitis
- Rheumatic fever prophylaxis

Contraindications: Penicillin-allergic patients

Adverse effects:
- Hyper-sensitivity reactions are common although most are not serious
  - the most frequent skin manifestations are urticarial or erythematous rashes or pruritis
  - erythema multiforme or the Stevens Johnson syndrome may occur occasionally.
- Serious anaphylactic reactions are more common with parenteral than oral penicillins.
- Toxic reactions to procaine may be shown by transient psychiatric disturbances, muscle twitching, seizures and cardio-respiratory problems (not anaphylaxis).

Dose:

Phenoxymethylpenicillin (penicillin VK)
- 1-9 years: 250 mg 2 x daily for 10 days
- 10 years and older: 500 mg 2 x daily for 10 days

Benzathine penicillin IM
- *Early syphilis:* 2.4 MU immediately as a single dose
- *Latent and late syphilis:* 2.4 MU once weekly for 3 weeks
- *Newborn exposed to syphilis in pregnancy:* 0.3 MU immediately as a single dose injected into the lateral thigh

PERMETHRIN (5% lotion)

Indications: Scabies and pediculosis

Contraindications: Pregnancy and lactation

Application:
- *Pediculosis capitus:*
  - apply lotion to towel-dried or dry hair
  - comb into hair repeatedly to cover all areas for ½ an hour while rinsing or wiping comb frequently
  - after combing wash permethrin lotion out with normal shampoo

- procedure should be repeated every 5 days for 3 weeks
- *Scabies:*
  - apply to the whole body from the neck to the feet
  - leave on overnight and wash off the next morning
  - repeat treatment after 1 week

PHENOBARBITONE

Indications: Epilepsy and convulsions, mainly in neonates and infants

Contraindications: Avoid in hyperactive children

Dose:
Children:
- *Epilepsy under 6 months of age*
  - 3.5-5 mg/kg at night
- *Convulsions (if no response to rectal diazepam)*
  - 20 mg/kg, oral by nasogastric tube, as a single dose

NB. Half life of 36 hours, so given only **once** daily

PHENYTOIN (Epanutin)

Indications:
- Generalised tonic-clonic seizures
- Complex and simple partial seizures
- Control of status epilepticus after initial control with diazepam

Contraindications: Dangerous in the porphyrias

Adverse effects:
- Coarsening of the facial features and gum hypertrophy (particularly in young individuals)
- Skin rashes, acne and hirsutism
- Can cause lethargy, ataxia, tremor, slurred speech and anaemia

Drug interactions:
- Phenytoin and phenobarb affect the elimination of one another.
- Induces liver enzymes and enhances metabolism of oral contraceptives, warfarin, doxycycline and furosemide.
- Sulphonamides increase phenytoin levels in the plasma.

Dose:
- *Adults:* 5 mg / kg / day
  NB. Half life of 24 hours, so only given **once** daily
- *Usual maintenance dose:* 300 mg at night
- *Loading dose in status epilepticus:*
  - 18 mg / kg IV by slow infusion in normal saline
  - rate of administration should not exceed 50 mg / min.
- Alternatively if the patient is conscious, an oral loading dose of 15-20 mg/kg can be given, divided into 3 doses, administered 2 hours apart.

POTASSIUM CHLORIDE (Slow-K)

Indications:
- Used to prevent or treat hypo-kalaemia.
- Mainly used together with furosemide in the treatment of heart failure.

Precautions and contraindications:
- Use with caution in patients with renal impairment and peptic ulcer disease.
- Contra-indicated in moderate or severe kidney failure.

Adverse effects:
Mainly GIT disturbance eg. epigastric pain, nausea and diarrhoea

Drug interactions:
Hyper-kalaemia may occur if potassium supplements are prescribed together with ACE-inhibitors or potassium sparing diuretics eg. spironolactone.

Dose:
- According to individual requirements
  - usual range 1-2 tabs
    2 x daily after meals.

POVIDONE IODINE (Betadine)

Therapeutic action:
Antiseptic (bacteriocidal, fungicidal and antiviral)

Indications: Skin infection, wounds, burns, chronic leg ulcers

Precautions and contraindications:
- Avoid in patients with non-toxic nodular goitre.
- Caution should be observed when applying to large areas of damaged skin because of possible systemic toxicity.

Adverse effects:
Local irritation if applied to surrounding healthy skin.

Application:
- Apply povidone iodine after cleaning the affected area.
- Apply sufficient to cover the affected area only.

PRAZIQUANTEL (Biltricide)

Indications:
- Treatment of choice for bilharzia
- Also used for intestinal tapeworm infestation, as well as cysticercosis

Precautions:
- Patients with cysticercosis are best treated in hospital.
- Treatment may result in the development of reactive cerebral oedema in patients with cerebral cysticercosis.

Adverse effects:
Malaise, headache, drowsiness and dizziness

Dose:
- *S. haematobium and mansoni:* 40 mg / kg in a single dose
- *Intestinal tapeworm:* 10 mg / kg as a single dose

PREDNISONE (Meticortin)

Indications *(clinic uses)*:
- Suppression of allergic and inflammatory disorders
- Moderate or severe asthmatic attack
- Inflammatory bowel disease
- Drug reactions

Precautions and contraindications:
- These are few with any short course (5-10 days)
- Avoid in active or suspected tuberculosis, mental instability, epilepsy or peptic ulcer disease.

Adverse effects:
- These are few with any short course (5-10 days)
- Acute reactions which might occur with high doses are:
  - hyperglycaemia
  - psychiatric reaction
  - worsening of epilepsy
  - peptic ulceration

Drug interaction:
The risk of peptic ulceration is increased if prednisone and the NSAIDs (including aspirin) are used together.

Dose:

Adults
- *Short course prednisone:* 40 mg daily for 7 days
  - there is no need to taper off the dose

Children: 1-2 mg / kg / daily for 7 days up to a maximum of 40 mg / day

PROMETHAZINE (Phenergan)

Therapeutic action:
Antihistamine with anti-emetic and marked sedative properties

Indications:
- Allergic conditions such as urticaria and angio-oedema
- Acute anaphylaxis
- Used to enhance sedation in acute psychosis
- Nausea and vomiting
- Prevention and treatment of motion sickness

Precautions and contraindications:
- Children are prone to paradoxical CNS stimulation with possible dystonic reactions, hallucinations and seizures
- Not recommended in children under 2 years.

Adverse effects:
- Drowsiness
- Paradoxical stimulation may occur in children eg. nervousness, restlessness, seizures, hallucinations

Dose:

Severe allergic reactions and anaphylaxis
- *Adults:*
  - 25-50 mg IMI or slow IVI
- *Children:*
  - under 2 years: not recommended
  - 2-5 years: 5 mg (0.2 ml)
  - 5-8 years: 10 mg (0.4 ml)
  - 8-12 years: 15 mg (0.6 ml)
  - over 12 years: 20 mg (0.8 ml)

PYRIDOXINE (Vitamin B6)

Indications:
- Prophlaxis and treatment of INH-induced peripheral neuropathy

Prophylaxis dose:
- *Adults:* 25 mg daily
- *Children:* 12.5 mg daily

Treatment dose:
- 50-200 mg daily for 3 weeks then 12.5-25 mg daily as a maintenance dose.

RIFAMPICIN

Indications:
- Treatment of tuberculosis (in combination with other agents)
- Leprosy

Drug interactions:
Phenytoin, theophylline, warfarin, sulphonylureas, oral contraceptives, digoxin, beta-blockers and verapamil may be less effective if taken with rifampicin.

Adverse effects:
- Hepatotoxicity
- Gastrointestinal upsets
  - nausea, vomiting and diarrhoea
- Urine coloured reddish-orange to reddish-brown
- Drowsiness, headache

Dose:
- 10 mg / kg in a single daily dose
- Maximum 600 mg / day

SALBUTAMOL (Ventolin, Venteze)

Therapeutic action: Beta-2 stimulant bronchodilator

Indications: Asthma, chronic bronchitis

Precautions:
Use with caution in patients with cardiac arrhythmias, ischaemic heart disease, heart failure and hyperthyroidism

Adverse effects: Fine tremor, headache, dizziness

Dose:
- *Adults and children over 10 years:*
  - aerosol inhalation 2 puffs (200 micrograms) 3 x daily as required
- *Children:*
  - under 10 years: aerosol inhalation 1 puff (100 micrograms) 3 x daily as required

SALMETEROL (Serevent)

Therapeutic action: Long-acting beta-2 stimulant bronchodilator (LABA)

Indications: Asthma, chronic bronchitis

Precautions:
- As for salbutamol
- Should be used in conjunction with inhaled corticosteroid therapy e.g. fluticasone with salmeterol (Seretide).
- Not suitable for relief of the acute attack as the onset of action is delayed.

Adverse effects: As for salbutamol and beclomethazone

Dose:
- *Adults and children over 8 years:*
  - salmeterol / fluticasone aerosol inhalation 2 puffs (50/250 mcg) 2 x daily
- *Children under 8 years:*
  - salmeterol / fluticasone aerosol inhalation 1 puff (25/125 mcg) 2 x daily

SELENIUM SULPHIDE (Selsun)

Therapeutic action: Antifungal and anti-seborrhoeic

Indications: Dandruff, seborrhoeic dermatitis, tinea versicolor

Application:
- *Dandruff:* use weekly; apply to wet hair and leave for 10 minutes; rinse off thoroughly.
- *Tinea versicolor:* lather on affected areas and leave for 30 minutes; use daily for 3 days only
  - or leave on overnight once a week for 3 weeks

SENNOSIDES A + B (Senokot)

Therapeutic action:
Irritant laxatives that stimulate colon motility (movement)

Indications: Constipation

Precautions and contraindications:
- Avoid in children and in patients with abdominal pain.
- Use only for short periods.

Adverse effects:
- Abdominal cramps
- Long term use may result in loss of normal bowel function with atony and laxative dependence
- Electrolyte disturbance including hypo-kalaemia, hypo-calcaemia

Dose: 2-4 tabs daily

SPIRONOLACTONE (Aldactone)

Therapeutic action: Diuretic and aldosterone antagonist

Indications:
- Resistant hypertension
- Cirrhosis with ascites and oedema
- Nephrotic syndrome
- Conjestive heart failure

Contraindications: Avoid in patients with renal impairment

Adverse effects:
- Hyperkalaemia usually associated with renal impairment and the use of potassium supplements or ACE-inhibitors
- Gynaecomastia (usually reversible), erectile dysfunction, loss of libido, menstrual irregularities.

Drug interaction:
Risk of hyper-kalaemia if an ACE-inhibitor or potassium supplements are used together with spironolactone.

Dose:
Resistant hypertension: 25 mg daily in combination with other antihypertensive medicines
- *Congestive heart failure:* 25 mg daily used after furosemide and an ACE-inhibitor.
- Provided the dose of furosemide is small or moderate there is usually no need to use Slow-K supplementation because of the potassium sparing properties of spironolactone.

TENOFOVIR (TDF)

Therapeutic action: Nucleotide reverse transcriptase inhibitor

Indications:
- The treatment of HIV infection in combination with at least 2 other anti-retroviral drugs.
- Tenofovir together with lamivudine or emtricitabine is recommended for hepatitis B co-infected patients.

Precautions:
- Renal impairment
- Severe acute exacerbation of hepatitis B on discontinuation of treatment

Drug interactions:
- Concurrent use with other nephrotoxic agents should be avoided.

Adverse effects:
- Nephrotoxic and can cause renal impairment (including acute kidney failure).
- Creatinine clearance should be calculated before initiation and 3-6 monthly thereafter.

Dose: *Adults:* 300 mg once daily

THIAMINE (Vitamin B1)

Indications:
- Beriberi cardiomyopathy
- Peripheral neuritis due to alcoholism and nutritional deficiencies
- Wernicke's encephalopathy

Precautions:
IV thiamine may cause a severe allergic reaction with
- Angio-oedema or respiratory distress
- Hypotension
- Vascular collapse

Dose: Usual dose 100 mg by mouth daily

TILIDINE (Valoron)

Therapeutic action: Opiate analgesic

Indications:
- Severe pain eg. burns
- As a pre-med for a procedure eg. incision and drainage, suturing

Contraindications: Avoid in infants under 1 year

Dose:
- *Children:* 1 drop for each year of age plus 2 drops to maximum 10 drops 3-4 x daily
  - not recommended for infants less than 1 year old
- Action can be reversed with
  - naloxone (Narcan) 0,01 mg / kg IVI up to maximum of 0,2 mg
  - repeat if necessary at 2-3 minute intervals

TRAMADOL

Therapeutic action:
Opiate analgesic

Indications:
- Moderate to severe pain e.g. burns, post-herpetic neuralgia

Contraindications:
Head injuries or increased intracranial pressure

Dose:
Adults:
- 50-100 mg 4 x daily
- Average dose: 50 mg 4 x daily
- Maximum 400 mg / day (elderly 300 mg / day)

UNG EMULSIFICANS (UE)

Indications:
- To moisturise the skin
- Mild eczema

Application: Apply 2 x daily or as often as necessary

UNG METHYL SALICYLATE (UMS)

Therapeutic action:
- Symptomatic relief of rheumatic and musculoskeletal pain
- Counter-irritant

Indications:
- Pain of arthritis and soft tissue rheumatism
- UMS is preferable to the NSAIDs if, by using, it can decrease the amount of NSAID used.

Cautions: Should not be applied to inflamed or damaged skin.

Application: Massage gently into affected areas 2-3 x daily.

VALPROATE

Indications:
- Generalised tonic-clonic seizures
- Simple and complex absence seizures (petit mal)
- Myoclonic and atonic seizures
- Preferred antiepileptic drug in HIV-infected children on ARV therapy because of fewer drug interactions
- Maintenance therapy following manic episodes of bipolar mood disorder

Contraindications:
- Should not be used in women of child-bearing age
- Female children on valproate should be switched to lamotrigine when they reach child-bearing age

Adverse effects:
- Nausea, vomiting, diarrhoea and constipation
- CNS effects (dose-related) - fatigue, ataxia, dysarthria
- Increased risk of congenial defects and developmental disorders in children

Drug interactions:
- Valproate may function as a hepatic enzyme inhibitor
    - metabolism of lamotrigine significantly reduced requiring reduction in lamotrigine dosage
    - serum levels of zidovudine are increased and may result in toxicity (severe anaemia)

Dose:
Adult (males only):
- Initially 300 mg 2 x daily
- If seizures are not controlled, increase by 100 mg 2 x daily at 2-weekly/monthly intervals
- Usual maintenance range 1-2 g/day

Children:
- Initially 7.5-10 mg/kg 12 hourly increasing according to response
- Maximum dose 15 mg/kg 12 hourly

VITAMIN K (Konakion)

Indications:
- Warfarin induced hypothrombinaemia
- Prophylaxis and treatment of haemorrhagic disease of the newborn
- Epistaxis in alcoholics

Dose:
- *Vitamin K deficiency and reversal of warfarin effect:*
    - IMI 1-3 mg if there is no bleeding; 5 mg IVI if there is haemorrhage injected into the IV line during an infusion of normal saline
    - resistance to oral anticoagulants may persist for as long as 2 weeks after administration of Vitamin K. If warfarin is to be continued, it is preferable to withdraw the anticoagulant temporarily and not to administer Vitamin K.
- *Neonates:* 1 mg IMI immediately after delivery.
- *Life threatening haemorrhage:* Fresh frozen plasma should be infused in addition to Vitamin K.

ZIDOVUDINE (AZT)

Therapeutic action: Nucleoside reverse transcriptase inhibitor

Indications:
- Used in HIV infection in combination with at least two other antiretroviral drugs
- Post-exposure prophylaxis

Contraindications:
- Neutropaenia
- Low haemoglobin

Precautions:
- Anaemia (mainly macrocytic) usually occurs after 4-6 weeks of therapy.
    - full blood counts are recommended at baseline
    - then monthly for the first 3 months
    - then 6 monthly.
- Oesophageal ulceration may occur unless adequate fluid is taken with the oral dose.

Adverse effects:
- Anaemia
- Neutropaenia, leucopaenia
- Nausea, headache, myalgia
- Insomnia
- Rarely lactic acidosis (stop treatment)
- Hepatoxicity

Dose:
Adults:
- 300 mg 12 hourly

Children:
- See dosage chart

ABBREVIATIONS

3TC	Lamivudine		EE	Ethinyloestradiol
AA	Alcoholics Anonymous Phone no. 086 143 5722		EEG	Electro-Encephalogram
			EFV	Efavirenz
ABO	Blood Grouping		ENT	Ear, Nose and Throat
ACE	Angiotensin Converting Enzyme (inhibitors)		ESR	Erythrocyte Sedimentation Rate
AFB	Acid-Fast Bacilli		ET	Endotracheal Tube
AGN	Acute Glomerulonephritis		EUA	Examination Under Anaesthetic
AIDS	Acquired Immune Deficiency Syndrome		EUM	External Urethral Meatus
ALT	Alanine Aminotransferase		FB	Foreign Body
ANC	Antenatal Clinic		FBC	Full Blood Count
APH	Ante Partum Haemorrhage		FHR	Foetal Heart Rate
ARC	AIDS Related Complex		FSH	Follicle Stimulating Hormone
AROM	Artificial Rupture of Membranes		FTA	Fluorescent Treponemal Antigen (for syphilis)
AZT	Zidovudine (for AIDS)		FTC	Emtricitabine
BG	Blood Glucose		g	Grams
BHCG	Beta Human Chorio-Gonadotrophin (Beta HG)		GA	General Anaesthetic
BOM	Burning on Micturition		GE	Gastroenteritis
BP	Blood Pressure		GIT	Gastrointestinal Tract
CCF	Congestive Heart failure (biventricular failure)		GPI	General Paralysis of the Insane
CD4	Lymphocyte cells		GTT	Glucose Tolerance Test
CMI	Cell Mediated Immunity		HAV	Hepatitis A Virus
CMV	Cytomegalo Virus		Hb	Haemoglobin
CNS	Central Nervous System		HBV	Hepatitis B Virus
COAD	Chronic Obstructive Airway Disease (same as COPD)		HELLP	Haemolysis, Elevated, Liver Enzymes, and Low Platelet count (syndrome)
CPR	Cardiopulmonary Resuscitation		HIV	Human Immuno Deficiency Virus
CSF	Cerebro Spinal Fluid		HPV	Human Papilloma Virus
CTG	Cardiotocography		I&D	Incision and Drainage
CVA	Cerebro Vascular Accident		IBS	Irritable Bowel Syndrome
CVS	Cardiovascular System		IBW	Ideal Body Weight
d4T	Stavudine		IDDM	Insulin Dependent Diabetes Mellitus
D&C	Dilatation and Curettage		IMI	Intramuscular Injection
DBP	Diastolic Blood Pressure		INH	Isoniazid
DC	Direct Current (electric-shock)		iu	International units
DD&C	Diagnostic Dilatation and Curettage		IUCD	Intra-Uterine Contraceptive Device
ddI	Didanosine		IUD	Intra-Uterine Death
DIP	Distal Inter-Phalangeal (joints)		IUGR	Intra-Uterine Growth Retardation
DOT	Directly Observed Therapy		IV	Intravenous
DPT	Diphtheria Pertussis Tetanus (Vaccine)		IVI	Intravenous Injection
DVT	Deep Venous Thrombosis		IVP	Intravenous Pyelogram
D/W	Dextrose Water		JVP	Jugular Venous Pressure
EBM	Expressed Breast Milk		KCl	Potassium Chloride
ECG	Electro-Cardiogram		KOH	Potassium Hydroxide
ECV	External Cephalic Version		LAP	Lower Abdominal Pain

LG	Levonorgestrel	PTB	Pulmonary Tuberculosis
LGV	Lymphogranuloma Venereum	PTSS	Post Traumatic Stress Syndrome
LH	Luteinizing Hormone	PUO	Pyrexia of Unknown Origin
LMP	Last Menstrual Period	PV	Per Vagina
LPC	Liquor Picis Carbonis (coal tar)	PVD	Per Vaginal Discharge
LPV/r	Lopinavir/ritonavir	PZA	Pyrazinamide
LTB	Laryngotracheo-Bronchitis	RAST	Radio Allergy Absorbent Test
LVF	Left Ventricular Failure	RDS	Respiratory Distress Syndrome
MAST	Medical Anti-Shock Trousers	Rh	Rhesus Factor
MC&S	Microscopic Culture and Sensitivity	RIF	Right Iliac Fossa
mcg	Micrograms	RPR	Rapid Plasma Reagin (syphilis test)
mg / kg	Milligrams per Kilogram	RVF	Right Ventricular Failure
mill	Million	SAIMR	South African Institute for Medical Research
ml	Millilitres	SAMF	South African Medicines Formulary
mm Hg	Millimetres of Mercury	SANCA	South African National Council on Alcoholism and Drug Dependence Phone no. 011 892 3829
mmol / L	Milli-mol per Litre		
MOH	Medical Officer of Health (local health authority)		
MSU	Mid-Stream Urine specimen	SB	Serum Bilirubin
MP	Metacarpo-Phalangeal (knuckle joints)	SBE	Sub-acute Bacterial Endocarditis
MVA	Motor Vehicle Accident	SBP	Systolic Blood Pressure
NB	Note well	SC	Subcutaneous (injection)
NE	Norethisterone	SFH	Symphysis Fundal Height
NG	Naso Gastric	SGA	Small for Gestational Age (babies)
NIDDM	Non-Insulin Dependent Diabetes Mellitus	stat	Statum (immediately)
NIV	National Institute of Virology	STD	Sexually Transmitted Disease
NSAID	Non-Steroidal Anti-Inflammatory Drug	subcut	Subcutaneous (injection)
NVP	Nevirapine	TB	Tuberculosis
OE	Otitis Externa	TBCo	Tincture of Benzoate Compound
OM	Otitis Media	TDI	Total Dose of Iron
OPD	Outpatient Department	TIA	Transient Ischaemic Attack
ORS	Oral Rehydration Solution	TNT	Glyceryl Trinitrate
PAP	Papanicolaou (cervical smear test)	TPA	Transvaal Provincial Administration
PCP	Pneumocystis Carinii Pneumonia	TPHA	Treponema Pallidum Haemagglutination Test
PCR	Polymerase Chain Reaction	TSH	Thyroid Stimulating Hormone
PEFR	Peak Expiratory Flow Rate	TTO	To Take Out (to take home)
PEM	Protein Energy Malnutrition	U&E	Urea and Electrolytes
PET	Pre-Eclamptic Toxaemia	u	Units
PHCN	Primary Health Care Nurse	UE	Emulsifying Ointment
PHCS	Primary Health Care Sister	UEA	Ung Emulsificans Aquosum (aqueous cream)
PID	Pelvic Inflammatory Disease	ug	Microgram
PIH	Pregnancy Induced Hypertension (also PET)	umol / L	Micro-mol per Litre
PIP	Proximal Inter-Phalangeal (joints)	UMS	Ung Methyl Salicylate (ung meth sal)
PMA	Paraff Molle Alb (white Vaseline)	URTI	Upper Respiratory Tract Infection
PMT	Premenstrual Tension	UTI	Urinary Tract Infection
POP	Plaster of Paris	UV	Ultraviolet (light)
PPD	Purified Protein Derivative	UWGA	Under Weight for Gestational Age
PPH	Post Partum Haemorrhage	VE	Vacuum Extraction
PR	Per Rectum	VL	Viral Load
PROM	Premature Rupture of Membranes	WCC	White Cell Count
PSGN	Post Streptococcal Glomerulonephritis		

INDEX

A

Abdomen 95–101
   anorexia 95
   children 95, 97, 98, 99–101
   colic, baby with 100–101
   constipation 98–99
   diarrhoea 99
   encopresis 100
   gastro-oesophageal reflux disease 101
   haematemesis 95–96
   hiccoughs 101
   incontinence of faeces 99–100
   loss of appetite 95
   nausea 95
   neonates 95, 98, 362–363
   pain 96–98
      burning 97
      chronic/recurrent 98
      colicky 96–97
      epigastric 96
      left iliac fossa 96
      left upper quadrant 96
      lower 179–180
      right iliac fossa 96
      right upper quadrant 96
      severe 97–98
      supra-pubic 96
      umbilical 96
      vague 97
   stab wounds 274–275
   vomiting 95–96
   wall, surgical problems with 285
Abortion *see* Miscarriage
Abrasions 277
Abscesses/pus formation
   Bartholin's 189–190
   breast 204–205
   dental 48
   drainage 280–281
   eye 242
   finger 281
   incisions into 280–281
   ischiorectal 124
   lungs 64
   meibomian 242
   neck 281
   in neck gland 40
   pelvic 198
   perianal 124
   periapical 48
   peritonsillar 43–44
   pilonidal 126
   pre-patellar 321
   quinsy 43–44
   retro-pharyngeal 45
   sebaceous 282
   septic arthritis 297
   submucous, of anal canal 124
   surgery 279–281
   toe 281
Absence seizures (petit mal) 214
Abuse
   alcohol 71, 228, 378
   analgesic 220
   child 193–195
   drugs 13–14, 377–378
   enemas 110, 123
   laxatives 123
   substance-related disorders 377–378
ACE-inhibitors (Angiotensin Converting Enzyme inhibitors)
   diabetes mellitus 131, 136
   enalapril (Renitec) 386
   heart disease 85
   heart failure 83, 84
   hypertension 73–74, 76–79
   kidney disease 150

Achilles
   bursitis 325
   para-tendonitis of tendon 324
Acne vulgaris 261–262
Acquired Immune Deficiency Syndrome *see* AIDS/HIV
Activated charcoal 13
Acute abdomen 105
Acute diarrhoea 99, 110, 158
Acute infection in spine (pyogenic spondylitis) 303
Acute kidney failure 149–150
Acute labyrinthitis 29
Acute lymphadenopathy 40
Acute mastoiditis 28
Acute necrotising ulcerative gingivitis 158
Acute otitis media 25–26, 28
Acute paronychium 281
Acute wry neck 303
Acyclovir 381
Addiction *see* Abuse
Adenoid hypertrophy 44
Adjustment disorder with depressed mood 377
Adnexal swelling 198
Aggressive behaviour 373-374
AIDS/HIV (Acquired Immune Deficiency Syndrome) 155–167
   acute necrotising ulcerative gingivitis 158
   in adults 155–161, 163–165
   antenatal problems 339–340
   antiretroviral therapy
      in adults 163–165
      in children 166–167
      epilepsy 216
   chest infections 156–157
      in children 161–163, 166–167
   chronic mucocutaneous ulceration 46
   cryptococcal meningitis 161
   diagnosis
      in adults 155–156
      in children 162
   diarrhoea 158, 162
   drug reactions 160
   epilepsy 216
   folliculitis 159
   Guillain-Barre Syndrome 161
   hair conditions 159
   headache 160
   health maintenance 156
   herpes simplex chronic mucocutaneous ulceration 159
   herpes zoster 159–160
   high-risk injuries 167
   HIV encephalopathy 161
   immune reconstitution inflammatory syndrome 164
   immunisation 156
   infections 156–161, 162–163, 164
   influenza vaccine 156
   Kaposi's sarcoma 160
   lymphadenopathy 160
   lymphoid interstitial pneumonia 162–163
   mental health 373
   molluscum contagiosum 160
   mother-to-child transmission 165
   mouth 158
   neonatal care 353
   neurological problems 160–161
   oesophageal candidiasis 158
   oral candidiasis 46, 158
   painful peripheral neuropathy 161
   papular pruritic eruption 159
   persistent generalised lymphadenopathy 155
   pneumocystis pneumonia 157, 162
   pneumonia 156–157, 162
   post-exposure HIV prophylaxis 167, 193, 195

   primary HIV infection 155
   prophylaxis 156, 167, 193, 195
   scabies 159
   seborrhoeic dermatitis 159
   seroconversion illness 155
   skin conditions 159
   testing 155, 167
   tuberculosis 156, 157, 162, 165
   viral infections 159–160
   WHO staging 155, 161–162
Airway *see also* upper airways
   babies 6–7
   burns 16
   children 6–7
   CPR 4
   obstruction 6–7
Akineton (biperiden) 375, 383
Albendazole (Zentel) 120, 381
Albinism 263
Alcoholism
   hypertension 71
   mental confusion 228
   withdrawel 378
Aldactone (spironolactone) 84, 395
Aldomet (methyldopa) 390
Allergex (chlorpheniramine) 384
Allergic reactions
   angio-oedema 256–257
   asthma 58
   atopic eczema 259
   children 8
   drug eruptions 258
   eczema 258–260
   endogenous eczema 259
   erythema multiforme 257–258
   erythema nodosum 257
   papular urticaria 257
   rash 248
   resuscitation 7–9
   rhinitis 32
   seborrhoeic dermatitis 259
   severe cutaneous adverse drug reactions 258
   skin 256–260
   Stevens Johnson syndrome 258
   toxic epidermal necrolysis 258
   urticaria 256–257
Allopurinol (Zyloprim) 295, 381
Alpha blockers 74
Aluvia (lopinavir/ritonavir) 390
Amenorrhoea 181–182
Amitriptyline (Tryptanol) 376, 381
Amlodipine (Norvasc) 382
Amoxicillin (Amoxil) 382
Anaemia 338
Analgesia
   abuse 220
   fractures 291
   headache 220
   in labour 346
   musculoskeletal system 290
Anaphylaxis 7–9
Angina pectoris 91–92
Angioedema 78, 256–257
Angiotensin Converting Enzyme inhibitors *see* ACE-inhibitors
Ankle 324
Anorectal conditions 121–126
   abuse of laxatives/enemas 123
   anal fissure 123
   bleeding from anus 121
   bowel habit change 122
   condylomata acuminata 125
   discharge near anus 122
   diseases 123–126
   fistula in ano 125
   haemorrhoids 124–125
   imperforate anus 363
   ischiorectal abscess 124
   itching anus 122

mass 122
painful natal cleft 122
perianal abscess 124
perianal fistula 125
physical examination 123
pilonidal abscess 126
pilonidal sinus 126
protrusion from anus 121
rectal prolapse 125
severe anal pain 121
submucous abscess of anal canal 124
ulcers around anus 122
Anorexia 95
Antenatal care, routine 331–334 see also pregnancy
check list 333
confirmation of pregnancy 331
first visit 331–332
gestational age 331
important aspects to assess 331–332
maternity record 331
normal pregnancy 331
risk factors 332
symphysis-fundal height 333–334
tests 331–332, 334
tetanus toxoid 332
ultrasound scanning 332, 334
urine pregnancy tests 331
visits 333–334
warning signs 332
Antenatal problems 335–343 see also pregnancy
AIDS/HIV 339–340
anaemia 338
antepartum haemorrhage 342
asthma 337
bacterial vaginosis 338
breech presentation 341–342
candidiasis 338
chlamydial cervicitis 338
congenital disorders 342
constipation 335
cystitis 340
diabetes mellitus
gestational 336–337
pre-gestational 337
epilepsy 337
gonorrhoea 338
heartburn (isilungulelo) 335
heart disease 336
hypertension 340–341
joint pain 336
multiple pregnancy 341
muscle pain 336
oedema 336
post-term pregnancy 342
pre-eclampsia 335, 336, 340–341
proteinuria 335
pulmonary tuberculosis 340
pyelonephritis 340
Rapid Plasma Reagin test 339
rashes 336
Rhesus incompatibility 343
sexually transmitted infections 338–340
syphilis 339
trichomoniasis 338
urinary tract infection 335, 340
vaginal discharge 338
varicose veins 336
vomiting 335
vulval warts 338–339
Antepartum haemorrhage (APH) 342
Antihistamine 7, 9
Antiretroviral therapy (ART)
in adults 163–165
in children 166–167
epilepsy and 216
Anus see Anorectal conditions
Anxiety
disorders 373, 378
hypertension 77
Apgar score 359
APH see Antepartum haemorrhage
Aphthous ulcer 45
Appendicitis 105–106
Appetite, loss of see Anorexia
Arc eye 239
Arm 311–316
change in sensation 227

elbow
in adults 313
in children 312–313
golfer's elbow 313
"pulled elbow" 313
supracondylar fracture 313
tennis elbow 313
tenosynovitis 313
finger
abscesses 281
crush injuries 276
extra digits 363
infections 281
swollen/painful 316
thumb pain 316
traumatic amputation of tip 276–277
forearm 313–314
in children 313–314
fractures 314
hand
eczema 259
injuries 276–277
swollen/painful 316
shoulder
bicipital tendonitis 311–312
dislocated 312
dystocia, in labour 347–348
fractured clavicle 312
fractured humerus 312
pain 311
rotator cuff syndrome 311
wrist
in adults 314
carpal tunnel syndrome 315
in children 314
Colles' fractures 314–315
Colles'-like fractures 314–315
De Quervain's tenosynovitis 315–316
ganglion 315
scaphoid fracture 316
ART see Antiretroviral therapy
Arteries 90–92
angina pectoris 91–92
atherosclerosis 90
cerebro vascular disease 90
clinical features 90
coronary artery disease 91–92
heart attack 92
myocardial infarction 92
pain below left breast 91
peripheral vascular disease 90–91
post-myocardial infarction 92
Arthritis
gonococcal 297
osteo- 293–294, 298, 304, 316, 321–322
rheumatoid 295–297, 298
septic 297
Artificial ventilation
babies 359–360
CPR 4
in emergencies 4
Ascabiol (benzyl benzoate) 383
Ascaris (round worm) 119
Asphyxia, birth 358–360
Aspirin (Disprin) **221, 382**
Asthma
antenatal problems 337
bronchial 57–61
acute 60–61
bronchodilators 58
children 59
classification 57
inhalers 59–60
management 57–61
medicine protocol 59–60
nebulisation 61
Atenolol (Tenormin) 382
Atherosclerosis 90
Athlete's foot (tinea pedis) 254
Augmentin (co-amoxiclav) 385
Aura
epilepsy 213–214
migraine 222
Avascular necrosis of hip 317
Azithromycin (Zithromax) 382–383
AZT see Zidovudine

B

Backache
acute 305–308
causes outside spinal column 305
chronic low 308–309
fibrositis 306
fracture of thoracic/lumbar spine 305
ligament damage in lower back 305
lumbar osteoarthritis 308
management 307–308
pelvis and 305
prolapsed intervertebral disc 306–307
slipped disc 306–307
slipped facet joint 306
spondylosis 308
X-rays 302
Bacterial vaginosis
antenatal problems 338
vaginal discharge 174, 191
Bactigras (chlorhexidine tullegras) dressing 275
Bactrim (co-trimoxazole) 385
Balanitis 169–170
genital candidiasis 169
secondary to genital ulceraton 169–170
Bartholin's
abscess 189–190
cyst 190
Beclomethazone 383
Bee stings 14
Bells Palsy 226
Benign paroxysmal positional vertigo (BPPV) 29
Benign prostatic hyperplasia (prostatism) 147
Benzoyl peroxide gel 383
Benzyl benzoate (Ascabiol) 383
Beriberi heart disease 85–86
Beta-blockers, treatment of hypertension 74
Betadine (povidone iodine) 393
Bicipital tendonitis 311–312
Bile duct stones 117
Bilharzia (schistosomiasis) 147–148
Biltricide (praziquantel) 120, 393
Biperiden (Akineton) 375, 383
Bipolar mood disorder 376–377
Biquanides 135
Birth asphyxia 358–360
Bites
animal 11
bee stings 14
human 11
snake 11–12
spider 14
Black hairy tongue 49
Blackout 228–229
Bladder
bilharzia (schistosomiasis) 147–148
cystitis 147
Blisters (bullous disorders) 264–265
Blood glucose management 135–136
Blood pressure see Hypertension
Blood tests, antenatal care 332
Body louse 255
Boil
ear canal furuncle 21–22
skin 250
BOM see Burning on micturition
Bone
diagnosis of orthopaedic problems 289
osteomyelitis 299
osteoporosis 299
Booking patients off work 292
Bowel see also constipation
atresia 363
habit, change of 122
Bow-legs (gonu varum) 323
BPPV see Benign paroxysmal positional vertigo
Bradycardia
CPR 5
hypertension 78
Breast
abscess 204–205
benign breast disease 285–286
blood-stained nipple discharge 205
breast feeding 203
cracked nipples 203
disease in males 286
engorged 204

fibroadenosis 286
gynaecomastia 286
lumps 285
lumps in pregnancy 205
malignant breast disease 286
mastitis 204
nipple discharge 205, 286
pain below left 91
post-pregnancy complications 203–205
surgery 285–286
Breathing, management in emergencies 4
Breech presentation 341–342
Bronchial asthma see Asthma, bronchial
Bronchiectasis 64
Bronchiolitis 56
Bronchitis 55
chronic 61–62
Brudzinski test 221
Brufen (ibuprofen) 388
Bruises (contusions) 277
Budesonide 383
Bullous disorders (blisters) 265
bullous pemphigoid 265
pemphigus vulgaris 265
porphyria 265
staphylococcal scalded skin syndrome 265
Bullous pemphigoid 265
Bumps, surgical 282–283
Bunion 328
Burning on micturition (BOM) 146
Burns 15–16
airway 16
children 15
classification
by depth 15
by extent 15–16
eyes 16, 240
feet 16
full thickness 15
hands 16
head 16
management 15–16
neck 16
partial thickness 15
perineal 16
Rule of Nine's 15–16
specific areas 16
superficial 15
Buscopan (hyoscine) 388

C

Calamine lotion 383
Calcium antagonists, hypertension 74
Calf
cramps 323
injuries to 323
severe pain 323
shin splints 323
Callosities 327
Cancer
carcinoma of cervix 192
carcinoma of oesophagus 103
carcinoma of pancreas 118
carcinoma of stomach 105
malignant breast disease 286
oral 47
pre-cancerous conditions 47
prostatic 147
squamous cell carcinoma 264
Candidiasis 253
antenatal problems 338
genital 169, 175
oesophageal 158
oral 158
Canestin (clotrimazole) 384–385
Caput succedaneum 358
Carbamazepine (Tegretol) 215–216, 383–384
Carbon monoxide poisoning 14
Carbuncle 250–251
Carcinoma
of cervix 192
of oesophagus 103
of pancreas 118
prostatic 264
squamous cell 264
of stomach 105
Cardiac disease see Heart disease

Cardiac failure see Heart failure
Cardiomyopathy 85
Cardiopulmonary resuscitation (CPR) 3–6
artificial ventilation 4
CAB 3–4
children 3
defibrillation 4–5
infants 4
management 3–5
Cardiovascular system 71–92
heart disease 85–87
heart failure 81–87
hypertension 71–80
palpitations 87
vascular disease 89–92
Carpal tunnel syndrome 315
Carvedilol 84
Cataracts 131, 242
Ceftriaxone 384
Cellulitis 250, 279
osteomyelitis 299
septic arthritis 297
Cephalexin 384
Cephalhaematoma 358
Cerebro vascular accident (CVA) 220–221
Cerebro vascular disease 90
Certificate of sickness 292
Cervical spine disease 223
Cervix
carcinoma of 192
cervicitis 191–192
diseases of 191–192
infections 175
Chalazion 242
Chancroid 172–173
Check list, antenatal care 333
Chest
AIDS/HIV 156–157
flail 278
infections 156–157
injuries 277–278
neonatal care 358–362
stab wounds 274
Chickenpox (varicella) 248
Child abuse 193–195
Chlamydial cervicitis 338
Chloasma 263–264
Chlorhexidine tullegras (bactigras) dressing 275
Chlorpheniramine (Chlortrimeton, Allergex) 384
Chlorpromazine 375
Chlortrimeton (chlorpheniramine) 384
Cholecystitis 117
Cholera 111
Chronic mucocutaneous ulceration 46, 252
Chronic obstructive airway disease (COAD) 61–62
Chronic otitis media with effusion 27
Chronic suppurative otitis media (CSOM) 27
Ciprofloxacin 384
Circulation
CPR 3–4
management in emergencies 3–4
Circumcision 152
Cirrhosis 116
Clavicle, fractured 312
Cleft palate 356
Clopixol depot (Zuclopenthixol decanoate) 375
Clotrimazole (Canestin) 384–385
Club feet 363
Cluster headaches 223
COAD see Chronic obstructive airway disease
Co-amoxiclav (Augmentin) 385
Colic, baby with 100–101
Colles' fractures 314–315
Colles'-like fractures 314–315
Colloids 271
Combined oral contraceptive 385
Compartment syndrome 278–279
Concussion 225
Condoms 207
Condylomata acuminata (genital warts) 125, 176
Confusion see Mental confusion
Congenital disorders 342
Congenital hip dislocation 363

Congenital syphilis 171–172, 246, 356
Conjunctivitis
allergic 237
bacterial 236
phlyctenular 237
spring catarrh 237
vernal 237
viral ("pink eye") 236
Consciousness, change in 228
Constipation see also bowel
acute 98–99
antenatal 335
chronic 99
Contact dermatitis 246
Contraception 207–210
additional, when to use 210
amenorrhoea 182
breakthrough bleeds 210
combined oral 385
condoms 207
in diabetes 210
for epileptics 210
in hypertension 210
injectable 208
intra-uterine contraceptive devices 207
oral 208–209, 385
post-coital 210
special situations 210
spotting 210
sterilisation 209–210
subdermal implants 207–208
Contusions (bruises) 277
Corneal ulceration 238–239
Corns 326
Coronary artery disease 91–92
Cor pulmonale 87
Corticosteroids 260
Cosmetic ochronosis 264
Co-trimoxazole (Purbac, Bactrim) 385
Coughing
hypertension 78
neonatal care 358
CPR see Cardiopulmonary resuscitation
Crab louse 255
Cramps in leg 323
Chronic paronychia 261
Chronic psychosis 375
Crooked
back 309–310
knees 322–323
Cross-eyes (strabismus/squint) 235
Cryptococcal meningitis 161
Crystalloids 271
CSOM see Chronic suppurative otitis media
Cutaneous larva migrans (sandworm) 120
CVA see Cerebro vascular accident
Cyclidox (doxycycline) 368, 386
Cysticercosis of brain 220
Cystitis 147, 340
Cysts
Bartholin's 190
eruption 48
gums 48
mouth 46
mucous 46
sebaceous 190, 282
thyroglossal 142
Cytotoxic poisons, snake bites 11–12

D

Daonil (glibenclamide) 135, 387
Deafness see also ear
causes of 19–20
children 19
conductive 19
sensorineural 19–20
tuning fork tests 19–20
Deep venous thrombosis (DVT) 89–90
Defibrillation
CPR 4–5
in emergencies 4–5
Delivery see Labour and delivery
Delusions 374
Dementia 229
Dental abscess (periapical abscess) 48
Dental disease 224
Depo-Provera (medroxyprogesterone) 390

Depressive disorders 376
De Quervain's tenosynovitis 315–316
De Quervain's thyroiditis (subacute thyroiditis) 142
Dermatitis
    contact 246
    eczema and 258
    pierced ears 24
    of pinna 24
    seborrhoeic 159, 259
Diabetes mellitus 129–139
    antenatal problems 336–337
    blood glucose management 135–136
    cataracts 131
    chronic kidney disease 150
    contraception 210
    diabetic foot 132
    diabetic nephropathy 131
    diabetic neuropathy 132
    diagnosis of 129
    dietary education 133–134
    gestational diabetes 336–337
    heart failure 84
    hyperglycaemia 130, 133, 137
    hypertension 77, 131
    hypoglycaemia 129–130, 133
    infections 131
    insulin 136–137, 139
    lifestyle education 134
    long-term complications 131–132
    management 133–134
    medicine protocol 135–139
    neonatal care 355
    pregnancy 336–337
    retinopathy 131
    short-term complications 129–131
    type 1 129, 136
    type 2 129, 134, 136–139
    vascular 132
Diaglim (glimeperide) 135, 388
Diarrhoeal conditions 107–113
    in adults 110
    in children 107–109, 110
    cholera 111
    diarrhoea 107–110
        acute 99, 110, 158
        AIDS/HIV 158, 162
        chronic 99, 158
    dysentery 111
    enema abuse 110
    giardiasis 111
    hydration 108–109
    intussusception 110
    malnutrition 112–113
    medicine management 109
    sugar salt solution 108–109
    typhoid 110–111
    vomiting 107–110
Diazepam (Valium) 217–218, 377–378, 385–386
Dietary education, diabetes mellitus 133–134
Diffuse otitis externa 21
Digoxin 84
Diphtheria 43
Disipal (orphenadrine) 392
Dislocated shoulder 312
Disprin (aspirin) 221, 382
Diuretics 83–84
Dizziness 20, 228–229
Dog bites 11
Dormicum (midazolam) 391
Doxycycline (Cyclidox, Doxyclin) 368, 386
Drips
    birth asphyxia 360
    in CPR 4–5
    in emergencies 4–5
    neonatal care 360
Drooping eyelid (ptosis) 236
Drowning 9–10
Drugs
    abuse 377–378
    AIDS/HIV 160
    in emergencies 4–5
    eruptions 258
    headache due to 225
    hypertension drug side effects 78
    overdose 13–14
    severe cutaneous adverse reactions 258

DVT see Deep venous thrombosis
Dysentery 111, 158
Dysmenorrhoea (pain with menses) 180–181
Dysphagia 39
Dysthymia 375

E

Ear 19–29
    acute labyrinthitis 29
    acute mastoiditis 28
    acute otitis media 25–26, 28
    acute trauma 28
    benign paroxysmal positional vertigo 29
    canal furuncle 21–22
    canal trauma 22–23
    causes of common symptoms 19–20
    children 23
    chronic otitis media with effusion 27
    chronic suppurative otitis media 27
    congenital abnormalities 24–25
    deafness 19–20
    dermatitis of pinna 24
    diffuse otitis externa 21
    discharge from, neonatal 357
    dizziness 20
    drops, insertion of 21
    dry mopping 26
    external 21–25
    foreign body in canal 23
    furuncular otitis externa 21
    glue ear 27
    grommet tubes 27
    haematoma 23
    headaches 224
    infection complications 28
    inner 29
    low set 25
    Meniere's syndrome 29
    middle 25–28
    neonatal care 357
    otitis externa 21
    painful 19
    perforated acute otitis media 26
    pierced 24
    pinna disorders 23–24
    pinnae protruding 25
    pre-auricular sinus 24
    pre-auricular tags 25
    syringing 22, 23
    vertigo 20, 29
    wax 22
ECG (electro-cardiogram)
    in CPR 5–6
    in emergencies 5–6
Ecthyma ("veld sores") 250
Ectopic pregnancy 201
    salpingitis and 197
Eczema 258–260
    atopic 259
    causes 259
    clinical features 258–259
    dermatitis and 258
    endogenous 259
    herpeticum 252
    intertrigenous 259
    management 260
    mummular 259
    seborrhoeic dermatitis 159, 259
Efavirenz (EFV) 386
Elbow
    in adults 313
    in children 312–313
    golfer's elbow 313
    "pulled elbow" 313
    supracondylar fracture 313
    tennis elbow 313
    tenosynovitis 313
Electric shock 10
Electro-cardiogram (ECG)
    in CPR 5–6
    in emergencies 5–6
Emergencies 3–16
    bites 11–14
    burns 15–16
    poisoning 11–14
    resuscitation 3–10

    stings 11–14
Emphysema 61–62
Empty scrotum 284
Enalapril (Renitec) 84, 386
Encopresis 100
Endocrine system 129–142
    diabetes mellitus 129–139
    thyroid gland 141–142
Endometriosis 198
Endometritis 196
Endomyometritis (puerperal sepsis) 202, 351
Endotracheal intubation
    birth asphyxia 359–360
    resuscitation 5–6
Enema abuse 110, 123
Enlarged thyroid gland (goitre) 142
Enuresis 152
Epanutin (phenytoin) 216, 393
    fibromatosis 48
Epididymo-orchitis 169
Epigastric hernia 285
Epiglottitis 54
Epilepsy 213–218
    absence seizures 214
    AIDS/HIV 216
    antenatal problems 337
    assessment of seizures 213–214
    "breakthrough fits" 216
    contraception and 210
    defaulters 216
    febrile convulsions 214
    generalised seizures 214
    headache 225
    Jacksonian 214
    lifestyle education 215
    management 214–217
    medicine management 215–217
    neonatal care 355
    partial seizures 214
    petit mal 214
    plasma level 216
    pregnancy 217
    status epilepticus 217–218
    Todd's paralysis 214
Epinephrine
    allergic reactions 8
    in CPR 5
    stab wounds 273
Episiotomy 202, 349
EPSEs see Extra pyramidal side effects
Eruption cysts 48
Erysipelas 250
Erythema multiforme 257–258
Erythema nodosum 257
Euglim (glimeperide) 135, 388
Euglucon (glibenclamide) 135, 387
Extra pyramidal side effects (EPSEs) 375
Eye 233–242
    abscesses 242
    allergic conjunctivitis 237
    bacterial conjunctivitis 236
    bilateral itchy 234
    bilateral red/painful 233
    burns 16
    cataract 242
    chalazion 242
    chemical burns 240
    children 233
    conjunctivitis 236–237
    corneal ulceration 238–239
    cross-eyes 235
    discharge from 357
    diseases of 236–240
    double vision 235
    drooping eyelid 236
    dry 235
    excessive lacrimation 235
    external hordeolum 242
    flashes of light 235
    "floaters" 235
    foreign body 241–242
    glaucoma 239–240
    headaches 223–224
    herpes zoster ophthalmicus 242
    inflamed pinguecula 238
    injuries 240–242
    itchy 234
    meibomian abscess 242

neonatal care 357
ophthalmia neonatorum 238
periorbital swelling 235
phlyctenular conjunctivitis 237
photophobia 236
"pink eye" 236
ptosis 236
referrals 233
red/painful 233
sensitive to bright light 236
snake venom in 12
spring catarrh 237
strabismus/squint 235
stye 242
swollen eyelid 235
symptoms 233–236
trauma to 240–241
unilateral itchy 234
unilateral red/painful 233
uveitis 239
vernal conjunctivitis 237
viral conjunctivitis 236
vision, difficulty with 234, 357

F

Face, stab wounds in 273
Facet joint, slipped 306
Fainting 213, 228–229
Falciparum malaria 367, 369
False labour 345
Febrile convulsions 214
Female reproductive system 179–210
 abortion 199–200
 contraception 207–210
 ectopic pregnancy 201
 genital tract diseases, lower 189–195
 genital tract diseases, upper 196–198
 gynaecological symptoms 179–188
 miscarriage 199–200
 post-pregnancy complications 202–205
Femoral epiphysis, slipped 318
Femur
 fractured 318
 fractured neck of 318
Ferrous sulphate 387
Fibroadenosis 286
Fibroids of uterus 196
Fibrositis 306
Finger
 abscesses 281
 crush injuries 276
 extra digits 363
 infections 281
 swollen/painful 316
 thumb pain 316
 traumatic amputation of tip 276–277
Fissured tongue 48
Fistula in ano (perianal fistula) 125
Flagyl (metronidazole) 391
Flail chest 278
Flat foot 326
Flexural 259
"Floaters" 235
Floppy child 355
Floxapen (flucloxacillin) 387
Fluanxol depot (Flupenthixol decanoate) 375
Flucloxacillin (Floxapen) 387
Fluconazole 387
Fluid therapy, in emergencies 6, 271–272
Fluoxetine (Prozac) 376
Flupenthixol decanoate (Fluanxol depot) 375
Fluphenazine decanoate (Modecate depot) 375
Foetal distress in labour 347
Follicular eczema 259
Folliculitis 159
Foot 325–328
 achilles bursitis 325
 bunion 328
 callosities 327
 corns 326
 diabetic 132
 eczema 259
 flat 326
 foreign bodies in 328
 fractured fifth metatarsal base 326
 fractured metatarsal bones 326

fracture of toe 327
gout of big toe 328
heel injury 325
heel pain in children 325
infections 327–328
metatarsalgia 327
pain 325–328
pain behind heel 325
painful first metatarsophalangeal joint 328
pain in children 325
pain underneath heel 325
pain under sole 326–327
plantar warts 327
Sever's disease 325
swelling 325–326
toes swollen/painful 327–328
Forearm
 in children 313–314
 fractures 314
Foreign bodies
 in ear 23
 in eye 241–242
 in foot 328
 inhalation, upper airways 54
 in nose 34
 in toe 328
Fractures
 ankle 324
 assessment of damage 290
 booking patients off work 292
 certificate of sickness 292
 clavicle 312
 clinical features 290
 Colles' 314–315
 Colles'-like 314–315
 femur 318
 fifth metatarsal base 326
 forearm 314
 humerus 312
 lumbar spine 305
 management 290–292
 metatarsal bones 326
 neck of femur 318
 neonatal care 363
 pelvis 317–318
 radius 314
 ribs 277–278
 scaphoid 316
 supracondylar 313
 thoracic 305
 toe 327
 ulna 314
Fungal diseases 253–255
 athlete's foot 254
 candidiasis 253
 infections 327–328
 kerion 254
 pityriasis versicolor 254
 ringworm 254
 tinea capitis 254
 tinea corporis 254
 tinea cruris 254
 tinea pedis 254
 tinea unguium 255
Furosemide (Lasix) 387
Furuncular otitis externa 21
Furunculosis 189
Fusospirochaetosis 174

G

Gall bladder problems
 bile duct stones 117
 cholecystitis 117
Ganglion 315
Gastric lavage 13
Gastritis 104
Gastrointestinal system 95–126
 abdominal symptoms 95–101
 anorectal conditions 121–126
  diseases 123–126
  physical examination 123
  symptoms 121–123
 diarrhoeal conditions 107–113
  children 107–109, 110
  cholera 111
  diarrhoea 107–110
  dysentery 111

 enema abuse 110
 giardiasis 111
 intussusception 110
 malnutrition 112–113
 typhoid 110–111
gall bladder 117
hypertension 78
intestinal infestations 119–120
intestines
 acute abdomen 105
 appendicitis 105–106
 irritable bowel syndrome 106
liver 115–116
pancreas 117–118
spleen 118
stomach
 carcinoma of 105
 gastritis 104
 peptic ulceration 104
upper gastrointestinal conditions 103–106
 carcinoma of oesophagus 103
 gastro-oesophageal reflux disease 103
 intestines 105–106
 oesophagitis 103
 oesophagus 103
 reflux oesophagitis 103
 stomach 104–105
Gastron (loperamide) 389–390
Gastro-oesophageal reflux disease (GORD) 101, 103
GCS see Glasgow Coma Scale
Genital candidiasis 169, 175
Genital herpes (herpes genitalis) 172, 189
Genital tract diseases
 adnexal swelling 198
 bacterial vaginosis 191
 Bartholin's abscess 189–190
 Bartholin's cyst 190
 carcinoma of cervix 192
 cervicitis 191–192
 cervix, diseases of 191–192
 child abuse 193–195
 endometriosis 198
 endometritis 196
 fibroids of uterus 196
 furunculosis 189
 genital herpes 189
 intertrigo 189
 labia, swellings of 189–190
 lower 189–195
 pelvic abscess 198
 pelvic inflammatory disease 197–198
 rape 192–193
 salpingitis 197–198
 sebaceous cyst 190
 trauma 192–195
 trichomonas vaginitis 191
 upper 196–198
 uterus 196
 vaginal discharge 190–191
 vulva infections 189
 vulvo-vaginitis 191
Genital ulceration 170–174
Genital ulcers 173–174
 scrotal swelling and 174
 urethritis and 174
 vaginal discharge and 175
Genital warts (condylomata acuminata) 125, 176
Genu valgum 322
Genu varum (bow-legs) 323
Geographic tongue 48
German measles (rubella) 247
Gestational age 331
Gestational diabetes 336–337
Giardiasis 111
Gingivitis 47
 acute necrotising ulcerative 47, 158
Glandular fever 43
Glasgow Coma Scale (GCS) 269
Glaucoma 239–240
 acute closed angle 239–240
 closed angle 223
 open angle 240
Glibenclamide (Euglucon, Daonil) 135, 387
Glimeperide (Diaglim, Euglim) 135, 387–388
Glossitis 49
Glucophage (metformin) 135, 390
Glucose check, in emergencies 6

Glucose Tolerance Test (GTT) 336–337
Goitre (enlarged thyroid gland) 142
Golfer's elbow (tenosynovitis) 313
Gonococcal arthritis 297
Gonococcal infection 175
Gonorrhoea 168, 338
GORD *see* Gastro-oesophageal reflux disease
Gout
    of big toe 328
        heart failure 83–84
        joints 294–295, 298
Granuflex 282
GTT *see* Glucose Tolerance Test
Guillain-Barre Syndrome 161
Gums
    acute necrotising ulcerative gingivitis 47
    dental abscess 48
    diseases of 47–48
    Epanutin fibromatosis 48
    eruption cysts 48
    gingivitis 47
    periapical abscess 48
    pericoronitis 48
    periodontal disease 47
    phenytoin fibromatosis 48
    Vincent's angina 47
Gynaecological symptoms 179–188
    abnormal uterine bleeding 183–185
        contact 185
        decreased menstruation 184
        dysfunctional 184
        increased menstruation 183–184
        inter-menstrual 184
        menorrhagia 183–184
        oligomenorrhoea 184
        post-coital 185
        post-menopausal bleeding 185
        pre-menstrual tension syndrome 185
    amenorrhoea 181–182
    decreased libido 186
    dysmenorrhoea 180–181
    dyspareunia 185–186
    infertility 186–187
    loss of interest in intercourse 186
    lower abdominal pain 179–180
    menopause 182–183
    menstrual bleeding changes 183
    pain on intercourse 185–186
    pain with menses 180–181
    sexual intercourse difficulty 185–186
    "something coming down"/"falling out" 187
    sores/ulcers of genitalia 186
    urinary incontinence 188
    vaginal discharge 180
Gynaecomastia 286

H

Haemaccel 271
Haematemesis (vomiting blood) 95–96
Haematuria 145
Haemoptysis 64
Haemorrhage
    antepartum 342
    postpartum 349
    secondary postpartum haemorrhage 351
    sub-aponeurotic 358
    sub-arachnoid 221
Haemorrhoids 124–125
Haemotoxic poisons, snake bites 12
Hair abnormalities, AIDS/HIV 159
Hairy leukoplakia 49
Hairy tongue, black 49
Hallucinations 374
Haloperidol 375, 388
Hand
    eczema 259
    injuries 276–277
    swollen/painful 316
HAV *see* Hepatitis A virus
HBV *see* Hepatitis B virus
HCV *see* Hepatitis C virus
Head
    injuries 269–271
    neonatal care 356–358
Headaches 219–225
    acute 219

    AIDS/HIV 160
    cerebro vascular accident 220–221
    cervical spine disease 223
    children 219
    chronic/recurrent 219–220
    clinical features 219
    closed angle glaucoma 223
    cluster 223
    dental disease 224
    ear diseases 224
    epilepsy 225
    eye disease 223–224
    hormonal 225
    hypertension 225
    hypoglycaemia 225
    malaria 224
    medicines 225
    meningeal irritation 224
    meningitis 221
    migraine 222–223
    nose diseases 224
    pain in maxilla/mandible 224
    post-concussion 225
    post-traumatic 225
    in pregnancy 225
    refractory errors 224
    sinusitis 224
    space-occupying lesion 223
    strokes 220–221
    sub-arachnoid haemorrhage 221
    subdural haematoma 225
    tempero-mandibular joint 224
    tension 221–222
    tick bite fever 224
    vision, difficulty with 224
Head louse 255
Hearing problem, neonates 357
Heart, stab wounds 274
Heart attack (myocardial infarction) 92
Heartburn (isilungulelo) 335
Heart disease 85–87
    antenatal problems 336
    beriberi 85–86
    cardiomyopathy 85
    cor pulmonale 87
    hypertensive 85
    palpitations 87
    rheumatic 86
    rheumatic fever 86
Heart failure 81–85
    ACE-inhibitors 83, 84
    acute pulmonary oedema 84–85
    anaemia 87
    congenital 87
    hypertension 76
    ischaemic 87
    left ventricular failure 76, 81
    management 82–84
    medicine management 83–84
    pericarditis 87
    pregnancy and 87
    right ventricular failure 81–82
    thyrotoxicosis 87
Heat rash (miliaria) 246
Heel
    injury to 325
    pain behind 325
    pain underneath 325
Hepatitis A virus (HAV) 115–116
Hepatitis B virus (HBV) 115–116
Hepatitis C virus (HCV) 115–116
Hepatitis E virus (HEV) 115–116
Hernia
    epigastric 285
    inguinal
        in adults 284
        in children 283–284
    para-umbilical 285
    umbilical 285
Herpangina 43
Herpes genitalis (genital herpes) 172, 189
Herpes labialis 45
Herpes simplex 45–46, 252
Herpes simplex chronic mucocutaneous ulceration 159
Herpes simplex keratitis 239
Herpes stomatitis 43
Herpes zoster 159–160, 251–252
Herpes zoster ophthalmicus 242

HEV *see* Hepatitis E virus
Hiccoughs (hiccups) 101
Hip
    avascular necrosis of 317
    bruising of thigh muscles 318
    congenital dislocation 363
    fractured femur 318
    fractured neck of femur 318
    osteo-arthritis of joint 317
    pain following injury 317–318
    pain in child/teenager 318–319
    pain in middle-aged/elderly adult 317
    pelvis, fractured 317–318
    Perthes' disease 318–319
    slipped femoral epiphysis 318
HIV and AIDS *see* AIDS/HIV
Hoarseness 39
Hookworm 119–120
Hormonal disorders
    headaches 225
    skin 262
Humerus, fractured 312
Hunch back 310
Hyaline membrane disease 361
Hydration 108–109
Hydrocele
    in adults 285
    in children 283
Hydrochlorothiazide 388
Hydrocortisone (Solucortef) 9, 21, 24, 159, 257, 258, 260–261, 283
Hyoscine (Buscopan) 388
Hyperglycaemia 130, 133, 137
Hyper-pigmentation 263
Hypertension 71–80
    angioedema 78
    antenatal problems 340–341
    anxiety 77
    bradycardia 78
    chronic kidney disease 150
    clinical signs of 71
    confirmation of 71
    contraception in 210
    coughing 78
    defaulters 73
    diabetes mellitus 77, 131
    drug side effects 78
    elderly patients 76
    gastrointestinal upsets 78
    headache 220, 225
    heart failure 76
    kidney disease 76–77, 150
    left ventricular failure 76
    letters 71, 80
    lifestyle management 72
    management in special conditions 76–77
    medicine management advice 72
    medicine protocol 72–75
    patients below 25 years 76
    postnatal patients 77
    pregnancy 77
    protocol 79
    referrals 73
    risk factors 71
    severe hypertension management 75
Hypertensive heart disease 85
Hyperthyroidism 141–142
Hypertrophic scar formation 283
Hypoglycaemia
    diabetes mellitus 129–130, 133
    fainting 213, 229
    headaches 225
    mental confusion 228
    syncope 213, 229
Hypo-pigmentation disorders 263
Hypothermia
    drowning 10
    neonatal care 355
Hypo-thyroidism 141
Hysteria 229

I

Ibuprofen (Brufen) 388
Immune reconstitution inflammatory syndrome (IRIS) 164
Immunisation 156
Imodium (loperamide) 389–390

Imperforate anus 363
Impetigo 249–250
Incontinence
    of faeces 99–100
    of urine 146, 152, 188
Infections
    AIDS/HIV
        in adults 156–161, 164
        in children 162–163, 164
    "blisters" 281
    diabetes mellitus 131
    knee 320–321
    pyogenic spondylitis 303
    in spine, acute 303
    surgery 279–281
    toe 327–328
Infectious mononucleosis 43
Infertility 186–187
Influenza vaccine 156
Infra-patellar bursae 320
Inguinal hernia
    in adults 284
    in children 283–284
Inguinal swellings 362
Inguino-scrotal region 283–285
    in adults 284–285
    in children 283–284
INH see Isoniazid
Injectable contraception 208
Insects 255–256
Insulin 136–137, 139
Intertriginous eczema 259
Intertrigo 189
Intestinal infestations 119–120
    ascaris 119
    cutaneous larva migrans 120
    hookworm 119–120
    pinworm 120
    round worm 119
    sandworm 120
    tapeworm 120
    whipworm 119
    worms 119–120
Intestines 105–106
    acute abdomen 105
    appendicitis 105–106
    irritable bowel syndrome 106
Intra-uterine contraceptive devices (IUCDs) 207
Intravenous therapy see Drips
Intussusception 110
Ipratropium 388
IRIS see Immune reconstitution inflammatory syndrome
Irritable bowel syndrome 106
Isilungulelo (heartburn) 335
Isoniazid (INH) 388-389
Isosorbide 389
Itching
    anus 122
    eye 234
IUCDs see Intra-uterine contraceptive devices
IV infusion see Drips

J

Jacksonian epilepsy 214
Jaundice 115, 354
Joints 293–298
    antenatal problems 336
    gonococcal arthritis 297
    gout 294–295, 298
    orthopaedic problems 289
    osteo-arthritis 293–294, 298
    pain 293
    rheumatoid arthritis 295–297, 298
    septic arthritis 297
    swelling 293
    tuberculosis 298
    viral infections 297

K

Kaletra (lopinavir/ritonavir) 390
Kaposi's sarcoma 160
Keloids 283
Keratosis, solar 264
Kerion 254
Kernicterus 354
Kernig's test 221
Kidney 148–150 see also urological problems
    acute failure 149–150
    chronic disease 150
    hypertension 76
    nephrotic syndrome 149
    post streptococcal glomerulonephritis 148–149
    pyelonephritis 148
    renal calculi 149
    stones 149
Knee 319–323
    bow-legs 323
    chronic pain/swelling 321–322
    crooked 322–323
    direct trauma 319
    genu valgum 322
    genu varum 323
    infection 320–321
    infra-patellar bursae 320
    injuries 319–320
    knock-knees 322
    lumps 320, 321
    Osgood Schlatter's disease 321
    osteo-arthritis 321–322
    pre-patellar abscess 321
    pre-patellar bursae 320
    twisting injury 319–320
Knock-knees 322
Konakion (vitamin K) 396
Kwashiorkor 112, 249

L

Labia
    Bartholin's abscess 189–190
    Bartholin's cyst 190
    sebaceous cyst 190
    swellings of 189–190
Labour and delivery 345–349
    analgesia 346
    common problems 346–347
    cord prolapse 347
    diagnosis of labour 345
    early labour 345
    episiotomy 349
    false labour 345
    foetal distress 347
    for low-risk women 345–346
    meconium staining of liquor 347
    partogram 345–346
    perineal tears 349
    postpartum haemorrhage 349
    pre-labour rupture of membranes 346
    pre-term labour 346
    retained placenta 348
    retained products of conception 348
    second stage of labour 347–348
    shoulder dystocia 347–348
    third stage of labour 348–349
Labryrinthitis, acute 29
Lacrimation, excessive 235
Lactose intolerance 108
Lamictin (lamotrigine) 216, 389
Lamivudine (3TC) 389
Lamotrigine (Lamictin) 216, 389
Lansoprazole (Lanzor) 389
Lanzor (lansoprazole) 389
Laryngotracheo-bronchitis (LTB) 53–54
Larynx see also mouth; throat
    diseases of 49–50
    hoarseness 39
    laryngitis
        acute 49
        chronic 49–50
Lasix (furosemide) 387
Laxatives, abuse of 123
Left ventricular failure (LVF) 57, 76, 81
Leg 317–328
    change in sensation 227
    foot 325–328
    knee 319–323
    lower 323–324
    ulcers 281–282
    upper 317–319
Leprosy 251
Leukoplakia 47
Levonorgestrel (Norlevo) 389
LGV see Lymphogranuloma venereum
Lice (pediculosis) 255
Lichen planus 261
Lifestyle education
    diabetes mellitus 134
    epilepsy 215
Ligament damage in lower back 305
Lightning 10
Limbs
    neonatal care 363
    paralysis 363
    stab wounds 275
LIP see Lymphoid interstitial pneumonia
Lipomas 283
Liver 115–116
    cirrhosis 116
    jaundice 115
    viral hepatitis 115–116
Loperamide (Imodium, Gastron) 389–390
Lopinavir/ritonavir (Kaletra, Aluvia) 390
LTB see Laryngotracheo-bronchitis
Ludwig's angina 40
Lumbar osteoarthritis (spondylosis) 308
Lumps
    breast 285
    knee 320, 321
    surgical 282–283
Lungs 57–68 see also tuberculosis
    abscesses 64
    bronchial asthma 57–61
        acute 60–61
        bronchodilators 58
        children 58–60
        classification 57
        inhalers 59–60
        management 57–61
        medicine protocol 59–60
        nebulisation 61
    bronchiectasis 64
    chronic obstructive airway disease 61–62
    emphysema 61–62
    haemoptysis 64
    pneumonia 62–64
        bronchopneumonia 63–64
        lobar 62
LVF see Left ventricular failure
Lymphadenopathy 160
    acute 40
    persistent generalised 155
Lymph node enlargement 303
Lymphogranuloma venereum (LGV) 173
Lymphoid interstitial pneumonia (LIP) 162–163

M

Maculopapular rashes 247–248
Major depressive disorder 375
Malaria 367–369
    cause 367
    complications 367
    diagnosis 367
    falciparum 367, 369
    headache 224
    management 369
    in pregnancy 369
    prevention 367–369
    vivax 369
Malignant melanoma 265
Mallory Weiss syndrome 96
Malnutrition 112–113
    kwashiorkor 112
    management 113
    marasmic kwashiorkor 113
    marasmus 113
    protein energy malnutrition 112–113
    underweight 112
Mandible, pain in 224
Mantoux test 65–66, 156
Marasmic kwashiorkor 113
Marasmus 113
Mastitis 204
Mastoiditis, acute 28

Maternity 331–363
   antenatal care, routine 331–334
   antenatal problems 335–343
   labour and delivery 345–349
   neonatal care 353–363
   puerperium 351
Maxilla, pain in 224
Maxolon (metoclopramide) 391
MDR (multidrug-resistant) tuberculosis 67–68
Measles 247
Mebendazole (Vermox) 390
Meconium aspiration 361
Meconium staining of liquor 347
Medroxyprogesterone (Provera, Depo-Provera) 390
Mefloquine 368
Meibomian abscess 242
Melanocytic naevi (moles) 264
Melanoma, malignant 264
Meniere's syndrome 29
Meningeal irritation 224
Meningitis
   cryptococcal 161
   headache 221
   meningococcal 221
   neck pain 303
Meningococcal meningitis 221
Menopause 182–183
   post-menopausal bleeding 185
Menorrhagia 183–184
Menstruation
   contraception 210
   decreased 184
   dysfunctional uterine bleeding 184
   dysmenorrhoea 180–181
   increased 183–184
   inter-menstrual bleeding 184
   menorrhagia 183–184
   oligomenorrhoea 184
   pain with 180–181
   post-menopausal bleeding 185
   pre-menstrual tension syndrome 185
Mental confusion 228
Mental health 373–378
   adjustment disorder with depressed mood 373, 378
   anxiety disorders 373, 378
     acute stress disorder 378
     panic attack 378
     panic disorder 378
     post-traumatic stress disorder 378
   drug abuse 377–378
   major groups 373
   mood disorders 373, 375–378
     bipolar mood disorder 375, 377
     classification 375
     clinical features 375–376
     due to medical condition 375
     dysthymia 375
     major depressive disorder 375
     management 376
     substance-induced 375, 377–378
   physical illness 373
   psychoses 373, 374–375
     acute 374
     chronic 374–375
     schizophrenia 374–375
   stress-related disorders 378
   substance-related disorders 377–378
     alcohol abuse 377–378
Metatarsalgia 327
Metformin (Glucophage) 135, 390
Methyldopa (Aldomet) 390
Meticortin (prednisone) 394
Metoclopramide (Maxolon) 390–391
Metronidazole (Flagyl) 391
Microval 209
Midazolam (Dormicum) 391
Migraine 222–223
Miliaria (heat rash) 246
Miscarriage (abortion) 199–200
   complete 200
   diagnosis 199
   incomplete 199
   inevitable 199
   legal 200
   septic 200
   threatened 199
   types of 199–200
   unsafe 200
Modecate depot (Fluphenazine decanoate) 375
Moles (melanocytic naevi) 264
Molluscum contagiosum 160, 176, 252
Mood disorders 373, 375–377
   bipolar mood disorder 376–377
   classification 375–376
   clinical features 376
   due to medical condition 376
   management 376
   substance-induced 377
Mother-to-child transmission, AIDS/HIV 165
Mouth *see also* larynx; throat
   AIDS/HIV 46
   aphthous ulcer 45
   chronic mucocutaneous ulceration 46
   diseases of 45–47
   dysphagia 39
   herpes labialis 45
   herpes simplex 45–46
   herpetic stomatitis 45
   HIV and AIDS 158
   leukoplakia 47
   mucous cysts 46
   mumps 47
   oral cancer 47
   oral candidiasis 46
   pre-cancerous conditions 47
   salivary glands 47
   sores 39
   swallowing, difficulty with 39
   swallowing, pain on 39
   swelling 39
Mouth breathing 31
Mucous cysts 46
Multidrug-resistant (MDR) tuberculosis 67–68
Mumps 47
Muscles
   antenatal problems 336
   injuries 278–279
   orthopaedic problems 289
   weakness 226
Musculoskeletal system 289–328
   arm 311–316
   bone disorders 299
   diagnosis of orthopaedic problems 289
   fractures 290–292
   general principles 289–292
   joints 293–298
   leg 317–328
   management of trauma 289–292
   spine 301–310
Mycostatin (nystatin) 392
Myocardial infarction (heart attack) 92
Myopathic disorders (muscle weakness) 226

N

Nappy rash 246
Nasal catheter, birth asphyxia 359
Natal cleft, painful 122
Nausea 95
Neck
   abscesses 281
   injuries 302, 303
   pain
     in adults 303–304
     in children 303
   stab wounds 273–274
   swelling 40
Neonatal care 353–363
   abdomen 362–363
   Apgar score 359
   birth asphyxia 358–360
   bleeding, abnormal 355
   bowel atresia 363
   breasts, swollen 362
   caput succedaneum 358
   cephalhaematoma 358
   chest 358–362
   cleft palate 356
   club feet 363
   congenital hip dislocation 363
   congenital syphilis 356
   cough 358
   diabetes mellitus 355
   discharge from ears 357
   discharge from eyes 357
   discharge from nose 357–358
   epilepsy 355
   extra digits 363
   floppy child 355
   fractures 363
   head, swelling of 358
   head problems 356–358
   hear, unable to 357
   HIV-exposed infant 353
   hyaline membrane disease 361
   hypothermia 355
   imperforate anus 363
   inguinal swellings 362
   jaundice 354
   kernicterus 354
   limb paralysis 363
   limb problems 363
   meconium aspiration 361
   oedema 354–355
   omphalocele 362
   pneumonia 361
   respiratory distress syndrome 360–361
   scrotal swellings 362
   sepsis of umbilical cord 362
   small for gestational age babies 356
   sub-aponeurotic haemorrhage 358
   subconjunctival bleeding 357
   tongue tie 356
   transient tachypnoea 361
   umbilical granuloma 362
   underweight for gestational age babies 356
   urine, difficulty passing 362–363
   vaginal bleeding 362
   vision 357
   vomiting 362
Nephrotic syndrome 149
Nerve disease (neurogenic disorders) 226
Nervous system 213–229
   epilepsy 213–218
   neurological problems 219–229
Neurogenic disorders (nerve disease) 226
Neurological problems 219–229
   AIDS/HIV 160–161
   Bells Palsy 226
   blackout 228–229
   change in sensation 227–228
   dizziness 228–229
   fainting 228–229
   headaches 219–225
   mental confusion 228
   syncope 228–229
   tremor 228
   weakness 225–226
Neuromuscular junction disorders 226
Neurotoxic poisons, snake bites 12
Nevirapine (NVP) 391
Niclosamide (Yomesan) 119
Nicotinamide (Vitamin B3) 391
Nipples *see also* breast
   blood-stained discharge 205
   cracked 203
   discharge 205, 286
Non-gonococcal urethritis 168–169
Nordette 209, 392
Norlevo (levonorgestrel) 389
Norvasc (amlodipine) 382
Nose 31–36 *see also* paranasal sinuses
   cauterisation 34
   chronic obstruction 31
   discharge from, neonatal 357–358
   drops, insertion of 31
   epistaxis 33–34
   foreign bodies in 34
   fractured 35
   furuncle 33
   headaches 224
   injuries 35
   mouth breathing 31
   neonatal care 357–358
   packing 34
   polyps 33
   rhinitis 31–32
     acute purulent 32
     acute viral 31
     allergic 32

newborns 32
septal abscess 36
septal deviation 35
septal haematoma 35
septal perforation 35
Nummular eczema 259
Nutritional skin diseases 249
NVP see Nevirapine
Nystatin (Mycostatin) 392

O

Ochronosis, cosmetic 263
OCs see Oral contraceptives
Oedema
 antenatal problems 336
 neonatal care 354–355
Oesophageal candidiasis 158
Oesophagitis 103
Oesophagus
 carcinoma of 103
 gastro-oesophageal reflux disease 103
 oesophageal candidiasis 158
 oesophagitis 103
 reflux oesophagitis 103
Oestrogen conjugated 392
Oestrogen therapy 183
Oligomenorrhoea 184
Omphalocele in neonates 362
Open wounds 275–276
Oral cancer 47
Oral candidiasis 158
Oral contraceptives (OCs) 208–209, 385
Orchitis 284
"Organic brain disease" 373
Organophosphate poisoning 14
Orphenadrine (Disipal) 392
Orthopaedic problems 289
Osgood Schlatter's disease 321
Osteo-arthritis
 of hip joint 317
 joints 293–294, 298
 of knee joint 321–322
 neck pain 304
Osteomyelitis 299
Osteoporosis 299
Otitis externa (OE) 21
Otitis media, acute 25–26, 28
Ovral 209

P

Painful peripheral neuropathy 161
Palpitations 87
Panado (paracetamol) 392
Pancreas 117–118
 acute pancreatitis 117
 carcinoma of 118
 chronic pancreatitis 118
Panic attacks 378
Panic disorder 378
PAP smear 176, 185, 190, 191, 192, 263
Papular pruritic eruption 159
Papular rashes 247–248
Papular urticaria 257
Paracetamol (Panado) 392
Paraffin poisoning 13
Paranasal sinuses 36–37 see also nose
 fractured mandible/maxilla 37
 sinusitis
  acute 36
  chronic 36–37
 tumours of maxillary sinus 37
Paraphimosis 176
Parasites 255–256
Para-tendonitis of achilles tendon 324
Para-umbilical hernia 285
Parkinsonism 228
Paronychium, acute 281
Partogram 345–346
Pediculosis (lice) 255
Pellagra 249
Pelvis
 abscesses 198
 backache 305
 fractured 317–318
 pelvic inflammatory disease 197–198

PEM see Protein energy malnutrition
Pemphigus vulgaris 265
Penicillin 392
PEP see Post-exposure prophylaxis
Peptic ulceration, suspected 104
Perianal fistula (fistula in ano) 125
Periapical abscess (dental abscess) 48
Pericoronitis 48
Perindopril 84
Perineum
 burns 16
 episiotomies 202
 lacerations 202
 tears 349
Periodontal disease (gingivitis) 47
Peripheral vascular disease 90–91
Peritonsillar abscess (quinsy) 43–44
Permethrin (5% lotion) 392–393
Persistent generalised lymphadenopathy 155
Perthes' disease 318–319
Petit mal (absence seizures) 214
Pharmacopoeia 381–396
Pharyngitis 41–43, 45
 viral 40–41
Phenergan (promethazine) 394
Phenobarbitone 393
Phenytoin (Epanutin) 216, 393
 fibromatosis 48
Phimosis 152
Phlyctenular conjunctivitis 237
Photophobia
 eye 236
 migraine 222
Phototherapy, jaundice 354
PID (pelvic inflammatory disease) 197–198
Pierced ears, problems with 24
Pigmentation disorders 263
 albino 262
 chloasma 263
 cosmetic ochronosis 263
 hyper-pigmentation 263
 hypo-pigmentation 262–263
 post-inflammatory depigmentation 263
 post-inflammatory hyper-pigmentation 263
 vitiligo 263
Pilonidal abscess 126
Pilonidal sinus 126
Pinguecula, inflamed 238
"Pink eye" 236
Pinworm 120
Pityriasis alba 259, 260
Pityriasis rosea 260–261
Pityriasis versicolor 254
Placenta, retained 348
Plantar warts 327
Plasma, management of shock 271
Plaster of Paris (POP)
 ankle 324
 fractures 291
PMT see Pre-menstrual tension syndrome
Pneumococcal keratitis 239
Pneumocystis pneumonia 157, 162
Pneumonia 62–64
 AIDS/HIV 156–157, 162
 bronchopneumonia 63–64
 children 64
 lobar 62
 lymphoid interstitial 162–163
 neonatal care 361
 pneumocystis 157, 162
Poisoning see also bites
 carbon monoxide 14
 identification of poison 13
 management 13
 organophosphate 14
 paraffin 13
 types of 13–14
Polyuria 146
POP see Plaster of Paris
Porphyria 265–266
Post-exposure prophylaxis (PEP) 167, 193, 195
Post-myocardial infarction 92
Postnatal patients, hypertension in 77
Postpartum haemorrhage (PPH) 349
 secondary 351
Post streptococcal glomerulonephritis

(PSGN) 148–149
Post-term pregnancy 342
Post-traumatic stress disorder 378
Potassium chloride (Slow-K) 393
Povidone iodine (Betadine) 393
PPH see Postpartum haemorrhage
Praziquantel (Biltricide) 120, 393
Prednisone (Meticortin) 393–394
Pre-eclampsia 335, 336, 340–341
Pregnancy see also antenatal care, routine; antenatal problems
 breast conditions 203–205
 confirmation of 331
 epilepsy during 217
 episiotomies 202
 headache in 225
 heart failure 87
 hypertension 77
 malaria in 369
 multiple 341
 normal 331
 perineal lacerations 202
 post-pregnancy complications 202–205
 puerperal sepsis 202
Pre-labour rupture of membranes (PROM) 346
Pre-menstrual tension syndrome (PMT) 185
Pre-patellar abscess 321
Pre-patellar bursae 320–321
Pressure bandages 282
Procaine reaction/mania 8
Prolapsed intervertebral disc (slipped disc) 306–307
PROM see Pre-labour rupture of membranes
Promethazine (Phenergan) 394
Prostate 146–147
 benign prostatic hyperplasia 147
 cancer 147
 prostatism 147
 prostatitis 146, 170
Protein energy malnutrition (PEM) 112–113
Proteinuria
 antenatal problems 335
 chronic kidney disease 150
 diabetic nephropathy 131
Provera (medroxyprogesterone) 390
Prozac (fluoxetine) 376
Pruritis ani 122
PSGN see Post streptococcal glomerulonephritis
Psoriasis 261
Psychoses 373, 374–375
 acute 374
 chronic 375
 schizophrenia 375
PTB see Pulmonary tuberculosis
Ptosis (drooping eyelid) 236
Pubic louse 255
Puerperal sepsis (endomyometritis) 202, 351
Puerperium
 discharge from clinic 351
 endomyometritis 351
 follow-up visits 351
 persistent vaginal bleeding 351
 postnatal problems 351
 puerperal sepsis 351
 routine postnatal care 351
"Pulled elbow" 313
Pulmonary tuberculosis (PTB) 340
Purbac (co-trimoxazole) 385
Pyelonephritis 148, 340
Pyogenic spondylitis (acute infection in spine) 303
Pyridoxine (Vitamin B6) 394

Q

Quinsy (peritonsillar abscess) 43–44

R

Radius, fractured 314
Rape 192–193
Rapid Plasma Reagin (RPR) test 339
Rashes 245–249
 allergic 248
 antenatal problems 336

assessment of 245
chickenpox 248
in children 245–246, 247–249
congenital syphilis 246
contact dermatitis 246
german measles 247
heat 246
maculopapular 247–248
measles 247
miliaria 246
nappy 246
papular 247–248
rubella 247
scabies 248
scarlet fever 247
streptococcal infection 247
varicella 248
vesicular 248–249
viral 248
RDS see Respiratory distress syndrome
Rectal prolapse 125 see also anorectal conditions
Red reflex test 234
Reflux oesophagitis (gastro-oesophageal reflux disease) 101, 103
Refractory errors (vision) 224
Renal calculi (kidney stones) 149
Renal function
heart failure 84
low set ears 25
Renitec (enalapril) 84, 386–387
Reproductive system see Female reproductive system
Resperidone 375
Respiratory distress syndrome (RDS) 360–361
Respiratory system 53–68
lungs 57–68
upper airways 53–56
Resuscitation 3–10
airway obstruction 6–7
allergic reactions 7–9
cardiopulmonary resuscitation 3–6
drowning 9–10
electric shock 10
lightning 10
Retinopathy 131
Retro-pharyngeal abscess 45
Rhesus incompatibility 343
Rheumatic fever 42, 86
Rheumatic heart disease 86
Rheumatoid arthritis 295–297
Rhinitis
acute purulent 32
acute viral 31
allergic 32
newborns 32
Ribs, fractured 277–278
RICE method 289–290
Rifampicin 394
Right ventricular failure (RVF) 81–82
Ringworm (tinea corporis) 251, 254
Rinne tuning fork test 20
Ritonavir/lopinavir (Kaletra, Aluvia) 390
Rotator cuff syndrome 311
Round worm (ascaris) 119
RPR (Rapid Plasma Reagin) test 339
Rubella (german measles) 247
Rule of Nine's, burns 15–16
RVF see Right ventricular failure

S

Salbutamol (Ventolin, Venteze) 394
Salivary glands 47
Salmeterol (Serevent) 394–395
Salpingitis 197–198
Sandworm (cutaneous larva migrans) 120
Scabies 159, 248, 255–256
Scaphoid fracture 316
Scarlet fever (streptococcal infection) 43, 247
Scars, hypertrophic formation 283
Scheuermann's disease 304
Schistosomiasis (bilharzia) 147–148
Schizophrenia 375
Scoliosis 309–310
Scrotum
empty 284
neonatal care 362
swelling 174, 362
Scurvy 249
Sebaceous abscess 282
Sebaceous cyst 190, 282
Seborrhoeic dermatitis 159, 259, 260
Selective serotonin re-uptake inhibitors (SSRI) 185, 376
Selenium sulphide (Selsun) 394
Selsun (selenium sulphide) 395
Sennosides A + B (Senokot) 395
Senokot (sennosides A + B) 395
Sensation, change in 227–228
Septic arthritis 297
Serevent (salmeterol) 394–395
Seroconversion illness 155
Sever's disease 325
Sexual intercourse
bleeding after 185
contact bleeding 185
decreased libido 186
difficulty with 185–186
dyspareunia 185–186
loss of interest in 186
pain on 185–186
post-coital contraception 210
Sexually transmitted infections (STIs) 153–176 see also AIDS/HIV
antenatal problems 338–340
bacterial vaginosis 174, 338
balanitis 169–170
candidiasis 338
cervical infections 175
chancroid 172–173
chlamydial cervicitis 338
epididymo-orchitis 169
fusospirochaetosis 174
genital candidiasis 169, 175
genital herpes 172
genital ulceration 170–174
genital ulcers 173–174, 175
genital warts 176
gonococcal infection 175
gonorrhoea 168, 338
herpes genitalis 172
lymphogranuloma venereum 173
molluscum contagiosum 176
non-gonococcal infection 175
non-gonococcal urethritis 168–169
paraphimosis 176
prostatitis 170
quality care for people with 168
secondary to genital ulceraton 169–170
syphilis 170–172
antenatal problems 339
congenital 171–172, 246, 356
latent 171
primary 170
rhinitis and 32
secondary 170–171
tertiary 171
trichomonas infection 174
trichomoniasis 338
urethritis 168–169
vaginal discharge 174–175, 338
vaginal infections 174
vulval warts 338–339
Sexual offences
AIDS/HIV 167
rape 192–193
sexual abuse 193–195
SFH see Symphysis-fundal height
SGA see Small for gestational age babies
Shin splints 323
Shock 271–272
Shoulder
bicipital tendonitis 311–312
dislocated 312
dystocia, in labour 347–348
fractured clavicle 312
fractured humerus 312
pain in 311
rotator cuff syndrome 311
Sinusitis 36–37
acute 36
chronic 36–37
complications 36
headaches 224
management 37
Skin 245–265
acne vulgaris 261–262
AIDS/HIV 159
allergies 256–260
bacterial conditions 249–251
boil 250
carbuncle 250–251
cellulitis 250
ecthyma 250
erysipelas 250
impetigo 249–250
leprosy 251
tuberculosis 251
"veld sores" 250
blisters 264–265
bullous disorders 264–265
fungal diseases 253–255
hormonal disorders 261–262
insects 255–256
lichen planus 261
nutritional diseases 249
parasites 255–256
pigmentation disorders 262–263
pityriasis rosea 260
psoriasis 261
rashes 245–249, 336
tumours 37, 263–264
viral conditions 251–253
herpes simplex 252
herpes zoster 251–252
molluscum contagiosum 252
warts 252–253
Slipped disc (prolapsed intervertebral disc) 306–307
Slow-K (potassium chloride) 393
Small for gestational age babies (SGA) 356
Snake bites 11–12
cytotoxic poisons 11–12
haemotoxic poisons 12
management 12
neurotoxic poisons 12
venom in eyes 12
Solar keratosis 264
Solucortef (hydrocortisone) 9, 21, 24, 159, 257, 258, 260–261, 283
Sores
genitalia 186
mouth 39
Spastic colon see Irritable bowel syndrome
Spider bites 14
Spine 301–310
backache 302
backache, acute 305–308
backache, chronic low 308–309
crooked back 309–310
fibrositis 306
hunch back 310
infection 303
neck injury 302
neck pain 303–304
osteo-arthritis 304
Scheuermann's disease 304
scoliosis 309–310
severe problems 301–302
slipped facet joint 306
spinal cord/nerves damage 301
thoracic pain 304
X-rays 302
Spironolactone (Aldactone) 84, 395
Spleen 118
Splenomegaly 118
Spondylosis (lumbar osteoarthritis) 308
Spring catarrh (vernal conjunctivitis) 237
Squamous cell carcinoma 264
Squint/strabismus (cross-eyes) 235
SSRI (selective serotonin re-uptake inhibitors) 185, 376
SSS see Sugar salt solution
Stab wounds 272–275
abdominal 274–275
chest 274
face 273
heart 274
limbs 275
management 272–273
neck 273–274
Staphylococcal scalded skin syndrome 265
Status epilepticus 217–218

Sterilisation (contraception) 209–210
Sterilising bottles and teats 107–108
Steristrip 273
Stevens Johnson syndrome 258
Stings, from bees 14
STIs *see* Sexually transmitted infections
Stomach 104–105
    carcinoma of 105
    gastritis 104
    peptic ulceration 104
Strabismus/squint (cross-eyes) 235
Streptococcal infection (scarlet fever) 43, 247
Stress
    neck pain 303
    -related disorders 378
Stridor 53
Strokes 220–221
Stye 242
Subacute thyroiditis (De Quervain's thyroiditis) 142
Sub-aponeurotic haemorrhage 358
Subconjunctival bleeding 357
Subdermal implants (contraception) 207–208
Subdural haematoma 225
Substance abuse *see* Abuse
Subungual haematoma 276
Sugar salt solution (SSS) 108–109
Sulphonylureas 135
Supracondylar fracture 313
Surgery 269–286
    abdominal wall 285
    abrasions 277
    abscesses 279–281
    acute paronychium 281
    amputation of finger tip 276–277
    benign breast disease 285–286
    breast 285–286
    breast disease in males 286
    bruises 277
    bumps 282–283
    cellulitis 279
    chest injuries 277–278
    children 283–284
    compartment syndrome 278–279
    contusions 277
    crush injuries of fingers 276
    empty scrotum 284
    epigastric hernia 285
    fibroadenosis 286
    finger abscesses 281
    finger infections 281
    flail chest 278
    fractured ribs 277–278
    gynaecomastia 286
    hand injuries 276–277
    head injuries 269–271
    hydrocele 283, 285
    hypertrophic scar formation 283
    infected "blisters" 281
    infections 279–281
    inguinal hernias 283–284
    inguino-scrotal region 283–285
    keloids 283
    leg ulcers 281–282
    lipomas 283
    lumps 282–283
    malignant breast disease 286
    muscle injuries 278–279
    neck abscesses 281
    nipple discharge 286
    open wounds 275–276
    orchitis 284
    para-umbilical hernia 285
    pus formation 279–281
    sebaceous abscess 282
    sebaceous cyst 282
    shock 271–272
    stab wounds 272–275
    subungual haematoma 276
    toe abscesses 281
    toe infections 281
    torsion of testis 284
    umbilical hernia 285
Suturing wounds 272–273
Swallowing
    difficulty with 39
    pain on 39

Swelling
    adnexal 198
    breasts, of babies 362
    eyelid 235
    finger 316
    foot 325–326
    hand 316
    head 358
    inguinal 362
    joints 293
    knee 319–322
    labia 189–190
    mouth 39
    neck 40
    neonatal care 358, 362
    periorbital 235
    scrotum 174, 362
    toes 327–328
Symphysis-fundal height (SFH) 333–334
Syncope 213, 228–229
Syphilis 170–172
    antenatal problems 339
    congenital 171–172, 246, 356
    latent 171
    primary 170
    rhinitis and 32
    secondary 170–171
    tertiary 171

T

Tachypnoea, transient 361
Tapeworm 120
TB *see* Tuberculosis
TDF *see* Tenofovir
Tegretol (carbamazepine) 215–216, 383–384
Tempero-mandibular joint 224
TEN *see* Toxic epidermal necrolysis
Tendons 289
Tennis elbow (tenosynovitis) 313
Tenofovir (TDF) 395
Tenormin (atenolol) 382
Tenosynovitis 313
Tension headaches 221–222
Tension pneumothorax 274
Testis, torsion of 284
Tetanus toxoid 332
Thiamine (Vitamin B1) 377, 395
Thiazide diuretic 73
Thigh muscles, bruising of 318
Thoracic pain 304
Thoracic spine backache 302
3TC (lamivudine) 389
Throat *see also* larynx; mouth
    acute streptococcal tonsillitis 41–42
    adenoid hypertrophy 44
    chronic causes 40
    diphtheria 43
    diseases of 40–45
    dysphagia 39
    glandular fever 43
    herpangina 43
    hoarseness 39
    infectious mononucleosis 43
    peritonsillar abscess 43–44
    pharyngitis 41–43
    quinsy 43–44
    recurrent tonsillitis 42–43
    retro-pharyngeal abscess 45
    rheumatic fever 42
    scarlet fever 43
    streptococcal tonsillitis 43
    swallowing, difficulty with 39
    swallowing, pain on 39
    swelling 40
    tonsil examination 42
    tonsillectomy 42
    tonsillitis 41–43
    viral pharyngitis 40–41
Thumb pain 316
Thyroglossal cyst 142
Thyroid gland 141–142
    De Quervain's thyroiditis 142
    enlarged thyroid gland 142
    goitre 142
    hyperthyroidism 141–142
    hypo-thyroidism 141
    single thyroid nodule 142
    subacute thyroiditis 142

    thyroglossal cyst 142
    thyroiditis 142
Tick bite fever 224
Tilidine (Valoron) 395
Tinea capitis 254
Tinea corporis (ringworm) 251, 254
Tinea cruris 254
Tinea pedis (athlete's foot) 254
Tinea unguium 255
Todd's paralysis 214
Toe
    abscesses 281
    bunion 328
    fractures 327
    gout of big toe 328
    infections 281, 327–328
    swollen/painful 327–328
Tongue
    black hairy 49
    diseases of 48–49
    fissured 48
    geographic 48
    glossitis 49
    hairy leukoplakia 49
    neonatal care 356
    tie 356
Tonsillitis 41–43
    acute streptococcal 41–42
    recurrent 42–43
    scarlet fever 43
    streptococcal 43
    tonsil examination 42
    tonsillectomy 42
Torsion of testis 284
Torticollis, acute 303
Toxic epidermal necrolysis (TEN) 258
Tracheitis 55
Tramadol 395
Transient tachypnoea 361
Trauma
    acute to ear 28
    child abuse 193–195
    to eye 240–241
    musculoskeletal system 289–292
    neck 40
    post-traumatic headache 225
    rape 192–193
Tremor 228
Trichomonas infection 174
Trichomonas vaginitis 191
Trichomoniasis 338
Tricyclic anti-depressants 106, 132, 376, 381
Triphasil 209
Tropical diseases 365–369
Tryptanol (amitriptyline) 376, 381
Tubal ligation 210
Tuberculosis 65–68
    in adults 66
    AIDS/HIV 156, 157, 162, 165, 166
    in children 65–66
    clinical features 65
    joints 297–298
    multidrug-resistant 67–68
    neck pain 303
    prevention 68, 156
    protocol for treatment 66–68
    pulmonary 340
    skin 251
Tubigrip sleeve 283
Tumours
    benign 263–264
    malignant 264
    malignant melanoma 264
    of maxillary sinus 37
    melanocytic naevi 264
    moles 264
    skin 263–264
    solar keratosis 264
    squamous cell carcinoma 264
    vascular naevi 263–264
Type 1 diabetes mellitus 129, 136
Type 2 diabetes mellitus 129, 134, 136–139
Typhoid 110–111

U

UE (UNG emulsificans) 396

Ulcers
    aphthous 45
    around anus 122
    genital 175, 186
    leg 281–282
Ulna, fractured 314
Ultrasound scanning, antenatal care 332, 334
Umbilical cord
    prolapse 347
    sepsis of 362
Umbilical granuloma 362
Umbilical hernia 285
UMS (UNG methyl salicylate) 396
Underweight 112
Underweight for gestational age babies (UWGA) 356
UNG emulsificans (UE) 396
UNG methyl salicylate (UMS) 396
Upper airways 53–56 see also airway
    bronchiolitis 56
    bronchitis 55
    epiglottitis 54
    foreign body inhalation 54
    laryngotracheo-bronchitis 53–54
    stridor 53
    tracheitis 55
Upper gastro intestinal conditions 103–106
    carcinoma of oesophagus 103
    gastro-oesophageal reflux disease 103
    intestines 105–106
    oesophagitis 103
    oesophagus 103
    reflux oesophagitis 103
    stomach 104–105
Urethritis 168–169
    genital ulcers and 174
    gonorrhoea 168
    non-gonococcal 168–169
Urinary tract infections (UTI) 150–152
    antenatal problems 335, 340
    in children 151–152
    recurrent 152
    in women 150–151
Urine pregnancy tests 331
Urine testing, antenatal care 332
Urological problems 145–152
    acute kidney failure 149–150
    benign prostatic hyperplasia 147
    bilharzia 147–148
    bladder 147–148
    burning on micturition 146
    chronic kidney disease 150
    circumcision 152
    cystitis 147
    difficulty passing urine 362–363
    diseases 146–152
    enuresis 152
    haematuria 145
    incontinence of urine 146, 188
    kidney 148–150
    kidney stones 149
    nephrotic syndrome 149
    phimosis 152
    polyuria 146
    post streptococcal glomerulonephritis 148–149
    prostate 146–147
    pyelonephritis 148
    renal calculi 149
    retention of urine 145–146
    schistosomiasis 147–148
    symptoms 145–146
    urinary tract infections 150–152
Urticaria 256–257
Uterus
    abnormal bleeding 183–185
    endometritis 196
    fibroids of 196
UTI see Urinary tract infections

Uveitis 239
UWGA see Underweight for gestational age babies

V

Vaginal bleeding
    neonatal 362
    persistent 351
Vaginal discharge 174–175, 180, 190–191
    antenatal problems 338
    bacterial vaginosis 174, 191
    genital candidiasis 175
    genital ulcer and 175
    management 190
    trichomonas infection 174
    trichomonas vaginitis 191
    vaginal infections 174–175
    vulvo-vaginitis 191
Vaginal infections 174–175
    bacterial vaginosis 174, 338
    genital candidiasis 175
    trichomonas infection 174
Valium (diazepam) 217–218, 377–378, 385–386
Valoron (tilidine) 395
Valproate 216, 396
Varicella (chickenpox) 248
Varicose veins 89, 336
Vascular disease 89–92
    arteries 90–92
        angina pectoris 91–92
        atherosclerosis 90
        cerebro vascular disease 90
        clinical features 90
        coronary artery disease 91–92
        heart attack 92
        myocardial infarction 92
        pain below left breast 91
        peripheral vascular disease 90–91
        post-myocardial infarction 92
    diabetes mellitus 132
    veins 89–90
        burst varicose 89
        deep venous thrombosis 89–90
        superficial thrombophlebitis 89
        varicose 89
        venous ulcers 90
Vascular naevi 264
Vasectomy 209–210
Vasodilators 84
Vasovagal attack 8
Veins 89–90
    burst varicose 89
    deep venous thrombosis 89–90
    superficial thrombophlebitis 89
    varicose veins 89
    venous ulcers 90
"Veld sores" (ecthyma) 250
Venous ulcers 90
Venteze (salbutamol) 394
Ventolin (salbutamol) 394
Ventricular fibrillation (VF) 4, 5
Vermox (mebendazole) 390
Vernal conjunctivitis (spring catarrh) 237
Vertigo 20, 29
Vesicular rashes 248–249
VF see Ventricular fibrillation
Vincent's angina 47
Viral hepatitis 115–116
Viral infections
    AIDS/HIV 159–160
    herpes simplex 252
    herpes zoster 251–252
    joints 297
    molluscum contagiosum 252
    pharyngitis 40–41
    rash 248
    skin 251–253
    warts 252–253
Vision
    at birth 357

    difficulty with 234
    double 235
    flashes of light 235
    "floaters" 235
Vitamins
    B1 (thiamine) 377, 395
    B3 (nicotinamide) 391
    B6 (pyridoxine) 394
    B Co 396
    K (Konakion) 396
    open wounds 276
Vitiligo 263
Vivax malaria 369
Vomiting
    abdominal symptoms 95–96
    antenatal problems 335
    blood (haematemesis) 95–96
    diarrhoea and 107–110
    neonatal care 362
Vulva
    furunculosis 189
    genital herpes 189
    infections of 189
    intertrigo 189
    vulvo-vaginitis 191
    warts 338–339

W

Warts 252–253
    common 252
    condylomata accuminata 253
    genital 253
    plane 253
    plantar 253, 327
    vulval 338–339
Wax in ear 22
Weakness 225–226
Weber tuning fork test 19–20
Whipworm 119
WHO staging, AIDS/HIV 155, 161–162
Worms 119–120
Wounds
    open 275–276
    stab 272–275
    suturing of 272–273
Wrist
    in adults 314
    carpal tunnel syndrome 315
    in children 314
    Colles' fractures 314–315
    Colles'-like fractures 314–315
    De Quervain's tenosynovitis 315–316
    ganglion 315
    scaphoid fracture 316
Wry neck, acute 303

X

X-rays
    backache 302
    backache, chronic low 309
    elbow 313
    fractures 290, 291
    neck injury 302
    pneumocystis pneumonia 157
    pneumonia 156
    tuberculosis 157

Y

Yomesan (niclosamide) 119

Z

Zentel (albendazole) 120, 381
Zidovudine (AZT) 396
Zithromax (azithromycin) 382–383
Zuclopenthixol decanoate (Clopixol depot) 375
Zyloprim (allopurinol) 295, 381

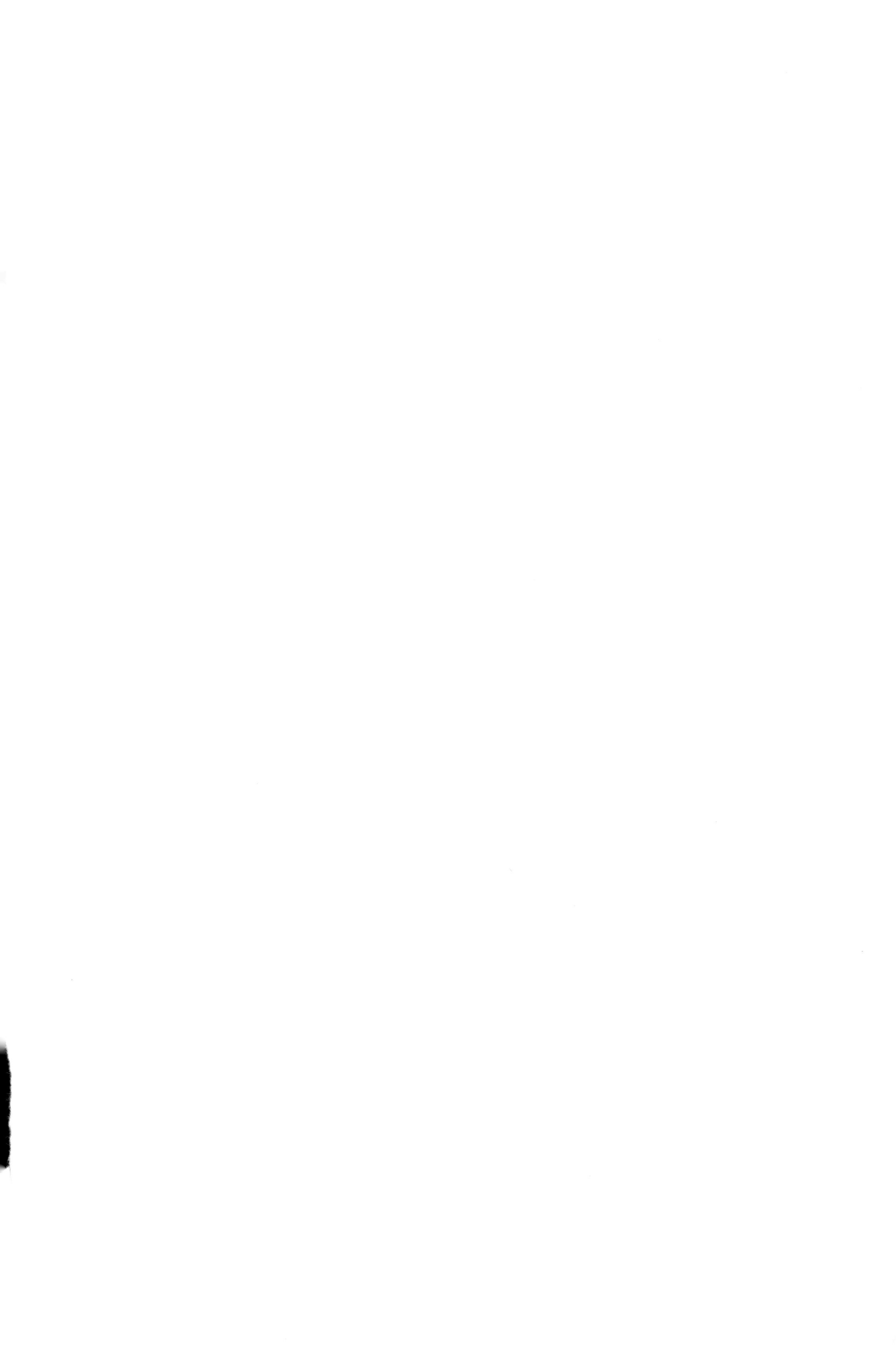